S0-CBI-735

Advances in tumour prevention,
detection and characterization

Vol. 2

Cancer detection
and prevention

303395

Excerpta Medica, International Congress Series

Advances in tumour prevention,
detection and characterization

Editor: C. Maltoni

Vol. 2

Cancer detection and prevention

Proceedings of the Second
International Symposium on
Cancer Detection and Prevention
Bologna, April 9-12, 1973

Editorial Board:
Cesare Maltoni (President)
Yves Fassin
Edward C. Hammond
Herbert E. Nieburgs
Ivan Vodopija
Massimo Crespi (Secretary)

Linguistic Editors:
M. S. Chesters
P. R. J. Burch

RC 255
A1
I 7
1974

1974
Excerpta Medica   Amsterdam
American Elsevier Publishing Co. Inc.   New York

302963

© *Excerpta Medica, 1974*

All rights reserved. No part of this publication may be reproduced, stored in a retrieval system or transmitted, in any form or by any means, electronic, mechanical, photocopying, recording or otherwise, without permission in writing from the publisher.

International Congress Series No. 322

ISBN Excerpta Medica 90 219 0228 1
ISBN American Elsevier 0 444 15058 7
Library of Congress Catalog Card Number 74-79159

Publisher: *Excerpta Medica*
　　　　　　335 Jan van Galenstraat
　　　　　　Amsterdam
　　　　　　P.O. Box 1126

Sole Distributors for the USA and Canada:
　　　　　　American Elsevier Publishing Company, Inc.
　　　　　　52 Vanderbilt Avenue
　　　　　　New York, N.Y. 10017

Printed in the Netherlands by Hooiberg, Epe

Second International Symposium on Cancer Detection and Prevention

The Symposium was held under the High Patronage of:
The President of the Italian Republic,
Sen. Prof. Avv. Giovanni Leone

Promoted by: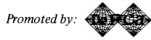

Under the Auspices of:
The International Agency for Research on Cancer
and
Union Internationale Contre le Cancer

In Collaboration with:
Istituto di Oncologia 'F. Addarii'
and
Centro Tumori di Bologna

President:
Carlo Rizzoli

Secretary General:
Cesare Maltoni

International Advisory Scientific Committee:

A. L. Abour Nasr	(Egypt)	D. Metcalf	(Australia)
N. Anchev	(Bulgaria)	N. Montero	(Chile)
Z. M. Bacq	(Belgium)	T. Mork	(Norway)
H. Berndt	(DDR)	A. Nagy	(Hungary)
D.A. Boyes	(Canada)	T. Nakayama	(Japan)
G. Chavanne	(France)	N. Napalkov	(WHO)
C. Craciun	(Rumania)	G. Notter	(Sweden)
P. F. Denoix	(France)	R.A.Q. O'Meara	(Eire)
J. Higginson	(IARC)	I. Padovan	(Yugoslavia)
M. Gaitan-Yanguas	(Columbia)	A. J. Phillips	(UICC)
D. J. Yussawalla	(India)	F. J. C. Roe	(UK)
A. Llombart	(Spain)	C. G. Schmidt	(BRD)
Z. Marinello	(Cuba)	Ph. Shubik	(USA)
L. Meinsma	(Holland)	G. Terzano	(Argentina)
A. Meisels	(Canada)	V. Thurzo	(CCSR)

Programme Committee:

F. Badellino	(Italy)
A. Caputo	(Italy)
M. Dargent	(France)
W. Davis	(IARC)
Y. Fassin	(Belgium)
C. Hammond	(USA)
H. Maisin	(Belgium)
C. Maltoni	(Italy) Ex officio
J. Martin-Lalande	(France)
H. E. Nieburgs	(USA)
M. G. Riotton	(Switzerland)
D. Schmahl	(Germany)
A. Tuyns	(IARC)
U. Veronesi	(UICC)
I. Vodopija	(Yugoslavia)
G. P. Warwick	(UK)
M. Crespi	(Italy) Secretary

Local Organizing Committee:

L. Cacciari
M. Campanacci
D. Carretti
R. Dal Zotto
G. Giamperoli
A. Palazzini
F. Pannuti
G. Pasquale
A. Rovinetti
A. Suppini
F. Vicini

Treasurer:
R. Dal Zotto

Italian Sponsoring Committee:

Pietro Bucalossi
  Società Italiana di Cancerologia

Leonardo Caldarola
  Società Italiana di Terapia
  Loco-Regionale del Tumori
  Associazione Italiana Centri Tumori

Antonio Caputo
  Associazione Nazionale
  Istituti Tumori

Giovanni D'Errico

Antelio Ficari

Luciano Gambassini

Silvio Garattini

Dino Merlini
  Lega Italiana
  per la Lotta contro I Tumori

Guido Moricca

Luigi Nuzzolillo
  Ministero della Sanità

Leonardo Santi

Mario Tortora
  Società Italiana di Citologia
  Clinica e Sociale

Foreword

At the present time much is expected from cancer detection and prevention in the fight against tumours.

The major aim of this Symposium has been to convene from all over the world scientists whose fields are the prevention and early detection of tumours, and with different approaches and disciplinary experiences (basic oncologists, epidemiologists, experimentalists, pathologists, clinicians, etc.) to present the results of their own studies, to point out the potentialities of operative tools, to exchange up-to-date information and to discuss future lines, programs and priorities.

The Editorial Board

Contents

Lectures

Panels

1. Gastric cancer
    Chairmen: N. Zamcheck, U. S. A. and G. Marcozzi, Italy

2. Cancer of the colon and rectum
    Chairmen: W. J. Burdette, U. S. A. and L. Barbara, Italy

3. Cancer of the lung
    Chairmen: R. Doll, United Kingdom and D. Campanacci, Italy

Symposia

6. Organizations of mass screening campaigns

7. Paraneoplastic manifestations and malignancy associated changes

8. *Tumour specific antigens*

Lectures

Developments in cancer prevention through environmental control

John Higginson

International Agency for Research on Cancer, Lyon, France

Introduction

While there are several approaches to the problem of cancer control, the present discussion is largely oriented to the role of the environment in human cancer.

Cancer prevention through the identification and subsequent removal of causative factors was clearly implied by the work of Potts in the late 18th century. This approach was later expanded in the occupational studies of the present century which provided the base for modern environmental carcinogenesis. However, the full potential of the epidemiological method in cancer control was only fully appreciated after the extensive studies on lung cancer and cigarette smoking in the fifties. Today the potentials and limitations of epidemiology and experimental carcinogenesis, which form the basis of environmental carcinogen studies in man have been established. Nonetheless, it has become increasingly clear that it may not be possible to initiate preventative measures following the identification of the cause of a cancer, in the absence of a suitable social and technological background. Thus, man has proved notoriously unwilling to change a pleasurable cultural habit, such as cigarette smoking, no matter how hazardous. The modern oncologist must therefore take into consideration both the legislative and the social aspects of prevention, in addition to the scientific problems.

The role of epidemiological studies

The major contributions of the epidemiological method to cancer control include the following areas:

1. The identification of environmental hazards to which man is already exposed, e.g. asbestos, cigarettes, occupational risks, etc.

2. The observation of changes in the incidence of a specific cancer, indicating the possible entry of a new carcinogenic agent into the environment. Such secular changes are illustrated by the associated increase in cigarette smoking with the rise in lung cancer, and the appearance of mesothelioma following exposure to crocidolite.

3. An improved understanding of the biology of human cancer can be used:

   (a) to explore the action of suspected environmental stimuli through the appropriate biochemical investigations, e.g. the development of comparative metabolic studies in human and animal tissues (Montesano and Magee, 1970);

   (b) to determine the nature of animal models best approximating to the situation in man as a basis for the establishment of systems for testing suspected carcinogens, e.g. selection of dog for testing aromatic amines as a bladder carcinogen;

   (c) to permit the application of sophisticated laboratory techniques to epidemiological studies on human cancer, e.g. endocrine studies in breast cancer (Bulbrook and Thomas, 1964; Bulbrook and Hayward, 1967); sero-epidemiological studies on African childhood lymphoma (Biggs et al., 1972).

4. The identification of levels of exposure to potential or known carcinogenic stimuli in the environment which do not apparently modify the incidence of cancer. Such studies

are invaluable in assessing whether or not an 'acceptable risk' level does exist for man.

More recently, in addition to investigations on the direct carcinogenic effects of external stimuli, changes in host susceptibility, e.g. nutritional and immunological status, as a result of exogenous stimuli, have received attention (Doll and Vodopija, 1973). The epidemiological method is equally suitable for such studies.

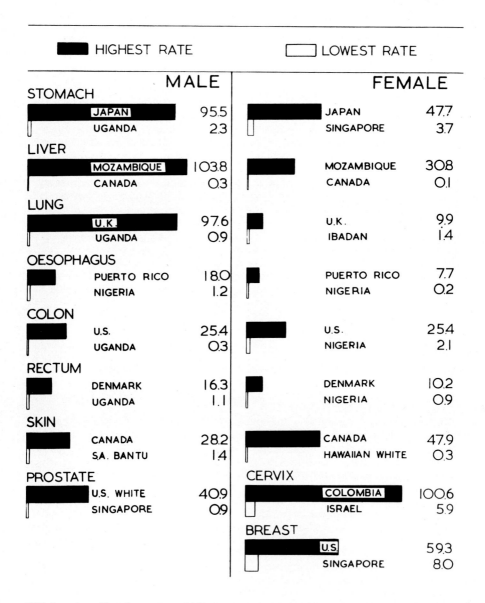

FIG. 1   *Age-adjusted cancer morbidity rates with theoretical low rates illustrating cancer incidence in areas of high and low cancer rates. Black bar represents areas with the highest known cancer rates; white bar represents those with the lowest reported rates.*

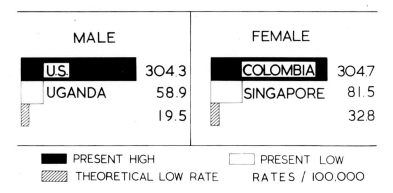

MALE		FEMALE	
U.S.	304.3	**COLOMBIA**	304.7
UGANDA	58.9	SINGAPORE	81.5
	19.5		32.8

■ PRESENT HIGH   □ PRESENT LOW
▨ THEORETICAL LOW RATE   RATES / 100,000

FIG. 2   *Age-adjusted cancer morbidity rates with theoretical low rates, indicating the theoretical low rate that could pertain if the lowest incidence rates were summated from all countries.*

Cancer and the environment

Amplifying earlier epidemiological studies, it has been calculated by various authors that the aetiology of approximately 80% of cancers in western industrialized countries are directly or indirectly dependent on environmental factors (Boyland, 1967; Doll, 1967; Higginson, 1969) (Figs. 1 and 2). That this calculation is a reasonable estimate is suggested by analysing the aetiology of individual cancers of known cause (Higginson, 1969). Thus, 90% of cancers of the mouth and lung are caused by factors which have already been identified. On the other hand, for cancers of other sites, such as colon, rectum, stomach and breast, no satisfactory hypotheses as to aetiology are available.

While individual susceptibility has an important role, even for such strong carcinogenic stimuli as cigarette smoking, non-hereditary factors, with a few exceptions, would appear of paramount importance (Haenszel, 1961; Haenszel and Kurihara, 1968) as suggested by studies on migrant populations. Although host factors may be of significance in relation to cancers of the breast and genital system, it cannot be excluded that such factors may not be wholly or partly dependent on environmental stimuli possibly often operating *in utero* or in very early life. From the viewpoint of practical prevention, Huebner's 'oncogene' hypothesis, if confirmed, would not reduce significantly the necessity to identify environmental factors, since the theory implies that the latter activate the 'oncogene'.

Identification of exogenous carcinogenic factors

While from a philosophical viewpoint carcinogenic stimuli may represent the interaction of a multitude of factors, e.g. historical, climatic, sociological, etc., such a vague approach to identification has so far led to few practical benefits. Thus, a distinction should be made between such distant and relatively immeasurable factors and 'intermediate' or 'immediate' stimuli (Fig. 3). These terms are not used here with the same connotation as 'proximate' or 'ultimate' carcinogen as in experimental carcinogenesis, but refer to stimuli which can be expressed in quantitative or qualitative terms for practical purposes, e.g. specific chemicals, cultural habits, etc.

Method of exposure

Man is most commonly exposed to exogenous carcinogens through *direct contact, inhalation, ingestion* or by the *parenteral route*. Direct contact occurs in certain occupations, e.g. shale oil workers, or as a result of a cultural habit, e.g. betel chewing. Occupational

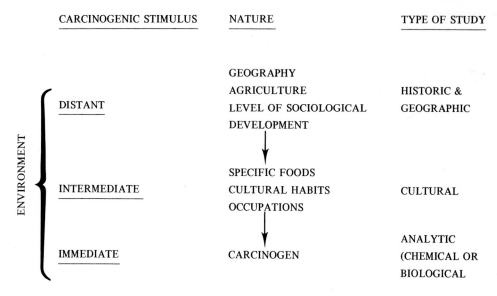

FIG. 3   *Relation between man and carcinogenic stimulus, showing various levels at which carcinogenic stimuli can be investigated in the environment.*

and cultural habits are also important in relation to inhalatory exposure, e.g. cigarettes and asbestos. Although dietary customs are believed to be of major aetiological consequence for certain cancers, e.g. stomach and large intestine, in only a few instances has a satisfactory causal relationship been established, e.g. over-indulgence in alcoholic beverages and carcinoma of the oesophagus.

There are several types of epidemiological studies which may contribute to the evaluation of aetiological stimuli in man.

Descriptive epidemiology

Sound data on the geographic distribution of cancers both within a country (micro-epidemiology) and at an international level provide the essential background to understanding the nature of the disease in man. In the early twentieth century descriptive epidemiology was largely dependent on mortality data (Segi and Kurihara, 1972) but today it is centred around the modern cancer morbidity registry. The latter permits adequate assessment of cancer incidence and eliminates the bias introduced by variations in cure rates, secondary risks. etc. Today, there are more than 60 registries covering a range of populations and environments around the world, many of which are members of the International Association of Cancer Registries (IACR). These registries provide age-specific cancer rates (Doll et al., 1970). While to date such a registration system has not been instrumental in identifying specific causes, it is essential for providing back-up data and will be necessary in any monitoring system. Moreover, some registries provide information permitting the identification of cancer patterns in high risk groups who show unusual cancer patterns or who are exposed to an unusual level of a suspected carcinogen and which can be studied. The record linkage system (Acheson, 1967) is the most sophisticated form of this activity, and will probably provide the basis for future cancer environmental monitoring studies, especially for high risk groups, e.g. woodworkers (Acheson et al., 1968).

Analytical epidemiology

The mere collection of cancer statistics per se is of little value unless it is directed to the identification of cancer causation. In the past, such studies have been either of the prospective or retrospective case-history type where it has been possible to identify either groups exposed to an unusual risk of a cancer, e.g. lung cancer, or to examine a group which has been exposed to an unusual environmental hazard, e.g. dye workers (Table 1). It is not my intention to discuss this aspect further, but only to emphasize that such investigations have been highly satisfactory in identifying an aetiological factor where the latter can be readily measured and the risk is considerable. Unfortunately, there are certain situations where such studies have so far proved unsatisfactory, notably homogenous modern societies exposed to a multiplicity of potential carcinogenic factors (Higginson, 1972). This may be due to the widespread exposure of the population to a carcinogen, tumours only developing in a limited number of slightly more susceptible individuals. Thus, case-history studies have so far failed to clarify adequately the aetiology of such cancers as breast, large intestine, cervix, etc.

TABLE 1   *Chemicals recognized as carcinogens in man*

Chemical	Site	Type of evidence*
Certain tars, soots, oils	Skin, lungs	C.R.
Cigarette smoke	Lungs	R.C.C.
2-Naphthylamine	Urinary bladder	C.H.
4-Aminobiphenyl	Urinary bladder	C.R.
Benzidine	Urinary bladder	C.H.
N,N-bis(2-chloroethyl)-2-naphthylamine	Urinary bladder	C.R.
Bis(2-chloroethyl)sulfide	Lungs	C.R.
Nickel compounds	Lungs, nasal sinuses	C.H.
Chromium compounds	Lungs	C.H.
Asbestos	Lungs, pleura	C.R.

* C.R.   – Case reports
    R.C.C.   – Retrospective case control
    C.H.   – Cohort study (non-concurrent prospective)

Correlation studies

A possible approach to the problem of carcinogens diffusely scattered in the environment is to investigate the incidence of cancers in communities exposed to the suspected factor at different dose levels. Theoretically, such communities should vary in cancer incidence according to the level of exposure and provide an opportunity for separating risk factors (Higginson, 1972). Unfortunately, although the statistical correlation may be strong, aetiological associations of this type are weak and do not necessarily permit identification of the factors concerned, especially if exposure to the suspected factor is difficult to measure accurately. However, if a suitable hypothesis is available and similar results are obtained in several geographical areas showing different environmental conditions, the causal relationship may become increasingly probable.

The greatest use of correlation studies would appear to be in the confirmation of hypotheses developed from case-history investigations or from animal studies. For example, good correlations have been demonstrated between the level of cigarette consumption within a country and the incidence of lung cancer. On the other hand, attempts to correlate the incidence of colon and rectal cancer with environmental factors have shown associations with so many environmental factors as to permit no firm conclusions (Day, unpublished data). An association with one factor may in fact only represent a secondary association with another parameter. On the other hand, where a reasonable aetiological hypothesis is consistently confirmed in several geographical areas, an aetiological relationship may be suspected to a degree justifying legislative action.

However, whereas positive correlations may not be very meaningful, a negative correlation may be of the utmost importance in suggesting that exposure at certain levels does not carry an appreciable risk. Thus, although many industrial societies show asbestos bodies in the lungs (Um, 1971) in a large proportion of the general population there is no evidence as yet that this low level of exposure has caused a significant increase in lung cancer, although there is good evidence that at higher levels asbestos has an additive effect with cigarette smoking (Selikoff et al., 1968) and is the cause of mesothelioma (Wagner, 1971).

Attempts to relate cancer frequency in several countries to such pesticides as DDT have so far indicated no major change in cancer patterns that can be readily ascribed to the utilization of this pesticide during the last 25 years. While this is not definitive proof of a non-effect in man, it would suggest that DDT is probably not a strong carcinogen at low levels of exposure.

Correlation studies however, provide the only base on which a cancer monitoring system may be developed, it being presumed that changes in cancer incidence would provide an index of the previous entrance of new risk factors into the environment (Higginson, 1972).

In addition to the statistical problem, there are many technical difficulties associated with correlation studies. Firstly, the problem of measurement is often compounded by the absence of suitable standardized analytical techniques for many potential carcinogens on a large-scale basis. Secondly, the large number of suspected carcinogens present in a single environment and which would require analysis presents a severe logistics problem. Thirdly, the differing biological action of such compounds makes assessment of the problem even more difficult to analyze in biological terms. Thus, for example, enzyme induction may imply inhibition or promotion according to the individual carcinogens present. Lastly, the amount of a compound present in the environment today may be very different from the situation 20 years earlier, at which time critical exposure may have occurred, thus rendering present-day correlations invalid.

The above problems of correlation studies are well illustrated by investigations on aflatoxin and liver cancer. The mycotoxin is widely distributed in Africa and has been suggested as the major cause of liver cancer there and in Asia (Wogan, 1973). Attempts to associate the frequency of liver cancer with contamination of foodstuffs, although suggestive, are far from unequivocal (Keen and Martin, 1971; Peers and Linsell, 1973). Thus, it has been necessary to determine how much aflatoxin people actually do eat. Preliminary studies do show a correlation between aflatoxin ingestion and liver cancer (Tables 2 and 3). However, there are other observations suggesting that the problem may be more complicated. Until the early sixties, it was believed that the virus of infectious hepatitis was the possible causative factor in liver cancer in Africa (Higginson, 1963). Recently, however, it has been shown that a very high percentage of primary liver cancers in Africa and Asia show evidence of being carriers of hepatitis B virus (Australia antigen) (WHO Scientific Group Report, 1973). Furthermore, the carrier rate among populations with a high frequency of liver cancer is also much higher than in North America or European populations. Thus, an aetiological association cannot be excluded and the possibility of multi-factorial origin must be considered. Future research will require the close integration of chemical and virological studies.

Measurement of the environment: individual exposure

In both correlation studies and case-history studies quantitative data on exposure is desirable at the individual level. Thus, Case (Case et al., 1954), in his classical studies on workers in the dye and rubber industries, was able to identify the level of exposure to

TABLE 2 *Study of aflatoxin exposure and liver cancer in Murang'a district, Kenya. Summary of principal results*

	High altitude area		Medium altitude area		Low altitude area		All areas	
	Males	Females	Males	Females	Males	Females	Males	Females
Total population (1962 census)	18,394	20,244	75,138	86,467	68,808	75,803	162,340	182,514
Population >16 years old (1962 census)	8,027	10,885	30,105	45,693	30,949	41,375	69,081	97,953
Frequency of aflatoxin-contaminated diets (mean level in µg/kg)	39/808 (0.121)		54/808 (0.205)		78/816 (0.351)		171/2,432 (0.226)	
Frequency of aflatoxin-contaminated beers (mean level in µg/l)	3/101 (0.050)		4/101 (0.069)		9/102 (0.167)		16/304 (0.095)	
Mean aflatoxin ingestion (ng/kg body weight per day)*	4.88	3.46	7.84	5.86	14.81	10.03	9.18	6.46
Primary liver cancer cases in population >16 years old, 1967/70	1	–	13	6	15	9	29	15
Annual incidence rates per 100,000, by sex	3.11	0	10.80	3.28	12.12	5.44	10.50	3.83

* Assuming a daily food intake of 2 kg, a daily beer intake of 2 litres (men only) and an average adult body weight of 70 kg (after: Peers and Linsell, 1973).

TABLE 3   *Geographical distribution of malignant hepatoma in Swaziland 1964-1968*

	Highveld	Middleveld	Lowveld
No. of cases	11	34	44
Crude rate/10^5/yr	2.2	4.0	9.7
Population ratios	1.0	1.7	0.9
Relative risk	1.0	1.8	4.5

Corresponding aflatoxin assays in groundnuts

% positive samples	20	57	60

(after: Keen and Martin, 1971)

certain carcinogens in these occupations. However, for most known, or even suspected carcinogens in the environment, only the concentration in the air or in isolated foodstuffs alone is available, and actual individual exposure is unknown.

The future of epidemiological investigations

Population laboratories

It is more than probable that future studies on the chronic degenerative diseases will require detailed investigations on individual population groups over long periods. Such 'population laboratories' should ideally cover several different environments and thus permit the separation of cancer risks. One such study has already been established in Japan. The IARC has also developed a study on oesophageal cancer in Iran which may provide guidance as to the potential value of such investigations (IARC Annual Report, 1972a). Along the Caspian Littoral there is an east/west gradient in the incidence of oesophageal cancer from 108.8 to 21.0 per 100,000 for males and from 174.1 to 14.7 per 100,000 for females, associated with significant changes in sex ratios from 0.6:1 to 3.1:1 (Kmet and Mahboubi, 1972). An aetiological role for alcohol and tobacco being unlikely, and in the absence of alternative hypotheses, an intensive study covering habits, diet, etc., of the communities along the Littoral has been developed. While logistic problems are great, such a multifactorial approach appears logical and, if possible, may provide a basis on which future population laboratories may be established.

Such an approach may also be suitable for the study of such cancers as colon, rectal, breast, etc., for which, as yet, we have no satisfactory hypotheses, possibly due to the fact that in modern industrial societies suspected carcinogens may be widely distributed through a relatively homogenous community. Case-history studies alone cannot demonstrate a dose relationship in such cases. On the other hand, striking geographical differences in incidence are observed between countries suggesting comparable variations in aetiological factors.

Monitoring

The studies described above have largely concentrated on carcinogens already present in the environment. There is now increasing interest in the possibility of developing a monitoring system for environmental carcinogens similar to that which has been reported as feasible for identifying environmental teratogens. The requirements for developing such a system include the following prerequisites:
    1. The existence of long-term cancer registration systems in certain key geographical

areas is essential in determining those secular changes in incidence which would indicate the introduction of a potential risk. Association with a record linkage system would enhance the value of such registries (Acheson, 1967). Few registries have been in operation sufficiently long to permit such studies.

2. Quantitative data must be available on the levels of potential environmental carcinogens. Since the latter are so numerous, priorities must be selected, based either on the degree of human exposure or on the suspected risk as indicated by circumstantial evidence or animal experimentation (IARC Monographs, 1972*b*). Problems will be least where the suspected factor is specific and readily measurable with available technology. In contrast, it will be difficult to relate future changes in cancer patterns to a past event in the absence of information on time and level of exposure. Simple situations such as a single exposure to ionizing radiation will be easiest to investigate. Indices of previous exposure, such as asbestos bodies within the lung, or DDT levels in body fat, represent another approach. Where exposure may be of short duration and the chemical rapidly metabolized, e.g. nitrosamines, no marker of exposure may be available. The situation is even more complicated if a carcinogen is formed in vivo by the interaction of two non-carcinogenic agents, as has been shown for secondary amines and nitrites (Sander, 1967).

3. Contrary to the case of congenital malformations, where the lesion can be referred back to an event occurring during the previous few months, some human cancers have latent periods of over 20 years; thus reference must be made to events many years earlier. The most helpful situation relates to childhood cancers with their relatively short latent periods, e.g. cancers induced by maternal diagnostic radiation or a transplacental carcinogen. Unfortunately, the trends in cancer patterns for childhood cancers in general do not show very prominent changes, nor in general are the same wide geographical variations observed as seen in adults (Table 4) (Doll et al., 1970).

4. Clearly, variations in human cancer rates may be very considerable and trends indicating an increase or decrease are sometimes of considerable magnitude. Thus, Table 5 gives the changes in cancer incidence that must occur over a period to permit identification of trends. The necessity to continue studies for periods of up to 15 years and the possibility that factors causing both increases and decreases may be present simultaneously would indicate that interpretation will be difficult, unless the effect of the agent is very obvious or unless it produces an unusual or rare cancer, e.g. mesotheliomas due to asbestos exposure (Wagner, 1971) or vaginal adenocarcinoma in the offspring of diethyl-stilboestrol treated mothers (Herbst et al., 1971).

TABLE 4   *Incidence of cancer in Connecticut 1935-1962. Age-specific rates per 100,000 per annum (0-14 years)*

	Males	Females
All sites	Increase up to 1955 then perhaps slight fall except in 10-14 age group	
Kidney	No increase	No increase
Eye	No increase	No increase
Brain	Slight increase up to 1955 then fall, except 10-14 age group	Slight increase up to 1950
Bone	No increase	No increase
Connective tissue	No increase	No increase
Lymphatic system	Steady increase in 10-14 age group but number small	No increase
Leukaemia	Slight increase up to 1955	Slight increase up to 1950

TABLE 5   *Average percentage change in rate which must occur each year to indicate a significant
trend over either 5- or 15-year period*

Absolute number of cases p.a.	5 yr*	5 yr**	15 yr*	15 yr**
500	4.5	8.4	0.5	0.8
50	14.2	26.4	1.6	2.4

Significance test
*   A one-sided test at 0.05% level
** A two-sided test at 1% level

Probably the greatest value of a monitoring system will lie in the potential of demonstrating marked changes in cancer patterns, thus providing a warning that some significant change has occurred in the environment. Its value as an identifying system will be much less satisfactory, and will probably be most successful in the following situations:

(a)   Childhood cancers, with their relatively short latent periods, as in transplacental carcinogenesis.

(b)   High-risk groups exposed to marked changes in the environment of a cultural or occupational nature, involving either an initiating or a promoting agent.

(c)   Large populations exposed to an unusual concentration of a carcinogen, e.g. atomic bomb.

(d)   Changes in rare cancers whose incidence may be rapidly appreciated, e.g. mesothelioma.

(e)   In providing additional evidence for safety of compounds to which man is exposed.

(f)   While the relationship between mutagenesis, teratogenesis and carcinogenesis is far from absolute, a registry for teratogenic effects might provide a useful indication of a possible later carcinogenic effect.

Cancer in an industrial society

A major problem exercising public health authorities reflects on the extent to which the nature of modern westernized states may expose the individual to a large number of carcinogens at low doses — the 'total carcinogenic load' — and thus be responsible for the high frequency of certain cancers in North America and Europe. Whereas the aesthetic results of air and water pollution are very obvious to the observer, it is far from clear to what extent such obvious pollution does in fact represent a carcinogenic risk. Thus, there is a surprising similarity in incidence rates for many sites between relatively non-industrialized rural Canada and New Zealand and the highly-industrialized United Kingdom. Nonetheless, there is evidence that striking geographical differences do exist, even within the same geographical area. Thus, the incidence of rectal cancer in Denmark is approximately twice that seen in Finland, although the frequency of colon cancer in the two countries is similar (De Jong et al., 1972). The carcinogenic stimuli to which individuals in these societies are probably exposed represent subtle changes in the environmental background, especially dietary factors, which are difficult to measure. It is thus necessary that such societies will require careful correlation investigations in which the levels of exposure are measured in many different communities.

Prevention of exposure to new carcinogens

Problems of extrapolation

Whereas the epidemiological method may prove of value in identifying the presence of a carcinogen already present in the environment, such studies cannot prevent the entry of new factors. For this we must rely on animal experimentation with all the difficulties of extrapolation to man.

Comparative studies on human and animal tissues   For only a few carcinogens do we have comparable data on their metabolism in man and animals. Furthermore, substances carcinogenic to animals show wide variations in their effects in different strains and species. The problem of evaluating rationally the production of cancer at one site in an animal as indicating carcinogenic activity at a second site in man remains insurmountable with our present limited knowledge.

Limitations of epidemiological data   Epidemiological data are insufficient to permit satisfactory comparisons in man and animals for many suspected chemicals, even those that have been in the environment for considerable periods, e.g. DDT. Moreover, while a number of carcinogenic stimuli in man are also carcinogenic to animals, the converse is not necessarily true. Thus penicillin G and isoniazid would appear non-carcinogenic in man from the available evidence, at present exposure levels.

Low dose carcinogenesis   Whereas in animals most carcinogens are tested at comparatively high dose levels, in man exposure in most cases is at very low dose levels. The action of a carcinogen at such low doses must be considered at two levels:
  (a)   the interaction between target cell and the 'ultimate' carcinogen;
  (b)   at the host level, where a large number of factors may modify the dose to which the target cell is exposed, e.g. rates of ingestion, absorption, detoxifying or activating mechanisms. Further, host protective mechanisms may modify actual tumour development.
    At present the interaction of a carcinogen at the cell level can best be studied in vitro and there does seem some evidence that below certain levels of exposure carcinogenic transformation does not occur. This could theoretically be due either to the fact that the dose per cell is below a critical mass level or that the interactions at the target cell level represent a series of molecular events occurring by hazard and that the chance of such an event occurring has become so low as to be unmeasurable. It should be noted that while single doses of certain chemicals produce cancer, this is not necessarily true for all chemical carcinogens. While theoretically there is no such thing as a completely safe dose level for carcinogens, experimental evidence would indicate that there could be a level below which exposure should be 'acceptable' in the context of the word as used by the average man.

Transplacental carcinogenesis

While theoretically it may be possible to establish acceptable low dose levels based on epidemiological evidence in adults, such levels might not be acceptable for the more susceptible tissues of the embryo e.g. vaginal adenocarcinoma in the offspring of stilboestrol-treated mothers (Herbst et al., 1971). If the latent period of transplacental-induced tumours extends beyond childhood or early adult life (Tomatis and Mohr, 1973) such situations will be exceedingly difficult to identify in man.

Role of promoters

Whereas direct-acting carcinogens (complete carcinogens) are of greatest concern at present, the potential role of promoters (incomplete carcinogens) must not be neglected.

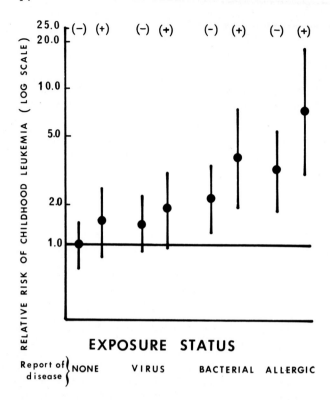

FIG. 4   *The effects of intra-uterine irradiation on increasing childhood susceptibility to leukaemia. (after: Bross and Natarajan, 1972).*

Their action has been established experimentally for mouse skin and possibly for bladder. Thus, it is possible that a stimulus which in one individual may be harmless, in another may induce cancer. This multifactorial situation in terms of promoting action has recently been ascribed to viral infection increasing susceptibility to leukaemia as a result of low-level radiation in utero (Bross and Natarajan, 1972) (Figure 4). It has also been suggested that aflatoxin and viral hepatitis may have a synergistic reaction.

Effect of host modifications

Whereas there has been a tendency to consider the influence of host factors only in terms of genetic or racial background, there is evidence that susceptibility may be modified by environmental factors. The potential epidemiological approaches to such studies were explored recently (Doll and Vodopija, 1973).

   Immunological and endocrinological mechanisms   The hypothesis of 'immune surveillance' has received considerable attention during the last decade. In addition to experimental data, the increased incidence of lymphomas in individuals receiving renal transplants has been ascribed to a reduction in the immune protective mechanism. It is also suspected that modifications in endocrine metabolism may modify susceptibility to neoplasia. Thus, the artificial menopause has been identified with an increased risk of breast cancer (Trichopoulous et al., 1972) and contraception through endocrines possibly with a decreased risk (Vessey et al., 1972). In both situations environmental factors could clearly be of importance.

Nutrition   It is well known that in experimental animals calorie and protein deficiency may reduce the incidence of spontaneous or induced tumours (Ross and Bras, 1965). Whether a similar situation occurs in man is unknown, but it is interesting to speculate whether the widespread protein and calorie deficiency in Africa may not be related to the low incidence of certain tumours on that continent. On the other hand, it is also interesting to speculate whether the deficiencies in immunity demonstrated in malnourished African children may not persist into adult life. Nutrition may also modify the internal milieu, e.g. bacterial flora of the bowel, which again may be a pertinent factor in human colonic cancer.

The profile of a susceptible individual

If individuals who are unduly susceptible to external carcinogens can be identified, this would be of potential value in prevention. Thus, if that tenth of the population who smoke two packets of cigarettes a day and who develop lung cancer can be identified as a high risk group, it is probable that control methods would have more chance of success if concentrated on those individuals. It would appear a highly desirable exercise to determine in what way the susceptible and non-susceptible groups differ biologically. As yet, studies in this area have been inadequately explored and the profile of the susceptible individual remains to be established (Doll and Vodopija, 1973).

An increased frequency of a second tumour, either at the same site, e.g. second breast, or at a different site in the same individual might suggest that a generalized increased susceptibility to cancer may exist. A full review of multiple tumours has been made by Lynch (1967) but many reports lack statistical control, rendering the distinction between genetic and environmental factors difficult to assess. Other studies (Bailar, 1963; Berg, 1967; Cook, 1966) suggest that while for certain endocrine-dependent cancers an increase of second tumours would appear to be present, the incidence is not high and for many sites is not present. The identification of situations where groups of individuals exposed to a common carcinogen show variations in incidence is likely to prove the most satisfactory situation for study, as being indicative of the existence of secondary factors. Such possibilities include not only geographical variations between countries, but also such situations as urban/rural differences within a country. Fraumeni (1969) has indicated some of the possibilities of cellular markers in relation to constitutional factors in predisposing to cancer. If similar cellular markers produced by environmental factors can be identified, they would be of great importance.

Legislation, education and prevention

From the above discussion it is clear that cancer prevention is far from being an exact science and that human data would appear essential to support definitive legislative proposals. Unfortunately, in practice it is necessary to take preventive action in a modern society in the absence of such data by making an educated guess as to the extent of the risk, based on degree of exposure and animal experimentation, but absolute safety can never be guaranteed. Where data are available it may be possible to imply that exposure at such and such a level is unlikely to be important in practice. A rule of thumb might be an incidence of risk of 1 per 1,000,000 individuals per annum. For common cancers, e.g. lung, an increase of this magnitude would not be identifiable, but for very rare cancers, e.g. mesothelioma, such a risk would be demonstrable, and therefore not acceptable.

Although it has been shown experimentally that certain carcinogens are active in a single dose, and while theoretically this may be true for all carcinogens, the fact that this is not the case is probably dependent on a wide variety of factors modifying the contact between the ultimate carcinogen and the target cell. Thus, differences between strong and

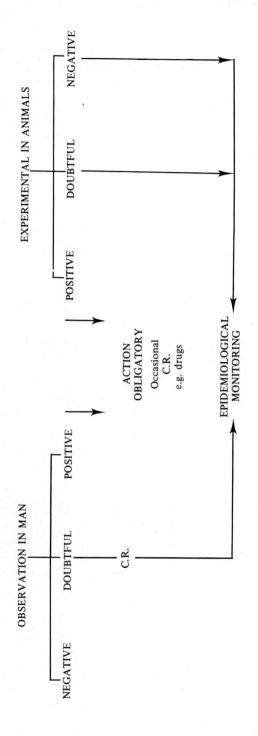

FIG. 5   *Criteria for legislation (C.R. = calculated risk implying some form of legislative control).*

weak carcinogens may be as much a reflection of host factors as an indication of their molecular format.

While theoretically there is no such thing as a completely safe dose level, clearly there is theoretically a level at which exposure should be considered acceptable.

In the absence of satisfactory methods of extrapolation the Delaney Clause would seem a reasonable approach in relation to new compounds where these offer no obvious human benefit. On the other hand, the situation is much more difficult in relation to substances utilized for many years without apparent ill-effect, e.g. GRAS list. Whereas it is not impossible that certain of these substances may in fact constitute a carcinogenic hazard, it might be argued that such a hazard may in fact be less than substitution by compounds for which we have as yet no human data, although apparently safe for animals.

In view of the complicated problems associated with legislation of cancer prevention through environmental control, there is no substitute for an adequately educated public to avoid hysterical decisions. It is desirable that the public be educated on the technical problems of environmental control and cost-benefit analysis, including the extent to which the calculation of human risks is an inexact science. There is considerable necessity to explore further the meaning of the term 'acceptable risk'. There are situations where a scientist may have to express an opinion as to the extent of the risk based on inadequate data. He may be wrong, but his opinion is less likely to be wrong than a decision made by someone with little experience in the field. On the other hand, a layman should be able to indicate the level of exposure he would accept in order to obtain certain benefits. Figure 5 illustrates in diagrammatical from the available criteria for legislation, indicating how observations in man and animals may be integrated to make some form of rational decision in relation to a calculated risk.

References

Acheson, E. D. (1967): Medical Record Linkage. Oxford University Press, Oxford.

Acheson, E. D., Cowdell, R. H., Hadfield, E. and MacBeth, R. G. (1968): Brit. med. J., 2, 587.

Bailar, J. C. III (1963): Cancer, 16, 842.

Berg, J. W. (1967): J. nat. Cancer Inst., 38, 741.

Biggs, P. M., De Thé, G. and Payne, L. N. (Editors) (1972): Oncogenesis and Herpes Viruses, IARC Scientific Publications Number 2. International Agency for Research on Cancer, Lyon.

Boyland, E. (1967): Proc. roy. Soc. Med., 60, 93.

Bross, I. D. J. and Natarajan, N. (1972): New Engl. J. Med., 287, 107.

Bulbrook, R. D. and Thomas, B. S. (1964): Nature (Lond.), 201, 189.

Bulbrook, R. D. and Hayward, J. L. (1967): Lancet, 1, 519.

Case, R. A. M., Hosker, M. E., McDonald, D. B. and Pearson, J. T. (1954): Brit. J. industr. Med., 2, 75.

Cook, G. B. (1966): Cancer, 19, 959.

De Jong, U. W., Day, N. E., Muir, C. S. et al. (1972): Int. J. Cancer, 10, 463.

Doll, R. (1967): Prevention of Cancer—Points for Epidemiology. The Rock Carling Fellowship 1967—Nuffield Provincial Hospitals Trust, 1967. Whitefriars Press Ltd., London.

Doll, R., Muir, C. and Waterhouse, J. (Editors) (1970): Cancer Incidence in Five Continents, Volume II. International Union Against Cancer, Geneva.

Doll, R. and Vodopija, I. J. A. (Editors) (1973): Proceedings of the Conference on 'Host-Environment Interactions in the Etiology of Cancer in Man—Implementation in Research', Primosten, Yugoslavia, 26 August to 2 September 1972. IARC Scientific Publications Number 7. International Agency for Research on Cancer, Lyon.

Fraumeni, J. F. (1969): Nat. Cancer Inst. Monogr., 32, 221.

Haenszel, W. (1961): J. nat. Cancer Inst., 26, 37.

Haenszel, W. and Kurihara, M. (1968): J. nat. Cancer Inst., 40, 43.

Herbst, A. L., Ulfelder, H. and Poskanzer, D. C. (1971): New Engl. J. Med., 284, 878.

Higginson, J. (1963): Cancer Res., 23, 1624.

Higginson, J. (1969): In: Proceedings, Eighth Canadian Cancer Conference, Honey Harbour, Ontario, 1968, pp. 40-75. Editor: J. F. Morgan. Pergamon Press, Toronto.

Higginson, J. (1972): In: Proceedings, 2nd International Symposium of the Princess Takamatsu Cancer Research Fund on 'Topics in Chemical Carcinogenesis', pp. 511-527. Editors: W. Nakahara, S. Takayama, T. Sugimura and S. Odashima. University of Tokyo Press, Tokyo.

IARC Monographs (1972a): Evaluation of the Carcinogenic Risk of Chemicals to Man. International Agency for Research on Cancer, Lyon.

IARC Annual Report (1972b): International Agency for Research on Cancer, Lyon.

Keen, P. and Martin, P. (1971): Trop. geogr. Med., 23, 44.

Kmet, J. and Mahboubi, E. (1972): Science, 175, 846.

Lynch, H. T. (1967): Hereditary Factors in Carcinoma. Recent Results in Cancer Research, Number 12. Springer-Verlag, Berlin-Heidelberg- New-York.

Montesano, R. and Magee, P. N. (1970): Nature (Lond.), 228, 173.

Peers, F.G. and Linsell, C.A. (1973): Brit. J. Cancer, 27, 473.

Ross, M. H. and Bras, G. (1965): J. Nutr., 87, 245.

Sander, J. (1967): Arch. Hyg. (Berl.), 151, 22.

Segi, M. and Kurihara, M. (1972): Cancer Mortality for Selected Sites in 24 Countries. No. 6 (1966-1967). Japan Cancer Society.

Selikoff, I. J., Hammond, E. C. and Churg, J. (1968): J. Amer. med. Ass., 204, 106.

Tomatis, L. and Mohr, U. (Editors) (1973): Transplacental Carcinogenesis. IARC Scientific Publications Number 4. International Agency for Research on Cancer, Lyon.

Trichopoulous, D., MacMahon, B. and Cole, P. (1972): J. nat. Cancer Inst., 48, 605.

Um, C.-H. (1971): Brit. med. J., 2, 248.

Vessey, M. P., Doll, R. and Sutton, P. M. (1971): Brit. med. J., 3, 719.

Wagner, J. C. (1971): J. nat. Cancer Inst., 46, No. 5.

WHO Scientific Group Report (1973): Viral Hepatitis. World Health Organization Technical Report Series Number 512. World Health Organization, Geneva.

Wogan, G. (1973): Assessment of Exposure to Aflatoxins. Proceedings of the Conference on 'Host-Environment Interactions in the Etiology of Cancer in Man—Implementation in Research'. Primosten, Yugoslavia, 26 August to 2 September 1972, pp. 237-241. Editors: R. Doll and I.J. A. Vodopija. IARC Scientific Publications Number 7. International Agency for Research on Cancer, Lyon.

Occupational carcinogenesis

Cesare Maltoni

Istituto di Oncologia 'F. Addarii' and Centro Tumori, Bologna, Italy

Occupational carcinogenesis is one of the most interesting, tragic, important and difficult fields in oncology.

It is interesting from the scientific point of view because it represents, dramatically, an experiment in carcinogenesis made on humans and it may teach us a lot about the natural history of tumours. It is tragic from a human point of view, because work which is per se a natural necessity of life, should not, at least, cause cancer. It is socially important because oncogenic factors increasingly are produced and diffused in occupational environments. Moreover from the factories they spread to the general environment, so that they come to be an ecological problem. Finally, occupational carcinogenesis is a difficult field to approach, because the care of the workers' health is often in conflict with the productive interests of the factories.

Industry has done a lot for experimental carcinogenesis, related to occupational cancer; often however the result is merely to prove the carcinogenic effect in animals of agents which have already proved to be carcinogenic for man: this is equivalent to saying that many people die of cancer but some make their living from cancer. On the other hand emotional arguments should be avoided. Thus I am aware that speaking on occupational carcinogenesis is a complex and difficult task.

Experimental carcinogenesis did not start with the experiment of Yamagiwa and Ichikawa in 1915, but rather in the 16th century with the observation of the so-called 'mountain disease' in miners of Joachimsthal. This disease was recognized at the end of the last century as pulmonary carcinoma, which we now know is due to radio-active pollution, present in those mines. In 1775 Percival Pott in 'Chirurgical Observations' described a cancer of the scrotum in chimney sweepers and he correlated it with the black soot. In 1894 Unna reported on the frequency of skin cancer found in maritime workers, and he considered it due to excessive exposure to sun light. In 1895 Rehn, a surgeon from Frankfurt, reported at the congress of the German Society of Surgeons, 3 cases of bladder tumours found among 45 workers from a factory which produced fuchsine. He thought that the tumours were caused by aniline, but in fact it was shown, several decades later, that they were due to other aromatic amines. In 1902 at a meeting of the Medical Society of Hamburg, Frieben presented a case of a cutaneous tumour found on the hand of an employee of a factory producing X-ray apparatus. This employee used his hand for radiological demonstrations.

The frequency of reports on occupational cancer has been increasing with the increase of industrialization, mainly due to the progress of chemistry. The most important thing to do in occupational carcinogenesis is to try to recognize occupations which may represent an oncogenic risk, and to identify the agent or agents which cause the risk, and also to try to assess the degree of risk. If the risk is related to an agent already known to be oncogenic for man, its detection in the occupational environment should be considered sufficient for undertaking preventive measures. On the other hand if the risk is related to agents, whose effects on workers have not yet been studied and are therefore not yet known, then we have to evaluate the risk they represent for workers. This can be done by means of epidemiological investigations and experimental testing. Most oncogenic occupational agents have been identified on the basis of retrospective epidemiological studies.

The progress in and the development of this branch of oncology should facilitate systematic experimental testing of agents heavily released in the occupational environment. In other words *the need of epidemiological evidence in man should be avoided.* Experimental tests on animals are the more relevant to man, the more they reproduce the conditions of human exposure and eventually induce in animals the same tumours that they induce in man. In this case, the results of experimental tests may be considered largely equivalent to epidemiological evidence in man.

On the other hand if an agent causes any kind of tumour in animals, in whatever experimental conditions, it should be considered potentially carcinogenic for man. To consider an agent definitely carcinogenic for man on such a basis, would be an excess, but no time should be lost before retesting it in more appropriate conditions. To reproduce experimentally the conditions of occupational exposure is often difficult and costly. Furthermore we have to consider that the number of agents in the occupational environment is large and increasing.

Thus, new agents to which workers may be exposed should be submitted first to the easiest and quickest tests, however incomplete those tests may be. Then, for those agents inducing tumours in the experimental animals in these conditions, more precise and sophisticated experimental tests should be devised. The validity of experimental testing and the prerequisites for validity have been a matter of long discussions in international

TABLE 1   *Incidence of subcutaneous sarcomas in rats, following local injection of some inorganic pigments*

Treatment	No. of animals	No. of tumours
Chromium yellow (lead chromate)	40	26
Chromium orange (lead chromate)	40	26
Molybdenum orange (lead chromate and molybdenum chromate)	40	36
Cadmium yellow (cadmium sulphide)	40	15
Iron red (iron oxide)	40	1
Iron yellow (iron oxide)	40	0
Controls	60	0

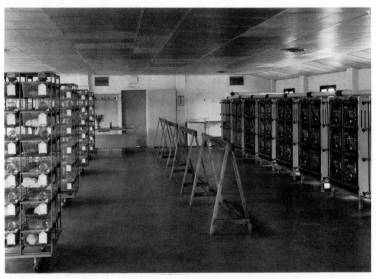

FIG. 1   *Apparatus for inhalation of controlled doses of gaseous compounds, in the Experimental Unit of the Istituto di Oncologia di Bologna.*

meetings and commissions, but of course, in the meantime the existing occupational exposure continues. Also, imperfect testing, for example the subcutaneous injection in the rat of compounds, to which man is exposed mainly by the respiratory route, may give some idea of their potential oncogenic risk.

In Table 1, data are reported on the induction of tumours (sarcomas) at the site of the subcutaneous injection of some inorganic pigments. From these data it clearly appears that chromium and cadmium pigments should be considered riskier than iron pigments. From what has been said before, the compounds shown to be carcinogenic in these conditions, should now be tested by inhalation. The latter way of exposure implies the availability of a complex apparatus for continuous inhalation of controlled doses. The apparatus is quite rare, as we discovered when we wanted to build one and we were not able to find any model in our own or any neighbouring country. Now an apparatus for inhalation of gaseous compounds has been functioning for more than two years in the experimental unit of our institute (Fig. 1).

With this apparatus we are now performing a carcinogenicity bioassay of vinyl chloride monomer (VC) and of vinyl acetate monomer (VA), which are (particularly the first) of great industrial importance. VC is used in the preparation of polyvinyl chloride resin, as a copolymer in saran and other plastics, as a solvent and as a chemical intermediate, and it is at present produced at a rate of 12,000,000 tons per year. Early results on these bioassays are shown in Table 2.

Zymbal glands carcinomas, nephroblastomas and liver angiosarcomas have never been observed as occurring spontaneously in our breed of Sprague-Dawley rats.

Only 3 cases of spontaneously occurring Zymbal glands carcinomas in rats (Sprague-Dawley) have been recorded in 1962. To our knowledge, no spontaneous nephroblastomas and liver angiosarcomas of rats have been reported in the literature. As far as we know, nephroblastomas have never been reported to be experimentally induced in rats; liver angiosarcomas have been induced in this species by diethylnitrosamine.

Although liver is the preferential site for onset of angiosarcomas, such kind of tumours have been observed in other tissues and organs: therefore VC should be considered in our experimental conditions generally cancerogenic for endothelia.

Zymbal glands tumours and nephroblastomas may be bilateral; liver angiosarcomas are often multiphocal.

Epidemiological investigations and medical controls should be undertaken on exposed workers. Would such neoplastic lesions of kidney and liver unhappily be found in man, given the rarity of these tumours in both animals and humans, it would be a precise indication of the high value of experimental testing in predicting the oncogenic potential of environmental agents and would strengthen the recommendation on the necessity of such bioassays before any new industrial compound is produced and widespread in large scale.

Another means of revealing the oncogenic risk of an agent is to examine the exposed working populations with methods which make it possible to assess the incidence of cancer precursors. The incidence of such precursors has been studied by us by exfoliative cytology among asymptomatic, apparently healthy workers exposed to risk, namely among workers exposed to aromatic amines (urine cytology), and among workers exposed to chromates (sputum cytology). The incidence of cellular atypias in these two groups of workers is shown in Tables 3 and 4. It far exceeds the expected incidence.

To evaluate in medical and legal terms the risks represented by occupational oncogenic agents, we must consider that:

1. a direct relation exists between dose (amount and length of exposure) and neoplastic response;

2. the oncogenic agents produce mainly non-reversible changes, which may continue to develop when the exposure is interrupted;

3. the oncogenic agents (occupational or generally environmental) may be additive in their effects.

According to our knowledge the occupational carcinogenic agents may be classified as:

(a) definite carcinogens, when epidemiological evidence exists,

TABLE 2   Preliminary results of carcinogenicity bioassay of vinyl chloride monomer (VC) and of vinyl acetate monomer (VA) (From C. Maltoni, G. Lefemine and L. Gualano, in press)

Groups and treatment	Animals (Sprague-Dawley rats)		Animals with tumours						
	Total	Survivors	Zymbal glands carcinomas (A) No.	Nephroblastomas (B) No.	Angiosarcomas Liver (C) No.	Angiosarcomas Other sites No.	Other type and/or site No.	Total No.
I VA 2,500 ppm.	96	15	–	–	–	–	–	–
II VC 10,000 ppm.	69	–	13	3	6	–	5 (H)	27
III VC 6,000 ppm.	72	5	5	3	8	1 (D)	1 (I)	18
IV VC 2,500 ppm.	74	16	2	4	6	3 (E)	1 (L)	16
V VC 500 ppm.	67	15	2	3	5	2 (F)	1 (M)	13
VI VC 250 ppm.	67	20	–	3	1	2 (G)	2 (N)	8
VII VC 50 ppm.	64	35	–	–	–	–	–	–
VIII No treatment	68	33	–	–	–	–	–	–
Total	577	139	22	16	26	8	10	82

(A) Metastases to lung. (B) Metastases to liver and/or to lung and spleen. (C) Metastases to lung. (D) Angiosarcomas in subcutaneous fibrosing angioma. (E) 2 intrabdominal angiosarcomas (1 next to spleen and 1 next to ovary); 1 ossifying angiosarcoma of neck. (F) 1 pulmonary angiosarcoma; 1 angiosarcoma of uterus. (G) 1 intrabdominal angiosarcoma (next to spleen); 1 intrathoracic ossifying angiosarcoma. (H) 2 Zymbal glands adenomas; 1 neurilemmoma of the ear; 1 mammary carcinoma; 1 cystoadenocarcinoma of ovary. (I) Sebaceous gland carcinoma of skin. (L) Zymbal glands adenoma. (M) Minimal deviation hepatoma. (N) 1 Zymbal glands adenoma; 1 salivary glands carcinoma.

TABLE 3   *Frequency of cellular atypias among workers exposed to aromatic amines in 4 North Italian dye-stuff factories*

Factory	No. of workers under control	Cytological classes (Papanicolaou)								
		I	I-II	II	II-III	III	III-IV	IV	IV-V	V
A	232	48	46	114	14	7	1	1	–	1
B	159	58	20	49	25	5	1	1	–	–
C	40	11	8	7	3	8	1	2	–	–
D	41	16	15	9	1	–	–	–	–	–
Total	472	133	89	179	43	20	3	4	–	1

TABLE 4   *Frequency of adenomatous typical and atypical hyperplasia, and of squamous metaplasia and dysplasia, in workers exposed to chromium compounds in one Northern Italian factory*

Type of occupation	Length of exposure (years)		Typical adenomatous hyperplasia		Atypical adenomatous hyperplasia		Squamous metaplasia		Squamous dysplasia	
	Length	No.	No.	%	No.	%	No.	%	No.	%
Production of chromates and dichromates	Up to 5	25	3	12	–	–	24	96	4	16
	6–10	14	3	21	1	7	12	86	3	21
	11–15	13	3	23	3	23	12	92	4	30
	Over 15	17	–	–	1	6	15	88	4	23
	Total	69	9	13	5	7	63	91	15	22
Production of chromium pigment	Up to 5	14	1	7	–	–	14	100	–	–
	6–10	17	1	6	–	–	14	82	2	12
	11–15	8	1	12	–	–	6	75	1	12
	Over 15	8	2	25	–	–	8	100	2	25
	Total	47	5	10	–	–	42	89	5	10

(b) highly suspected carcinogens, when strong experimental and/or some epidemiological evidence is present,

(c) potential carcinogens, when experimental data give some indication of carcinogenic action of a compound on an experimental animal.

According to their effects, the carcinogenic agents may be classified as strong or medium.

The agents, which have been definitively proved or are suspected to be oncogenic for man on an epidemiological basis, are listed in Table 5, together with the target tissues and the degree of evidence. The list of the agents present in the occupational environment, which, on an experimental basis should be considered highly suspect or potentially carcinogenic for man, is reported in Table 6.

TABLE 5   *Agents proved or suspected to be oncogenic for workers on an epidemiological basis*

Agents	Evidence	Tumours
U.V. radiations	+	Skin carcinomas
X-rays	+	Skin carcinomas Leukaemias
Uranium ore	+	Pulmonary carcinomas
Arsenic	(+)	Skin carcinomas (lung carcinomas) (liver tumours)
Asbestos	+	Lung carcinomas Pleural mesotheliomas (abdominal malignancies)
Chromium	+	Lung carcinomas
Nickel	+	Lung carcinomas Carcinomas of nasal and paranasal cavities
Iron ore	(+)	Lung carcinomas
Bis-chloromethyl ether	+	Lung carcinomas
Benzene	+	Leukaemias
Isopropylic oil	(+)	Carcinomas of paranasal cavities
Soot, tars, mineral oils, cutting oils	+	Skin carcinomas
Carbon black	+	Lung carcinomas
Mustard gas	+	Laryngeal carcinomas
Aromatic amines	+	Bladder and upper urinary tract carcinomas

TABLE 6   *Agents suspected to be carcinogenic for workers on an experimental basis*

Beryllium	Pesticides (DDT, aldrin, dieldrin, Aramite, DMDT, Amizol, Thiuram)
Cadmium	
Cobalt	Thiourea and related compounds
Lead	Tannins
Selenium	Detergents
Zinc	Alkylating agents
Carbon tetrachloride	Nitrosamines
Chloroform	Azo-dyes
Vinyl chloride	Oestrogens

In Italy carcinogenic occupational risk exists for workers who are:

(a) exposed to chromates, mainly the ones working in factories where chromates are produced;

(b) exposed to nickel, mainly the ones exposed to nickel-carbonyl;

(c) exposed to asbestos, mainly the ones who extract it from its natural source, or workers in factories where asbestos is used for manufacturing;

(d) in factories making shoes, purses and raincoats, exposed to benzene;

(e) in factories producing carbon black from mineral oils; and

(f) in the dye and rubber industries, exposed to aromatic amines.

In our country occupational tumours have been observed in many of the above mentioned workers. 21 lung carcinomas have been found among less than 200 workers in a chromate factory in Northern Italy. Pleural mesotheliomas have been discovered among workers in asbestos mines. A number of leukaemias have been found among shoe-makers, who were heavily exposed to benzene, in factories in Lombardy (Vigevano), Bologna Province and Tuscany. The incidence of bladder and other urinary tract carcinomas among workers in 5 Italian dye-stuff factories are shown in Table 7. In these factories workers had been exposed to β-naphthylamine, benzidine, α-naphthylamine, Auramine, fuchsine, 3,3'-dichlorobenzidine. Now in our country the production of β-naphthylamine and benzidine has been withdrawn. One may conclude that prevention of occupational carcinogenesis is a very urgent problem.

TABLE 7   *Frequency of carcinomas of the urinary tract among workers of 5 Italian dye-stuff factories exposed to aromatic amines*

Factory	Total No. of exposed workers	No. of workers with carcinoma		
		Bladder	Renal pelves and ureters	Total
A	286	17	1	18
B	386	87	5	92*
C	213	44	–	44
D	135	4	–	4
E	135	7	1	8
Total	1,155	159	7	166

* In 1 case bladder and upper urinary tract tumours were coexistent.

The methods of prevention may be summarized as follows:

1. correct experimental testing of all newly used agents;

2. up to date epidemiological data from various categories of workers exposed to risk;

3. legislative measures forbidding the production and the utilization of agents which have been shown to be oncogenic on an epidemiological and/or an experimental basis, especially if the said agents are strong carcinogens;

4. measures of technical protection, when weak or doubtful carcinogens continue to be produced or employed; these protective measures should be periodically examined by Public Health Inspectors;

5. specific medical checks to make possible, on the one hand, the early detection of preneoplastic lesions and tumours, and on the other, the quantitative evaluation of the risks through the incidence of these changes.

It is my opinion that the value of medical checks is mainly to evaluate the risk that is epidemiological. Early detection of occupational tumours which, as already shown, are mainly located in the respiratory and urinary tract, has been, I think, over-emphasized. We know that these tumours are multicentric. In other words all the target apparatus is in some way affected by the carcinogenic process.

Concerning the urinary tract, in a systematic histological study, I have seen that in patients with bladder tumours, dysplastic and cancerous foci may be detected from renal pelvis to urethra. Therefore it is obvious that in such conditions early diagnosis can achieve very little. We may diagnose some tumours quite early, but on the basis of 15 years' experience with periodic checks of workers exposed to high risk, I doubt that periodical medical examination has a real bearing in saving people with occupational cancer although detected early, or in prolonging their life span. Thus my position is in sharp contrast with those who claim to 'protect' (!) workers exposed to carcinogenic risk with medical examinations. *I do believe that the potentialities of medical examinations should be evaluated at an international level.*

In conclusion, I would like to emphasize the need of a close collaboration among scientists, public health services, workers unions and industries, to evaluate the risks and to devise preventive measures for avoiding or minimizing occupational tumours.

References

Frieben (1902): Fortschr. Röntgenstr., 6, 106.
Pott, P. (1775): In: Chirurgical Observations, relative to the Cataract, the Polypus of the Nose, the Cancer of the Scrotum, the Different Kinds of Ruptures, and the Modification on the Toes and Feet. Hower, Clarke and Pollins, London.
Rehn, L. (1895): Arch. klin. Chir., 50, 588.
Unna, P. G. (1894): In: Histopathologie der Hautkrankheiten, p. 719. Hirschwald, Berlin.
Yamagiwa, K. and Ichikawa, K. (1915): Mitt. med. Fak. Tokyo, 15, 295.

Aspects of experimental carcinogenesis related to cancer prevention in children

N. P. Napalkov

Petrov Research Institute of Oncology, Leningrad, U.S.S.R.

Until recent years, only a few isolated experimental observations have been reported on so-called transplacental carcinogenesis. However, investigation of the problem of immediate and late effects of blastomogenic agents on the organism during prenatal life has more than theoretical importance for understanding the inter-relations between teratogenesis and blastomogenesis. Now that the reality of transplacental carcinogenic action of chemical agents has been firmly proved, not only by animal experiments but also by observations on man, the need to characterize the main modes of transplacental carcinogenesis becomes obvious. This need is closely connected with the search for aetiological factors and with the elaboration of measures for preventing tumours in children (Napalkov, 1971).

Malignant tumours have already become one of the main causes of mortality in children under 15 in most of the industrially-developed countries (Ariel and Pack, 1960; Marsden and Steward, 1968). According to WHO figures (1967-70) tumours stood second in children's death toll, (next to accidents) in the age bracket of 5-14 years; and fourth for children aged 1-4. The existing proximity of morbidity and mortality rates for malignant tumours in children is, unfortunately, determined by many factors. There is no established programme for clinical prevention of malignancies; there is also a lack of epidemiological data on tumours in children.

The problem was tackled systematically only 6-7 years ago, and the efforts of researchers, clinicians and epidemiologists working in this field have not yet reached that stage of integration which can promise tangible success. However, the intensive studies which have recently been carried out, mainly by Dr R. Miller and his colleagues (1966-71), as well as by some other investigators working in the field of epidemiology of tumours in children, have already yielded many interesting data and could provide oncopaediatricians with means for determining groups at high risk of tumours. Moreover, clinico-epidemiological observations (Miller, 1968) and mathematical evaluation (Emanuel et al., 1969) of growth dynamics of such malignant neoplasmas in children as Wilms's tumour, neuroblastoma, rhabdomyosarcoma and some others have indicated that tumour growth might be induced as early as embryogenesis. There are indirect indications which, however, seem to make it logical to assume that many tumours found in children may result from exposure to blastomogenic chemicals during embryogenesis (Peller, 1960). Direct clinico-epidemiological observations in this field also have already become available due to the work of Herbst et al. (1971). They have revealed the association between the administration of stilboestrol to mothers during pregnancy and the development of clear-cell vaginal carcinomas in their daughters. Since accumulation of such experience is apparently complicated, the solution of the problem may be aided by extrapolation to humans of the experimental results obtained from the studies of blastomogenic effect of substances during embryogenesis in various animals.

Fragmentary data on immediate and, particularly, late effects of treatment of pregnant animals with some blastomogenic substances available until recently, have grown considerably within the last 2 or 3 years. For instance, until 1968, the possibility of inducing tumours in the progeny of animals treated during gestation was proved in the experiments involving 6-7 compounds only, as seen from the reviews by Di Paolo and

Kotin (1966), Napalkov and Alexandrov (1968). Later, more than 10 other chemicals have extended the list of substances capable of exerting transplacental blastomogenic effect in experimental animals (Druckrey et al., 1968, 1969, 1970; Tomatis and Goodall, 1969; Tomatis et al., 1970).

At the very early stages of research in the field of transplacental carcinogenesis, it becomes apparent that serious recommendations for prevention of malignant tumours in children based on experimental observations could evolve only after study of relationships of embryotoxic, teratogenic and blastomogenic effects of prenatal treatment with carcinogenic substances. Without knowledge of these relationships and a number of other regularities of transplacental blastomogenesis, it would be hard to say whether this experimental model is adequate to the ultimate goal of the experiments — the study of pathogenesis and feasibility of cancer prevention in children.

For this purpose, since 1965 our laboratory has been systematically studying the primary response of the embryo (embryotoxic and teratogenic effects) and late (carcinogenic) effect of some chemicals on the organism at the embryonic period of its development.

In experiments on rats, we have studied the embryotoxic and teratogenic properties of the following highly-blastomogenic compounds: nitrosodimethyl-, -diethyl-, -dipropyl-, and -dibutylamine (NDMA, NDEA, NDPA and NDBA), nitrosomethyl- and -ethylaniline (NMA, NEA); nitrosomethyl-, -ethyl-, -propyl-, and -dimethylurea (NMU, NEU, NPU, NDMU); nitrosomethyl-urethane (NMUt); 2-fluorenylacetamide (FAA) and 7,12-dimethylbenz(a)anthracene (DMBA). Nearly 1,000 pregnant rats have been used in these experiments and changes in about 6,000 fetuses have been followed.

These experiments have shown that symmetrical dialkylnitrosamines applied in different doses and administered for varying lengths of time, by different routes and at different stages of embryogenesis, do not produce malformations in rats, exerting an embryotoxic effect only. The effect proved non-specific and the mortality of fetuses showed a slight rise as compared against controls, occurring after NDMA administration in the last third of embryogenesis only, when administration of the same substance results in inducing renal adenosarcomas in the offspring. It should be noted that these tumours were not frequent and were found mostly in old rats. The absence of a teratogenic effect in these experiments may be due to the failure of activation of the original compounds to occur at teratogenesis-sensitive stages (organogenesis) because of the immaturity of the relevant embryonic enzymatic systems. At the same time, the alkylating metabolite formed in the mother fails to reach the embryo, because it is very reactive and is utilized at the site of formation. This conjecture, however, cannot provide a satisfactory explanation of the observations of the blastomogenic effect of NDMA when administered at later stages of embryogenesis.

Nitrosoalkylureas were shown to have a strong embryotoxic and teratogenic effect, particularly when administered during organogenesis (Kreybig, 1965; Napalkov and Alexandrov, 1968). However, antenatal administration resulted not only in malformations but in various tumours occurring in the progeny with fairly high frequency (Alexandrov, 1969). The occurrence of either effect of NMU and its extent are closely related to the stage at which the embryo is treated. These observations of stage dependence of the effect corroborated the results of our above-mentioned experiments with NDMA and similar findings of the study of transplacental effect of NEU (Ivankovic and Druckrey, 1968).

The embryotoxic effect of NMU was very high when administered during the first week of prenatal life and it was associated with a reduction of the embryoblast. This, as well as atrophy of the allantois, and placentation disorders, may account for the high mortality of embryos when the substance was administered in smaller doses but throughout embryogenesis. The teratogenicity of NMU was manifested in the induction of hydro- and microcephaly in the fetuses, following treatment during the 2nd and 3rd weeks of gestation, or throughout embryogenesis. The worst and most frequent malformations, however, arose after treatment at the stages of organogenesis (the 8th-14th days after conception).

A late effect, i.e. tumour formation in the offspring, was observed in the experiments involving NMU administration to females at all stages of pregnancy, the highest incidence of neoplasms being registered in cases of treatment during the last third of embryogenesis. Furthermore, treatment during the 1st and 2nd weeks of gestation resulted exclusively in mammary and pituitary tumour formation in the progeny, whereas administration of NMU during the last third, or within the whole period of intrauterine development, produced tumours, chiefly, in the nervous system and kidneys of survivors.

These findings are in good agreement with the results of subsequent experiments designed to determine the relationship of NMU teratogenic and transplacental blasto-mogenic effects with the dose of NMU. A single injection of 5 mg/kg on the 21st day of gestation did not produce any apparent malformations and its effect was confined to formation of tumours in the nervous system, kidneys and mammary gland in 27% of animals.

Similar tumours were found in 51% of the descendants of those mothers that were treated with 20 mg/kg at the same stage of gestation; also, all offspring were found to have cerebellar malformations. A further increase in NMU dosage up to 40 mg/kg in-variably resulted in a higher tumour incidence in the offspring (85%) and a more pro-nounced cerebellar hypoplasia in all descendents. Although all the animals used in these experiments had congenital cerebellar defects, none was found to have a tumour at this site. However, neoplasms occurred in other parts of the nervous system.

Thus, it was shown that congenital defects may be induced even at the latest stages of embryogenesis. The doses required, however, were much larger than those needed to produce teratogenic effect at earlier stages: the sites of malformations and tumours were also different between early and late stage treatment.

The next series of experiments was aimed at determining the stages of embryogenesis with the highest sensitivity to various types of transplacental blastomogenic substances. These experiments followed the lives of approximately 300 mother rats treated with single doses of NMU or NEU at different stages of gestation, and of about 1,000 of their descendants. The results of these experiments appeared to agree with previous observa-tions that administration of blastomogenic substance during the 1st week of embryo-genesis results chiefly, in a strong embryotoxic effect; during the 2nd week, a teratogenic effect; and during the 3rd week, the induction of tumours in descendants. Furthermore, two periods were found during which the embryo is highly sensitive to the lethal effect. They are the 3rd-4th and 9th-10th days of gestation in the case of NEU. The highest teratogenic effect was shown to follow NEU-treatment on the 10th day of embryogenesis. This treatment produced disorders of neurulation affecting the formation and closure of the neural tube which led to such malformations as hydrocephaly, exencephaly, cerebral hernia, cleft spine and lip and anophthalmia.

The blastomogenic activity of NEU after its transplacental administration was observ-ed beginning from the 11th day of embryogenesis, the survivors having mostly multiple tumours of the nervous system. Among 8 substances which have been tested in rats, including the experiments with combined application of ethylurea and sodium nitrite, we found NEU, NMUt and DMBA to be the most effective agents in inducing primary multiple tumours. It has been found that in rats, tumours arise most frequently in different portions of the nervous system, or in the kidneys.

Experiments on rats establish that the type of transplacental effect of substances such as NMU or NEU, whose blastomogenic activity does not depend on metabolic enzymatic transformation, is determined mostly by the stage of embryogenesis and, to a certain extent, by the dosage of the compound. Recent experiments showed that with larger doses of NEU (as was formerly found with NMU), malformations could be induced by injection of the substance even on the 21st day of pregnancy.

Transplacentally-induced tumours were of the same types, and arose at the same sites, as those produced by postnatal treatment with NMU, NEU and NDMA.

To what extent are the parameters of transplacental blastomogenesis found in rats inherent to this particular species? When NEU is administered transplacentally in ham-sters, it induces tumours which are not confined (as they are in rats) to the nervous system

(Ivankovic and Druckrey, 1968). However, in our laboratory treatment of pregnant hamsters with 100 mg/kg NEU, 2-3 days prior to delivery, produced tumours only in the peripheral nervous system in 61% of the descendants. Treatment of pregnant mice with NEU in experiments of Rice (1969) showed that induced adenomas of the lungs and tumours of the liver are similar to those arising after postnatal administration of NEU. The highest transplacental blastomogenic effect was recorded in these experiments when animals were treated during the last days of pregnancy. Treatment of mice with NDMA, NMU and NEU in similar experiments induced only lung adenomas and adenocarcinomas in 71-74% of animals. Hence, for the time being, it can be said that when animals of different species are subjected to the transplacental action of the same blastomogenic substance, differences in types of induced tumours and sites of their occurrence are similar to those observed with postnatal treatment. This conclusion is also borne out by the results of the few available comparisons of the effects of postnatal and prenatal treatment of different species with such substances as NDMA, NDEA and MC. As in the case of nitrosoureas, the tropism of the blastomogenic effects of each of these substances shows the same species-specificity for both prenatal and postnatal treatments.

However, data which have been obtained recently in our experiments with transplacental carcinogenesis in rats treated with DMBA, differ significantly from earlier observations. DMBA applied transplacentally in rats is able to induce tumours mainly of the nervous system. Therefore, these experiments revealed that in transplacental carcinogenesis a tropism can occur that is not identical with that observed when the carcinogen is given at later stages of ontogeny.

Important results have been obtained in the experiments with nitrosomethyl-urethane (NMUt) conducted in our laboratory. This substance produced neither teratogenic, nor transplacental blastomogenic effects when administered to pregnant rats by conventional routes, i.e. intraperitoneally or intravenously. These negative results are supposed to be due to a much lower stability of NMUt — as compared with NMU and NEU — and to the inability of its blastomogenic metabolite to reach the embryo. This suggestion was confirmed when a direct injection of NMUt intraplacentally produced a marked teratogenic effect and induced neurogenic, renal and pituitary tumours which were found in almost 40% of the rats some time later in postnatal life.

A comparison of transplacental effects of NDMA, NMU and NMUt on rats leads to a conclusion that teratogenesis and tumour development in the offspring depend, to a large extent, on those characteristics of the metabolism of the substance administered in pregnancy that are associated with the formation of genuine blastomogenic products and their transport to the embryo in quantities sufficient to exert an effect.

So far, we have treated the problems of transplacental blastomogenesis proper, that involve exposure during prenatal life only. However, other aspects of the problem gain in importance, particularly in the light of our knowledge of the irreversible nature of the blastomogenic influence and the combined effect of blastomogenic agents and modifying factors (Druckrey, 1967; Likhachev, 1968; Neiman, 1968; Berenblum, 1969). It seems likely that the organism exposed to blastomogenic substances in prenatal life is more likely to come in contact with them during postnatal life, which is much longer than embryogenesis. Therefore, an assessment of the combined effect of transplacental and postnatal blastomogenic exposures seems to be of vital importance.

The first attempts of experimental studies in this field were undertaken in our laboratory by Drs A. J. Likhachev and O. P. Saveljeva who studied the results of the combined exposure to NDEA, NMU, 6-methylthiouracil (MTU) and 2-fluorenylacetamide (FAA). Thus, Likhachev treated non-inbred mice with NDEA during the last days of embryogenesis and repeated the treatment with the same agent during postnatal life after puberty. The prenatal treatment with NDEA alone more than trebled the tumour incidence in mice, increased the occurrence of primary multiple tumours and induced neoplasms in the liver, fore-stomach and oesophagus, i.e. at sites unaffected in controls (Likhachev, 1971a). A similar effect, though caused by much larger doses of NDEA, was observed in mice treated during postnatal life only. This shows the mouse embryo to be more sensitive to the blastomogenic effect of NDEA.

Finally, the group of animals subjected to the combined action of NDEA, both in pre- and post-natal life, revealed the summation of blastomogenic effects. This phenomenon found its expression in a statistically-significant rise in multiple tumour incidence and development of neoplasms at the sites which are typical of the blastomogenic effect of NDEA in mice of the colony used (Likhachev, 1971*b*).

Another series of experiments on mice revealed that transplacental exposure to NMU induced lung tumours in 71% of the animals, which was 3 times the tumour incidence observed in controls. When transplacental treatment with NMU was complemented with exposure to NDEA in postnatal life, the lung adenocarcinoma incidence was 3 times the relevant value for treatment with NDEA alone. Another characteristic feature observed was that the tumours appeared very early. Thus, the transplacental treatment with NMU exerted its intrinsic blastomogenic effect which was additive to the action of NDEA whose characteristic influence was as fully-manifested in the incidence and locations of the induced tumours.

An even more striking manifestation of the combined effect of pre- and post-natal exposure to different blastomogenic substances was observed by Saveljeva (1971). In her experiments, pregnant rats were treated with MTU which, in addition to its thyreostatic activity, has a direct blastomogenic effect (Napalkow, 1967). Some descendants of the treated rats and the control females were exposed to FAA in postnatal life. While the doses of MTU administered during embryogenesis and FAA administered in postnatal life separately failed to induce tumours of the thyroid epithelium, the combined exposure to these two agents in pre- and post-natal life induced adenomas and adenocarcinomas of the thyroid gland in 29% of the rats.

The above data permit us to draw the following conclusions on relationships between teratogenesis and oncogenesis revealed under experimental conditions:

Transplacental treatment of the embryo with carcinogenic compounds may induce tumours in postnatal life without any additional influences causing the neoplastic growth.

The organotropism of chemical blastomogenic agents inherent in their action in the adult organism, proves generally to be the same in the offspring of the animals treated with these substances during gestation. In contrast, the teratogenic reaction of the embryo to carcinogenic chemicals is determined by the stage of embryogenesis at which they are applied, rather than by the organotropic properties of the agents. The embryo is found to exhibit the highest response to the carcinogenic effect of chemicals at relatively late stages of development in the period of histogenesis; to the teratogenic effect during organogenesis; and to the lethal effect at the earliest stages (cleavage of zygote, implantation of embryo and formation of placenta).

An exposure of the organism to carcinogenic substances in antenatal life may lead to the induction of congenital defects as well as of tumours. The experimental observations available at the moment serve to indicate that both congenital defects and tumours are different outcomes of the same, or various, causes rather than consecutive stages of one and the same process. The occurrence of congenital defects or tumours and their characteristic features in the case of treatment of the embryo with carcinogenic substances, depend on the species-sensitivity, peculiarities of the chemical metabolism, its dosage and the period of embryogenesis at which exposure is made.

The risk of tumour development in the descendants of the mothers exposed to carcinogenic compounds during pregnancy is also determined by the passage of these substances, or their active metabolites, through the placental barrier and embryonic membranes in concentrations sufficient to exert an effect. Of particular interest in this connection is the report of vigorous enzymatic hydroxylation of blastomogenic polycyclic hydrocarbons in the human placenta (Welch et al., 1969). High activity of the detoxifying enzymatic systems of the placenta, which is determined not only by the enzyme-inducing agent but the individual genetic characteristics of the maternal organism as well, may serve as a safe shield for the embryo, warding off the hazards of transplacental blastomogenesis. Nevertheless, high permeability for DMBA of the placental barrier in rats and mice, which has been already demonstrated in experiments of Shendrikova et al. (1973), Alexandrov and Shendrikova (1972), warns us not to overestimate the safety of this shield.

Congenital defects, abnormal development and tumours may result from factors other than exposure of the maternal organism to genuine blastomogenic substances. Recent experiments (Ivankovic and Preussmann, 1970; Alexandrov and Jänisch, 1971) showed that the separate treatment of pregnant rats with ethylurea and sodium nitrite to be sufficient to induce malformations and tumours in the offspring as a result of the endogenous synthesis of NEU.

In conclusion, I would like to emphasize again that epidemiological studies, in conjunction with experiments on transplacental blastomogenesis in animals, may lead to the discovery of environmental factors, an exposure to which during embryogenesis may result in tumour growth in children.

Summary

Data available in the literature, and results obtained in the author's laboratory since 1965 in animal experiments with transplacental carcinogenesis, are considered in connection with epidemiological observations on tumours in children and oncogenic defects. Animal experiments have revealed several general regularities of transplacental carcinogenesis. The most important is the finding that even a single shot of a carcinogenic chemical during pregnancy either leads to tumour development in the offspring, or increases the sensitivity of the progeny to subsequent repeated exposure to carcinogenic agents during postnatal life.

The discovery of the dependence of the type of predominant response of the embryo (lethal, teratogenic, carcinogenic) on the stage of prenatal development, and on the dose of the chemical, leads to a better understanding of the relationship between carcinogenesis and teratogenesis. Analysis of these and other observations made in experiments with transplacental carcinogenesis gives rise to the hope that many of the experimental findings could be successfully applied to a better understanding of the aetiology and pathogenesis of tumours in children and to an elaboration of criteria for defining high risk groups.

References

Alexandrov, V.A. (1969): Vop. Onkol., 15, 55.
Alexandrov, V.A. and Jänisch, W. (1971): Experientia (Basel), 27, 538.
Alexandrov, V.A. and Shendrikova, I.A. (1972): Vop. Onkol., 18, 56.
Ariel, I.M. and Pack, G.T. (1960): Cancer and Allied Diseases of Infancy and Childhood. Little, Brown and Co., New-York-Boston-Toronto.
Berenblum, I. (1969): Progr. exp. Tumor Res. (Basel), 11, 21.
Di Paolo, J.A. and Kotin, P. (1966): Arch, Path., 81, 3.
Druckrey, H. (1967): In: Potential Carcinogenic Hazards from Drugs, Vol. 7, p. 60. Editor: R. Truhaut. UICC Monograph Series, Springer-Verlag, Berlin-Göttingen-Heidelberg-New York.
Druckrey, H., Ivankovic, S., Sandschütz, C., Stekor, J., Brunner, U. and Schagen, B. (1968): Experientia (Basel), 24, 561.
Druckrey, H., Kruse, H., Preussmann, R., Ivankovic, S. and Sandschütz, C. (1970): Z. Krebsforsch., 74, 241.
Druckrey, H., Preussmann, R. and Ivankovic, S. (1969): Ann. N.Y. Acad. Sci., 163, 676.
Emanuel, N.M., Evseenko, L.S., Korman, N.P. and Korman, D.B. (1969): Viniti (Moscow), 27, 7.
Fraumeni, J.F., Miller, R.W. and Hill, J.A. (1968): J. nat. Cancer Inst., 40, 1087.
Herbst, A.L., Ulfelder, H. and Poskanzer, D.C. (1971): New Engl. J. Med., 284, 878.
Ivankovic, S. and Druckrey, H. (1968): Z. Krebsforsch., 71, 320.
Ivankovic, S. and Preussmann, R. (1970): Naturwissenschaften, 57, 460.
Kreybig, T.V. (1965): Z. Krebsforsch., 67, 46.
Likhachev, A.J. (1968): Vop. Onkol., 14, 114.
Likhachev, A.J. (1971a): Vop. Onkol., 17, 45.
Likhachev, A.J. (1971b): Vop. Onkol., 17, 64.

Marsden, H.B. and Steward, J.K. (1968): In: Recent Results in Cancer Research, Vol. 13. Springer-Verlag, Berlin-Göttingen-Heidelberg-New York.

Miller, R.W. (1966): New Engl. J. Med., 275, 87.

Miller, R.W. (1968): J. nat. Cancer Inst., 40, 1079.

Miller, R.W. (1971): J. nat. Cancer Inst., 46, 203.

Miller, R.W., Fraumeni, J.F. and Hill, J.A. (1968): Amer. J. Dis. Child., 115, 253.

Napalkov, N.P. (1967): In: Potential Carcinogenic Hazards from Drugs, Vol. 7, p. 172. Editor: R. Truhaut. UICC Monograph Series, Springer-Verlag, Berlin-Göttingen-Heidelberg-New York.

Napalkov, N.P. (1971): Vop. Onkol., 17, 3.

Napalkov, N.P. and Alexandrov, V.A. (1968): Z. Krebsforsch., 71, 32.

Neiman, J.M. (1968): Europ. J. Cancer, 4, 537.

Peller, S. (1960): Cancer in Childhood and Youth. John Wright and Dons, Ltd., Bristol.

Rice, J.M. (1969): Ann. N.Y. Acad. Sci., 163, 813.

Saveljeva, O.P. (1971): Vop. Onkol., 17, 53.

Shendrikova, I.A., Ivanov-Golitsyn, M.N., Anisimov, V.N. and Likhachev, A.J. (1973): Vop. Onkol., 19, 75.

Tomatis, L. and Goodall, C.M. (1969): Int. J. Cancer, 4, 219.

Tomatis, L., Turusov, V., Guibbert, D., Duperay, B. and Pacheco, H. (1970); In: Abstracts, X International Cancer Congress, Houston, Tex. 1970, p. 43. Editor: R.W. Cumley. Medical Arts Publishing Co.

Welch, R.M., Harrison, Y.E., Gommi, B.W., Poppers, P.J. and Conney, A.H. (1969): Clin. Pharmacol. Ther., 10, 100.

WHO (1967): World Health Statistics Annual 1963, Vol. 1. Vital Statistics and Causes of Death. (Russian Ed.).

WHO (1970): World Health Statistics Annual 1964, Vol. 1. Vital Statistics and Causes of Death. (Russian Ed.).

Carcinogenic hazards from drugs

D. Schmähl

The Institute of Toxicology and Chemotherapy, German Cancer Research Center, Heidelberg, Federal Republic of Germany

The increasing use of drugs requires special regard to the potential hazards of these drugs. A typical example of an iatrogenic carcinogen is arsenic which was suspected as carcinogenic in man already in the middle of the nineteenth century. Observations in man and experimental studies during the last decades have shown that some other drugs must be regarded as potentially carcinogenic in man (Clayson, 1972; Schmähl, 1970). The purpose of this lecture is to describe a few examples of such drugs and to point out toxicological aspects in this connection.

In respect to the principle of nil nocere in therapy adverse effects of drugs are of special concern. Side effects, which occur shortly after application can be discovered readily by the toxicological methods in use or at least in clinical treatment, but it is difficult to attribute side effects that occur after a long delay to the previously administered drug. From research in occupational cancer we know that chemically induced cancer in man – e.g. bladder cancer following β-naphthylamine exposure – has an induction period of many years or even decades. Because of the long induction period of these tumors animal experiments are necessary to detect substances possessing such dangerous side effects.

It is certainly impracticable to examine all drugs for carcinogenic effects which are in clinical use. But long-term experiments must be carried out when (1) a drug is suspected to be carcinogenic due to its chemical structure or reactivity (e.g. alkylating properties) and when (2) a drug is to be given to pregnant women or children, in a high dosage over a long time (Schmähl, 1972). The examination, of course, must be done before clinical use.

In Table 1, I have compiled a list of drugs which are assumed to be potentially carcinogenic in man. Only chemical substances are described; radiation and the plastics sometimes used for implantations are omitted. The potential carcinogenic hazard of these drugs has been estimated from the data so far available. Under the heading 'certain or probable', I have listed only those substances which either clinical or epidemiologic studies have proved to be carcinogenic or which have had regular carcinogenic effects in many species of animals when given in dosages which are also used in human therapy. Since the time available does not permit the discussion of all the drugs which are listed in Table 1, I have to restrict myself to a few examples.

The first example is arsenic. This substance, which was formerly used as a pesticide, particularly in the German and French vine growing areas, caused tumors in a relatively high percentage of the vineyard workers. Skin carcinomas following arsenic melanosis, carcinomas of the bronchi, and liver carcinomas following liver cirrhosis are characteristic tumors that appear after previous exposure to arsenic. The same kind of tumors were observed after long-term treatment with high dosages of arsenic – e.g. when patients had received Fowler's solution for therapy of psoriasis. We have for quite some time stopped using arsenic as a pesticide, but it is still comparatively often prescribed as a drug, especially in dermatology – that is, in doctors' surgeries, but not in hospitals (Ehlers, 1968). German toxicologists and clinicians have warned against the use of arsenic as a drug in the future.

Alkylating agents used in cancer chemotherapy and as immunodepressives must also be regarded as potentially carcinogenic in man (Schmähl and Osswald, 1970). Our team as

TABLE 1 *Drugs to be regarded as potential carcinogens in man on the basis of animal tests or case histories*

Carcinogenic effect of drugs in man

Certain/probable	Possible	Improbable/not assessable
Alkylating agents (Compounds of mustard gas, i.e. cyclophosphamide, ethylenimine, i.e. thiotepa) Arsenic Diethylstilboestrol (transplacental) Procarbacine	Antimetabolites Chinolin derivatives Furium Halogenated paraffins Hydantoin derivatives Lysergides Nitrofuran derivatives Phenacetine Phenylbutazone Streptozotocine Tannins (epicutan) Tar salves Thiourea Urethane	Cantharidine Cyclamate Iron-dextran Griseofulvin Hexamethylenetetramine INH 'Pill' Potassium perchlorate Lactames Metronidazole Paraffin oils (orally) Polyvinylpyrrolidone and similar plasma expanders Pronethalol Safrole Tannins (orally)

well as other examiners have been able to prove that alkylating cytostatics have considerable carcinogenic effects in rats and mice, in dosages — scaled in proportion to kg body weight — such as are given to patients in hospitals. The results of our investigations are listed in Tables 2 and 3. Table 3 shows the results obtained when the substances were applied only 5 times, as recommended in postoperative chemoprophylaxis today. The incidence of tumors in those animals, which had been treated with the cytostatics, was increased 4-6 fold compared with the controls. We observed a great number of malignant tumors in various organs that did not appear in the control animals. Therefore we have suggested that such drugs should be administered in therapy only if their use is vital, a suggestion which clinicians now support also (Hartwich, 1973). In the chemotherapy of tumor disease the use of those substances cannot be renounced, but in postoperative chemoprophylaxis consideration should be given to the use of therapeutics, especially when the operation may be curative, as e.g. in the case of the mammacarcinoma Steinthal I.

We have also warned against the use of alkylants as immunodepressives, particularly since a correlation between carcinogenic and immunodepressive action does not appear to exist (Scherf et al., 1970). These results may suggest to the pharmacotherapist that he be very wary in the application of those substances — except, of course, when vitally necessary.

Occupational studies have also described the carcinogenic effects of alkylating cytostatics of the mustard gas and ethylenimine type in man, inducing tumors mainly of the respiratory system (Schmähl and Osswald, 1970). Workers who had previously been exposed to such substances and people who had endured acute mustard gas poisoning developed tumors of these organs. But carcinogenic effects to other organs of man (e.g. the bladder) have been recently suggested (Weiss, personal communication).

Some authors have recommended the use of alkylating compounds for the treatment of multiple sclerosis and collagenosis. Procarbacine, which is also an alkylant according to its chemical reactivity, was recommended for the therapy of Dupuytren's contracture. But therapy of these diseases with alkylating drugs carries a high risk to the patient and should be done only if other therapeutic efforts do not prove successful. Furthermore its efficiency in these cases is quite uncertain.

A specially instructive example of carcinogenic hazards due to alkylating drugs is

TABLE 2   *Survey on carcinogenesis experiments in male BR 46-rats injected intravenously with 7%*
            of the LD_{50} of different cytostatics once weekly over a period of 52 weeks

Experiment	Number of animals		Malignomas (%)	Induction time t_{50} (months)
	N_0	$N_{1.Tu.}$		
Control	89	65	6	23±5
Alkylating agents [a]	391	271	24	15±4
Antimetabolites [b]	148	73	4	16±5
Natural substances [c]	200	121	3	16±4
X-rays [d]	120	114	22	14±4

[a] Substances tested: Myleran, Degranol, Dichloren, Mitomen, Endoxan, thiotepa, Trenimon, Natulan.
[b] 6-mercaptopurine, 5-fluorouracil, methotrexate.
[c] Colcemid, A-Blastomase, Proresid, vinblastine.
[d] Whole body irradiation (together with E. Stutz, Freiburg).

TABLE 3   *Survey on carcinogenesis experiments with some cancer chemotherapeutics in male*
            BR 46-rats injected intravenously with 17% of the LD_{50} five times at fortnightly intervals

Experiment	Number of animals		Malignomas (%)	Induction time t_{50} (months)
	N_0	$N_{1.Tu.}$		
Control	89	65	6	23±5
Vinblastine	96	31	3	24
Endoxan	96	66	24	18±4
Mitomycin C	96	79	34	18±4

chlornaphazine (I), formerly used mainly in the therapy of polycythemia (Thiede et al., 1964; Thiede and Christensen, 1969) (Fig. 1).

Chlornaphazine   (I)   FIG. 1

This substance induced bladder carcinoma in a high percentage of patients after an unusually short induction period (Table 4). The formula shows a bis-β-chlorethylamine group in position 2 of the naphthaline ring system which is presumably split off in the organism providing the bladder carcinogen β-naphthylamine. β-Naphthylamine is well-known to be a potent bladder carcinogen in man. It is interesting that the induction period of bladder tumors induced by chlornaphazine was only about 3 years, whereas tumors induced by β-naphthylamine have an induction period ranging from 15 to 25 years. This may be due to the fact that the naphthaline ring system directs the carcinogenic effect of chlornaphazine to the bladder as target organ. The induction period of only a few years can be explained by the chemically highly reactive mustard function at the naphthaline molecule.

It was thought possible that immunodepressive treatment predisposes to the formation of tumors since it had been noted that patients, who had received organ transplants (e.g.

TABLE 4   *Bladder tumors induced by chlornaphazine in polycythemic patients*

	No. of patients	No. with carcinoma of bladder	Also received ^{32}P
Received chlornaphazine	61	10	9
Received > 100 g chlornaphazine	20	7	6
No chlornaphazine	40	0	–
^{32}P but no chlornaphazine	46	0	–

(According to D. B. Clayson, *Drug Induced Diseases, Vol. 4*, Excerpta Medica, Amsterdam (1972), p. 91-109)

of the kidney), developed malignant lymphomas as well as solid carcinomas after short induction periods (Penn et al., 1969, 1971). It had also been observed that the recipients developed tumors of the transplanted organ when its donor had suffered from cancer. The histology of the tumors in both the recipient and the donor was the same. From these observations it was concluded that the organ transplantation caused an inoculation of latent tumor cells which proliferated in the recipient organ. The immunodepressive treatment to prevent rejection was assumed to be responsible for the proliferation of these tumor cells in the recipient organ. Genuine immunodepression is presumably responsible for the increased tumor rate (particularly of malignant lymphomas) in children who have been born with immune insufficiency; characteristic diseases are ataxia teleangiectasia, Wiscott-Aldrich syndrome and agammaglobulinemia.

Immunodepressive drugs are used in the therapy of many diseases today. Adverse consequences of such treatment, however, must be expected. The fact that immune-insufficient individuals have an increased incidence of malignant tumors indicates that there may exist unknown immunologic control mechanisms which possibly influence the formation of tumors. This is certainly an open question for future research (Schmähl, 1971).

The same is true for diethylstilboestrol, which has been used as a synthetic estrogen for many years. Recent reports suggest that this drug possibly has diaplacental carcinogenic effects in man (Miller, 1971). In America it was noted that some young women aged from 16 to 23 years had developed adenocarcinomas of the vagina, a kind of tumor which is extremely rare at this age. The case histories of these women showed that their mothers had received diethylstilboestrol during the second and the third month of pregnancy to prevent abortion. Diethylstilboestrol had been administered in high dosages without addition of gestagen. In a control population without that treatment these tumors were not observed. American epidemiologists agree that from these data a correlation between the occurrence of these tumors and the treatment of pregnancies with diethylstilboestrol is evident. Transplacental carcinogenic effects of chemical carcinogens are well known experimentally (Ivankovic, 1972).

Similar observations in Europe have not been reported. As far as I know, in the European area estrogens have never been applied alone in abortion prophylaxis, but always in combination with gestagens. It is also a question whether the estrogen effect of stilboestrol is responsible for the transplacental carcinogenic action or whether the substance per se is carcinogenic due to its chemical structure and reactivity. This, however, seems very unlikely in respect to what is known about the relationships between constitution and effect of estrogens (Schmähl, 1957).

I will now point out by a few examples how difficult it is to classify drugs which have only possible carcinogenic effects in man (Table 1). As is well-known, the abuse of phenacetine, which is contained in many analgesics, leads to interstitial kidney diseases. Swedish examiners (Angervall et al., 1969) now report that about 10% of patients whose case records showed heavy abuse of phenacetine developed carcinomas of the kidney. Phena-

TABLE 5   *Survey on carcinogenesis experiments in Sprague-Dawley rats with cyclamate, saccharin, the combination of cyclamate and saccharin and cyclo-hexylamine*

Experiment	d (mg/kg)	D (g/kg)	Number of animals		Malignant tumors			MIT (days)	MLE (days)
			N_0	N_1.Tu.	Total	$N_0\%$	1.Tu.		
Control (untreated)	–	–	104	98	13	13	13	725±141	791±152
Cyclamate 2%	1000	882	104	97	16	15	17	692±198	805±208
Cyclamate 5%	2500	2188	104	101	20	19	20	742±174	884±170
Cyclamate + Saccharin 2%	909 91	750 83	104	102	12	12	12	655±188	820±180
Cyclamate + Saccharin 5%	2270 227	1852 195	104	95	11	11	12	689±176	823±210
Saccharin 0.2%	100	83	104	94	11	11	12	691±189	769±207
Saccharin 0.5%	250	210	104	93	17	16	18	686±185	760±224
Cyclohexylamine	200	177	104	68	6	6	9	877±164	801±230

MIT = medium induction time; MLE = medium life expectation; d = single dose; D = total dose.

cetine is, therefore, suspected of being carcinogenic in man. Some years ago we tested phenacetine because of its chemical similarity to Dulcin, which was used as a sweetener. In these animal tests phenacetine was found to be without any carcinogenic effect, even when given in extremely high dosages (Schmähl and Reiter, 1954). However, the possibility exists that man in this case may be more sensitive than laboratory animals. Even though the reports from Sweden have not yet been supported by similar observations in other countries, the possibility cannot be excluded that there is a link between excessive consumption of phenacetine and kidney cancer in man.

I will now describe a few examples of those drugs which I have listed in Table 1 under the heading of 'improbable or not assessable'. The first instance is cyclamate which was used as a synthetic sweetener. In 1970 American examiners reported a carcinogenic effect of cyclamate in the bladders of rats. The use of cyclamate was therefore abandoned in America and also in some European countries. In order to reproduce the above results we have carried out investigations in more than 800 Sprague-Dawley rats which received extremely high dosages of the sweetener. The animals received cyclamate at two different dose levels, cyclohexylamine (which is the main metabolic product of cyclamate), saccharine and a combination of cyclamate + saccharine. As can be seen from Table 5 a bladder carcinogenic effect of the sweeteners could not be established (Schmähl, 1973). As far as I know investigations in other countries have also shown negative effects. This example may show that a drug should be prohibited only when reproducible results are present.

A particularly instructive example of how careful we have to be in the evaluation of potentially carcinogenic drugs is INH (isonicotinic acid hydrazide). This substance is a highly potent drug in the therapy of tuberculosis. Hungarian and Italian investigators have now reported that INH has induced lung adenomas, lymphosarcomas and leukemias in mice. In rats and hamsters, however, INH was not effective (Schmähl, 1970). Therefore, in Table 1, I have listed INH under the heading of 'improbable/not assessable'. But it is difficult to forecast if man in his type of reaction to a specific substance will resemble the mouse rather than the rat and the hamster. Epidemiological investigations have not yet given evidence for carcinogenicity of INH in man, but due to the limited duration of observation it is not yet possible to decide whether INH is carcinogenic in man or not. On the other hand, INH has such beneficial tuberculostatic effects that we can hardly renounce its use. This example may show that the therapeutic effect of a drug must be balanced against its potential risk in every individual case.

With only a few words I will mention the possibility of the formation of 'nitroso drugs' from amines which can be nitrosited by NO_2-compounds. Since nitrates are commonly present in our food and our saliva 'nitroso drugs' can be synthesized in our body when the precursors are present. Since the experimental data are relatively small up to now I only want to say that there is a large field for research in the future. Pioneer work has been done by Lijinsky.

The present clinical and epidemiologic data give clear evidence that some drugs in use today have carcinogenic effects in man. The awareness of these hazards may enable the pharmacotherapist to balance the benefit of a drug against its potential risk in every individual case. Further research in preventive medicine is necessary to identify drugs which have adverse and possibly carcinogenic effects.

References

Angervall, L., Bengtsson, U., Zetterlund, C.G. and Zsigmond, M. (1969): Brit. J. Urol., 41, 401.
Clayson, D. B. (1972): In: Drug-Induced Diseases, Vol. 4, pp. 91-109. Editors: L. Meyler and H. M. Peck. Excerpta Medica, Amsterdam.
Ehlers, G. (1968): Z. Haut-Geschl. Krankh., 43, 763.
Hartwich, G. (1973): Fortschr. Med., 91, 357.

Ivankovic, S. (1972): In: Topics in Chemical Carcinogenesis, pp. 463-475. Editors: W. Nakahara, S. Takayama, T. Sugimura and S. Odashima. University Press, Tokyo.

Miller, R. W. (1971): J. nat. Cancer Inst., 47, 1169.

Penn, I., Hammond, L. Brettschneider, L. and Starzl, T. E. (1969): Transplant. Proc., 1, 106.

Penn, I., Halmgrimson, C. G. and Starzl, T. E. (1971): Transplant. Proc., 3, 14.

Scherf, H. R., Krüger, C. and Karsten, C. (1970): Arzneimittel-Forsch., 20, 1467.

Schmähl, D. (1957): Arzneimittel-Forsch., 7, 211.

Schmähl, D. (1970): Entstehung, Wachstum and Chemotherapie maligner Tumoren, 2nd ed. Editio Cantor, Aulendorf.

Schmähl, D. (1971): Dtsch. med. Wschr., 96, 1771.

Schmähl, D. (1972): Verh. dtsch. Ges. Path., 56, 133.

Schmähl, D. (1973): Arzneimittel-Forsch., 23, 1466.

Schmähl, D. and Osswald, H. (1970): Arzneimittel-Forsch., 20, 1461.

Schmähl, D. and Reiter, A. (1954): Arzneimittel-Forsch., 4, 404.

Thiede, T., Chievitz, E. and Christensen, B. C. (1964): Acta med. scand., 75, 721.

Thiede, T. and Christensen, B. C. (1969): Acta med. scand., 185, 133.

The possible importance of nitrosamines as carcinogens in humans

P. N. Magee

Courtauld Institute of Biochemistry, Middlesex Hospital Medical School, London, United Kingdom

The present widespread interest in the carcinogenic nitrosamines arose from clinical evidence of liver injury in men exposed to dimethylnitrosamine while working on a pilot plant involving the use of this compound as a solvent. Dimethylnitrosamine was shown to be a powerful and specific liver poison in rats, mice, rabbits and dogs (Barnes and Magee, 1954) and later to induce malignant liver tumours in rats when added to their diet (Magee and Barnes, 1956). These observations were, however, preceded several years earlier by a detailed account of the clinical picture and postmortem appearances of dimethylnitrosamine poisoning in man reported by Freund in 1937. This paper had the title 'Clinical manifestations and studies in parenchymatous hepatitis' which gave no indication that the hepatitis was caused by exposure to dimethylnitrosamine and explains the failure for some years of most authors to quote it. This paper is of considerable importance since it provides the essential evidence that human subjects are susceptible to a similar type of hepatotoxic action after ingestion of dimethylnitrosamine to that seen in experimental animals similarly treated.

During the following years various aspects of the biological actions of the nitrosamines were studied by several groups of investigators without any clear recognition that they might cause any hazard to man apart from the small numbers of industrial workers exposed to the compounds in the course of their work. The formation of amounts of dimethylnitrosamine which were acutely toxic to sheep in fishmeal preserved with nitrites was reported by Ender and his colleagues (Ender et al., 1964) and initiated the present period of disquiet concerning the possible formation of dangerous amounts of nitrosamines in food preserved with nitrites.

In what follows there will be a brief account of the toxicity and carcinogenicity of the N-nitroso compounds followed by a discussion of their possible modes of action. Recent work on the occurrence of carcinogenic nitrosamines in food for human consumption will be surveyed and the formation of these compounds from amine precursors and nitrites in the stomach and elsewhere in the body will be discussed with consideration of the possible importance of bacteria in these nitrosation reactions. Evidence of toxic injury and carcinogenesis in various organs resulting from simultaneous feeding of various amines, together with nitrites and the sources of these nitrosamine precursors in the human environment will be discussed. Finally an attempt will be made to assess the possible human hazard from nitrosamines present in food and the environment.

General articles on nitrosamine carcinogenesis which are relevant to the possible hazard for man have been provided by Barnes (1973); Lijinsky and Epstein (1970); Magee (1971, 1972); Wolff and Wasserman (1972).

Toxic and carcinogenic actions of nitrosamines

There are, broadly speaking, two kinds of N-nitroso compounds. The nitrosamines, as exemplified by the simplest of the dialkyl series, dimethylnitrosamine $(CH_3)_2NNO$, and the nitrosamides, as exemplified by N-nitrosomethylurea, $NH_2 CO- \underset{NO}{N} -CH_3$. Both types of compound undergo photodecomposition on exposure to U.V. light but the nitrosamines are chemically stable while the nitrosamides are unstable and decompose at alkaline pH to give gaseous nitrogen and the corresponding diazoalkane. Although the nitrosamides are more stable at neutral pH, some may decompose quite rapidly under physiological conditions and the rate of decomposition in some cases, e.g., N-nitrosomethylurethane, may be accelerated by the presence of sulphydryl compounds such as cysteine (Schoental and Rive, 1965). These differences in chemical stability are associated with marked differences in toxicity. In general the dialkyl nitrosamines and some cyclic nitrosamines, such as N-nitrosomorpholine, are strongly hepatotoxic, producing little or no toxic damage in other organs. In contrast, the nitrosamides have powerful local tissue damaging actions at the site of application and they tend to injure tissues with a high rate of cellular turnover, including the small intestine, the bone-marrow and the lymphoid tissues. These differences in biological behaviour are thought to be determined by the requirement for enzymic activation by the nitrosamines and the lack of this requirement by the nitrosamides. The tissue injury appears to be caused by a chemically reactive metabolic product, the amount formed from the nitrosamines being determined by the level of enzyme activity present in the tissue. The toxicity of the N-nitroso compounds has been discussed by Magee and Swann (1969). The carcinogenic action of the nitroso compounds has been discussed in several reviews (Magee and Schoental, 1964; Magee and Barnes, 1967; Druckrey et al., 1967). Largely due to the work of Druckrey, Preussmann, Schmähl and their colleagues, with contributions from many other laboratories, about a hundred N-nitroso compounds are known to be carcinogenic in one or more experimental animal species. The rat has been more extensively tested than the others and remarkable specificities for different organs by nitrosamines of different chemical structures, the organotropic effects of Druckrey, have been revealed. Examples of these effects are the selective carcinogenic action on the bladder by di-*n*-butylnitrosamine and 4-hydroxybutylbutylnitrosamine and on the oesophagus by phenylmethylnitrosamine and other unsymmetrical nitrosamines (Druckrey et al., 1967). This organ specificity is not confined to the rat. Another remarkable property of some nitrosamides, notably N-nitrosoethylurea, is to induce cancer transplacentally in the offspring of mother animals treated with the compound during pregnancy. Doses of this nitrosamide well below the lethal level are known to induce tumours of the brain or other parts of the nervous system in the offspring. These tumours may not become apparent until many months after birth. Unlike some chemical carcinogens the nitrosamines are effective in a wide range of species (Schmähl and Osswald, 1967), including birds, amphibia and fish (see Table 1). It seems highly probable, therefore, that man is susceptible to the carcinogenic action of the nitroso compounds. This conclusion is supported by the observation that human liver slices metabolise dimethylnitrosamine at a comparable rate to rat liver slices and that

TABLE 1   *Species susceptible to carcinogenesis by nitrosamines*

Mammals	Birds
Monkey	Fowl
Rat	Grass parakeet
Mouse	
Guinea-pig	*Fish*
Syrian hamster	Rainbow trout
Chinese hamster	Aquarium fish – *Brachydanio rerio*
European hamster	
Rabbit	
Dog	*Amphibia*
Pig	Newt – *Triturus helveticus*

similar methylation of nucleic acids occurs (Montesano and Magee, 1970). Although some of the nitroso carcinogens persist in the body as such for periods of minutes or hours only, they are capable of producing tumours after only one dose (Magee and Barnes, 1967; Druckrey et al., 1967). It is clear, therefore, that the nitrosamines are a group of highly potent chemical carcinogens and must be considered to represent a potential hazard to human subjects exposed to amounts comparable to those used in the experimental work briefly outlined above.

Mechanism of action of nitroso carcinogens

The mechanism of action of the carcinogenic nitroso compounds is not yet understood but it seems probable, as stated above, that the active or ultimate carcinogen as defined by Miller and Miller (1966) is a metabolic product rather than the unchanged parent carcinogen. There is good evidence for the formation of alkylating intermediates by metabolism or spontaneous decomposition of the nitroso carcinogens (see Magee and Barnes, 1967) but the role of these intermediates, possibly carbonium ions, in the induction of cancer is not clear. Other active metabolites may be formed (Süss, 1965; Neunhoeffer et al., 1970). The alkylating intermediate reacts with nucleophilic centres in the cell to give various alkylated products. In the case of the nucleic acids the predominant site of action is at the 7-position of guanine. Although it is now thought rather unlikely that alkylation at this position has important biological consequences, the detection of its presence may be a valuable indicator of sites in the body where metabolism or decomposition of the nitroso compound has occurred. This method was used by Montesano and Magee (1971) to demonstrate that nitrosation of methylurea had occurred in rats given this compound simultaneously with sodium nitrite (see later).

Formation and occurrence of nitrosamines in foods

As mentioned above, the possibility of nitrosamine formation in foods preserved with nitrites has been recognized since the reports by the Norwegian workers (Ender et al., 1964; Sakshaug et al., 1965) of toxicity, sometimes fatal, in sheep fed fishmeal containing added nitrite as a preservative and the demonstration of dimethylnitrosamine in this meal. Early investigations of food for human consumption were greatly handicapped by lack of adequate analytical methods for the reliable detection and estimation of nitrosamines in trace amounts. Great advances in methods have been made in recent years and recommendations have been made by the International Union of Pure and Applied Chemistry (IUPAC, 1972) and by the International Agency for Research on Cancer (IARC, 1972). The IUPAC report gives details of procedures for extraction, cleanup and concentration of the nitrosamines from the foodstuff under investigation and for their detection. Critically discussing the various methods for estimation of nitrosamines in foods Crosby et al. (1972) conclude that methods employing thin-layer chromatography, gas-liquid chromatography, polarography or nitrite-release can be ambiguous. In their view gas-liquid chromatography and mass-spectrometry provide more reliable characterization of individual N-nitrosamines. The results of a number of studies on the nitrosamine content of a variety of foods, beverages and other sources indicate that very small amounts of carcinogenic nitrosamine may be present in hams, various other cured meats, fried bacon, sausages, various smoked and dried fish, some cheeses and in some tobacco smoke condensates. The concentrations determined by reliable methods are usually in the parts per billion range. The reported formation of nitrosamines in food by the Maillard reaction (Devik, 1967) has not been confirmed (Heyns and Koch, 1971). Since the amounts of nitrosamine present in foods may be dependent on the amount of nitrites added as preservatives, the question of the safety of nitrites as food additives has become one of great immediate concern. The use of nitrites has been restricted in Norway and powerful groups are pressing for similar action in the United States. Withdrawal of nitrites or drastic reduction in their permitted use might lead to increased risk of botulism since nitrite is thought to have a powerful action against *Clostridium botulinus*, the organism responsible for the production of botulinus toxin. Opinions differ on the efficacy of nitrites in the control of botulins but recent publications (Christiansen et al., 1973; Hustad et al., 1973) confirm the value of these additives in the preservation of cured meats and wieners. It must be remembered that some cured meats are not exposed to temperatures sufficiently high to destroy the toxin producing bacteria. Nitrites are also known to contribute to the characteristic flavours of cured meats. In a long-term toxicity experiment rats were fed a diet containing 40% canned meat treated with either 0.5% or 0.02% sodium nitrite, with or without the addition of glucono-δ-lactone. Special attention was paid to the detection of any carcinogenic effect but none was found (Van Logten et al., 1972).

Formation of carcinogenic nitrosamines in the body

Any evaluation of nitrites as food additives must take into account the contribution made by this source to the total nitrite intake from all sources, which include drinking water and various vegetables (see below). This is extremely important because it is now well established that nitrosamines can be formed in the body, particularly in the acid medium of the stomach, following the simultaneous ingestion of various amine precursors and nitrites. This phenomenon was first reported by Sander (1968) and has subsequently been reviewed in detail (Sander, 1971). Simultaneous oral administration of N-nitroso-$[^{14}C]$-methylurea and sodium nitrite to rats gave rise to methylation of nucleic acids in the liver and other organs of rats which did not occur when the nitrite was omitted. These findings indicate that N-nitrosomethylurea must have been formed in the body (Montesano and Magee, 1971). It is now clear that not only secondary amines but also tertiary amines are capable of nitrosation to give carcinogenic nitrosamines. Only those secondary amines with low or moderate basicity are readily nitrosated and this may explain the failure of Druckrey et al. (1963) to induce tumours in rats fed diethylamine and nitrite simultaneously for their life span. Mirvish (1970) has studied the kinetics of nitrosation of dimethylamine, showing that the rate of nitrosamine formation was greatest at pH 3.4 and that it was proportional to the concentration of dimethylamine and to the square of the nitrite concentration. The nitrosation of secondary amines is, of course, a very well known reaction but nitrosation of tertiary amines, although reported as long ago as 1906 by Solonina has only recently been studied further (Hein, 1963; Smith and Loeppky, 1967). The formation of dimethylnitrosamine from nitrite and tetramethylammonium chloride and some naturally occurring quaternary ammonium compounds has also been recently demonstrated (Fiddler et al., 1972). The biological implications of tertiary amine nitrosation have been recognized by Lijinsky and his colleagues (Lijinsky et al., 1972). Nitrosation of tertiary amines may occur, generally speaking, in two ways as shown in Figure 1. The mechanism in which the N-dialkyl group is cleaved from the parent molecule and converted to the corresponding dialkylnitrosamine may have important implications. This process was first demonstrated to occur in the reaction of aminopyrine with sodium nitrite at pH 2.4, to give rise to a high yield (up to 70% of the theoretical) of dimethylnitrosamine (Lijinsky and Greenblatt, 1972). Subsequent work showed that a number of other tertiary amino compounds also gave simple carcinogenic dialkyl nitrosamines on reaction with nitrite. The tertiary amines tested included the drugs oxytetracycline (antibiotic), disulfiram (antialcoholic), nikethamide (respiratory stimulant) and tolazamide (oral hypoglycaemic) as well as piperine, a component of pepper. Nitrosation of oxytetracycline by nitrite was greatly reduced by the simultaneous administration of ascorbic acid which appeared to react preferentially with the nitrite (Mirvish et al., 1972). The possible use of ascorbic acid to reduce the nitrosation of drugs by nitrites in the stomach has been suggested. Since many alkaloids and other natural products as well as drugs are tertiary amines, as are some surfactants and agricultural chemicals which may be ingested by man incidentally, the implications of these observations are obvious.

1)

$$>N-R \xrightarrow[\text{N}_2\text{O}_3]{\substack{\text{HONO} \\ \text{or}}} >N-NO$$

2)

$$> -N \begin{smallmatrix} R \\ R \end{smallmatrix} \xrightarrow[\text{R N}_2\text{O}_3]{\substack{\text{HONO} \\ \text{or}}} \begin{smallmatrix} R \\ R \end{smallmatrix} N-NO$$

Nitrosation of N-methylmorpholine   Nitrosation of oxytetracycline

FIG. 1   *Nitrosation of tertiary amines. (From W. Lijinsky et al., 1972, J. nat. Cancer Inst., 49, 1239; by courtesy of the editors.)*

All the above examples of nitrosation of amines occurred in acid media. There is evidence, however, that bacteria can catalyse nitrosation reactions at neutral pH (Sander, 1968) which has been supported by Hawksworth and Hill (1971) and by Klubes et al. (1972), the last authors noting some residual non-enzymic nitrosation, even at pH 7. Non-enzymic in vitro formation of nitrosamines by bacteria isolated from meat products has been reported by Collins-Thompson et al. (1973).

The first attempt to demonstrate the production of pathological changes in animals treated simultaneously with an amine and nitrite was made by Druckrey et al. (1963) who administered diethylamine and sodium nitrite to rats in a life-time study. No liver tumours or other tumours were produced, probably because of the relatively high basicity of the secondary amine. Schweinsberg and Sander (1972) carried out a similar experiment with triethylamine and nitrite in rats and also failed to induce tumours which was not surprising since the production of diethylnitrosamine was considerably smaller than from diethylamine. There have been, however, several examples of tumour induction by simultaneous administration of nitrite and various amines and amides including morpholine, N-methylbenzylamine, N-methylaniline, 2-imidazolidone, methylcyclohexylamine, methylurea, dimethylurea and ethylurea (see Sander, 1971). Increased incidence and number of lung tumours was observed after simultaneous oral administration to mice of various amines and amides including piperazine, morpholine, N-methylaniline, methylurea and ethylurea (Greenblatt et al., 1971). It is of interest that similar concurrent administration of the amino acids proline, hydroxyproline and arginine with nitrite failed to induce tumours in mice (Greenblatt and Lijinsky, 1972). Acute liver necrosis has been induced in rats by oral administration of nitrite and secondary amines, including dimethylamine (Asahina et al., 1971) and similar liver necrosis was produced by oral treatment with aminopyrine and nitrite, which is known to give rise to the production of dimethylnitrosamine (Lijinsky and Greenblatt, 1972). Long term administration of aminopyrine with nitrite to rats induced malignant liver tumours similar to those induced by dimethylnitrosamine (Lijinsky et al., 1973). It is therefore of interest that ascorbic acid, which inhibits nitrosation reactions as described above, exerted a protective effect against the hepatotoxic effects of nitrite plus aminopyrine (Kamm et al., 1973). It is clear, therefore, that simultaneous administration of nitrite and a variety of secondary or tertiary amines may give rise to the formation of carcinogenic nitrosamines in the body which, under certain experimental conditions, are produced in sufficient quantity to exert acute toxic and carcinogenic effects.

Sources of nitrites and amines

Nitrites may be ingested in the form of preservatives which are permitted in many countries in cured meats and certain cheeses. They may also be formed in the body after ingestion as nitrates and subsequent reduction by microorganisms of the alimentary tract or infected urinary bladder (Hawksworth and Hill, 1971) which contain the appropriate nitrate reductase enzymes. Nitrates are present in most drinking water supplies and the amount may vary considerably from geographical area to area. Some well waters have very high nitrate content, sufficient to induce methaemoglobinaemia in infants after reduction to nitrite following ingestion (Lee, 1970). Some vegetables, including spinach, beets and carrots may contain high concentrations of nitrates. Nitrite is present in the saliva of most human subjects in the concentration range 1–10 p.p.m. (Tannenbaum and Weisman, personal communication). Nitrite appears to be absent from ductal saliva and is probably formed by reduction of nitrate by organisms present in the mouth (Goaz and Biswell, 1961). Since the average output of saliva per individual per day is 1 to 1.5 l, the contribution made by saliva to the total nitrite intake from the environment may be important. It is also of interest that nitrosation reactions are catalysed by thiocyanate which is present in saliva (Boyland et al., 1971).

A variety of amines may be present in food (Table 2) and many drugs and other environmental chemicals are secondary or tertiary amines (see above). Dimethylamine, pyrrolidine and piperidine are known to occur in normal human urine (Asatoor and Simenhoff, 1965) but their origin is not clear.

It seems, therefore, that there are ample possibilities for the formation of carcinogenic nitrosamines from amine precursors and nitrite in the human body but it is not possible, at present, to form any realistic estimate of the amounts involved.

TABLE 2 *Some secondary amines which may occur in food*

Adrenaline	4-Hydroxyproline
Agmatine	Methylguanidine
Anabasine	Pipecolinic acid
Arginine	Piperidine
Azetidine carboxylic acid	Proline
Canavanine	Pyrrolidine
Dimethylamine	Sarcosine
Ephedrine	Spermidine
Glycocyamine	Spermine
	Spherophysine

Conclusions

There can be no reasonable doubt that very small amounts of carcinogenic nitrosamines are present in some foods consumed by man and that these carcinogens may also be formed in the body from amine precursors and nitrites. It is not possible in the present state of knowledge to form a realistic estimation of the possible hazard to man that may arise from absorption of these nitrosamines. Further work is needed to enable better estimates to be made of the total intake of different nitrosamines from all sources, to clarify the effects of simultaneous exposure to several nitrosamines and to determine the nature of the dose-response relationships at low dose levels of administered nitrosamines.

References

Asahina, S., Friedman, M. A., Arnold, E., Millar, G. N., Mishkin, M., Bishop, Y. and Epstein, S. S. (1971): Cancer Res., 31, 1201.
Asatoor, A. M. and Simenhoff, M. L. (1965): Biochim. biophys. Acta (Amst.), 111, 384.
Barnes, J. M. (1973): In: Essays in Toxicology, Vol. 5. Editor: W. Hayes. Academic Press, New York, N.Y.
Barnes, J. M. and Magee, P. N. (1954): Brit. J. industr. Med., 11, 167.
Boyland, E., Nice, E. and Williams, K. (1971): Food Cosmet. Toxicol., 9, 639.
Christiansen, L. N., Johnston, R. W., Kautter, D. A., Howard, J. W. and Aunan, W. J. (1973): Appl. Microbiol., 25, 357.

Collins-Thompson, D.L., Sen, N.P., Aris, B. and Schwinghamer, L. (1973): Canad. J. Microbiol., 18, 1968.
Crosby, N. T., Foreman, J. K., Palframan, J. F. and Sawyer, R. (1972): Nature (Lond.), 238, 342.
Devik, O. G. (1967): Acta. chem. scand., 21, 2302.
Druckrey, H., Preussmann, R., Ivankovic, S. and Schmähl, D. (1967): Z. Krebsforsch., 69, 103.
Druckrey, H., Steinhoff, D., Beuthner, H., Schneider, H. and Klarner, P. (1963): Arzneimittel-Forsch., 13, 320.
Ender, F., Havre, G., Helgebostad, A., Koppang, N., Madsen, R. and Ceh, L. (1964): Naturwissenschaften, 51, 637.
Fiddler, W., Pensabene, J. W., Doerr, R. C. and Wasserman, A. E. (1972): Nature (Lond.), 236, 307.
Freund, H. A. (1937): Ann. int. Med., 10, 1144.
Goaz, P. W. and Biswell, H.A. (1961): J. dent. Res., 41, 355.
Greenblatt, M. and Lijinsky, W. (1972): J. nat. Cancer Inst., 48, 1389.
Greenblatt, M., Mirvish, S. and So, B. T. (1971): J. nat. Cancer Inst., 46, 1029.
Hawksworth, G. M. and Hill, M. J. (1971): Brit. J. Cancer., 25, 520.
Hein, G. E. (1963): J. chem. Educ., 40, 181.
Heyns, K. and Koch, H. (1971): Z. Lebensmitt.-Untersuch., 145, 76.
Hustad, G.O., Cerveny, J.G., Trenk, H., Deibel, R.H., Kautter, D.A., Fazio, T., Johnston, R.W. and Kolari, O.E. (1973): Appl. Microbiol., 26, 22.
I.A.R.C. (1972): In: IARC Scientific Publications No. 3, pp. 140. Editors: P. Bogovski, R. Preussmann and E. A. Walker. International Agency for Research on Cancer, Lyon.
I.U.P.A.C. Information Bulletin (1972): A Survey of Analytical Procedures for Traces of N-nitrosamines in foods. Technical Reports No. 5, pp. 1-18.
Kamm, J. J., Dashman, T., Conney, A. H. and Burns, J. J. (1973): Proc. nat. Acad. Sci. (Wash.). 70, 747.
Klubes, P., Cerna, I., Rabinowitz, A. D. and Jondorf, W. R. (1972): Food Cosmet. Toxicol., 10, 757.
Lee, D. H. K. (1970): Environmental Res., 3, 484.
Lijinsky, W. and Epstein, S. S. (1970): Nature (Lond.), 225, 21.
Lijinsky, W. and Greenblatt, M. (1972): Nature New Biol., 236, 177.
Lijinsky, W., Keefer, L., Conrad, E. and Van De Bogart, R. (1972): J. nat. Cancer Inst., 49, 1239.
Lijinsky, W., Taylor, H. W., Snyder, C. and Nettesheim, P. (1973): Nature (Lond.), 244, 176.
Magee, P. N. (1971): Food Cosmet. Toxicol., 9, 207.
Magee, P. N. (1972): Ann. occup. Hyg., 15, 19.
Magee, P. N. and Barnes, J. M. (1956): Brit. J. Cancer, 10, 114.
Magee, P. N. and Barnes, J. M. (1967): Advanc. Cancer Res., 10, 163.
Magee, P. N. and Schoental, R. (1964): Brit. med. Bull., 20, 102.
Magee, P. N. and Swann, P. F. (1969): Brit. med. Bull., 25, 240.
Miller, E. C. and Miller, J. A. (1966): Pharmacol. Rev., 18, 805.
Mirvish, S. S. (1970): J. nat. Cancer Inst., 44, 633.
Mirvish, S. S., Wallcave, L., Eagen, M. and Shubik, P. (1972): Science, 177, 65.
Montesano, R. and Magee, P. N. (1970): Nature (Lond.), 228, 173.
Montesano, R. and Magee, P. N. (1971): Int. J. Cancer, 7, 249.
Neunhoeffer, O., Wilhelm, G. and Lehmann, G. (1970): Z. Naturforsch., 25b, 302.
Sakshaug, J., Sognen, E., Hansen, M. A. and Koppang, N. (1965): Nature (Lond.), 206, 1261.
Sander, J. (1968): Hoppe-Seylers Z. physiol. Chem., 349, 429.
Sander, J. (1971): Arzneimittel-Forsch., 21, 1572-1580, 1707-1713, 2034-2039.
Sander, J., Schweinsberg, F. and Menz, H. P. (1968): Hoppe-Seylers Z. physiol. Chem., 349, 1691.
Schmähl, D. and Osswald, H. (1967): Experientia (Basel), 23, 497.
Schoental, R. and Rive, D. J. (1965): Biochem. J., 97, 466.
Schweinsberg, F. and Sander, J. (1972): Hoppe-Seylers Z. physiol. Chem., 343, 1671.
Smith, P. A. and Loeppky, R. N. (1967): J. Amer. chem. Soc., 89, 1147.
Solonina, V. A. (1906): J. Russ. Phys. Chem. Soc., 38, 1286.
Süss, R. (1965): Z. Naturforsch., 20b, 714.
Van Logten, M. J., Dentonkelaar, E. M., Kroes, R., Berkvens, J. M. and Van Esch, G. J. (1972): Food Cosmet. Toxicol., 10, 475.
Wolff, I. A. and Wasserman, A. E. (1972): Science, 177, 15.

Recent advances and perspectives of automation in cytology

O.A.N. Husain

Regional Cytology Centre, St. Stephen's Hospital, Chelsea, London, United Kingdom

The potential for automated scanning of malignant cells is vast, as cytology is now examining cells from lungs, kidneys, bladder, prostate, breast, the whole of the alimentary tract and, by virtue of needle puncture, numerous other sites, but none so thoroughly as the female genital tract, especially the cervix uteri. The tremendous task of screening normal female populations by microscopy, when the reward rate to the cyto-technician is 5 positive smears per thousand for the first test, which may drop to 5 or even 2 per 10,000 on repeat yearly examination, can only be viewed with apprehension when the work load in Great Britain alone is of the order of 3 million smears per year, and in America over 30 million at the present time.

Table 1 shows that the approach to such a task has been comprehensive. We have been associated with the first two categories before settling to fixed cell pattern recognition.

The use of enzyme titres, mainly of the pentose shunt and especially that of the 6-phosphogluconate dehydrogenase, following Bonham and Gibbs' original communication (1962), demonstrated a remarkable success in separating the malignant from the benign case. This was investigated by Cameron and Husain (1965). Our results of about 10,000 comparative tests showed that though raised enzyme titres were obtained from the vaginal posterior fornix mucus samples in all invasive cancers, only about half the cases with carcinoma in situ demonstrated any activity. There was a high false positive rate even when potassium was used as a measure of cellular content and was often related to the presence of certain cells and inflammatory states. This does not preclude the use of such a technique as we may need to seek for the elusive endometrial cancer after the menopause in this way.

We then became interested in the claims for the Coulter Counter following Ladinsky's (1964) original account from Wisconsin. Here, cells in saline are passed through an aperture across which there is an electronic field. A pulse wave proportional to the 'non-conductive' cell volume is registered on an oscillograph. By means of a size distribution plotter with upper and lower limit threshold settings, a range of cell volumes can be recorded at 50 μ^3 intervals.

Ladinsky showed that aspirate samples of posterior fornix mucus produced simple parabolic curves of diminishing numbers as the cell size increased from 50 to 1400 μ^3 in the benign case, but that a secondary peak around 500 to 700 μ^3 occurred, she presumed, from the existence of large malignant cells in samples from cancer cases.

Ladinsky's results, however, demonstrated a false positive rate from 0 to 20% amongst the benign cases, and a false negative rate from 15 to 17% in the pre-invasive group though none of the invasive carcinomas were missed.

We and a number of others (Husain and Cameron, 1966; Iverson et al., 1966) failed to reproduce these figures. We found that we could obtain secondary peaks in only some malignancies and often produced some in non-malignant, sometimes infective cases where we felt that neutrophil clusters were the main cause of the secondary peaks. Perhaps we have not finished with this approach as I am sure that with the biological cell sample we are not just measuring particle size but something of the interrelationship of cell to substrate. Also, improved cell presentation techniques may well reduce the false positive rate.

Still on the cell flow systems we should look at 2 or 3 other instruments, the first being a rather historic one of Dr. Louis B. Kamentsky, working in the IBM laboratory at Columbia University, New York (Kamentsky et al., 1965).

This very sophisticated instrument sends a fluid cell stream through a 100μ wide

TABLE 1   *Automated techniques for malignant cell detection*

Technique	Type	Instrument
Enzymes	6 Phosphogluconate dehydrogenase	Auto-analyser
	Glucuronidase	
	Mannosidase	
Cell suspension scanners	Cell volume measurement	Electronic counter (size) distribution plotter (Coulter)
	Differential light absorption systems	
	Selective wavelength spectrophotometry	Rapid spectrophotometry Cytofluorograf (Kamentsky)
	DNA profile scanners	Impulscytophotometer (PHYWE)
Fixed cell scanners	*Visible light scanners*	
	Source plane scanner	Cathode ray tube systems
	Object plane scanner	Slit scanners/rotating mirror (Vickers): multiple channel photomultipliers (Birmingham)
	Image plane scanner	Television (Quantimet/Cytoscreen)
	Ultraviolet light scanners	
	Cytophotometric absorbance	Integrating microdensitometer (modified Deeley)
	Cytophotometric fluorescence	Leitz M.P.V. (basis)
Cell separators	Electronic	Electrostatic (Fulwyler)
	Biological	Wheat germ agglutinins
	Flow systems	NCI, IBM cell sep.
	Electrophoretic	Free curtain electrophoresis
Cell presentors	Film (35mm) with electromagnetic signals	Tetronics 'Cytotrack'
	Melinex tape (ICI)	Vickers scanning machine
Other techniques	Laser beam	Laser beam/crossed nicol prism microscope
	Tetracycline fluorescence	Simple UVL source

quartz channel at the rate of 5000 cells per sec. Light from a Hanovia low pressure mercury source is passed through the cell stream into the objective lens of a microscope. The transmitted light is then split by a dichroic mirror to direct the 4000 to 6000 Å component on to a photomultiplier, while the shorter wavelengths are reflected at 90°. The latter are then passed through a quartz cell containing 1,4-diphenylbutadiniene dissolved in ethanol in order to isolate the 2537 Å line which is near the absorption maximum of nucleic acid. This is then imaged on to a solar blind photomultiplier.

The two components thus give an indication of the nucleic acid/total cell volume ratio — one of the most fundamental criteria in identifying a malignant cell, and these are presented as scattergrams on the oscillograph. Further refinements were to involve up to 4 photomultipliers and include the recording of certain fluorescent dye stain properties. Another is a high speed electronic pulsing device which deflects the cell stream when a cell with a high nuclear-cytoplasmic ratio passes by. These cells are collected in a side channel and fed periodically on to a micro-millipore membrane for staining and visual observation. The instrument showed great potential. Unfortunately, Dr. Kamentsky left Columbia before this was made commercially available to create another series of instruments designed more for differential blood cell counting than malignant cell detection.

His latest instruments are the Cytograf and the Cytofluorograf, utilising a focussed laser beam (red helium in the Cytograf and a blue argon-ion laser in the Cytofluorograf) (Adams and Kamentsky, 1971). The cells flow through at 5000 per sec and can be counted by particle number and size from 1μ to 100μ diameter. Here, many dyes can be excited by the 4880 Å light and the instrument has two additional sensors to detect fluorescence at two different wavelengths. There is insufficient time to detail the sensor systems and photometric parameters used, but Dr. Kamentsky has utilised the red and green fluorescence of the acridine dyes and fluorescein. Scattergrams have been produced for blood and for cervical cytology but much less work has been done on the latter.

Another similar flow-through system is being perfected in Freiburg by Sprenger et al. (1971). Based on the Leitzmicroscope photometer (MPV) with a high pressure Zenon arc HBO 100 epi-illumination light source, they are passing cells stained by 0.01% Acriflavine Schiff through the focal plane of the objective at the rate of 100—1050 cells per sec. *The cells* are flushed off by a horizontal water current and the fluorescent light pulses of the cells are classified and stored by an impulse height discriminator where they may be recalled analogically as a histogram, or digitally as a series of numbers. The latest publications do provide some interesting plots of their instrument with histograms in the benign and malignant cases showing the DNA content equivalent of di-, tetra-, and hexaploid sets of chromosomes. However, in a recent series of 60 cases, though there were no false negatives, 10% were false positive and a third were unsatisfactory (Sprenger et al., 1972).

Another example of DNA assessment in a flow-through method is that of PHYWE with their Impulscytophotometer (Reiffenstuhl et al., 1971). The technique of cell preparation is simple. They are fixed in absolute alcohol at −30°C which is later replaced by tris buffer and subsequently incubated in 0.1% ribonuclease in order to destroy the RNA before staining. The cells are stained by Ethidium Bromide (1:20,000 in tris buffer) for 2 hr, each cell absorbing an amount of stain proportional to its DNA content. After washing and diluting and sieving off large particles by a 70μ sieve the cells are drawn up by a pump and flushed across an 100μ aperture by a further stream of particle-free liquid. Light from a powerful source is fed downstream by means of a dichroic mirror. The scatter of fluorescent light emanating from a cell in the measuring aperture is reflected up again and directed at a series of photomultipliers.

Electrical signals with amplitudes proportional to the intensities of scattered or fluorescent light from the cells are sent from the photomultipliers to a multichannel analyser which classifies the signals as a function of amplitude visualised on the oscilloscope and stored, to be recorded as a histogram. It is too early to give an assessment of such an instrument, the success of which will depend on the proportion of cells in the test sample possessing increased DNA content to provide a distinctive alteration of profile.

Cell separators or sorters

A word about other forms of approach to this problem would not be out of place here.

(a) Electronic

The apparatus developed by Van Dilla et al. (1967) in California works by fractionating a mixture of microscopic particles according to small differences in their volume. A dilute suspension of cells passes through a sensor within which the volume of each cell is electronically measured and subsequently discharged into the air as a liquid jet. This is broken into a large number of minute droplets, some containing suspended cells. These are electronically charged and then electrostatically deflected into suitable receptacles. Successful so far in separating blood cells, it is being applied to the problem of cancer cell sorting.

(b) Biological separator

Cell separation by wheat germ agglutinins also has been demonstrated by Prof. E. J. Ambrose of London (Ambrose et al., 1968). He has shown that there are certain sugars on the surface of malignant cells such as sialic acid and N-acetylglucosamine, and that the latter combines specifically with wheat germ agglutinin and certain poly-electrolytes such as polyethyleneimine. Using a monolayer of HeLa cells grown on a coverslip he has obtained agglutination of added malignant cells together with many of the parabasal cells by means of wheat germ extract. One of the most significant features of this process is that it serves to exclude the polymorphs which bedevil the whole of automated malignant cell scanning. His latest work includes culture of cells in vitro to identify cell formation which seeks to distinguish if they are invasive or not.

(c) Cell separation by continuous free curtain electrophoresis

Using the Elphar VaP$_2$ apparatus it has been somewhat successful in separating blood cells and some mice tumour preparations, but is not likely to provide rapid automated separation.

Fixed cell scanners

The most intensely-followed field of malignant cell scanning is that of the fixed cell scanner reading from slide or film strip. The rationale for these procedures resulted from the work of Tolles, Horvath and Bostrom in 1961 who demonstrated that the presence of large and atypical and densely-staining malignant nuclei could serve to distinguish malignant cell patterns from the normal as shown in their graphs plotting nuclear size against density (Tolles et al., 1961). Much of this early work was put to the test by Tolles and his colleagues on the Cytoanalyser (Spencer and Bostrom, 1962). This was an image plane scanner converting optical information on grey density levels by high speed microphotometry into electrical analogues — amplitude and time. Both measurements and control circuits existed, the latter to eliminate or cancel out false measurements such as cell clusters and debris. The whole exercise was intended to divide up a series of cell samples into malignant and benign groups. As everyone knows, the resultant clinical trials proved disappointing. An apparent 36.6% false positive and 10.3% false negative rate was obtained.

We have approached this problem a little differently in England. Spriggs et al. (1968) set out to confirm the thesis that malignant smears always contain large nuclei. Diamond assessed nuclear size by traditional Papanicolaou-stained cervical smears but did not register the problem of stain density levels to signal effectively the enlarged malignant nucleus distinct from its background of cytoplasm, non-malignant nuclei, mucus and debris. He found in a small series that all malignant cases contained at least 12 nuclei over 12μ and most contained some over 16μ, a finding I think we have to a large extent confirmed (Diamond, 1967).

Their work stimulated the Vickers company to create the Vickers Cytology Screening Apparatus where, using a rotating mirror, a narrow 5μ slit scan of the field occurs registering density, or light absorption, over a given threshold on a slit length of over 12 and under 20μ.

The cells collected in solution from scrape smears were spread on to thin, transparent Melinex tape and stained by the Papanicolaou technique, covered by a mountant and Scotch tape. There are three modules:

1. The tracking or graphing instrument.
2. The staining apparatus.
3. The scanner.

The instrument scans the cell sample and punches a hole in the tape when it registers a dense particle of the right size. As it would continue to punch for the whole of a dark mass and thus shred the tape, a negative phase has to occur for about 1cm which therefore may miss some good nuclear signals.

This instrument possessed a rather unrefined scanning system, and though some have demonstrated a better than random punching selection of fields it has no pattern recognition ability and cannot discriminate between malignant nuclei or a cluster of polymorphs, or other nuclei, or heavily-stained cytoplasm overlaps or mucus, or, where no punching is occurring, that there are any cells present at all. The principle of approach here was excellent but improved pattern recognition is necessary to make it an economic possibility.

A more refined instrument is being constructed in Great Britain at Birmingham University by Dr. Skinner and his colleagues (Skinner, personal communication). Here the principle is the detection of enlarged cell nuclei by analysis of size and shape of dense objects by a scanning slit or wedge passing across the microscope field with light signals fed by a rotating mirror to a bank of 16 photomultipliers, providing considerable data for computation. The hardware logic system uses parallel processing in a number of similar channels to attain a high speed. Here the basic region scanned is 28μ wide $\times$ $300\,\mu$ long in a time of $250\,\mu sec$. With 140,000 regions per slide it is calculated to be about a minute per specimen including printout. There has been initial success using ordinary Papanicolaou-stained scrape smears and we await with interest more substantial results.

We ourselves have been developing a more elaborate fixed cell scanning instrument, the Quantimet, or Image Analysing Computer (Husain and Henderson, 1970). Developed originally for assessing metal impurities, the pore size in ceramics and the size of powder particles, this instrument was converted to use with a transmission light microscope to scan suitably-presented cell samples.

It is an image plane scanner using a single spot scan with a one-line memory. The spot scans the whole of the microscopic field imaged on the surface of the vidicon tube and is displayed on the television monitor. By using a bright light signal on the monitor image potentiometers vary density thresholds and minimum chord intersects (which is the time the spot takes to pass across a dense particle along the horizontal television lines) the Quantimet can size out and register the density of suitably-stained nuclei.

Using this instrument we surveyed large numbers of Papanicolaou-stained cervical scrape smears to assess both the nuclear size and density content of various types of cases. These, when plotted with size against nuclear density, demonstrate sufficient separation of malignant and dyskaryotic from the non-malignant nuclei to make it possible to scan at certain thresholds to seek for malignancy. Moreover, there appeared a graded separation where the larger malignant nuclei could be selected at a less densely stained level than the smaller darker nuclei suggesting a differential size-density acceptance register.

What bedevils the whole problem is the fact that these pattern-recognition instruments, scanning monochromatically, cannot distinguish nuclei from cytoplasm if they approach each other in stain density or light transmission and also if the nuclei are too close together. The result is a mass of 'lost signals' or malignant nuclei buried in unresolvable clusters which can vary from 10 to 50% of the abnormal cells. Our task has been to liberate these hidden nuclei and a large scale effort has been mounted by us to disperse cells and suitably stain both nucleus and cytoplasm, preferably at opposite ends of the spectrum.

We have investigated numerous fixatives with and without post-fixation techniques, a range of dispersal agents such as polymers and polyvinyl alcohol, various enzymes including cytolytic systems and physical methods of mucus- and cell-cluster disruption such as ultrasonics, vibrators, syringing and differential centrifugation. Finally, the layering of cells on both glass slides and film strips, the latter suitably coated with a range of hydrophilic substances. As the Papanicolaou stain presents stain densities in some cytoplasmic areas as high as with nuclei, we have experimented widely with numerous nuclear and cytoplasmic stains. These include the polychromes such as methylene blue, a variety of haematoxylins, the nuclear or DNA stains such as Feulgen and Gallocyanin chrome alum and differing cytoplasmic stains presenting more uniform density for densitometric scans. Time does not permit us to dwell on any of these techniques in particular but a measurable degree of success has resulted with the very complex cell suspensions presented from both scrapes and aspirates.

From our experience with the Quantimet, the company IMANCO has built us the Cytoscreen, the design of which is a compromise between what we felt were the best parameters to seek for in assessing malignancy, and what the manufacturers could achieve practically. We kept in mind the cardinal features of a malignant cell as listed on the next slide, and saw what parameters would be practical to use.

We had to keep in mind the basic principles of its use: that the Cytoscreen would scan, sort and select in real time suspect cells which would alert a microscope field for review by eye, and thus the cell presentation and staining should be usable by both machine and cytologist − a somewhat restricting compromise. For instance, the complete disruption of cell clusters would liberate more cells but would probably strip them of cytoplasm and would certainly remove much of the inter-cellular relationships which the cytologist depends on to make a diagnosis. There is a happy mean to be achieved.

The Cytoscreen was further restricted to an economic rate of scan. 40 to 50,000 epithelial cells normally found on a scrape smear must be scanned in 2 to 3 min, which places a limit on the magnification of the system. We have chosen a ×25 Zeiss objective with a 0.65 NA, which gives a picture point or resolution of 0.7μ.

Using a special plumbicon tube scanning a 704 line system, each line is divided into 832 picture points. The analysed image area is, however, 640 × 624 picture points and there are two speeds of scan, one at 5.5 and one at 11 frames per sec. The computer therefore is handling information at the rate of 4.4×10^6 picture points per sec.

It is equipped to accept two forms of cell presentation systems, on slide or tape, the latter either 16 or 35 mm film strips tracked centrally with a 1 to 2mm wide band of cells. Both Vickers and Tetronics tape systems are utilised.

There is a binocular head with ×16 eyepieces for visual checking, and an automatic slide scan stage. Various colour filters can be introduced into the light path before or after the object. The automatic slide stage is controlled by a drive module providing both X and Y movement co-ordinate control register and recall facilities. Automatic focussing is incorporated.

There are 2 methods of illumination; tungsten light for ocular viewing, and a short duration flash to freeze the field of view for television scanning and to permit erasure before the next field is scanned. It has 3 modes of action: (1) Manual − where single field data acquisition can occur; (2) semi-automatic where the specimen moves automatically but the equipment is pre-programmed to stop for an operator decision whenever fields of view contain features of interest; and (3) fully automatic for assessment of large series of specimens.

The computer facilities include 5 nuclear sizing banks, all with upper and lower threshold limits controlled by potentiometers with a maximum size of 22μ, large enough to contain most large single malignant nuclei and 4 density banks, one for cytoplasm and 3 for the nuclei, all with upper and lower thresholds. These thresholds can be bright-light signalled on the monitor.

There are thus 15 different size and density categories, and with 14 data channels one can accumulate valuable information for *any specific cell* or presentation system.

Having categorized the nuclei, the use of parameter selectors eliminates the unnecessary. These include:

(1) Minimum chords

Elimination of short chords will clean up a background without too greatly altering the shape of a particle.

(2) Re-entrant and convex curvature criteria

These reject artefacts having sharply angled or undulating edges or nuclear clusters such as polymorphs, though the individual polymorph is too small to be rejected by this parameter. We would have liked to have used the irregularity of the malignant nuclear membrane as an acceptance criteria but this is a very fine irregularity and only recordable at a much higher resolution of about 0.25μ or even 0.1μ needing a magnification of $\times 1000$ or above. The same applies to the assessment of the irregular chromatin condensation, so characteristic of malignancy.

(3) Form factor

This parameter may well have to be used at 1:2, or 1:3 ratio, as in malignancy there is often considerable fusiform distortion of the nucleus. Beyond a certain ratio we may find it better to exclude, as much distorted debris and mucus strands will need to be rejected, though there again one would lose the fibre cell characteristic of invasive squamous cancer.

(4) Cytosurround

This is one of the most interesting and valuable parameters. The more valuable register of nucleo-cytoplasmic ratio is not easily assessed by this scanning technique using our present methods of cell presentation, as it is difficult to avoid cytoplasmic overlap without uneconomical wide dispersals. We have therefore made use of the register of cytoplasmic density on one or other side of the nucleus at various picture point intervals away from the nuclear margin. This, in effect, cancels the simple debris and artefacts, and though it may also exclude the stripped malignant nuclei in a cell sample it will be worth it. Moreover, it is a valuable way of rejecting the bulk of the polymorph neutrophils or pus cells.

The apparatus will be completed by incorporating automatic cell register selector and recall equipment which will be optico-electronic for tape and for slides, probably a sensed area on one half of the slide permitting coincident co-ordinate reference coding for recall purposes.

The ultimate intention is to scan automatically and code probably no more than 1 to 3% of the fields normally looked at by eye, and that such film strips or slides will be check-scanned by a cytotechnologist either on the parent instrument or, more economically, on microscopes with specially attached decoding devices. This would result in 5 to 10 times more cell samples being screened per cytotechnician with accompanying relief of boredom, fatigue and cost.

A rather similar instrument, where the principle of a 2 phase image analyser utilising similar criteria and an on-a-line computer is used, is being developed in Edinburgh by J.H. Tucker. Various other instruments are being developed in the United States, Canada and Japan.

Finally, I would like to say a word about the much more refined densitometric analysis of cell nuclei. The work on more detailed high-powered scanning has been performed for some years now by Drs. G.L. Wied, G. Bahr and P. Bartels using the Zeiss Cytoscan, already presented to this Conference by Dr. Wied. This is the successor to the Universal Microspectrophotometer (UMSP1) connected on-line to a linc 8 (now 10) computer. They have created the method of cell identification called Taxonomic Intracellular Analytic System (TICAS) (Wied et al., 1968). Using slow but accurate high resolution scan with a picture point of 0.25 at various wavelengths they are creating algorhythms and histograms of different parameter selections and coming very close to identifying cell types and changes within cell types.

It will be a logical outcome to link a rapid pre-screening apparatus such as the Cytoscreen to a Zeiss Cytoscan and in a two-step process achieve a diagnostic procedure commensurate with human ability. I say this with caution as it is obvious that a machine will not be able to register anything like the amount of background detail that a cytotechnician can do, and in any case such a link is in the somewhat distant future. There are compelling reasons for creating and using a first and even second generation machine which will serve as a most valuable technical aid in an ever expanding field of work.

References

Adams, L.R. and Kamentsky, L.B. (1971): Acta cytol. (Philad.), 15, 289.

Ambrose, E.J., Smith, W.J. and Forrester, J.A. (1970): In: Proceedings, Second Tenovus Symposium, Cardiff 1968, p. 100. Editor: D.M.D. Evans. E. and S. Livingstone, Ltd., Edinburgh-London.

Bonham, D.G. and Gibbs, D.F. (1962): Brit. med. J., 2, 823.

Cameron, C.B. and Husain, O.A.N. (1965): Brit. med. J., 1, 1529.

Diamond, R.A. (1967): Cytological Criteria Applicable to Automatic Scanning of Cervical Smears for Malignancy. Thesis, Oxford.

Husain, O.A.N. and Cameron, C.B. (1966): Proc. roy. Soc. Med., 59, 982.

Husain, O.A.N. and Henderson, M.J. (1970): In: Proceedings, Second Tenovus Symposium, pp. 214-227. Cardiff, 1968. Editor: D.M.D. Evans. E. and S. Livingstone, Ltd., Edinburgh-London.

Iverson, S., Gordon, W.J., Cowell, M.A.C. and Watson, E.R. (1966): Brit. med. J., 1, 1209.

Kamentsky, L.A., Melamed, M.R. and Derman, H. (1965): Science, 150, 630.

Ladinsky, J.L., Sarto, G.E. and Packham, B.M. (1964): J. Lab. clin. Med., 64, 970.

Reiffenstuhl, G., Severin, E., Dihrich, W. and Gohde, W. (1971): Arch. Gynäk., 211/4, 595.

Spencer, C.C. and Bostrom, R.C. (1962): J. nat. Cancer Inst., 29, 267.

Sprenger, E., Sandritter, W., Bohm, N., Schaden, M., Hilgarth, M. and Wagner, D. (1971): Beitr. path. Anat., 143, 323.

Sprenger, E., Sandritter, W., Bohm, N., Wagner, D., Hilgarth, M. and Schaden, M. (1972): Acta cytol. (Philad.), 16, 297.

Spriggs, A.I., Diamond, R.A. and Meyer, E.W. (1968): Lancet, 1, 359.

Tolles, W.F., Horvath, W.J. and Bostrom, R.C. (1961): Cancer (Philad.), 14, 437, 455.

Van Dilla, M.A., Fulwyler, M.J. and Boone, I.U. (1967): Proc. Soc. exp. Biol. Med., 125, 367.

Wied, G.L., Bartells, P.H., Bahr, G.F. and Oldfield, D.G. (1968): Acta cytol. (Philad.), 12, 180.

The evaluation of cancer control measures

A. J. Phillips*

Committee on Cancer Prevention and Detection, International Union Against Cancer, Geneva, Switzerland

The activities of the International Union Against Cancer are carried out through 6 Commissions, one of which is the Commission on Cancer Control. Within this Commission are 4 committees and one of these is the Committee on Prevention and Detection. The Union holds a Congress every 4 years and in general Committees plan their programmes from one Congress to the next. During the period 1970-1974 the Committee on Prevention and Detection planned its programme to include a symposium on the evaluation of screening procedures for various sites of the disease and this was held in Sheffield, England on Sept. 12th – 15th, 1972. Twenty-seven scientists were invited from 8 countries and presented results of screening programmes covering cancer of the breast, cervix, stomach, colon and liver. In addition a session was held on methodologic principles in evaluating cancer control through early detection and one on control through Health Education. This report of the symposium presents excerpts from the submissions presented, which are gratefully acknowledged, and summarizes the conclusions reached by the delegates.

The philosophy of cancer screening

We believe that cancers begin as changes in the mode of activity of a small number of cells, in many instances probably a single cell, and that the clinical effects of the lesion result from an increase in the number of tumour cells and physical extension of the tumour both locally and by metastasis to distant organs. It follows therefore, that if the lesion can be identified when it is confined to a small group of cells it can be extirpated and the clinical manifestations of malignancy can be averted. For any form of screening to be contemplated, we must accept the concept that there is a stage in the life of the neoplasm at which a small localised group of cells can be recognised by clinical, cytological, chemical or radiological means. The validity of this concept is a function of the natural history of the disease particularly when there are differences between the form of the disease recognised at screening and the form seen in the clinical setting.

From a 'purely' scientific point of view there are two basic issues which must be resolved. The first of these is in the field of the natural history of the disease. Is there a stage of the tumour at which a small localised group of neoplastic cells can be identified? Ideally this would be a small mass of tissue which, when sectioned, showed histological appearances which were identified by pathologists unanimously as being identical with those of the clinically apparent lesion. Sometimes this is the case, but it is not necessary that this should be the case. In some circumstances histological entities can be identified which differ from the cancer which they precede, yet such a lesion is an acceptable basis for a screening exercise.

The second basic issue is that there should be a test available by which a localised form of the disease can be recognised. This test may be clinical, simple inspection or palpation; it may be cytological, chemical or immunochemical or radiological. At this level of consideration two parameters are to be applied to the test. The first of these is specificity,

* National Cancer Institute of Canada, Toronto, Canada.

the test should be 'positive' in cases of the disease, and negative in patients who do not have the lesion for which the test is devised. The degree of specificity is measured by the proportion of false 'positive' results which is obtained, and a great deal of research and development often has to be undertaken to determine the specificity of a test and to refine it so as to increase this desirable characteristic. The second parameter is sensitivity, the capacity of the test to detect all patients in whom the disease exists. This parameter is in some ways the converse of the first, and is measurable by estimation of the false 'negative' rate. Regrettably these two sources of error usually act in opposite directions, if the specificity is increased by refinements of technique the sensitivity is affected adversely and vice versa.

Finally the test must be assessed in terms of reduced mortality or morbidity. The simplest way to achieve such an assessment would be to select a population to whom the test is to be applied and a matched control population to whom the test would not be applied and then await results for a period of one or even two generations. This is not a generally acceptable procedure so it becomes necessary for some other experimental design, with probably somewhat less accurate criteria, to be applied. Included in these new criteria will be the usefulness of the test, i.e. that the clinical action to be taken will reduce the morbidity and mortality.

The effectiveness of cancer screening

The hypothesis that early detection reduces the chance of invasive cancer has been widely adopted and has resulted in a variety of mass screening programmes for specific sites of the disease. However, increasing skepticism of the effectiveness of such measures has been expressed, ranging from reasonable certainty that some, such as radiography for lung cancer, are not, and are not likely to be, effective; through dilemmas hinging upon uncertainties about the natural history of the disease as in cervical cytology; to the cost-benefit problems which arise when a procedure is shown to be implemented only at great cost, as in proposals for breast cancer screening. These doubts, sometimes expressed as a challenge, have been reinforced by the seeming incompatibility of changes in incidence rates but not in mortality in certain sites, together with the uncertainties inherent in all programmes which screen apparently healthy people.

After careful study of the evidence presented and recognizing the sincerity of the skepticism regarding the effectiveness of mass screening programmes the Symposium reached a consensus on the value of screening for cancers of the breast, cervix and stomach.

The evidence is summarized as follows:

(a) Screening for cancer of the breast

The experience of the Cancer Detection Centre, under Dr. V. Gilbertsen of the University of Minnesota in Minneapolis, U.S.A., showed that of 8649 women screened, 110 breast cancers were found whose survival at 15 years was as favourable as that for Minnesota women without breast cancer.

A randomized clinical trial, under the direction of Mr. S. Shapiro, Dr. P. Strax and Dr. L. Venet, has been conducted to determine if repetitive screening for breast cancer with clinical examinations and mammography lowers the mortality from breast cancer. The population consists of women aged 40 to 64 years, enrolled in a prepaid group practice plan in a large urban area, New York City. Randomization techniques were applied to allocate 31,000 of these women to a study group, which was invited to screening examinations, and the same number to a control group, which was not invited. Close comparability exists between the study and control groups in a broad spectrum of demographic characteristics. Also, mortality from all causes other than breast cancer is almost identical for the two groups.

About two-thirds of the women in the study group accepted the invitation to have an initial screening examination and a large majority of these women appeared in one or more of the 3 successive rounds of annual screening examinations. A high degree of selectivity occurred in deciding whether to participate in the screening programme. Those who did, had a higher breast cancer incidence rate and considerably lower general mortality than those who refused screening. In view of this, the primary comparisons to test the underlying hypothesis of the investigation utilize the experience of the total group of study women, including those who refused screening.

The screening examinations resulted in a higher proportion of breast cancers being detected with no evidence of axillary node involvement in the study group as compared with the control group. Both mammography and clinical examination of the breast contributed to the improved picture of early detection. At ages 50 and over, omission of either one of the modalities would have resulted in a significantly lower breast cancer detection rate on screening. Mammography led to detection of only a small proportion of additional cases at ages 40 to 49 years. Treatment of breast cancer cases does not appear to have been affected by whether the woman was in the study or in the control group.

The evidence on the impact of repetitive screening on breast cancer mortality is now quite convincing. Over the short run period of 5 years of follow-up, women offered screening have about a one-third lower mortality from breast cancer than those in the control group. This holds whether the comparison is based on deaths due to breast cancer during the 5 years following entry to the investigation (63, control vs. 40, study) or on case fatality rates for the 5 years of follow-up after diagnosis (42%, control vs. 28%, study). The screening programme appears to have resulted in a reduction in breast cancer mortality at ages 50 and over but not at ages 40 to 49 years.

The differential between control and study cases in their fatality rates is almost entirely due to the exceptionally low rate (17%) among the cases detected through screening. Both the clinical examination and mammography contributed to this favourable situation but mammography, with a fatality rate of only 2% among cases it detected in the absence of a positive clinical finding during screening, was especially important. Whether the picture that seems to be emerging about the role of mammography in reducing mortality among women with breast cancer being a short-term phenomenon remains to be determined. A point to be borne in mind is that the gain of 1 year's lead time that enters into the calculation of case fatality rates for breast cancers detected on screening is an average and the possibility that this average is longer for mammography detected cases than for those detected clinically is in fact part of the underlying assumptions in introducing mammography in the screening programme. However, it is of interest that in the age group 40-49, in which the case fatality rate did not change as a result of screening, mammography was relatively ineffective.

Another issue for which longer periods of follow-up are needed concerns the lower case fatality rates observed among the study group of women as compared with the control group's rates regardless of the stage of the disease at time of diagnosis. The differentials are not statistically significant and widely diverse cases are included in each of the two categories, 'no evidence of axillary node involvement' and 'evidence of metastases' used in this study. However, persistence of the differentials over a long period of time would affect the point of view concerning the gain to be made through earlier detection even in cases where metastases have already occurred. In any event, the need for continuing to follow-up the breast cancer cases to determine whether the study group women, as a whole, and the screened group as a component, continue to have a lower case fatality rate than the control group over the long run is clear and plans have been made for this activity. The delegates at the Symposium agreed that there was evidence supporting screening for cancer of the breast but there were serious problems in operation — as yet we just do not know how to do it.

(b) Screening for cancer of the cervix

The project in British Columbia, under the direction of Dr. D. A. Boyes, has reached the point where approximately 80% of the females over the age of 20 have been screened.

The population in question is made up of approximately 690,000 women over the age of 20 and about 550,000 of these have been screened. In the year 1970, 297,000 patients were screened, 27% for the first time and 73% as repeat screenings. The principal means of evaluation of the project have been observations as to the change in mortality and incidence of clinical carcinoma of the cervix in the population.

It should be recalled that in this project there is one central laboratory to which slides are sent from doctor's offices throughout the province so there is uniform reporting of cytology. All of the histology is reviewed at the central laboratory so this reporting is uniform as well. The mortality and incidence data are collated with the help of the Division of Vital Statistics of the Province of British Columbia and a registry for these two rates is maintained in the laboratory.

Mortality data are meticulously scrutinized and a 'refined' rate is obtained by removing all cases known never to have had a carcinoma of the cervix and searching vital statistics' reports of near-by sites of disease to check for cases known to be cancer of the cervix but incorrectly labelled. This 'refined' rate has shown a significant decline through the period 1958-1971.

A steady decline in the incidence of clinical squamous carcinoma of the cervix has been observed, the actual rate per 100,000 women over the age of 20 has dropped from 28.4 to 12.3 in the past 15 years. The experience of the screened and unscreened segments of the population, in terms of the incidence of clinical disease, shows that the screened population (80% of total population) produces one-seventh of the clinical carcinoma of the original unscreened population. While there are certain differences between these two populations it must be remembered that all patients attending family planning clinics, outpatient departments, venereal disease clinics or are being sent to jail, have Papanicolaou smears taken. The data suggest that the maximum possible benefit to a population is a reduction of clinical disease to about one-seventh of its previous rate and that a voluntary programme can probably not exceed this by very much. Of those patients who develop clinical carcinoma in the screened population, the commonest reason was that they entered the population 15 or 20 years ago, had one smear and have never been seen again until they developed their disease. The second most common reason was screener error, thirdly physician error and that the smear appeared to be of poor quality and was not taken from the cervix, fourthly, a small group of rapidly growing tumours that represent the lower end of a spectrum of activity such as one expects in all biological phenomena. Thus, even if one refuses to admit the worth of a screening programme to the whole population, one can certainly say that if the patient wishes to join such a programme she places herself in a group with a rate of disease that is significantly lower than that of the unscreened group. The annual mortality rate in the screened population (approximately 1.5 per 100,000) is extremely low and has been so over the years. The rate in the unscreened population is approximately 22.0 per 100,000.

A second experience presented at the Symposium was that of Dr. W. M. Christopherson who had organized a screening programme in Jefferson County, Kentucky, U.S.A. in 1956. The female population over the age of 20 is approximately 200,000 and over 90% have been screened at least once. During the past 15 years 2,809 cases of cancer of the cervix were diagnosed (97.7% histologically proved) of which 1339 (47.7%) were in situ. Over the years the incidence rates for uterine cancer first increased, attributable to the detection of asymptomatic cases, followed by a decrease. The decrease has been more pronounced in women under 50 years of age and the highest rate occurred in the lowest income group. This socio-economic status is considered to be an important measure of risk of cervix cancer. The lowest income area had a risk 2.5 times the affluent area. The study showed that a major problem was persuading older women to be screened. From age 40 on, they not only have a high incidence rate but the percentage of cases with Stage I disease decreases with each decade, reaching a low of 15% for those 70 and older. It was also found that in addition to a decrease in rates there was a remarkable increase in early diagnosis over the years and it was concluded that, given two facts, death rates from the disease must decrease following an intensive cytologic screening programme.

A third experience which began in 1957 was presented by Dr. Elizabeth MacGregor for the north-east region of Scotland with a population of 125,000 married women of all ages of whom 85% have been screened at least once. Among these women 649 cases of pre-clinical cancer have been detected of which 495 (76.3%) were in situ. The detection rate and the mortality ratio are almost 4 times as high in the lowest social groups as in the highest. In addition the detection rate of pre-clinical cancer corresponds exactly with the incidence of cervical cancer in the city of Aberdeen − population 60,000 with a detection rate of 6.7 per 1,000 or 402 expected cases in 20 years. The actual number of clinical cases diagnosed was 415 between 1946 and 1965. From the beginning of the screening programme in 1957 up to 1963 there was a rise in the number of cases of clinical cancer of the cervix − mostly in the 40-49 year age group. Since 1963, however, there has been a steady fall in the number of cases of clinical cancer of the cervix − mostly in those under 60 years of age. It is considered early to estimate progress in terms of reduction in mortality of cervical cancer but an increase in the 5-year survival rate among cases diagnosed by screening has occurred.

In the discussion of these presentations various factors were considered important, e.g. population, migration, dysplasia, inconsistencies in diagnosis, the time-scale for in situ lesions to progress to invasive, laboratory standards, public education and selection of high risk groups. The delegates were agreed that,

1.   cervical cytology screening is of value;

2.   skilled cytologists are essential for any screening programme;

3.   in situ carcinoma is an important precursor of invasive carcinoma, and does progress to invasive carcinoma in a substantial proportion of patients with the lesion;

4.   further information is required in order to define the particular population groups on which screening should be concentrated; and

5.   given the appropriate data from studies currently in progress, mathematical models are likely to be of considerable assistance in deciding on the appropriate courses of action to ensure the best use of available resources.

(c)   Screening for cancer of the stomach

The only organized mass screening programme for cancer of the stomach is in Japan where, in 1969 and 1970, some 4,000,000 adults (mostly over 40 years of age) were examined by photofluorography. Out of these 0.12% were found to have cancer of the stomach, 0.20% gastric polyps and 1.5% gastric ulcers. In 1966-1967 the crude mortality rates for males and females in Japan were 59.6 and 35.9 compared to Canada 16.9 and 9.0, United States (white) 10.5 and 6.7, England and Wales 31.9 and 22.5, and France 26.9 and 21.2. The screening programme shows that cancer of the stomach can be divided into two histological types − diffuse or undifferentiated stemming from the gastric mucosa and intestinal or differentiated arising from intestinal metaplasia. The undifferentiated type is more predominant in females and in younger age groups.

Although the mortality rate has shown little decrease there have been significant declines of approximately 20% in those Prefectures where extensive mass screening has been carried out. The 5-year survival rate is over 90% in cases of early gastric cancer, both intramucosal and submucosal.

In view of these data, presented by Dr. S. Ishikawa of the National Cancer Centre in Tokyo, there was unanimous agreement that mass screening for cancer of the stomach had a significant effect on the morbidity and mortality attributed to this site of the disease.

(d)   Screening for cancer of the colon

This presentation, by Dr. A. B. Miller of the National Cancer Institute of Canada, described an investigation of the value of the carcinoembryonic antigen test (CEA), originally proposed by Gold and Freedman of Montreal, as a mass screening procedure. In the study patients were admitted from 5 centres in Canada and the United States and the CEA levels were measured both in the local laboratory and in the reference laboratory in

Montreal. Good reproducibility of the results from the reference laboratory was obtained in all but one of the participating laboratories. The correlation coefficients were 0.84, 0.75, 0.73, 0.72 and 0.39.

The study has confirmed the results obtained in other studies from single laboratories concerning the levels of CEA in patients with colo-rectal cancer. In the present investigation, by averaging the results of the local and reference laboratories it was found that 64% of patients with proven colo-rectal cancer had CEA levels of 2.5 ng/ml or more and 75% had levels of 1.0 ng/ml or more.

A significant number of patients with gastrointestinal polyps, ulcerative and granulomatous colitis, diverticulitis, alcoholic cirrhosis and miscellaneous gastrointestinal diseases had elevated levels of CEA. However, since this study was planned, other investigators as well as the Montreal group have also shown that elevated levels of CEA, or of antigens that cross-react with CEA, can occur in the serum of patients with conditions other than digestive system cancer.

A test which is positive in 60-70% of patients with a given disease is likely to become part of the diagnostic work-up of patients with suspicious symptoms. Nevertheless, positivity is lower in patients with less advanced local lesions (Duke's A and B) than in those with spread to regional nodes (Duke's C). The value of the test as a screening procedure for cancer in asymptomatic patients remains to be assessed in large-scale studies. The findings have also pointed an important direction for continuing research in the detection of cancer by immunological methods.

(A full report on this study was published in the *C. M. A. Journal*, July 8th, 1972, *Vol. 107.*)

(e) Screening for primary liver cancer

The use of the alpha-foetoprotein test as a tool for early detection of primary liver cancer was presented by Dr. A. J. Tuyns of the International Agency for Research on Cancer. A population survey was initiated in Dakar covering over 9,000 adult males working in the major factories in that city. Nine cases of primary liver cancer were detected, 6 being found or suspected at clinical examination and 3 being picked up by the AFP test only at the presymptomatic stage. All 9 cases died after a few months survival. The view of the Symposium was that the test is an excellent tool for diagnosing primary liver cancer; it is reproducible, highly specific and fairly sensitive and can be used for screening. However, there is no evidence supporting the usefulness of the test in detection programmes as it does not alter the fatal course of the disease.

Health education in cancer screening

The evaluation of the contribution of Health Education to cancer control was presented by Dr. Leila Watson, Senior Medical Officer, Edinburgh and Dr. J. Wakefield, Department of Social Research, Christie Hospital, Manchester. It was emphasized that to be successful, a programme in health education must recognize the importance of 3 factors — communication, evaluation and participation. Communication via the mass media, the printed word, graphics etc. prepares the way for the implementation of a programme but can never be assumed to have reached everyone in the target group. More experimentation with methods of communication is necessary so that greater success in total communication may be achieved. This was illustrated with 'If I do not hear you, I cannot do what you ask'. Evaluation was considered the most important of the 3 factors and it was recommended that it start 'at home'. It was suggested that, for true evaluation to be possible, every programme must have declared objectives before it begins. Otherwise honest measurement is later impossible. The final factor, participation, measures the success of any health education approach to cancer control and although it is difficult to identify any single reason for near perfect participation there are certain influences to be recognized; e.g. doctors form one of the most effective groups to involve in health education activities and television is the media with greatest impact.

It was recognized that certain defects existed in Health Education, e.g. too little research has been undertaken on which to base a programme, some methods of communication such as pamphlets and posters are of unknown value and studies of attitudes are sorely needed. Nevertheless the Symposium agreed that Health Education played an important role in cancer control and every effort should be made to increase the number of specialists in this field.

Summary

The assessment of a screening procedure falls into two parts. The first is the development of a test and the establishment of criteria of specificity and sensitivity. The second stage is that of the application of the test to the general population, demanding attention to the natural history of the disease and to the usefulness and simplicity of the test itself. The decision to organize a screening programme has usually to be taken on the basis of incomplete information and in the setting of a population subjected to constant change. It is the hope of the Committee on Cancer Prevention and Detection of the UICC that the conclusions from the Symposium will prove helpful to all who face such decisions.

Problems in the detection of early malignant tumors of the locomotor system

M. Campanacci

Clinica Ortopedica Università di Bologna, Istituto Ortopedico Rizzoli, Bologna, Italy

Primary malignant tumors of bone (excluding multiple myeloma) can be classified into 6 principal categories. The experience of the tumor service of the Rizzoli Orthopaedic Institute of Bologna, which is one of the largest in the world, covering over 800 malignant primary bone tumors, indicates that the survival rate varies widely from one category to the other. A malignant tumor of bone cannot be considered to be cured for 10 years at least following the therapeutic procedure.

Any malignant localized bone tumor can be cured. The principal factors enhancing the probability of a cure are early detection and immediate therapy. Early detection is seldom accomplished, not only in this country but in any region of the world. Among the difficulties which cause this dramatic situation and deserve immediate attention, are the following:

1. There is no reliable test applicable to large groups of the population which can detect early asymptomatic bone sarcomas.

2. The initial symptoms and signs are usually mild and frequently misleading. The main symptom is a moderate pain; when a local swelling appears the tumor has already reached a rather advanced stage of development.

As primary bone sarcomas frequently occur in children or young people, in perfectly good general health, these early symptoms are easily related to some sort of trauma, or they are interpreted and treated as 'rheumatic' conditions.

3. It is unusual for an X-ray to be taken at the onset of the symptoms. The X-ray picture is the first and the most important evidence which permits one to diagnose or to suspect the presence of a tumor. An arteriogram is useful for the detection of soft tissue tumors.

4. Tumors of the skeleton are comparatively infrequent; a great majority of practitioners and even specialists are not familiar with them. So not at all infrequently the first X-ray gives rise to doubtful and equivocal opinions. If the possibility of an amputation is mentioned, quite often the patient or the family seeks another opinion. This causes a further waste of time.

5. When finally a biopsy is performed, there are 3 possibilities: (a) wrong histological diagnosis, leading often to inadequate treatment; (b) exact histological diagnosis, but delayed and/or inadequate treatment; (c) exact histological diagnosis and prompt adequate treatment.

We think that generally speaking, the last is not the most frequent case.

6. As a matter of fact, the hospitals and institutions really qualified to make a reliable diagnosis and to provide adequate therapy are still few in number, in Italy and abroad.

7. If pitfalls in diagnosis are to be avoided, the diagnosis should always rely upon an accurate and comprehensive appraisal of the clinical history and signs, the radiographic picture, the gross pathology and histopathology.

A few examples are presented to illustrate some diagnostic errors mainly due to 'blind' evaluation of the histological slide only.

The first case refers to a boy, 11 years old, with a swelling in the left thigh. A biopsy was taken elsewhere and a histological diagnosis of osteosarcoma was made. As a matter of fact there was an actively proliferating tissue producing an osteoid. This histological picture may suggest an osteogenic malignant growth. But if one considers also the X-ray picture, the diagnosis of myositis ossificans becomes quite obvious. The threatened dis-articulation of the hip changed into . . . nothing. No treatment at all was undertaken and the boy healed satisfactorily.

In the second case too, a biopsy led to the diagnosis of osteosarcoma, and the leg was amputated. It was instead a benign osteoblastoma, and inspection of the X-ray would have been of help in making an exact diagnosis, because the cortex was not broken by the tumor, as it would have been if the tumor were an osteosarcoma.

Other diagnostic errors depend on a wrong impression gained from the X-ray picture alone, without a biopsy.

In the first case, a diagnosis of Ewing sarcoma was made based on the X-ray evidence alone, and consequently the femur was heavily irradiated. It was instead an osteomyelitis, and the wrong treatment eventually caused necrosis of the bone, pseudo-arthrosis and a shortening of 23 cm.

In the second case, the radiologist felt quite sure of a diagnosis of osteomyelitis. This girl was treated with antibiotics for a long period of time. When we took a biopsy it was a Ewing sarcoma.

The third case, presenting a large osteolytic defect in the upper tibia, was considered to be a tumor of bone. Without a previous biopsy the upper tibia was resected. Then it was found to be a chronic abcess of bone.

This huge osteolytic lesion of the pelvis was considered to be a malignant tumor from radiographic evidence. The biopsy proved it was a benign lesion, an aneurysmal bone cyst to be precise, which healed following X-ray therapy at moderate doses.

Both, radiographic and histopathologic detection, may be difficult in cases of early osteosarcoma.

Nowadays it is becoming more and more common to observe cases of osteosarcoma in an initial stage of evolution. From the X-ray picture alone, in such cases, it may be difficult to identify an osteosarcoma. In some cases, the tumor is mainly osteolytic. Its malignancy is suggested by an initial disruption of the cortex and by a little bulging of the periosteum. In cases like these, though the X-ray alone is not very characteristic, micro-scopic examination usually allows an easy diagnosis of osteosarcoma.

Sometimes, the X-ray picture is even more equivocal suggesting a benign tumor. In this case, for example, the presence of a small nidus set in an area of bone sclerosis and cortical thickening may even suggest an osteoid osteoma, though there is an osteolytic area which does not fit such a diagnosis. Microscopic examination failed to show the more characteristic features of osteosarcoma. As a matter of fact, in the heavily ossifying area of the osteosarcoma, the cells are sparsely distributed and, imbedded in the abundant osseous matrix, they tend to become smaller, with dark nuclei. In a word, the more evident and typical features of cellular malignancy are lacking. The correct diagnosis is mainly suggested by the histological architectural pattern of the neoplastic tissue and by the fact that this tissue fills the marrow spaces and surrounds the spongy trabeculae of the bone.

In the second case, the first X-ray picture showed a large area of radio-opacity with fuzzy limits, containing a small osteolytic focus. At the biopsy, we found a small, round-ish, rather soft nodule imbedded in a shell of eburnated bone and sharply delimited. The macroscopic appearance is almost typical of the osteoid osteoma. The tissue of this nidus is composed of osteoid and bone, where the signs of malignancy are not striking. The slide was seen by 3 pathologists, and 2 of them said it was an osteoid osteoma or a benign osteoblastoma. Studying the surrounding bone, it is evident that the neoplastic tissue fills the marrow spaces and surrounds the original spongy trabeculae, and therefore it is an osteosarcoma. Three weeks after the biopsy, the X-ray showed the initial erosion of the cortex and the fuzzy periosteal ossification, typical of osteosarcoma.

In the third case in point, the X-rays showed a focus of heavy radio-opacity in the epiphysis. This area is rather well limited; there is no penetration of the cortex. The microscopic pattern, again, fails to show the more striking features of cellular malignancy. However, the original bony trabeculae are surrounded by the neoplastic tissue, and this makes the diagnosis of osteosarcoma quite sure. One month later, the epiphyseal eburnated mass appeared enlarged, with erosion of the intercondylar cortex. The gross pathology is characteristic of the osteosarcoma, though the neoplastic focus has relatively well defined limits.

What can be done to improve early detection of malignant bone tumors?

1. Institute and develop specialized centres where correct diagnosis and appropriate treatment can be obtained.

2. Make medical practitioners and the population aware of the fact that bone tumors occur frequently in young people, and that any persistent osteo-articular complaint not due to any obvious cause makes X-ray examination mandatory.

3. Multiple exostoses, chondromatosis, osseous Paget's disease, giant cell tumor, and previously irradiated bone are known to be possible presarcomatous conditions.

In these cases patients should be taught to seek medical advice at the first appearance of pain or swelling.

4. Patients with a suspected or proved bone tumor should be referred for ultimate diagnosis and appropriate therapy only to the specialized centres.

Panels

Contents

1. Gastric cancer

Introduction to the panel on gastric cancer

Norman Zamcheck

*Department of Medicine, Harvard Medical School; Mallory GI Research
Laboratory, Boston City Hospital; Department of Pathology, Boston University
School of Medicine, Boston, Mass., U.S.A.*

It is a great pleasure and privilege for me to Chair the Panel on Gastric Cancer. Dr. Hammond will introduce us to the key geographical and epidemiological facts known about gastric cancer. Rates are highest in the poorer classes suggesting that dietary deficiencies, food contamination, or carcinogens may play important roles. Despite the declining rates in some developed countries, the rates in Japan continue to be high. That environmental factors are important appears certain. Genetic influence is suggested by the more frequent occurrence of stomach cancer in patients with blood group A and in patients with pernicious anemia.

Most workers agree that the most effective way to improve our present unsatisfactory results in this disease is by earlier detection. Dr. Crespi will present a summary of his approach to detection based on endoscopy, cytology, and biopsy, and will discuss the possible application of his findings to screening, suggesting that screening be directed toward identifying those patients with gastric atrophy, intestinal metaplasia, gastric ulcer, polyps and long-term resected cases, conditions in which a high incidence of cancer occurs. The importance of histologic and cytologic alterations of the gastric mucosa for understanding the pathogenesis of malignancy and for making early diagnosis will be reviewed by Dr. Nieburgs.

Early detection is presently heavily dependent upon roentgen and endoscopic diagnosis. Japanese workers have the largest experience in the use of roentgen diagnosis. Dr. Yamada will summarize experiences using combined double-contrast radiography and endoscopy, including the extraordinary 5-year survival rates of cases diagnosed early. The fiber-gastroscope has greatly improved the early diagnosis of gastric cancer and we will hear examples of its possible application for mass survey.

Three leading investigators will summarize for us the present status of newer techniques for immunologic detection of gastric cancer. Dr. Hakkinen will review his studies of the use and limitations of fetal sulphoglycoprotein antigen in the detection and diagnosis of gastric cancer. Dr. Hollinshead has reported previously delayed hypersensitivity reactions to intradermal skin tests of specific soluble antigens from human colon cancer and will report her findings using soluble membrane antigens obtained from fetal stomach cells and from normal and malignant gastric cells. Dr. Tee will summarize his experiences with another test based upon the measurement of transient erythema resulting from intradermal injections of antigens extracted from human tumor. Whereas these basic studies may have only limited immediate clinical application, the promise they hold for the future warrants our continued interest.

We are indebted to our hosts for the opportunity to hear these distinguished speakers.

Epidemiology of gastric cancer

E.C. Hammond and H. Seidman

Department of Epidemiology and Statistical Research, American Cancer Society, Inc., New York, N.Y., U.S.A.

Whatever may be the cause of gastric cancer, it is certainly not place of residence per se, or place of birth or date of birth or socio-economic status per se or anything of the sort. Yet the majority of epidemiological studies of the disease have been concerned with just such factors. The justification is that if gastric cancer death rates or incidence rates vary greatly in respect to such a factor, then that factor must in turn be associated with some other factor or set of factors of importance in the etiology of the disease. Thus, in theory,

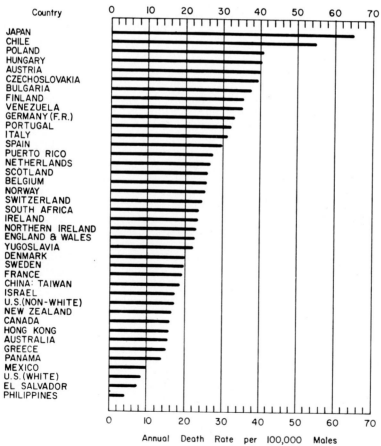

FIG. 1   *Age standardized male stomach cancer death rates for various countries, 1966–1967. (Source: Segi and Kurihara, 1972; WHO Statistics Annual, 1968, 1970).*

such studies might perhaps give a hint which could lead to the discovery of some causative factor. So far, they have been disappointing in this respect; but not wholly so.

Figure 1 shows age-standardized gastric cancer death rates for *males* as reported from various countries in the period 1966-1967 (Segi and Kurihara, 1972; WHO Statistics Annual, 1968, 1970) Japan heads the list followed by Chile, Poland, Czechoslovakia and Hungary. At the bottom of the list we find the Philippines, the United States (white population), Mexico, El Salvador, Panama, Australia, Greece and New Zealand.

In almost all countries, the rates for females are considerably lower than the rates for males (Fig. 2). However, the rank order of countries in relation to the rates is similar for the two sexes. What factors of possible importance in the etiology of gastric cancer do the high risk countries, such as Japan, Chile and Poland, have in common? How do they differ from low risk countries such as the Philippines, the United States, Mexico, Greece and New Zealand? And what do the low risk countries have in common?

These questions are more easily asked than answered. Probably the variation in reported gastric cancer death rates between countries is due at least in part to differences in accuracy and completeness of diagnosis and reporting. However, it is extremely unlikely that gastric cancer rates are grossly over-reported in *all* of the high rate countries and grossly under-reported in *all* of the low rate countries. Nor can such great differences in

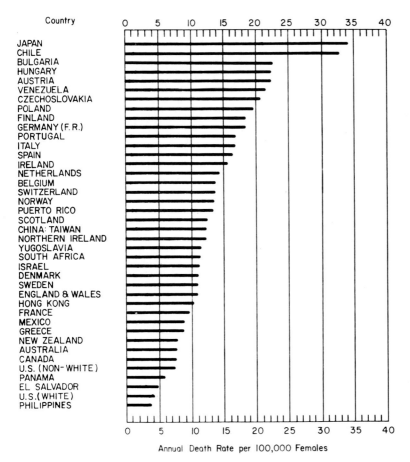

FIG. 2 *Age standardized female stomach cancer death rates, various countries, 1966-1967. (Source: same as Fig. 1).*

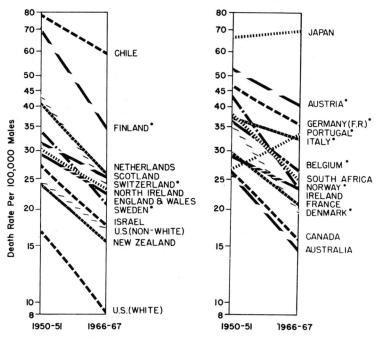

FIG. 3   *Trend lines in age-standardized male stomach cancer death rates, various countries, 1950-51 to 1966-67. (* Data not available for 1950, 1951. Trend line computed from data that are available).*

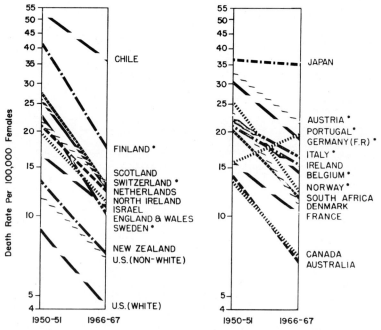

FIG. 4   *Trend line in age-standardized female stomach cancer death rates, various countries, 1950-51 to 1966-67. (* Data not available for 1950, 1951. Trend line computed from data that are available).*

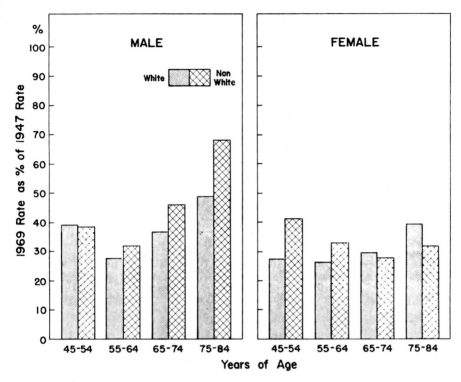

FIG. 5   *Change in incidence rates of stomach cancer by sex, age and race. U.S. Cancer morbidity surveys, 1947-1969. (Source: Dorn and Cutler, 1959; Biometry Branch, National Cancer Institute, 1971).*

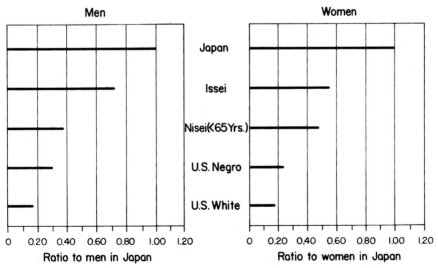

FIG. 6   *Stomach cancer mortality ratios by sex – Japan (1960, 1961), Issei and Nisei (1952-1962) and U.S. Whites and Negroes (1956-1961). Note: Rates are age-adjusted by indirect method as ratio of rates for Japan. Issei are migrants from Japan to Continental U.S. and Hawaii. Nisei are U.S. born children of Issei. (Source: Segi and Kurihara, 1972; Haenszel and Kurihara, 1968).*

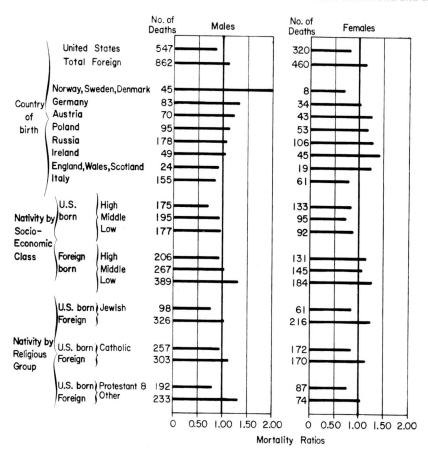

FIG. 7   *Stomach cancer mortality ratios among various subgroups of the 25-64 year old white population of New York City, 1949-1951. Note: Rates age-adjusted by indirect method as ratio of annual rates per 100,000 citywide 25-64 year old white males of 23.4 and females of 12.9. (Source: Seidman, 1971.)*

death rates be attributed to differences in cure rates since gastric cancer cure rates are very low in all countries.

Now let us turn to time trends in reported male gastric cancer death rates. Figure 3 shows trend lines age standardized death rates between 1950-51 and 1966-67 (Segi and Kurihara, 1972). In most countries from which figures are available, gastric cancer death rates appear to have declined dramatically. This applies to high rate countries such as Chile, Finland and Austria as well as low rate countries such as the United States, New Zealand, Canada and Australia. Exceptions are Portugal (where the rates rose considerably) and Japan where male rates rose slightly.

The picture for females is similar except for Japan (Fig. 4). In Japan, the rates reportedly increased somewhat for males but declined slightly for females.

As Clemmesen (1965) and others have pointed out, the validity of diagnosis of gastric cancer is often dubious; and, conversely, many cases may escape diagnosis. In Denmark, he found many deaths attributed to gastric cancer which were actually due to other causes as well as the reverse. In a study made in the United States in the 1950's we found that in a large proportion of deaths reported as due to gastric cancer the diagnosis was made on the basis of inadequate evidence (Hammond and Horn, 1958). Accuracy of

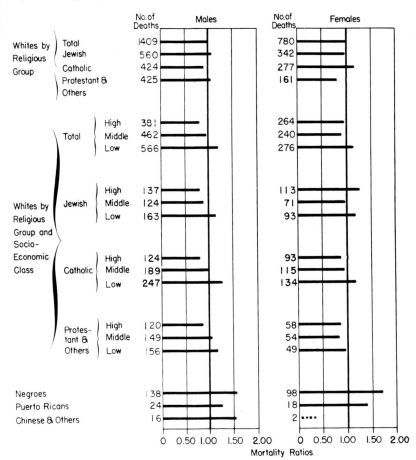

FIG. 8   *Stomach cancer mortality ratios among various subgroups of the 25-64 year old population of New York City, 1949-1951. Note: Rates age-adjusted by indirect method as ratio of annual rates per 100,000 citywide 25-64 year old white males of 23.4 and females of 12.9.*

diagnosis of cancer has improved since that time. Some of the apparent decline in gastric cancer death rates is almost certainly an artifact resulting from improvement in diagnosis.

Evidence on trends in gastric cancer are not entirely limited to mortality statistics. For example; surveys were made of the incidence of gastric cancer in the United States in 1947 (Dorn and Cutler, 1959) and in 1969 (Biometry Branch, National Cancer Institute Report, 1971), (Fig. 5). In both sexes and in each of various age groups for both whites and Negroes, the incidence of diagnosed gastric cancer was far lower in 1969 than in 1947. The percent decline was greater for females than for males and greater for whites than for Negroes. Figures from the Connecticut and New York State cancer registries also show great declines in incidence rates.

Almost everyone who has examined the data closely is now convinced that there has been a real and considerable decline in gastric cancer in the United States — although improvement in diagnosis probably accounts for a part of the apparent decline.

What caused the decline?

This is one of the greatest puzzles in the whole field of cancer research.

One of the most interesting set of studies on the epidemiology of gastric cancer has been carried out by Smith (1956) and by Haenszel, Kurihara (1968) and their associates.

TABLE 1   *Factors reported to be associated with high stomach cancer incidence*

Soil	*Climate*
acidic soil	northern countries
meadow soil	heavy rainfall
peat soil	low temperature
low-lying clay areas	
igneous rocks near the surface	*Environment*
deep ground water	rural areas
mineral balance high zinc/copper ratio	grain dust
inorganic dust with free silica	iron dust
Occupation	*Dietary factors*
farmers	irregular meal times
workers in quarries	excess zinc, copper
low social class	deficiency in iron,
	molybdenum
Diseases	deficiency in vitamins A, B_1,
stomach ulcer	B_{12}, C.
chronic gastritis	tobacco
adenomatoid polyps	alcohol
intestinal metaplasia	liquid paraffin (purgative)
hyposecretion	
pernicious anemia	*Diet*
Plummer Vinson	high intake of starchy foods rice,
dental caries	cereals, potatoes
	highly brined food, homecured bacon,
Heredity	salami sausage
blood group A	smoked food, salted food, fried food
race (Mongolian, Japanese, Finnish	hot food
etc.)	low protein diet
	low consumption of fruit and fresh
	vegetables

(*Source*: Saxen and Hakama, 1967)

They ascertained gastric cancer deaths of Japanese living in Japan; Japanese who migrated to the Continental United States and Hawaii (Issei) and the first generation of Japanese born in the United States (Nisei). As shown in Figure 6, death rates were highest among Japanese living in Japan and lowest in non-Japanese Americans. The rates for Issei were lower than the rates for Japanese in Japan; and the rates for Nisei were still lower — but not quite as low as the rates for non-Japanese Americans.

More recent data collected and published by Haenzel, Kurihara and their associates confirm these relative figures and provide additional information (Haenzel et al., 1972). The findings are widely interpreted as conclusive evidence that the occurence of gastric cancer is dependent primarily upon environmental factors than genetic factor. How else is one to explain the fact that the rates for migrants changed in the direction of the rates for the population in their new country? Differences in accuracy of diagnosis? Perhaps, but then why would not this apply equally to Issei and Nisei?

Case control studies by these same authors suggested the possibility that certain changes in diet might be responsible; but the picture is neither clear nor consistent and would in any event have to be substantiated by findings in other population groups.

Seidman has reported on relative gastric cancer death rates of various different migrant groups living in New York City in 1949 to 1951 (Fig. 7). This period was selected for study because up to that time people of the same ethnic background and socio-economic levels tended to live in well demarked neighborhoods and were thus easily identified (Seidman, 1970).

Gastric cancer death rates were roughly 30% or 40% higher in foreign born whites than in native born whites living in New York. This was found for both males and females.

TABLE 2 Expected* and observed number of deaths among 625 New York-New Jersey asbestos insulation workers, Jan. 1, 1943-Dec. 31, 1971, twenty or more years after onset of first exposure to asbestos

	1943–1947		1948–1952		1953–1957		1958–1962		1963–1971		Total	
	Expected	Observed	Expected	Observed	Expected	Observed	Expected	Observed	Expected	Observed	Expected	Observed
Total cancer: all sites	5.7	13	8.1	17	13.0	26	9.7	39	15.7	94	52.2	189
Lung cancer	0.8	5	1.4	8	2.0	12	2.4	17	4.8	42	11.4	84
Pleural mesothelioma	**	1	**	0	**	1	**	1	**	5	**	8
Peritoneal mesothelioma	**	0	**	1	**	2	**	1	**	20	**	24
Cancer of stomach, colon, rectum	2.0	4	2.5	4	2.6	7	2.3	14	3.1	12	12.5	41
Cancer all other sites	2.9	3	4.2	4	8.4	4	5.0	6	7.8	15	28.3	32
Asbestosis	**	0	**	1	**	4	**	7	**	21	**	33
All other causes	34.0	15	42.7	36	43.6	55	44.8	42	69.5	53	236.3	201
Total all causes	39.7	28	50.8	54	56.6	85	54.4	88	85.0	168	288.5	423
Person years of observation:	1,912.0		2,478.0		2,336.5		2,011.0		2,520.0		11,257.5	

632 members were on the Union's rolls on Jan. 1, 1943. Seven died before reaching 20 years from first employment. All others entered these calculations after reaching the 20-year-from-first-exposure point

* Expected deaths are based upon death rate data reported annually by the U.S. National Office of Vital Statistics. Rates for 1968–1971 were extrapolated from age-specific rates for 1961–1967

** U.S. death rates not available, but these are rare causes of death in the general population

(*Source*: Selikoff et al., 1972)

TABLE 3   *Expected* and observed deaths among 17,800 asbestos insulation workers in the United States, Jan. 1, 1967–Dec. 31, 1971*

| | Total | | Distribution by duration from onset of exposure | | | |
| | | | Less than 20 years | | 20 years and more | |
	Expected	Observed	Expected	Observed	Expected	Observed
Total deaths	805.63	1,092	178.94	211	626.69	881
Cancer: all sites	144.09	459	26.31	51	117.78	408
Lung cancer	44.42	213	7.03	22	37.39	191
Pleural mesothelioma	**	26	**	2	**	24
Peritoneal mesothelioma	**	51	**		**	48
Cancer of stomach	6.62	16	0.97	1	5.65	15
Cancer of colon, rectum	17.51	26	2.51	3	15.00	23
Cancer of esophagus	3.21	13	0.44	1	2.77	12
All other cancers	72.33	114	15.36	19	56.97	95
Asbestosis	**	78	**	5	**	73
All other causes	661.54	555	152.63	155	508.91	400
Number of men	17,800		12,681		5,119	
Person-years of observation	86,300		62,673		23,627	

  * Expected deaths are based upon age specific death rate data of the U.S. National Office of Vital Statistics. Rates for 1968–1971 were extrapolated from rates for 1961–1967

** U.S. death rates not available, but these are rare causes of death in the general population

(*Source*: Selikoff et al., 1972)

Interestingly, the highest rates for males occurred in migrants from Norway, Sweden and Denmark which are not high risk countries. Male migrants from the same countries had the lowest relative death rates from cancer of the colon. The gastric cancer death rates of females from the 3 Scandinavian countries were, if anything, lower than the rates for native born white females.

Seidman also reported on gastric cancer death rates in relation to socio-economic class and religion (Seidman, 1970, 1971). In white males, the rates were about 40% higher in the lowest socio-economic group than in the highest socio-economic group. The rates were especially low for Jewish and Catholic males in the highest socio-economic group (Fig. 8).

The picture was different for females. The highest rates were for upper economic class Jewish females and the lowest rates were for middle class white Protestant females.

Why these differences in gastric cancer death rates among various segments of the population of the same city? No one yet knows the answer.

Table 1, taken from a paper by Saxen and Hakama (1967), based on Clemmesen's compilations (Clemmensen, 1965), lists various specific factors which have been suggested as possibly related to the etiology of gastric cancer. Many studies have shown a somewhat elevated rate of the disease among persons with blood group A (Aird et al., 1953); and this suggests that heredity plays a role in susceptibility. Various environmental factors are shown; but proof of their significance in relation to gastric cancer is not strong. The causes of the disease remain obscure.

Epidemiological studies of workers with occupational exposure to various substances may provide some clues.

TABLE 4   Expected* and observed deaths among 933** amosite asbestos factory workers first employed 1941–1945, and observed to Dec. 31, 1971

	Before 1952		1952–1961		1962–1971		Total, 1941–1971	
	Expected	Observed	Expected	Observed	Expected	Observed	Expected	Observed
Total deaths	69.98	88	108.27	146	121.24	250	299.49	484
Total cancer: all sites	9.81	15	18.72	44	21.63	84	50.16	143
Lung cancer	1.49	3	3.71	23	6.21	47	11.41	73
Pleural mesothelioma	***	1	***	0	***	2	***	3
Peritoneal mesothelioma	***	0	***	0	***	4	***	4
Cancer of stomach	1.45	3	1.84	4	1.29	4	4.58	11
Cancer of colon, rectum	1.56	2	2.61	5	2.88	8	7.05	15
Cancer of esophagus	0.27	0	0.45	0	0.51	0	1.23	0
All other cancers	5.04	6	10.11	12	10.74	19	25.89	37
Asbestosis	***	3	***	7	***	17	***	27
All other causes	60.17	70	89.55	95	99.61	149	249.33	314

* Expected rates are based upon age-specific death rate data of U.S. National Office of Vital Statistics from 1949–1967. Rates were extrapolated 1941–1948 from rates for 1949–1955 and for 1968–1971 from rates for 1961–1967

** 933 men were employed. In 5 cases, ages were not known and these men have been excluded from these calculations. 877 men were traced to death or to Dec. 31, 1971. 51 men were partially traced and remain in the calculations until being lost to observation

*** U.S. death rates are not available, but these are rare causes of death in the general population

(*Source*: Selikoff et al., 1972)

Table 2 shows the mortality experience among a relatively small number of N.Y. and N.J. asbestos insulation workers from 1943 through 1971. For stomach and colon-rectum cancer combined the ratio to 'expected' deaths was about 2.5 to 1.

For the period 1967-1971 data are available requested on all U.S. and Canadian members of asbestos workers union, a much larger group. Stomach cancer is shown separately. The ratio to 'expected' deaths was about 2.5 to 1 (Table 3).

Some findings in asbestos insulation factory workers are shown in Table 4. The stomach cancer mortality ratio to expected was about 2.5 to 1.

In summary: There is relatively little definitive information on the causes of gastric cancer. Indeed it is a difficult problem. We hope it will be resolved in the not too distant future.

References

Aird, Il., Bentall, H. H. and Roberts, J. A. F. (1953): Brit. med. J., 1, 799.
Biometry Branch, National Cancer Institute (1971): Preliminary Report, Third National Cancer Survey. 1969 Incidence, DHEW Publication No. (NIH) 72-128. U.S. Government Printing Office, Washington, 1971.
Clemmesen, J. (1965): Statistical Studies in Neoplasms. Review and Results, pp. 343-407. Munksgaard, Copenhagen, 1965.
Dorn, H. F. and Cutler, S. J. (1959): Morbidity from Cancer in the United States. Public Health Service Monograph No. 56. U.S. Government Printing Office, Washington, 1959.
Haenszel, W. and Kurihara, M. (1968): J. nat. Cancer Inst., 40, 43.
Haenszel, W., Kurihara, M., Segi, M. and Lee, R. K. C. (1972): J. nat. Cancer Inst., 49, 969.
Hammond, E. C. and Horn, D. (1968): J. Amer. med. Ass., 166, 1159 and 1294.
Saxen, E. A. and Hakama, M. (1967): In: Proceedings, Ninth International Cancer Congress, 1966, UICC Monogr. Ser., vol. 10, pp. 49-55. Editor: R. J. C. Harris. Springer Verlag, New York, N.Y.
Segi, M. and Kurihara, M. (1972): Cancer Mortality for Selected Sites in 24 Countries, No. 6 (1966-1967). Japan Cancer Society, Nagoya, Japan, 1972.
Selikoff, I. J., Hammond, E. C. and Seidman, H. (1972): Cancer Risk of Insulation Workers in the United States. A paper presented at the meeting of the Working Group to Assess Biological Effects of Asbestos, Conference of the International Agency for Research on Cancer. Lyons, France, October 4, 1972.
Seidman, H. (1970): Environ. Res., 3, 234.
Seidman H. (1971): Environ. Res., 4, 390.
Smith, R. L. (1956): J. nat. Cancer Inst., 17, 459.
World Health Organisation (1968, 1970): World Health Statistics Annual, 1966 and 1967. Geneva, 1968 and 1970.

Prevention and detection of gastric cancer

M. Crespi

Cancer Detection Center, Regina Elena Institute for Cancer Research, Rome, Italy

Gastric cancer represents one of the best examples, a model, of how unrewarding can research on the etiology and pathogenesis of tumors be.

As Dr. Hammond has already pointed out, up to 10 years ago extensive research had been devoted to the primary factors that might be involved in gastric carcinogenesis. Nevertheless, nothing more than sparse and even inconclusive correlations, such as 'potato consumption' or 'smoked-food intake' can be drawn from years and years of this kind of effort. Moreover, the incidence and mortality-rates of stomach cancer showed during the last 20 years a marked decrease in one of the countries, the United States, which mainly contributed and could further contribute to this kind of etiological-pathogenic study. This trend allowed epdemiologists and public health services to foresee an autonomous solution of this problem as a consequence of the continuously improving socio-economic conditions. Unfortunately, the trend has not proved so favourable in other countries with a high incidence of gastric neoplasms, such as Japan and European countries, including Italy.

As demonstrated by a thorough study some years ago (Sotgiu, 1967), stomach cancer is the major killer in our country, representing 22% of all cancer deaths. What is even more interesting is the regional distribution which ranges from 70 per 100,000 deaths in regions with the highest socio-economic level, versus 12 per 100,000 deaths in the poorest rural areas. The trend in Italy thus seems to be opposite to the one observed in the United States and other countries. Because of these facts, it seems clear that the problem of the etiology and pathogenesis of gastric cancer, far from being obsolete, requires instead a multidisciplinary approach and further attention. I will now try to rationalize what alternative guidelines may be exploited with the aim of stomach cancer control.

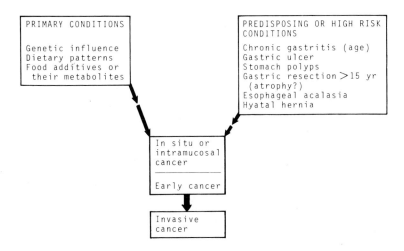

FIG. 1   *Factors in gastric carcinogenesis.*

Figure 1 shows the already known, or suspected, factors involved in gastric carcinogenesis and the different steps in the natural history of gastric malignancies.

It is highly probable, and clearly established in some instances by epidemiological data, that some unknown environmental or genetic factors play an important role in the incidence of stomach cancer (Gregor et al., 1969; Haentszel et al., 1972). This may be due to a direct action of environmental or dietary carcinogens, but the results of some scanty clinical investigations point more and more to the possible role of some predisposing conditions, such as chronic gastritis, in which the physiology of gastric mucosa is completely upset. In fact, chronic gastritis is found as the basic illness in most of the high risk or predisposing conditions (see Fig. 1) and is present in 85 to 90% of cases of stomach cancer, its incidence increasing with age, with patterns similar to those of gastric cancer. Moreover, some relationship exists between the incidence of chronic gastritis and that of gastric cancer in different countries (Imai et al., 1971). A very high incidence of stomach neoplasms (around 10%) was found in the long-term follow-up of individuals with histologically-confirmed chronic gastritis (Siurala et al., 1966; Hanik and Gregor, 1970; Walker et al., 1971).

All these possible correlations are very well known by research workers in the field and we may say that it is hard to find a cancer localization in which there exists a more clearly-established 'predisposing condition' than for gastric cancer. It is nevertheless surprising, if one considers the social impact of the high mortality-rates of stomach cancer in different countries, how few and unco-ordinated up to now, have been the studies devoted to elucidating the mechanisms by which chronic gastritis facilitates the onset of malignant tumors.

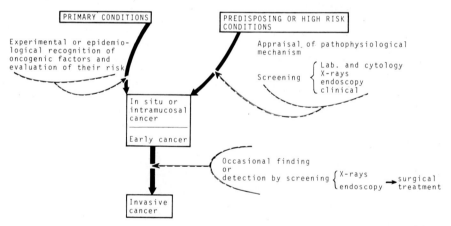

FIG. 2   *Possibilities in achieving gastric cancer control by interference in its pathways at different levels.*

However, with what we know today we can try to plot the different theoretical and practical possibilities in achieving gastric cancer control by interfering with its pathways (Fig. 2). The kind of approach devised by Japanese researchers, i.e. the detection of cancer in its earliest phases by mass X-rays and endoscopy (see bottom of Fig. 2), was very fruitful in developing the modern endoscopic techniques and in giving us a better understanding of the pathology and gross appearance of stomach tumors in the earliest phases of their development. The survival figures published up to now as a result of such a large screening campaign are astonishingly high and not at all comparable with the figures obtained in the Western world (Kennedy, 1970) using the same strict criteria. Basic differences in the minimal requirements to send a suspected case to the surgeon may be responsible for these divergent patterns.

The highly expensive 'Japanese Approach' lacks, in our opinion, more than one of the basic requirements for a mass screening:

it is not simple: the procedures employed are highly specialized and sophisticated;

it does not have a pyramidal structure, because specialized procedures have to be employed from the beginning, without selection, resulting in an unacceptable budget in terms of money, time and skills;

the procedures employed are not easily accepted by an unselected population of 'healthy' individuals, especially in a different social and cultural background, as in Western countries.

Even in Japan, no published data show whether a significant proportion of the pre-selected population groups was reached and if a reduction of the mortality figures in these groups was achieved.

Because of these considerations it is mandatory to search for an approach which could better answer the general requirements for a screening campaign. It is our conviction that this kind of approach must be based on the screening and strict follow-up of cancer precursors (see top right of Fig. 2), because up to now we lack tests to detect, by simple, cheap and acceptable procedures, gastric cancer in its earliest phases of development.

For these reasons, a pilot study was begun 4 years ago, and gradually implemented, with the following aims:

1. To determine the importance of chronic gastritis as a possible precursor to gastric carcinoma.

2. To assess the prevalence and incidence-rate of chronic gastritis in various age-groups.

3. To establish the relationship between incipient gastric carcinoma and the duration of chronic gastritis.

4. To evaluate the technical feasibility, the reliability and the cost figures of the screening procedures adopted.

5. To maintain under strict control all pathological conditions of the stomach found during screening, in order to assess their possible role as precursors of gastric cancer.

The general outline of the diagnostic steps employed by us is summarized in Fig. 3. All the individuals mentioned are participating in a multi-phasic cancer screening on a self-selected population of 'healthy' people. As one may see from the Figure, two inputs were assessed for the gastro-intestinal consultation: a clinical one, being a general physical

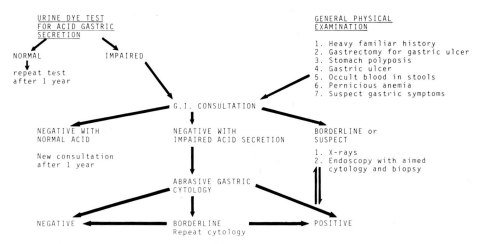

FIG. 3   *Gastric cancer screening: Diagnostic steps.*

examination and an epidemiological inquiry as part of our screening, and a second one based on laboratory techniques. The procedures employed are of increasing complexity, depending on the degrees of risk, and this in line with the generally-accepted prerequisites for screening.

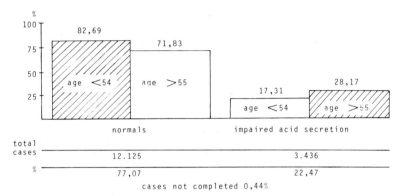

FIG. 4   *Results of the dye urinary test for acid gastric secretion.*

TABLE 1   *Results of the dye urinary test for acid gastric secretion*

	Age 45	46–49	50–54	55–59	60–64	over 64	Total
Normals	330	2,458	3,362	2,810	1,759	1,406	12,125
	83.75%	84.75%	81.62%	78.29%	70.61%	62.82%	77.07%
Borderline results suggesting impaired acid secretion	28	148	285	263	217	221	1,162
	7.10%	5.10%	6.91%	7.32%	8.71%	9.87%	7.38%
Impaired acid secretion	35	286	466	501	496	590	2,374
	8.88%	9.86%	11.31%	13.95%	19.91%	26.36%	15.09%
Not completed	1	8	6	16	19	21	70
	0.25%	0.27%	0.14%	0.41%	0.76%	0.93%	0.44%
Total	394	2,900	4,119	3,589	2,491	2,238	15,731

Up to now, 15,731 individuals have been examined. Figure 4 shows the results of the dye resin test for the assessment of gastric acidity (Segal et al., 1955), which is part of our procedure. A more detailed display of the results, arranged by age-group, is given in Table 1. Previous research was done by pH radiotelemetry in order to assess the reliability of the method (Crespi et al., 1969). In fact, it turned out to be consistent in screening normo-secreting individuals from those with impaired secretion, but unreliable in telling us the degree of impairment. This is, in our opinion, fully acceptable for screening purposes, because it ensures the broadest possible basis for further, more complex examinations. In our group 3,536 individuals showed an impaired acid secretion, presumptive of some degree of chronic gastritis.

The subsequent step was abrasive gastric cytology, performed with a special brush, in order to achieve a morphological documentation of the degree of gastritis and the alloca-

TABLE 2   *Progressive cellular alterations in chronic gastritis*

─ Increase in the average nuclear diameter and in N/C ratio
─ Anisonucleosis
─ Chromatin content progressively decreased
─ Chromatin irregularly disposed, with numerous small chromocenters
   connected by chromatin bands outlining achromatic areas
─ Multiple and prominent nucleoli
─ Nuclear membrane sometimes broken.

tion of each person to different risk categories. This has been done, up to now, in 2,784 cases. The interpretation of smears followed special criteria (Table 2) of progressive cellular alteration (Nieburgs et al., 1965; Crespi et al., 1970), which were previously checked by double-blind cross-filing with multiple gastric suction biopsies (Crespi and Bigotti, 1971). The smears were classified in 4 grades (Fig. 5).

At the beginning of 1973 a follow-up schedule was established in order to recall gradually all individuals in the high risk group, i.e. those showing a certain degree of cytological alteration in the smears performed at the periodic examination by blind abrasive gastric cytology.

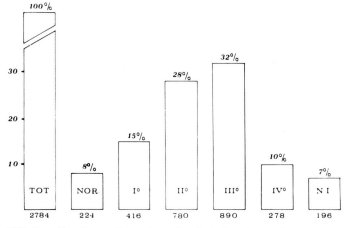

FIG. 5   *Abrasive gastric cytology: Cytological grading at the first examination.*

All these patients were subjected to gastroscopic control and it is of interest to consider the surprisingly high stomach pathology found in the 60 subjects checked so far (Table 3).

In order to make a comprehensive judgement on the value of our program, one must take into consideration that a similar protocol is running in parallel for early detection of large bowel cancer and that a major input of cases in our Unit consists of suspected individuals referred by our Out-Patients Department. Table 4 summarizes all the cases of oncological interest found in 4 years of activity.

We cannot end this short report on our activities without giving some cost figures on

TABLE 3   *Screening of high risk cases for gastric cancer, on the basis of impaired acid secretion*

No. of cases with impaired secretion	3536
No. of cytological examinations on this group	2784
No. of cases with cytological alterations	629

Preliminary results of 60 gastroscopic controls on this group

1 ca in situ
1 polyp with morphological atypia
2 gastric ulcers
24 severe atrophic gastritis
3 early cancer

TABLE 4   *Gastrointestinal tract pathology of oncological interest (From 1969 to 1973)*

— Resected stomachs for gastric ulcer	10	— Gallbladder, benign tumors	9
— Gastric ulcer	14	— Large bowel polyps	175
— Gastric cancer	67	— Large bowel cancer	64
— Gastric cases under follow-up (erosions, Menetrière, polyps)	20	— Ulcerative colitis	5
— Esophageal cancer	36	— Large bowel cases under follow-up	13
— Esophageal cases under follow-up (diverticula, mega-esophagus, esophagitis, acalasia, hernia)	12	— Large bowel diverticula	15

our first level screening. The expenses for material and personnel, plotted against the maximal theoretical capacity of patient-input of 12,500/year, gives us a cost per case screened of two U.S. Dollars and a theoretical cost per case of gastric cancer of U.S. Dollars 10,000. Both figures may be considered acceptable.

Conclusions

What conclusions can be drawn from all the reported or discussed evidence?

First, that much epidemiological and experimental research is needed to make a breakthrough in gastric carcinogenesis. We may say that even the first step has yet to be taken.

Despite its complexity, the interesting approach under trial in Japan has not shown, so far, a real reduction of mortality from gastric cancer. Moreover, the approach is not feasible in Western countries.

Our approach, which can be better defined as a 'pilot study', is of some interest, however frustrating it may appear at present. But this is a common experience in all prospective studies. Anyway, it is very inexpensive and is based on acceptable procedures, especially in the population group under examination. But what can be said beyond doubt is that more comprehensive multidisciplinary studies, beyond the reach of single laboratories, are urgently needed for gastric cancer, which in many countries is still a top priority.

It is our firm conviction that the time has come for international agencies to devote more effort and to aim it at this and other fields of cancer research that are closely related to the curbing of morbidity and mortality in human beings. And, of course, a special effort should be made giving priority to cancer localizations showing, by their incidence, a consistent social impact on the population in different countries.

References

Crespi, M., Bani, U., De Meo, S. and Carnevali, C. (1969): In: Proceedings, 8th International Congress of Gastroenterology, p. 170. Editors: G. Marcozzi and M. Crespi. Schattauer Verlag, Stuttgart.

Crespi, M., Bigotti, A. and Di Matteo, S. (1970): In: Proceedings, 2nd World Congress of Gastro-intestinal endoscopy, p. 227. Editors: G. Marcozzi and M. Crespi. Piccin, Padova.

Crespi, M., and Bigotti, A (1971): Gazz. Sanitaria (English Issue) 20, 77.

Gregor, O., Toman, R. and Prusova, F. (1969): Rev. Med., 13, 741.

Haentszel, W., Kurihara, M., Segi, M. and Lee, R. K. C. (1972); J. nat. Cancer Inst., 49, 969.

Hanik, L. and Gregor, O. (1970): Abstracts, 4th World Congress of Gastroenterology, p. 262, Copen-hagen. Editors: P. Riis, P. Anthonisen and H. Baden. Danish Gastroenterological Association.

Kennedy, B. J. (1970): Cancer (Philad.), 26, 971.

Imai, T., Kubo, T. and Watanabe, H. (1971): J. nat. Cancer Inst., 47, 179.

Nieburgs, H. E., Rubio, C. and Oppenheim, A. (1965): Amer. J. dig. Dis., 10, 485.

Segal, H. L., Miller, L. L. and Plumb, E. J. (1955): Gastroenterology, 28, 402.

Siurala, M., Varis, K. and Wiljasalo, M. (1966): Scand. J. Gastroent., 1, 40.

Sotgiu, G. (1967): In: Proceedings, 3rd World Congress of Gastroenterology Vol. 1, p. 20, Tokyo.

Walker, I. R., Strickland, R. G., Ungar, B. and Mackay, I. R. (1971): Gut, 12, 906.

Roentgen diagnosis of gastric cancer

Tatsuya Yamada, Heizaburo Ichikawa and Hidetaki Doi

National Cancer Center, Tokyo, Japan

Introduction

In order to improve the 5 year survival rate of gastric cancer, it is important to employ methods for early detection. Today, X-ray and endoscopic examination are playing a great role in the early detection of gastric cancer. In the National Cancer Center Hospital, Tokyo, more than 500 cases of early gastric cancer have been successively detected, mainly by X-ray examination and endoscopy, during the last 10 years since the opening of the hospital. The definition in Japan of early gastric cancer is carcinoma where infiltration is limited to the mucosa or the mucosa and the submucosa. The early gastric cancer cases operated on in the hospital have shown extremely good results, as the 5 year survival rate is as high as 90%.

The purpose of this paper is to explain the X-ray diagnostic method in detecting early gastric cancer, especially the double contrast method which has been playing a vital role in X-ray diagnosis of early gastric cancer.

Early gastric cancer in the National Cancer Center

1. Frequency of occurrence

532 cases of early gastric cancer have been detected and operated in the National Cancer Center, from May, 1962, up till the end of 1972. The incidence of early gastric cancer was 21.6% of a total of 2463 cases of resected gastric cancers.

Early gastric cancer is classified in Japan, into three types macroscopically, that is, Type I (protruded type), Type II (superficial type) and Type III (excavated type). Type II is further divided into three subtypes, that is, Type IIa (superficial elevated type), Type IIb (superficial flat type) and Type IIc (superficial depressed type). According to this classification, the 532 cases of early gastric cancer were divided into 62 cases (11.7%) of Type I, 84 cases (15.8%) of Type IIa, 9 cases (1.7%) of Type IIb, 310 cases (58.2%) of Type IIc, 47 cases (8.8%) of Type III and 20 cases of multiple lesions which had more than two early gastric cancers in a stomach.

2. Diagnostic success by X-ray

X-ray diagnostic rates were calculated for 512 cases of the 532 cases of early gastric cancer; those excluded were 20 cases with multiple lesions. 451 cases (88.1%) of early gastric cancer were correctly diagnosed radiologically. In 50 cases, suspected diagnoses of early gastric cancer were made and 11 cases were misdiagnosed radiologically, but they were diagnosed by endoscopy or biopsy.

3. 5 year survival rate

Table 1 shows the 5 year survival rate in relation to the depth of the cancerous invasion of all resected cases seen at the National Cancer Center. When the invasion is limited to the mucosa or the mucosa and submucosa, the 5 year survival rate is 94.2% and 82.5%,

TABLE 1   *5 year survival rate in relation to the degree of depth of invasion*

	Invasion	Deaths	Survivors	Survival rate (%)
Early Cancer	Mucosa	7	113	94.2
	Submucosa	21	99	82.5
Advanced cancer	Muscularis propriae	42	56	57.1
	Subserosa	109	96	46.8
	Serosa	532	157	22.8

respectively. However, when the invasion extends to·the muscle layer, the subserosa or the serosa, the 5 year survival rate is reduced to 57.1%, 46.8% and 22.8%, respectively.

Double contrast method

For the routine X-ray examinination of the stomach, a series of required positions will be suggested as shown in Table 2. Skilful application of the conventional techniques, including the barium filled method, the compression method, mucosal study and the double contrast method, is important for early detection of gastric cancer. However, the double contrast technique is particularly important in demonstrating the minute changes associated with early gastric cancer. This technique is easy to practise. Even beginners can master this technique after 6 month training.

Now, the details of the double contrast technique, that is, the positioning, the barium meal, the amount of air and the introduction of additional air, will be explained.

TABLE 2   *Positioning the patient*

1. Spot X-ray of cardiac portion on first swallowing.

2. Fluoroscopy and spot X-ray with compression.

3. Mucosal study in prone position.

4. Spot X-ray of esophagus.

5. Barium filled. Upright position:
   i) Postero-anterior.
   ii) Right anterior oblique.
   iii) Left anterior oblique.

6. Barium filled. Prone position.

7. Double contrast in supine position.
   i) Postero-anterior.
   ii) Right anterior oblique.
   iii) Left anterior oblique.

8. Double contrast in 45° semi-erect position.
   Left anterior oblique.

9. Double contrast in upright position.
   i) Postero-anterior.
   ii) Right anterior oblique.
   iii) Left anterior oblique.

10. Double contrast in prone position.

11. Spot X-ray with adequate compression.

1. Positioning

(a) Upright position (postero-anterior)   The examination table is vertical. The patient is placed in a postero-anterior and upright position. A picture of the barium filled stomach with 300 ml of barium is taken in this position. Subsequently, the amount of air is confirmed by checking the size of the fornix. If it is not sufficient for the following double contrast examination, additional air should be added with a gastric tube or with a gas producing powder. (The method of introducing air will be explained later in this paper).

(b) Supine position (postero-anterior)   The examination table is in a horizontal position. The patient is placed in a postero-anterior and supine position. Before taking a picture, the patient should be rotated left and right in order to get a nice coating of barium on the gastric mucosa. The double contrast picture in this position can demonstrate the angular region, lower gastric body and antrum.

(c) Supine position (right anterior oblique)   The patient is placed in a right anterior oblique and supine position for taking a double contrast picture of the antrum and prepyloric region. In this position, it is important that radiographs are taken when the antrum is sufficiently expanded.

(d) Supine position (left anterior oblique)   The patient is placed in a left anterior oblique and supine position. In this position, the upper gastric portion can be clearly demonstrated in the double contrast picture.

(e) Semi-erect position (left anterior oblique)   The patient is placed in a left anterior oblique and semi-erect 45° position. In this position, the upper gastric body and the fornix can be nicely demonstrated in the double contrast picture. Furthermore, this position is most important for demonstrating the cardia in the en-face view. Quite a large amount of air is required for this position.

(f) Prone position (antero-posterior)   So far, the double contrast technique for the examination of the posterior wall has been described. Now, the technique for the anterior wall will be explained.

After swallowing about 30 ml of barium and introducing about 300 ml of air, the patient is put in a prone position with a tilt of about 10° in the Trendelenburg position. The double contrast picture taken in this position can demonstrate the anterior wall clearly.

2. Barium meal

300 g of commercial barium powder in 300 ml of barium meal is recommended for the double contrast examination. 300 ml of barium meal per case is required. By using a thick and large amount of barium, the gastric juice and mucus are almost completely washed away, and the gastric wall is nicely coated with barium. This is a very important point for getting good results. The distension of the gastric wall with a large amount of barium is also helpful.

3. Amount of air

It is almost impossible to get a nice picture using the double contrast method without having enough air in the stomach. Approximately 300 ml of air is usually necessary. If the amount of air is not enough, the double contrast picture cannot demonstrate minute lesions on the gastric wall satisfactorily. After putting in additional air, the double contrast picture can adequately demonstrate a wide area of the posterior wall of the stomach.

4. Introduction of air

There are two ways to introduce additional air into the stomach. The first one is by a gastric tube. In order to regulate the exact amount of air in the stomach, the gastric tube is easier for the radiologist but not easier for the patient. For this reason, a second way of introducing air is suggested. One or two packages of gas producing powder are administered followed by a small amount of water with a drop of silicon.

Case study

Finally, two early gastric cancer cases with minimal findings are shown in Figures 1 and 2, demonstrating typical double contrast X-ray picture. One is a depressed and the other is an elevated lesion.

Case 1   This is a minimally depressed lesion, Type IIc (see Fig. 1). No abnormalities were found in the barium filled stomach. However, the double contrast radiograph demonstrates a small irregular patchy mucosal depression with converging and abruptly interrupted mucosal folds on the posterior wall of the lower gastric body. The pre-operative diagnosis of this case was early gastric cancer, Type IIc.

On the respected specimen, the lesion was so small and located among mucosal folds that it could be overlooked on the surgical specimen. The lesion was 2. 0 x 2. 0 cm in size. The cancerous invasion is limited to the mucosa with no lymph node metastasis.

Case 2   This is a minimally elevated lesion, Type IIa (see Fig. 2). The double contrast radiograph demonstrates clearly an irregular oval tumor consisting of numerous small, irregular shadows, near the cardia. As shown in this case, lesions near the cardia can be satisfactorily demonstrated in the double contrast method. Diagnosis by the compression method is impossible in this area. The pre-operative diagnosis in this case was early gastric cancer, Type IIa.

On the resected specimen, a small sessile mucosal elevation was seen near the cardia. The lesion was 2.5 x 2.0 cm in size. The cancerous invasion extended partially into the submucosa.

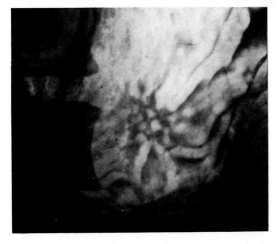

FIG. 1   *Case 1. A minimally depressed lesion, Type IIc.*

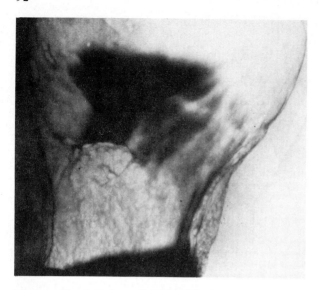

FIG. 2   *Case 2. A minimally elevated lesion, Type IIa.*

Conclusion

1. The most important approach towards improving the 5 year survival rate of gastric cancer concerns the detection of the lesion at as early a stage as possible.

2. For this purpose, the double contrast technique has been applied with satisfactory results and 532 cases of early gastric cancer have been detected in the National Cancer Center, during the last 10 years.

3. It is not difficult to become proficient in the double contrast technique, even for the beginner in X-ray diagnosis.

4. The authors hope that the double contrast technique will be widely used since many cases of early gastric cancer should be detected by this method.

Summary

532 cases of early gastric cancer, defined in Japan as carcinoma where infiltration is limited to the mucosa or the mucosa and submucosa have been detected mainly by X-ray and endoscopy in the National Cancer Center, Tokyo, during the last 10 years. The early gastric cancer cases have shown excellent results with respect to the 5 year survival rate which is as high as 90%.

The use of double contrast radiography has played a major role in X-ray diagnosis for detection of early gastric cancer cases. In this paper, the double contrast technique has been described together with 2 cases with minimal findings of early gastric cancer.

References

Ichikawa, H., Yamada, T. and Doi, H. (1964): Praxis of X-ray Diagnosis of the Stomach (in Japanese). Bunkodo Co., Tokyo. (English edition to be published).
Kuru, M. (1967): Atlas of Early Carcinoma of the Stomach. Nakayama Shoten, Tokyo.

Shirakabe, H. (1971): Double Contrast Studies of the Stomach. Bunkodo Co., Tokyo.
Shirakabe, H., Ichikawa, H. et al. (1966): Atlas of X-ray Diagnosis of Early Gastric Cancer (in Japanese). Igaku Shoin, Tokyo. (English edition, J. B. Lippincott Co., Philadelphia, 1969; Spanish edition, Editorial Científico Médica, Barcelona, 1969; Italian edition, Società Editrice Universo, Rome, 1969).
Shirakabe, H., Ichikawa, H. et al. (1969): Frühcarzinom des Magens. Georg Thieme Verlag, Stuttgart.

Foetal sulphoglycoprotein antigen (FSA) as a possible precursor of alimentary canal cancers*

I. P. T. Häkkinen

Departments of Pathology and Medical Microbiology, University of Turku, Turku, Finland

Introduction

Earlier opinions about sulphated polysaccharides in human gastric juice were re-evaluated in the early sixties on the basis of evidence concerning the glycoprotein nature of acid gastric macromolecules (Häkkinen et al., 1965). These molecules, when not split by enzymatic hydrolysis, were found to be of considerable size, ranging from 7 to 20 S in normal gastric juice from young subjects (Häkkinen, 1966). The mean sulphation ratio was 0.32 calculated on the basis of their aminosugar content but variations in the ratio were common, the lower sulphated fractions prevailing. We can say that in normal human gastric secretion, highly sulphated macromolecules tend to disappear so that there are difficulties in the histochemical demonstration of sulphate, the picture being the opposite of that in embryonic gastric mucosa (Häkkinen et al., 1968b; Hakkinen and Virtanen, 1970).

Due to diverse extrinsic stress factors the gastric mucosa frequently shows more or less profound alterations. The biochemical parameters, for example variations in mucosubstances, are less well known. Polydispersivity in size and elevated sulphate-amino sugar ratios were, however, often observed in gastric diseases such as peptic ulcer, pernicious anemia and especially gastric cancer (Häkkinen, 1966, 1967).

The possible immunogenicity or antigenicity of acid gastric glycoproteins was investigated simultaneously with the above physico-chemical studies and forms the basis of our understanding of the role of foetal sulphoglycoprotein antigen (FSA) considered in the following pages (Häkkinen, 1966, 1967; Häkkinen et al., 1968a).

Immunochemical detection of sulphoglycoprotein antigens in cancerous gastric juice

The guiding principle throughout our immunochemical studies on alimentary canal glycoproteins has been the utilization of the partial purification made by Nature itself i.e. the use of gastric juice instead of gastric tissue as the starting material. Gastric glycoproteins appear to be consistently immunogenic in laboratory animals such as rabbits but the immunogenicity is not very marked – immunization with natural or concentrated but unfractionated gastric juice seldom raises the desired antibodies.

The acid glycoproteins of gastric juice can be separated from the rest of the macromolecules – neutral glycoproteins and proteins – by using the cationic detergent cetyl pyridinium chloride. Details of the procedure have been described earlier (Häkkinen,

* This work has been supported by grants from the J.K. Paasikivi Foundation and the Finnish Medical Research Council and by a research contract with the Finnish Cancer Society.

1966, 1972*a*). Acid glycoproteins separated in this way usually give rise to considerable antibody formation in rabbits. The family of acid glycoproteins is not necessarily homogeneous in its antigenic structure. As a rule young healthy people secrete only one kind of antigen in their acid glycoproteins and this we have called N_O-antigen (Häkkinen et al., 1968*a*). Many patients with peptic ulcer and pernicious anemia secrete besides N_O, another glycoprotein antigen called I, which is the normal antigen of the colon and the lower part of the intestine.

The above antigens can be looked upon as being organ-bound structures since they can be detected only in organs of endodermal origin, having a secretional function. In the foetus I and N_O can be found both in the colon and in the stomach (Häkkinen et al., 1968*b*), the reappearance of I in the adult stomach perhaps reflecting a less differentiated state than before its secretion.

It soon became apparent that glycoproteins with N_O and I also show serological specificity in the ABH blood group system (Häkkinen and Virtanen, 1970). Cancerous gastric juice always contains N_O and I but also another antigen which differs from them in immunological properties. The antigen was called FSA since it was regularly found in the embryonal gut and stomach (Häkkinen, 1966, 1967; Häkkinen et al., 1968*b*).

In the preparation of anti-FSA the antisera to I and N_O are used to absorb acid glycoproteins derived from cancerous gastric juice. The supernatant, after absorption with an excess of anti-I and anti-N_O, is used for immunization. The procedure has been described elsewhere (Häkkinen, 1966, 1967, 1972*a*). Antiserum prepared in this way gives one precipitation line with acid glycoproteins of cancerous gastric juice. Absorption with non-cancerous gastric acid glycoproteins does not abolish the specific reaction, nor does absorption with salivary glycoproteins.

In the first study, the non-cancerous material was obtained from healthy students and in all cases a negative result was obtained when the samples were tested against anti-FSA in Ouchterlony plates. Out of 116 cases with non-cancerous gastric diseases there were 14 with a positive result, thus indicating that FSA cannot be considered strictly cancer-specific. In the same study, 75 out of 78 verified gastric cancer cases were FSA secretors.

Immunohistological studies on the occurence of FSA

Immunohistological study of gastric cancer and non-cancerous mucosa outside an existing

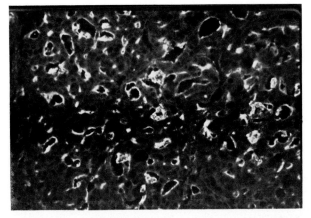

FIG. 1   *Photomicrograph of gastric cancer tissue. Specific fluorescence in cell surfaces and secretions. Rabbit anti-FSA serum and anti-rabbit sheep gammaglobulin fluorescein isothiocyanate.*

tumour revealed that FSA is always present in the surface and secretion of gastric cancer cells (Fig. 1), but can occasionally be found in circumscribed areas of superficial mucosal cells outside the tumour. In 4 cases out of 29 in stomachs with peptic ulcer there were areas in the superficial antral mucosa showing specific fluorescence with anti-FSA.

FSA could not be found in the intestinal mucosa. In the case of the colon we restricted the study to strictly normal juvenile samples where, as expected, FSA was not found. Pilot experiments with normal colonic tissue in connection with colonic cancer seem, however, to suggest the presence of FSA or an antigen cross-reacting with it. Since normal colon material is difficult to obtain systematically the question of the existence and re-appearance of FSA in the colon remains unresolved.

TABLE 1   *Occurrence of 3 alimentary canal glycoprotein antigens in various human organs and tumours outside the gastro-intestinal tract as detected by the immunofluorescence technique*

Sample	Number of samples	Immune sera		
		N_O	I	FSA
Lung	2	−	−	−
	3	+	+	−
Sublingual gland	2	+	+	−
Cervix uteri	6	+	+	−
Pseudomucinous ovarian cyst	6	+	+	−
Cancer of cervix uteri	2	+	+	−
	3	−	−	−
Pancreatic cancer	6	+	+	−

Negative: Spleen (5), kidney (5), liver (5), skin (3), uterus (6), mammary gland (6), prostate (5), parotic gland (5), pancreas (2).

Serous ovarian cyst (6), cancer of corpus uteri (5), ovarian cancer (5), renal cancer (5), prostatic cancer (6), cancer of urinary bladder (6).

+ = positive finding; − = negative finding

Using the same fluorescence technique as described above (Häkkinen et al., 1968a) the most important tissues of the body and tumours arising from them have been studied. Table 1 gives the results concerning the presence of the glycoprotein antigens N_O I and FSA in tissue samples. Except in the case of colonic cancer, which has been studied separately (see section 4) FSA could not be found in any of the samples.

Immunochemical relationship of FSA to other glycoprotein antigens in the alimentary canal

Perchloric acid extraction, described by Gold and Freedman (1965) for the preparation of glycoprotein samples from colonic cancer and colonic mucosa produces material which reacts with anti-FSA in both cases. Evidence has recently been provided that the CEA of colonic cancer shares a common antigenic determinant (Häkkinen, 1972a) with FSA. This is, however, different from the colon cancer specific part of the CEA molecule. The same FSA specificity without colon cancer specificity can be found in colonic mucosa outside a tumour (Häkkinen, 1972a). CEA seems to be very complex in its antigenic structure, one of the latest observations being that by Mach and Pusztaszeri (1972) concerning the cross-reactivity of a lung glycoprotein (NGP) with CEA. NGP did not cross-react with FSA in our experiments. FSA shares a common determinant with some of the salivary glycoproteins, different from that which cross-reacts with CEA. This was detected when in some immunizations, especially at an early stage in the production of anti-FSA sera, the antibodies giving the reaction with FSA were eliminated by absorption with salivary glycoproteins. Such a serum gave rise to spur formation with absorbed standard serum against FSA (Fig. 2) thus indicating that there might be FSA molecules in the gastric juice both with and without the salivary determinant. Hence, when preparing anti-FSA sera it is necessary to absorb the sera with salivary glycoproteins before the immune sera can be used for analyses of FSA of gastric origin.

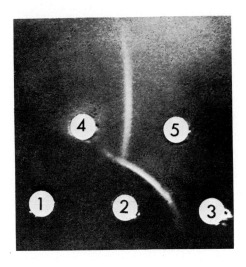

FIG. 2 *Ouchterlony plate of cancerous gastric sulphoglycoproteins, anti-FSA antiserum and an antiserum specific to salivary glycoprotein antigen, using a microtechnique. 2= anti-FSA, 4= anti-salivary glycoprotein serum, 5= sulphoglycoproteins of cancerous gastric juice.*

FSA in normal healthy population

A sample of gastric juice needed for the preparation and analysis of acid glycoproteins can be taken with an oral tube by first introducing buffered saline and then withdrawing the gastric contents with a syringe. The procedure usually takes some 3 min and is of little discomfort to the person being tested when well trained personnel collect the sample.

We have collected over 1,700 samples from industrial workers in Turku, Finland. The prevalence of FSA in this group and the clinical findings for FSA secretors have been presented earlier (Häkkinen, 1972b). The overall prevalence of FSA in the age group 40 to 64 in both sexes was ca.3%. After a one year follow-up, one case of superficial ulceration, symptomless but slowly growing, was operated on as an early gastric malignancy.

Later on a second population study was made, in which over 10,000 samples were collected. Table 2 shows the age distribution and the results of FSA analyses, which again indicate an overall prevalence of ca. 3% for FSA positives. The clinical findings, including one symptomless gastric cancer, are shown in Table 3.

Blood group glycoprotein and FSA

N_O and I glycoproteins of gastric origin contain blood group specific structures. This indicates that the structural details of blood group active glycoproteins are apparently not yet fully known and perhaps vary according to whereabouts in the body they are taken

TABLE 2   *A screening examination of 10,151 workers over 40 years for detection of foetal glycoprotein antigen in gastric juice. Age distribution and percentage of positive findings*

Age (years)	Number investigated	Number of positive findings	%
Females			
40–44	1052	34	3.2
45–49	1091	24	2.2
50–54	984	21	2.1
55–59	802	24	2.9
60–64	601	21	3.5
Total	4530	124	Mean 2.8
Males			
40–44	1371	39	2.8
45–49	1387	42	3.0
50–54	1115	38	3.4
55–59	928	32	3.4
60–64	820	19	2.3
Total	5621	170	Mean 3.0

from. The FSA of cancerous gastric juice does not usually include blood group antigens of known specificity, nor does anti-FSA sera have blood group antibodies. This has been tested with the haemagglutination technique and with Ouchterlony plates, using both human and rabbit anti-A and anti-B sera with precipitating specific antibodies and Ulex europeus extract. As controls, blood group substances of ovarian cyst origin were tested, and absorptions with appropriate human red cells performed.

In the course of our population study, however, samples were analyzed which contained both FSA-specific and compatible blood group antigens, apparently in the same molecules, as can be seen in Figure 3 in the Ouchterlony runs. Among the FSA positive samples in the population study some gave rise to 2 to 3 precipitation lines against compatible blood group antibodies of human origin, thus strongly indicating the polydispersivity and the importance of physico-chemical properties in Ouchterlony runs of gastric glycoproteins (Fig. 4). By using FSA it was also possible to detect duplication and triplication of precipitation lines.

Molecules with both FSA and blood group specificity and those with FSA specificity alone were occasionally observed in the same sample as is sometimes the case with gastric cancer.

The above data suggest a relationship between FSA and blood group substances. Most probably the FSA is an uncompleted blood group glycoprotein. In some instances some of the carbohydrate side chains are fully synthesized, the blood group specificities being the last and most superficial in the chain (Watkins, 1966). Some of the other chains must be incomplete, lacking serological specificity but having an open structure to which rabbits respond by forming anti-FSA.

Significance of FSA

In the light of the foregoing data we can infer that structures like FSA hardly participate

TABLE 3   Clinical findings of 294 FSA–positive cases

Case No.	Gastroscopy									No gastroscopy	History			
	U	D	R	E	G	M	A	P	None		U	C	Epig. pain	No symptoms
1–6	6			1	1								1	5
7–15		9			2						3		5	4
16–27			12	4	1						11	1		12
28–31				4	1									4
32–34						3*	1							3
35–68					34		1				4		6	28
69–81					4		13						3	10
82–89								8						8
90–269									180		6		12	168
270–294										25	1		3	22

U = Ulcer; D = Deform. of pylorus; R = Resection; E = Erosion; G = Gastritis; M = Malign. susp.; A = Atrophy; P = Polyp; C = Gastric cancer.

* One of cases has been operated on and gastric cancer verified.

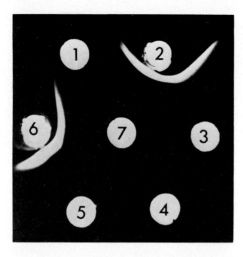

FIG. 3   *Ouchterlony plate of sulphoglycopro-*
          teins of gastric juice, anti-FSA anti-
          serum and anti-A serum of human
          origin, using a microtechnique. 2 and
          6 = samples of gastric sulphoglyco-
          proteins from the population study
          (see text). 3 and 5= anti-A serum of
          human origin. 7= anti-FSA.

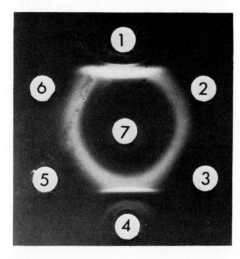

FIG. 4   *Ouchterlony plate of sulphoglycopro-*
          teins of gastric juice, bloodgroup sub-
          stance of ovarian cyst origin and hu-
          man anti-A serum, using a microtech-
          nique. 1,3,4 and 6 = FSA- positive
          samples of gastric sulphoglycoprotein
          from the population study (see text).
          2 and 5 = Bloodgroup substance A.
          7 = Human anti-A serum.

in the process leading to tumour immunity in the host. The same thing might be true in the case of CEA (Lejtenyi et al., 1971) which, it has been suggested, is also related to blood group glycoproteins (Simmons and Perlmann, 1973).

The significance of FSA seems to be on the diagnostic side. In the FSA analysis of gastric juice as described above, two results emerge both of which have previously been found to be associated with gastric cancer: (1) The re-appearance of glycoprotein structures charged with SO_4-groups, which has been shown histochemically (Lev, 1965; Järvi, personal communication). (2) The disappearance of blood group specificity from glycoprotein structures (Davidsohn et al., 1966; Sheahan et al., 1971; Häkkinen, 1970). These two results are consistent and the molecule called FSA thus reflects some of the biochemical properties of malignant transformation.

We may suppose that cells producing glycoproteins with both FSA and blood group antigens are somewhat altered, perhaps reversibly. By measuring the FSA/blood group antigen ratio we could perhaps draw a standard curve to illustrate the degree of risk of cells developing which produce acid molecules with FSA specificity only. Our population study shows that large groups can be examined using the method described. The potential importance of our method and the anticipated improved method (in which FSA and blood group antigens are quantitatively determined) is — as I see it — that we may be able to foresee the course of events and so discover early cases of gastric malignancy.

References

Davidsohn, I., Kovarik, S. and Lee, C. (1966): Arch. Path., 81, 381.
Gold, P. and Freedman, S. (1965): J. exp. Med., 122, 467.
Häkkinen, I. (1966): Scand. J. Gastroent., 1, 28.
Häkkinen, I. (1967): Scand. J. Gastroent., 2, 39.
Häkkinen, I. (1970): J. nat. Cancer Inst., 44, 1183.
Häkkinen, I. (1972a): Immunochemistry, 9, 1115.
Häkkinen, I. (1972b): Scand. J. Gastroent., 7, 483.
Häkkinen, I., Hartiala, K. and Terho, T. (1965): Acta chem. scand., 19, 797.
Häkkinen, I., Järvi, O. and Grönroos, J. (1968a): Int. J. Cancer, 3, 572.
Häkkinen, I., Korhonen, L. and Saxén, L. (1968b): Int. J. Cancer, 3, 582
Häkkinen, I. and Virtanen, S. (1970): Int. Arch. Allergy, 39, 272.
Lejtenyi, M., Freedman, S. and Gold, P. (1971): Cancer (Philad.), 28, 115.
Lev, R. (1965): Lab. Invest., 14, 2080.
Mach, J. and Pusztaszeri, G. (1972): Immunochemistry, 9, 1031.
Sheahan, D., Horowitz, S. and Zamcheck, N. (1971): Amer. J. dig. Dis., 16, 961.
Simmons, D. and Perlmann, P. (1973): Cancer Res., 33, 313.
Tyrkkö, J., Häkkinen, I. and Rimpelä, U. (1968): Brit. J. exp. Path., 49, 371.
Watkins, W. (1966): Science, 152, 172.

Skin testing with soluble membrane antigens obtained from fetal stomach, and normal and malignant gastric cells

Ariel Hollinshead and R.B. Herberman

Laboratory for Virus and Cancer Research, Department of Medicine, George Washington University, Washington, D.C., and Cellular and Tumor Immunology Laboratory of Cell Biology, National Institutes of Health, Bethesda, Md., U.S.A.

In previous studies, we have reported delayed hypersensitivity reactions to intradermal skin tests of specific soluble antigens from human intestinal cancers and from first and second trimester fetal intestinal cells (Hollinshead et al., 1970, 1972). These antigens which produced delayed skin reactions (SRA) were found to be separate from another carcinoembryonic antigen (CEA) described by Gold (Gold and Freedman, 1965). Our methods used for the separation of membranes, for obtaining the soluble membrane antigens by stepwise sequential sonication followed by partial separation by Sephadex G-200 column chromatography followed by further separation using a special method of gel electrophoresis are described in detail elsewhere (Hollinshead et al., 1970, 1972; Hollinshead and Stewart, 1974). We now report the differences in the structure and chemistry of fetal glycoproteins (FGP) and SRA associated with gastric cancer. As shown in Figure 1, a single Sephadex separation of the gastric cancer cell membranes sonicate from 10^9 gastric cancer cells gives a profile, when monitored at 280 mμ, which is very similar to the profile of the separations of intestinal cancer sonicates. Since there is a 'trailing' of the first peak, the separated materials were pooled into 4 fractions (a,b,c,d) as indicated in Figure 1. When these individual pooled fractions of the crude Sephadex separations were each analyzed by gel electrophoresis, FGP was seen to be present in the high molecular weight region (a) and was also present in fraction b. A comparison was made with the gel electrophoretic profile of the membrane sonicate prior to separation over Sephadex. Gels were stained individually for protein, carbohydrate and lipid bands (see Figure 1). The FGP bands stained for the presence of carbohydrates, and this is consistent with the known chemistry of the intestinal cancer CEA, which is a high molecular weight glycoprotein. However, instead of one large band, the gastric cancer FGP is composed of at least 2, and perhaps 3 glycoprotein bands.

Thus, the FGP is quite different for gastric cancer, and these antigens must be studied in detail. It is of considerable interest to study fractions b and c electrophoretic profiles. The skin reactive antigen is composed of two bands, and the upper band stained with Oil Red O indicating the presence of lipids. Upon further analysis, this band was found to contain phospholipids using a previously described method (Hollinshead et al., 1969; Randerath, 1965). Therefore, the skin reactive antigen of gastric cancer is present in the same region and is comparable to the SRA of intestinal cancer. However, the gastric cancer antigens have a higher molecular weight, and one of the bands is a phospholipoprotein.

The same SRA bands were found in first trimester fetal gastric cells but not in second trimester. This is again in contrast to the intestinal cancer SRA which was found in first and second trimester fetal intestinal cells. Counterpart normal adult gastric mucosa cells were carefully studied, and do not contain FGP or SRA. However, the normal gastric

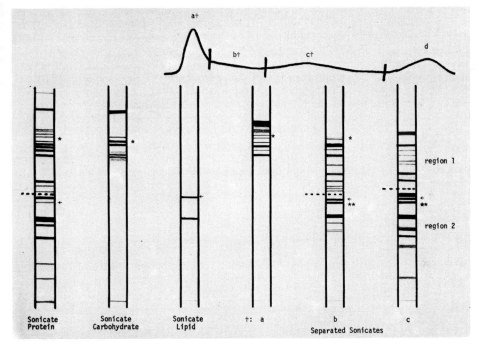

FIG. 1   *Separation by polyacrylamide gel electrophoresis (using 4 stacked gels; 10%, 7%, 4.75% and 3.5%). Profiles shown are: analysis of gastric cancer cell soluble membrane antigens obtained in the crude sonicate after stepwise sequential sonication of the separated membranes. The sonicate was stained with Coomassie Brilliant Blue for protein bands, with PAS Schiff Stain for carbohydrate and with Oil Red O for lipid containing bands. The sonicate was separated over Sephadex G-200, as shown in the elution profile diagram at the top of the figure. Fractions containing CEA or SRA, or both, are shown in the figure. The area marked by an asterisk (*) contains CEA. The areas marked by a double asterisk (**) contain SRA. The band marked with an arrow is a phospholipoprotein and is one of the SRA antigens.*

mucosa cells do contain a band in the same position as that seen just above the phospholipoprotein band fraction c of the gastric cancer separated sonicates (see Fig. 1). This normal antigen is found in the region above two SRA antigens of intestinal cancer.

The crude sonicate, and the separated sonicate fraction b and c were sliced (see dotted line Fig. 1) into two different regions and the gels eluted, the protein concentrated, dialyzed and filtered for skin testing. Fraction d was also skin tested. Only region 2 of fraction b and region 2 of fraction c gave positive skin tests, which were biopsied and shown to be a typical delayed hypersensitive reaction at 48 hr with indurations greater than 5 mm. Likewise, region 2 of separated fetal stomach cell sonicate gave a positive skin test.

We have shown with many different types of cancer, that the crude soluble cell membrane sonicate does not produce skin reactivity. We have defined a blocking factor present in the cancer cell sonicate (Hollinshead and Herberman, in preparation). It is likewise true that whole sonicate as well as gel region 2 (Fig. 1) of the gastric cancer sonicate does not produce a positive skin test. By careful examination of the bands in the sonicate (Fig. 1) it is clear that one of the SRA bands is missing and the other is barely discernible. There are 3 possible explanations. (1) Either the heavier molecular weight material present in the unseparated sonicate prevented part of the antigen from migrating from the upper portion of the gel, or (2) the antigens were blocked somehow, perhaps by other antigens or antibodies present in the membrane pellet, and the material either sedimented at 100,000 × g during the sequential sonication prodedure, or (3) remains in an inactive form in the sonicate. The second explanation is unlikely, since during gel filtration and later gel electrophoresis the SRA separates from the sonicate. Both explanations 1 and 3 may apply. Incubation of the SRAs of leukemia or lung cancer with sonicates of equivalent protein content from several different types of cancer blocked the cancer type-specific delayed hypersensitive skin reactions produced by unmasked SRAs. Sonicates from a normal cell membrane preparation had no effect upon SRA reactivity, but sonicates from counterpart 'normal' cell membrane preparations from the cancer patients did. A standard recall antigen SKSD (streptokinase-streptodornase) was not masked after incubation with each of several cancer cell membrane sonicates. Conversely, when each of several SRAs were mixed with 3× crystallized bovine albumin in solutions of equivalent protein content the skin reactions were not blocked. It would thus appear that there is a general blocking factor present in some cancer patient cell membranes.

Acknowledgements

We are grateful for the excellent technical assistance of O.B. Lee, K. Tanner, P. Jones, M. Dannbeck, L. Seigal and P. Pugh. This work was supported by USPHS Contract number NIH-NCI-G-69-2176, National Cancer Institute.

References

Gold, P. and Freedman, S. (1965): J. exp. Med., 122, 467.
Hollinshead, A., Bunnag, B. Alford, T. and Cusumano, C. (1969): J. gen. Virol., 4, 433.
Hollinshead, A., Glew, D. and Bunnag, B. (1970): Lancet, 1191.
Hollinshead, A. C., McWright, C. G., Alford, T. C. and Glew, D. H. (1972): Science, 177, 887.
Hollinshead, A. C. and Stewart, T. H. M. (1974): J. nat. Cancer Inst., 52, 327.
Hollinshead, A. C. and Herberman, R., In preparation.
Randerath, K. (1965): Thin Layer Chromatography. Verlag Chemie Academic Press, New York-London.

Role of skin responses to tumour-associated macromolecules in the diagnosis of neoplasia

D. E. H. Tee

Department of Experimental Pathology, King's College Hospital Medical School, London, United Kingdom

Using the Schultz-Dale technique, Makari (1955, 1958*b*) demonstrated in tumours and in the serum of patients with malignant or benign tumours the presence of antigens that were not detectable in the absence of tumour. Makari (1958*a*) obtained evidence that these were either polysaccharidal or glycoprotein in nature which was subsequently supported by Smith (1963) and Jeanloz (1971). The antigens are referred to as tumour polysaccharidal substances (TPS).

Since, for technical reasons, the Schultz-Dale test was not suitable for general diagnostic testing, Makari sought to develop a more practical procedure. The reaction of the skin to pneumococcus capsular polysaccharide antigen and the apparent polysaccharidal nature of the TPS antigens prompted Makari to investigate the development of an intradermal skin test. Makari (1960, 1962) was able to show that TPS antigens derived from carcinoma, sarcoma and lymphoma were capable of inducing immediate erythematous reactions when injected intradermally. These reactions were potentiated if the antigens were pre-incubated with either untreated or trypsinized serum from the patient being tested. In the skin test as developed by Makari, a positive result consists of an erythematous reaction of any of the antigens whose mean diameter compared to that given by a control injection without antigen is greater than 1.35. A positive result was stated to occur either in the presence of a benign or malignant tumour or in the presence of one or more of a group of diseases which included hepatic cirrhosis, ulcerative colitis, diverticulitis and peptic ulcer.

Makari (1969) demonstrated that the test was positive in all patients with early non-metastatic carcinoma of a wide variety of organs; in patients with metastases, however, an appreciably lower incidence was seen. The apparent success of this work suggested the need for confirmation or rejection of the validity of these findings. The present paper describes the results of a completely independent study in which possible investigator bias was eliminated by means of a double-blind controlled procedure. The initial results of this trial have been reported elsewhere (Tee, 1972*a, b*).

Materials and methods

Performance of the test

In this study the antigens (TPS) were prepared by subjecting extracts from lung carcinoma, sarcoma and lymphoma to degradative chemical and physical separative procedures (Makari, 1958*a*). An extract of normal lung tissue (NPS) was employed as one control, together with others consisting of isotonic saline and untreated or trypsin-treated serum.

The test preparations were prepared aseptically; 0.1 ml diluted serum was pipetted into each of 10 sterile tubes labelled 1-10, 0.1 ml isotonic saline was added to each of Tubes 1, 2, 3, 4, 9 and 11, and 0.1 ml of the trypsin working solution (0.02 mg/ml) was added to each of Tubes 5, 6, 7, 8 and 10. The rack was shaken gently and left at 5° C for 30 min. Then 0.1 ml sterile isotonic saline was added to Tubes 1 and 5, 0.1 ml TPS-1 to Tubes 2 and 6, 0.1 ml TPS-2 to Tubes 3 and 7, 0.1 ml TPS-3 to Tubes 4 and 8 and 0.1 ml NPS to Tubes 9 and 10. The rack was shaken gently and placed in the refrigerator for 24 hr. Then 0.1 ml aliquots were injected into the patient's skin on either side of the spinal column starting 3 inches (76 mm) below the prominence of the 7th cervical vertebra. After an interval of 2 min from the first injection the longest diameter of the erythema and the diameter at right angles were measured at each injection site sequentially.

The study was carried out on a double-blind controlled basis. The syringes were coded by an assistant according to a table of random numbers. Thus the physician administering the injections knew neither which material had been injected into any site, nor the patient's diagnosis.

Diagnosis of disease status

The definitive diagnosis of carcinoma or other type of tumour was arrived at only after histological examination of the tumours. If no definitive histological categorization could be made the patient was assigned to the 'questionable tumour' group.

The carcinomas were classified into 4 stages: (1) tumour less than 2 cm diameter or the mucosa only involved; (2) tumour between 2 and 3 cm diameter or muscularis mucosa involved; (3) tumour greater than 3 cm diameter or serosa involved; and (4) lymph nodes involved or metastasis in other organ or tissue.

Results

The results are summarized in Table 1 according to diagnostic category. The non-neoplastic patients were divided into 3 categories, healthy subjects, non-inflammatory, and inflammatory and reactive. The latter consisted of patients with fibrocystic disease of the breast, peptic ulcer, prostatic hyperplasia and other inflammatory diseases. The neoplastic patients were divided into those with malignant or benign tumours; the former were further divided (Table 1) into carcinomas, carcinomas in situ, skin tumours (including carcinomas and melanomas), malignant tumours (other than carcinomas) and multiple tumours (when more than one tumour was present). The carcinomas group was further subdivided according to the stage of advancement of the disease.

The overall summary (Table 1) showed that of the non-neoplastic patients, those with inflammatory and reactive disorders gave a higher proportion of positive results than either the healthy subjects or non-inflammatory group (40.7, 5.6 and 18.2% respectively). Patients with localised carcinomas exhibited a considerably higher incidence of positive tests (Stage I 66.7% and Stage II 57.1%), but those with advanced or disseminated disease had incidences (Stage III 20.9% and Stage IV 32.0%) that approximated to that of the non-inflammatory group. These results emphasize the stage dependency of the skin test. It is of interest that the carcinoma treated-no recurrence group gave comparable results to those of the healthy subjects.

Statistical analysis of the overall data showed that there was a highly significant difference between the incidence of positive results in early localised carcinomas (Stages I and II) when compared with those in the healthy, non-inflammatory and inflammatory and reactive groups (P <0.001; <0.001; and <0.05 levels respectively). In contrast, when the carcinomatous process was more advanced (Stages III and IV) the percentage of positives was marginally greater than that of the healthy subjects (P <0.10), and was not significantly greater than in the non-inflammatory group but indeed was below that of the inflammatory group (P <0.025).

An analysis of the results by organ system (Table 2) showed that the incidence of positive skin tests in the carcinoma groups did not differ appreciably in different organ systems. However, there were some differences between organ systems with respect to the

TABLE 1   *Results of intradermal test in 584 subjects*

Diagnostic category	No. of cases	No. positive	% positive
Non-neoplastic			
Healthy subjects	18	1	5.6
Non-inflammatory disorders	33	6	18.2
Inflammatory and reactive disorders	172	70	40.7
Neoplastic			
Benign tumours	26	11	42.3
Malignant tumours*	284	97	34.2
Carcinomas:			
Stage I	12	8	66.7
Stage II	35	20	57.1
Stage III	67	14	20.9
Stage IV	100	32	32.0
Questionable stage	13	5	38.5
Treated. Possible recurrence	7	2	28.6
Treated. No recurrence	28	3	10.7
Multiple carcinomas	10	3	30.0
Carcinoma in situ	7	3	42.9
Skin tumours (including carcinomas and melanomas)	14	4	28.6
Malignant tumours (other than carcinomas)	11	4	36.4
Multiple tumours (including malignant and benign)	8	2	25.0
Questionable tumours	23	11	47.8

* This group does not include (1) carcinomas treated with no recurrence, and (2) questionable tumours.

TABLE 2   *Analysis of results by organ system*

Organ system	Diagnostic category											
	Non-inflammatory			Inflammatory and reactive			Carcinomas Stages I and II			Carcinomas Stages III and IV		
	No.	Pos.	%	No.	Pos.	%	No.	Pos.	%	No.	Pos.	%
Breast	0	0	–	114	53	46.5	23	11	47.8	60	16	26.7
Digestive	8	1	12.5	31	15	48.4	7	4	57.1	40	12	30.0
Genito-urinary	8	1	12.5	11	1	9.1	13	9	69.2	29	9	31.0
Respiratory	1	0	–	8	0	00.0	4	4	–	32	7	21.9

Percentages were not calculated when the number of cases was less than six.

incidence of positives in inflammatory and reactive disorders. The significance of these in terms of the clinical value of the test must be further evaluated but strongly suggests that the test is not limited to a particular organ or organ system. In patients with gastric disorders (Table 3) no appreciable difference in the incidence of positive tests was seen in those having, respectively, duodenal ulcer, gastric ulcer or oesophagitis and gastric reflux, nor with the clinical stage of the lesion. These conclusions must, however, be tentative in view of the small numbers involved.

The gastric carcinoma groups showed the typical decrease in percentage positivity as the disease became more advanced. Within the group of Stage IV patients, no difference in the incidence of positive tests could be observed between those with lymph node involvement as compared to those with distant metastases. There were insufficient patients with Stages I and II carcinomas to permit a comparison with comparable disease in the remainder of the digestive tract. No difference was discernible between the test results in gastric or other digestive tract carcinomas of Stages III and IV.

Discussion

The data demonstrates that there is a high degree of association between positive Makari intradermal test results and early neoplastic change in a wide range of different organs including those of the digestive, genito-urinary and respiratory systems. The results given by the test, subject to exclusion of inflammatory and reactive disorders, could usefully assist the clinician, since although early cancer is difficult to diagnose, it is the most likely to respond favourably to treatment.

Clinically it is a disadvantage that the test is positive in a proportion with inflammatory and reactive disorders. However, in the majority of patients with a positive test, it should be possible to exclude such conditions as peptic ulceration, diverticulitis, cirrhosis of the liver and ulcerative colitis by other investigations. Nevertheless, a positive result with the skin test in a patient with any of these disorders does not exclude the coexistence of neoplastic disease.

Other applications of the test which could be of particular value are the monitoring of postoperative response to treatment and the early detection of recurrence. In these situations the incidence of complicating inflammatory disease are likely to be lower than the rate of tumour recurrence. There is evidence (Makari and Hayton, 1965; Makari, 1972, personal communication) that patients treated surgically and subsequently re-

TABLE 3   *Results of intradermal test in 161 patients with gastric disorders from United Kingdom series and from France, Japan and U.S.A.*

Diagnostic category	U.K. series		Other series		All series		
	No. of cases	No. positive	No. of cases	No. positive	No. of cases	No. positive	% positive
Non-neoplastic							
Peptic ulceration	17	8	34	18	51	26	51.0
Other	2	0	14	1	16	1	6.3
Neoplastic							
Carcinomas:							
Stage I	0	0	4	4	4	4	100.0
Stage II	1	1	3	3	4	4	100.0
Stage III	4	1	8	7	12	8	75.0
Stage IV	13	3	61	33	74	36	48.7
Questionable stage	1	1					
Treated. No recurrence	2	0					
Benign tumours	1	0					
Questionable tumours	1	0					

sponding positively and negatively to the test formed two separate populations with different incidences and rates of appearance of recurrent tumours; the positive reactors showing a higher incidence and a faster rate of recurrence of tumours.

The present findings are in broad agreement with those of trials carried out in the U.S.A. (Makari, 1969), France (Boisivon, 1973) and Japan (Honda et al., 1973) covering the testing of 920 patients in all. With the present trial, the aggregate number of patients tested is 1,504. The lower incidence of positive Makari intradermal tests results (66.7%) in subjects with early carcinoma (Stage I) in the present series, as compared with the 100% observed by Makari, Honda and Boisivon respectively may be a reflection of the greater prevalence of carcinoma of the breast in our series and the difficulties inherent in the classification of this type of carcinoma rather than a lack of sensitivity of the test. In contrast with the other studies, half of the subjects with early localised carcinomas (Stages I and II) in my series had carcinoma of the breast. Classification of carcinoma of the breast according to size only, as was done here, may not be entirely satisfactory as other factors such as anatomical location, microscopic structure and hormone dependence may be significant. The results reported in Table 2 support this contention, thus of the 23 subjects with early localised carcinomas (Stages I and II) of the breast 47.8% were positive, while of the 24 subjects with early (Stage I and II) carcinoma of other organs 70.8% were positive. Currently an attempt is being made to reclassify all our cases with carcinoma to include criteria other than size so that a more accurate picture of the sensitivity of the test can be obtained.

Apropos the safety in use of the test, it is relevant to note that in none of these studies have signs of general toxicity or carcinogenicity been observed. Animal tests (Perkins, 1971; Wells Laboratories Inc., 1972) have also failed to demonstrate any evidence of toxicity or carcinogenicity.

In our study, considerable care was exercised to ensure objectivity. The precautions included measures to ensure that the physician administering the injections did not know which injection sites received particular preparations. Also, neither the patient's diagnosis nor which investigations had been previously performed were known to the physician carrying out the test. Indeed the diagnosis was not finally established in the majority of patients until exploratory surgical procedures had been performed and the resulting histological specimens had been examined. It is therefore reasonable to believe that these results were not influenced by observer bias and that they derive from the operation of a valid biological phenomenon.

Since different components of the oncogenic process, or the host's response to it, may be assayed by different tests, combined testing may provide the physician with fuller and more valid information than that from a single test. A consideration of the CEA data (Laurence et al., 1972) suggests that joint use of the CEA and Makari tests could be of advantage in particular situations. In very early cases, where the prospects for successful treatment is best, the Makari technique may be somewhat more sensitive as a diagnostic indicator. However, with progression of the disease, the incidence of positives seen with the CEA test rises whereas the positive Makari results fall to around 20%.

Summary

A double-blind controlled evaluation of the Makari intradermal test was performed in 584 patients in order to confirm or refute the results of previous trials. Positive results were seen in the majority of patients with early carcinomas. Statistical analysis showed that, compared to the non-neoplastic groups, the incidence of positive responses to the test was highly significantly associated with the presence of early carcinomas ($P < 0.001$). In the latter stages of the disease, this association was not statistically significant. An appreciable but lower incidence of positive responses was seen in patients with conditions associated with inflammatory and reactive processes. The results of this trial broadly confirmed those previously reported. It was concluded that the test was not of value in mass population screening but may have a useful place in the differential diagnosis and staging of tumours, in monitoring response to treatment and in the detection of tumour recurrence.

References

Boisivon, A. (1973): Trans. N.Y. Acad. Sci., 35,380.
Honda, K., Hoshishima, K., Kato, K., Okazaki, T., Higuchi, Y. and Ikeda, M. (1973): Trans. N.Y. Acad. Sci., 35,368.
Jeanloz, R. (1971): Communication to M. Goer.
Laurence, D. J. R., Stevens, U., Bettelheim, R., Darcy, D., Leese, C., Turberville, C., Alexander, P., Johns, E. W. and Munro-Neville, A. (1972): Brit. med. J., 3, 605.
Makari, J. G. (1955): Brit. med. J., 2, 1291.
Makari, J. G. (1958a): Brit. med. J., 2, 355.
Makari, J. G. (1958b): Brit. med. J., 2, 358.
Makari, J. G. (1960): J. Amer. Geriat. Soc., 8, 675.
Makari, J. G. (1962): Ann. N.Y. Acad. Sci., 101, 274.
Makari, J. G. (1969): J. Amer. Geriat. Soc., 17, 755.
Makari, J. G. and Hayton, T. (1965): Trans. N.Y. Acad. Sci., 28, 198.
Perkins, F. T. (1971): Communication to R. S. Forrest.
Smith, F. (1963): Communication to Food and Drug Administration, USA.
Tee, D. E. H. (1972a): Proc. roy. Soc. Med., 65, 638.
Tee, D. E. H. (1972b): J. Amer. Geriat. Soc., 20, 305.
Wells Laboratories Inc. (1972): Communication to Ormont Drug and Chemical Co. Inc.

2. Cancer of the colon and rectum

The etiology of cancer of the large bowel

Ernest L. Wynder and Bandaru S. Reddy

Naylor Dana Institute for Disease Prevention, The American Health Foundation, New York, N.Y., U.S.A.

Any investigation of the etiology of a given cancer should begin with logical reasoning. Thus, if we consider causative factors of skin cancer, we should think about factors which come into contact with the skin; if we investigate cancer of the lung, we should give primary attention to factors which are inhaled; and if we explore the etiology of cancer of the large bowel, we should focus on the food that is ingested.

When we take a look at the distribution of cancer in the colon, we note significant differences in its incidence in various parts of the world (Doll, 1969). Generally, colon cancer is relatively uncommon in developing countries and common in industrial societies, a notable exception being Japan (Fig. 1). On the other hand, the Japanese are not genetically immune to colon cancer which is evidenced by the fact that the rate of colon

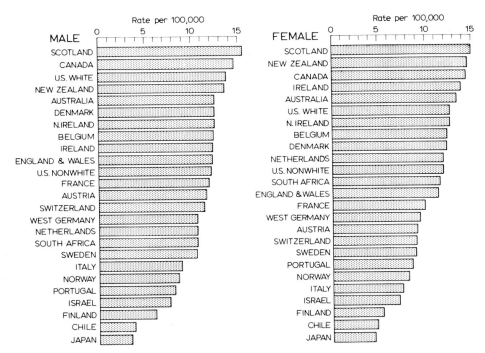

FIG. 1   *Age-adjusted mortality rate from cancer of the colon in various parts of the world. (From Segi and Kurihara, Jap. Cancer Soc., 1972, 6, 137. By courtesy of the Editors.)*

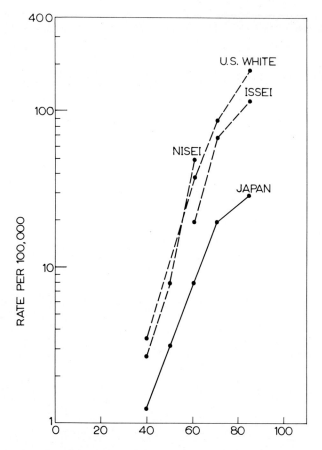

FIG. 2   *Specific mortality rates of colon cancer among Japanese immigrants to Hawaii. Issei, 1959-1962; Nisei, 1959-1962; U.S.Whites, 1959-1961; Japan, 1960-1961. (From Haenszel and Kurihara, J. nat. Cancer Inst., 1968, 40, 43. By courtesy of the Editors.)*

cancer appears to increase very rapidly among Japanese immigrants to Hawaii (Haenszel and Correa, 1971) (Fig. 2).

As a working hypothesis we may, therefore, state that large bowel cancer, particularly cancer of the colon, is related to a factor or factors which we ingest, is more common in developed countries than in developing societies, and is uncommon in Japan but common among Japanese immigrants to the United States.

In this regard we should also emphasize that these factors are likely to affect the colon part of the large bowel more than the rectal part since rectal cancer is about equally as common in Japan and the United States. Some caution should be given in respect to the recto-sigmoid area which may be grouped differently in various vital statistics. Our findings suggest that epidemiologically it should be listed with the colon rather than the rectum. Unfortunately, vital statistics tend to group recto-sigmoid lesions with those of the rectum.

Case control studies

Large-scale case control studies by our group and several other investigators have failed to identify factors which differ between study and control cases (Wynder and Shigamatsu,

1967). To the extent that diet might be a factor, this could have been expected at least in the United States where dietary intake in terms of broad food categories — though not in terms of food sources — of most people is roughly the same. In addition, accurate dietary information is difficult to obtain. On the other hand, data from Japan indicate patients with colon cancer have a more westernized diet than their respective controls (Wynder et al., 1969).

Specifically, our studies showed no relationship of large bowel cancer with such factors as constipation, weight, tobacco and alcohol usage, nor to any large bowel diseases with the exception of ulcerative colitis. In this regard, the relative variety of large bowel cancer among patients with Crohn's disease deserves special attention (Farmer et al., 1971). A suggestion that large bowel cancer is related to a history of appendectomy could not be confirmed by our studies (Hyams and Wynder, 1968).

In Japan, large bowel cancer was somewhat more common among people of higher socio-economic status, which is in line with their more westernized diets. In New York, cancer of the colon is more common among our Jewish population.

Largely on the basis of (*a*) the distribution of large bowel cancer in various parts of the world and (*b*) data dealing with migrant populations, we have proposed that dietary factors (particularly in terms of dietary fats and cholesterol and high animal protein) play an important part in large bowel carcinogenesis (Wynder and Shigematsu, 1967). We do not believe that transit time of the stool as suggested by Burkitt (1971) is an important factor because whatever bacterial conversion which takes place in the stool components has already taken place even in the relatively rapid transit time which is reported to occur among Africans.

Metabolic epidemiological studies

These facts raise the question as to specifically which dietary factors play a role in the etiology of colon cancer. The important endogenous compounds secreted into or present in the gut and as dietary components include acid and neutral steroids, bile pigments, digestive enzymes, amino acids, fatty acids, to cite a few. Lacassagne et al. (1961, 1966) and other investigators (Cook et al., 1940; Haddow, 1958, 1970) found that several bile acids could induce sarcomas at the site of injection in the laboratory animals. Some investigators have become interested in the potential carcinogenic activity of certain bile acids because of their overall structural and steric similarity to carcinogenic polycyclic hydrocarbon. Hill et al. (1971) showed a strong correlation between high concentrations of acid and neutral steroids in the feces and the incidence of colon cancer based upon geographic distribution. Fecal microflora was found to be different among groups with different rates of colon cancer incidence (Hill et al., 1971; Aries et al., 1969). We now have some information leading to the concept that the effects of diet may be mediated through changes in the composition of the intestinal microflora, and also through changes in the composition of intraluminal compounds secreted into the gut. Several ways by which the intestinal microflora could play a significant role are (*a*) the microflora could convert dietary components such as select proteins, peptides, or amino acids and lipids into biologically active compounds, cocarcinogens and/or carcinogens, (*b*) it could metabolize endogenous secretions, themselves controlled by diet, into such compounds, and (*c*) it could produce carcinogenic compounds from suitable precursors. The importance of the microflora and microbially modified endogenous compounds in colon carcinogenesis is supported by the fact that the incidence of cancer of small intestine, which has a low bacterial count compared to large intestine, is very, very low.

On the basis of the above hypothesis and conclusions, we analyzed the feces of various groups with diverse dietary habits for a variety of chemical constituents and for microbial activity (Wynder and Reddy, 1973). The fecal microflora of Americans consuming a mixed western diet were able to hydrolyse glucuronide conjugates more than those of American vegetarians, and Seventh-Day Adventists, and Japanese and Chinese (Reddy and Wynder, 1973) and thus suggesting an increase in microbial activity in Americans on a

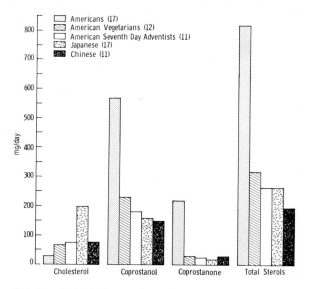

FIG. 3   *Daily fecal neutral sterol excretion in different populations. Number of subjects are shown in parenthesis. Coprostanol and coprostanone are microbial metabolites of cholesterol.*

mixed western diet. Bacterial β-glucuronidase activity was also higher in stools of subjects during the period of high-meat, high-fat diet than during the period of non-meat diet (Reddy et al., unpublished data). This increase in microbial activity could amplify the biologic activity of many exogenous and endogenous compounds. The daily fecal excretion of coprostanol and coprostanone (microbial metabolites of cholesterol), and of lithocholic acid, deoxycholic acid, and other microbially modified bile acids was higher in Americans on a mixed western diet than in other groups (Figs. 3 and 4). Our data also indicate that fecal bile acids were much more extensively modified in Americans on a mixed western diet than in other groups. Our explanation for this difference in acid and neutral

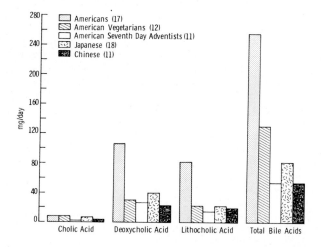

FIG. 4   *Daily fecal bile acids excretion in different populations. Number of subjects are shown in parenthesis. Total bile acids include cholic acid, deoxycholic acid, lithocholic acid, and other microbially modified bile acids.*

steroid excretion is obviously related to dietary composition. The quantitative aspects of intestinal microflora are also affected by the composition of the diet, and the effects of diet on the extent to which cholesterol and bile acids are transformed into these microbial metabolites depend on changes in the composition of intestinal microflora. In vitro parallel studies also indicate that bile acids and cholesterol were much more extensively degraded to various metabolites by anaerobes isolated from Americans on a high-meat western diet compared to a non-meat diet.

Future studies

It now needs to be shown that the association between cholesterol metabolites and/or bile acid metabolites to the incidence of cancer of the colon is of causative significance. Towards this end, we are currently testing a variety of bile acid metabolites for tumorigenic activity in experimental animals. Similarly, cholesterol metabolites need to be tested. We also need to determine whether carcinogens can be formed through the interaction of bacteria, and acid and neutral steroids and the like.

In the area of large bowel carcinogens, we obviously need to consider the possibility that (either because of tissue differences or because lower forms of animals are unable to develop a bacterial flora similar to man or because their bile acids are considerably simpler than man's) we are dealing with a situation in which the human environment cannot be duplicated in the laboratory setting unless we are prepared to work with higher forms of animals, especially monkeys.

In our Institute, through close collaboration of epidemiologists and laboratory investigators, we intend to pursue the dietary hypothesis linking overnutrition (especially in terms of fats and cholesterol) to large bowel cancer. A confirmation of this hypothesis has obvious preventive implications.

References

Aries, V., Crowther, J. S., Drasar, B. S., et al. (1969): Gut, 10, 334.
Burkitt, D. P. (1971): Cancer, 28, 3.
Cook, J. W., Kennaway, E. L. and Kennaway, N. M. (1940): Nature (Lond.), 145, 627.
Doll, R. (1969): Brit. J. Cancer, 23, 1.
Farmer, R. G., Hawk, W. A. and Turnbull, R. B. (1971): Cancer, 28, 289.
Haddow, A. (1958): Brit. med. Bull., 14, 79.
Haddow, A. (1970): In: Abbottempo, Bk. 4, pp. 8-11. Abbot Universal Ltd.
Haenszel, W. M. and Correa, P. (1971): Cancer, 28, 14.
Haenszel, W. M. and Kurihara, M. (1968): J. nat. Cancer Inst., 40, 43.
Hill, M. J., Drasar, B. S., Aries, V., et al. (1971): Lancet, 2, 95.
Hyams, L. and Wynder, E. L. (1968): J. chron. Dis., 21, 391.
Lacassagne, A., Buu-Hoi, N. P. and Zajdela, F. (1961): Nature (Lond.), 190, 1007.
Lacassagne, A., Buu-Hoi, N. P. and Zajdela, F. (1966): Nature (Lond.), 209, 1026.
Reddy, B. S. and Wynder, E. L. (1973): J. nat. Cancer Inst., 50, 1437.
Segi, M. and Kurihara, M. (1972): Jap. Cancer Soc., 6, 137.
Wynder, E. L., Kajitani, T., Ishikawa, S., et al. (1969): Cancer, 23, 1210.
Wynder, E. L. and Reddy, B. S. (1973): J. nat. Cancer Inst., 50, 1099.
Wynder, E. L. and Shigematsu, T. (1967): Cancer, 20, 1250.

Proliferation and differentiation of colonic epithelial cells in lesions of man and rodent*

Martin Lipkin

Memorial Sloan-Kettering Cancer Center, New York, N. Y., U.S.A.

The main point that I would like to describe in this presentation relates to the changes that develop in colonic epithelial cells in several neoplastic diseases. These develop in areas of cell metabolism that influence the synthesis of DNA and the proliferation of the cells. The preceding discussion in this symposium described the fact that suspected carcinogens most likely contribute to the development of neoplasms in the colon of man. However, the mode of operation of these carcinogens, and indeed exactly what the carcinogens may be, are not known.

An area that we have investigated concerns the evaluation of proliferative and differentiation-specific defects in colon cells as neoplasms develop. The latter are very likely influenced by the suspected carcinogens. We have found similar molecular changes to develop affecting the proliferative behavior of the cells in several groups of patients: those with the precancerous disease familial polyposis, and also patients in the general population who develop isolated neoplastic lesions of the colon. In addition, we have observed similar findings in the colons of mice after administration of the potent chemical carcinogen, 1,2-dimethylhydrazine.

The abnormal characteristics in colonic epithelial cells that have been found lead to a failure of the cells to repress DNA synthesis and to undergo normal differentiation. The cells develop an enhanced ability to proliferate.

The simplest characteristic affecting the proliferative behavior of the cells appears in patches of mucosa in man where colonic epithelial cells fail to repress DNA synthesis (demonstrated with microautoradiography) during their migration to the surface of the colonic crypts. (The repression of DNA synthesis during migration to the mucosal surface and maturation is an important feature of normal cells.) These epithelial cells thus begin to develop an enhanced ability to proliferate. This abnormal characteristic develops while the overall or net cell proliferation kinetics are normal (number of cells born = number of cells extruded from the mucosa). The abnormality remains hidden and cannot be seen on conventional morphological examination. It has been called a *Phase 1* proliferative lesion of colonic epithelial cells (Lipkin, 1973a).

The fact that it appears in 3 neoplastic conditions of the colon is of particular interest: in patients with familial polyposis (Deschner and Lipkin, 1973) and after administration of a chemical carcinogen to rodents (Turnherr et al., 1973). As noted above, the lesion also appears in patients in the general population who develop isolated neoplasms of the colon (Lipkin, 1973b).

At another stage of abnormal development, colonic epithelial cells with persistent DNA synthesis also develop other properties that enable them to be retained in the colonic mucosa in increasing numbers. Their net proliferation becomes abnormal, with the birth rate of cells greater than the extrusion rate, and cells begin to accumulate in the

* This work was supported by National Cancer Institute grants — Ca 14991; Ca 08748, and Contract NCI 72-2041.

various morphologically recognizable excrescences. The beginning accumulation of cells with persistent DNA synthesis has been termed a *Phase 2* proliferative lesion of colonic epithelial cells (Lipkin, 1973a).

In addition to the above, other evidences of impaired differentiation have been observed in colon cells during the development of polypoid lesions. RNA and protein synthesis remain elevated in colonic epithelial cells as they develop a *Phase 2* proliferative lesion and accumulate in colonic excrescences. Well differentiated and mature normal colonic epithelial cells incorporate less leucine into protein and uridine into RNA than immature colon cells. However, in the cells of colonic polypoid lesions incorporation of leucine and uridine remains high, comparable to that seen in immature cells (Deschner and Lipkin, 1970).

Activity of the important DNA precursor enzyme thymidine kinase also remains elevated in cells of polypoid lesions as in immature colon cells (Peterson and Lipkin, 1974). The result is that the cells of precancerous lesions retain important characteristics of immature proliferative cells that enable them to continue to synthesize DNA and to proliferate. Metabolic pathways leading to continued DNA synthesis persist in the cells of polypoid lesions in the colon.

Our findings also indicate that the cellular changes described above are accelerated in familial polyposis, for reasons that are still unknown (Deschner and Lipkin, 1973). The findings support the likelihood that these are common changes leading to the neoplastic transformation of colon cells. They also support the concept that a chemical carcinogen contributes to colon cancer in man, since the same proliferative changes develop in rodent after a chemical carcinogen, as develop in man. At this time it is important to understand the complete sequence of molecular events leading to the persistent DNA synthesis and associated abnormalities in these cells, and to determine which carcinogenic influences may be contributing to these cellular defects. Information of this type will be of interest in connection with the detection and prevention of developing neoplasms in the colon, and also in considerations of possible therapy.

References

Deschner, E. and Lipkin, M. (1970): J. nat. Cancer Inst., 44, 175.
Deschner, E. and Lipkin, M. (1973): Proc. Amer. Ass. Cancer Res., 14, 59.
Lipkin, M. (1973a): Cancer (Philad.), in press.
Lipkin, M. (1973b): Physiol. Rev., 53, 891.
Peterson, A. and Lipkin, M. (1974): Proc. Amer. Ass. Cancer Res., 15, 28.
Thurnherr, N., Deschner, E. H., Stonehill, E. H. and Lipkin, M. (1973): Cancer Res., 33, 940.

Precancerous changes in ulcerative colitis and its association with carcinoma of the colon

Chr. Åhrén, L. Hultén and J. Kewenter

Department of Pathology, and Department of Surgery II and III, Göteborg Universitet, Sahlgrenska Sjukhuset, Göteborg, Sweden

The existence of precancerous changes in the colonic or rectal mucosa, analogous to carcinoma in situ of the uterine cervix and the bronchus, has been suggested in occasional cases by a number of authors e.g. Dawson and Pryse-Davies (1959). Morson and Pang (1967) gave a more detailed description of this mucosal lesion in a study of some cases of total colitis with carcinoma and furthermore stressed the possibility of using rectal biopsies as a screening test for patients at risk. Even if they are only a small fraction of all cases of colitis one cannot neglect the fact that in cases of long-standing total colitis the risk of developing carcinoma increases dramatically with time. Any possibility of selecting those patients that are at risk and offering them the opportunity of a prophylactic procto-colectomy must be of great importance, particularly as carcinoma of the colon or rectum in ulcerative colitis usually occurs at an early age. It is well known that in young people carcinoma of the colon is highly malignant and the prognosis is bad. Due to a mainly conservative policy in the treatment of ulcerative colitis in the past decades cases of long standing total colitis are comparatively common in Sweden. As a consequence we have studied the described precancerous mucosal lesion.

Histopathology of 'precancer' of the colon and rectum

Precancerous change in the mucosa appears, either as a diffuse continuous change of the whole mucosa, or as patchy lesions irregularly spread mainly over the recto-sigmoid or the

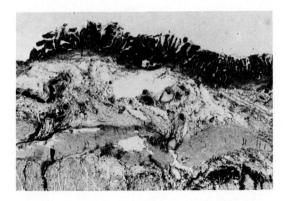

FIG. 1   *Precancerous change of a low villous growth pattern throughout the entire mucosa. vanGieson X 5. Reduced for reproduction 36%.*

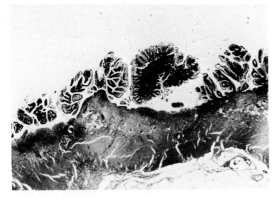

FIG. 2 *Villous precancerous change of a polypoid pattern. There are no true adenomas. vanGieson* **X** *5. Reduced for reproduction 36%.*

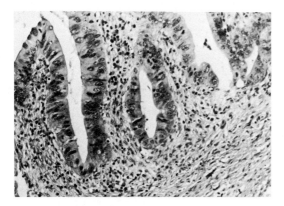

FIG. 3 *Precancerous change at the cellular level. The epithelium has lost its mucus-producing activity. The nuclei are stratified, showing some variation in size and shape and in several areas loss of polarity. Mitoses are frequent and the nucleoli are prominent. The inflammatory reaction in the propria is only moderate. vanGieson* **X** *190. Reduced for reproduction 36%.*

whole large bowel. 'Precancer' occurs in two forms: (1) 'precancer' of flat mucosae (Fig. 1), and (2) 'precancer' of a polypoid pattern (Fig. 2). In both groups the mucosa has a villous surface, sometimes visible macroscopically.

Histologically 'precancer' of the rectal mucosa shows the same cellular changes as carcinoma in situ of other mucous membranes (Fig. 3). The cell nuclei are stratified, enlarged, hyperchromatic, sometimes with prominent nucleoli and furthermore show polymorphism and in focal areas loss of nuclear polarity. The epithelium at the base of the crypts proliferate causing lateral budding (Fig. 4) while the surface epithelium often shows a rather marked increase in mucus production. Epithelial crypts may also be found in the submucosal layer probably due to proliferations through normal defects of the muscularis mucosa or defects following ulcerations. However, in cases where precancerous change is connected with invasive carcinoma it is quite impossible to decide which epithelial crypt is only misplaced and which is truly invasive.

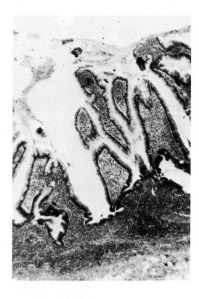

FIG. 4   *'Precancer' of a low villous growth pattern with heavy mucus production in the superficial part and lateral budding of the dark epithelium with hyperchromatic nuclei at the base of the crypts. vanGieson X 30. Reduced for reproduction 36%.*

The validity of individual criteria given for the diagnosis of 'precancer'

The chief difficulty in the diagnosis of precancer in rectal biopsies lies in the risk of confusion with *reactive hyperplasia* which is a common finding even in Crohn's disease and non-specific chronic colitis. Reactive hyperplasia includes many of these cellular changes described as typical of precancer. To evaluate the individual criteria suggested by Morson and Pang (1967) we made a comparative study of 10 cases of Crohn's disease in the colon and 10 cases of subtotal ulcerative colitis of short duration. We also studied nuclear polarity, as loss of polarity is thought to play an important part in carcinoma in situ in other mucous membranes. As can be seen from Table 1 all the individual criteria for the presence of 'precancer' can be readily demonstrated in most of these cases. However, loss of nuclear polarity was never found and neither was true villous splitting of the mucous membrane. Furthermore usually only one or two of these individual criteria were found in one and the same area which means that the 'full picture' of precancerous lesion was never demonstrated. Thus our policy in practice is never to give a clear cut diagnosis of 'precancer' unless all the criteria are found in one and the same area including villous splitting of the membrane and loss of nuclear polarity. This policy may lead to a number of false negative diagnoses but we prefer that to false positive diagnoses, as long as our experience is limited.

TABLE 1   *Occurrence of cellular atypia in operation specimens from 10 cases of Crohn's disease in the colon and 10 cases of subtotal ulcerative colitis of 1 to 4 years' duration*

	No. of cases	Loss of nuclear polarity	Nuclear stratification	Variation in nuclear size and shape	Hyper-chroma-tism	Lateral budding	Increase in number of Paneth cells
Crohn's disease in the colon	10	0	9	9	10	5	5
Subtotal ulcerative colitis of short duration	10	0	10	9	9	2	9

Using the above criteria we confirmed the existence of 'precancer' in 23 out of 25 cases with ulcerative colitis and carcinoma, and in about 50%, continuity between 'precancer' and invasive carcinoma could be demonstrated (Hultén et al., 1972).

TABLE 2   *Occurrence of cellular atypia and/or precancer in rectal biopsies and in operative specimens from 50 patients with ulcerative procto-colitis. Within brackets the number of patients with carcinoma*

Rectal biopsy	Operative specimen			
	No atypia or precancer	Atypia	Precancer	Total
No atypia or precancer	14	9	1	24
Atypia	1	5	10	16
Precancer	0	0	10(5)	10
Total	15	14	21	50

Diagnostic value of rectal biopsies

Being convinced that carcinoma in situ really exists as an entity in the colon and rectum we have also started a pilot study of preoperative rectal biopsies, in patients about to undergo procto-colectomy for total ulcerative colitis, at Sahlgrens hospital in Gothenburg, Sweden. The results are given in Table 2. 'Precancer' was found in 21 out of 50 operation specimens. 5 out of the 21 had early carcinoma although 4 of the 5 were detected only in microscopic sections. In half of these cases 'precancer' was clearly diagnosed from the rectal biopsy. 10 showed only cellular atypia, but most of these were classified as probably precancerous. One case showed no cellular atypia. This high number of false negative diagnoses is in part due to the relative lack of experience of the pathologist, in part due to the fact that we wanted to avoid false positive diagnoses of 'precancer' and furthermore due to the fact that 'precancer' in many cases is patchy and that the rectal biopsy therefore may not be representative. However, this can probably be avoided to a certain degree by increasing the number of rectal biopsies. As can be seen there was no false positive diagnosis.

One may conclude that routine examination of rectal biopsies is of great value in selecting patients at risk with respect to carcinoma. The method is simple and fast and with a proper biopsy technique there is very little risk of complications for the patient. It is of great importance, however, that the biopsy specimens are so mounted, fixed and correctly sectioned as to provide good orientation and that the pathologist is familiar with the diagnostic problems.

Other methods of diagnosing 'precancer' in the colon and rectum.

We have already mentioned the routine examination of multiple rectal biopsies which has proved to be reliable and is, no doubt, the simplest and easiest method available.

Attempts have been made to apply other techniques in the differential diagnosis of inflammatory diseases of the intestinal tract and in the study of carcinoma and precancerous intestinal polyps (Table 3). All these methods are still, however, at the level of basic research and have shown no definite characteristics or patterns so far which could be employed in a routine diagnostic method. Some interesting results have been reported concerning changes in the secretion of acid and neutral mucosubstances in papillomas and

TABLE 3   *Diagnostic methods in precancer of colon and rectum*

1. Rectal biopsy

    (a) routine examination
    (b) histochemistry
    (c) immunofluorscence
    (d) autoradiography (in vitro)

2. Exfoliative cytology

    (a) conventional
    (b) 'forced' (brushing)

in familiary polyposis (see Filipe, 1969; Gad, 1969; Greco et al., 1967). Studies with an immunofluorescence technique, based on the presence of CEA in carcinoma of the colon, have not been encouraging. Earlier studies on CEA in plasma give no reason to believe that detection of the antigen would be of any diagnostic value in the precancerous stage of ulcerative colitis, as the amount of antigen increases only when the carcinoma has grown larger or metastasised.

Some interesting results have been published of in vitro studies on rectal mucosa labeled with tritiated thymidin. Certain differences have been found between mucosa, adenomas and epithelial cells adjacent to an adenoma. So far we know of no investigations of 'precancer' in ulcerative colitis using these techniques, but such investigations would be of great interest.

Attempts have been made to use the conventional *exfoliative cytology* technique in the detection of carcinoma in situ in ulcerative colitis, by Galambos et al. (1956) and Boddington and Truelove (1956), but the method did not prove reliable. However, exfolative cytology has proved of great value in e.g., female genital carcinoma of the urinary bladder. Using a small brush 'forced' exfoliative cytology has proved valuable in the diagnosis of malignant disease of the stomach. In a preliminary study we have tried this technique on the rectal mucosa in ulcerative colitis with 'precancer' and in some cases of large villous papillomata with a suspected focus of malignancy. The study is too preliminary to allow any assessment of the usefulness of the technique. However, it is quite possible to get good material for cytology. The technique gives not only exfoliated, dissociated cells in the smear but also groups of cells. Normal epithelial cells as well as atypical cells with large hyperchromatic nuclei can be demonstrated. An advantage of this technique compared with the conventional rectal biopsy is that brushing a larger surface, of e.g. a large villous papilloma, or rectal mucosa with patchy 'precancer', increases the chance of catching the precancerous cells or hitting the focus of malignancy.

Final remarks

Our studies have lead us to the conclusion that routine examination of rectal biopsies provides a simple and, if correctly handled, reliable method for the diagnosis of 'precancer' in the colon and rectum in ulcerative colitis. We also think that together with other indications, such as long standing total colitis, the demonstration of 'precancer' strongly indicates that prophylactic proctocolectomy should be performed. In the last 3 years we have pursued this policy in Gothenburg and during this time 4 cases of very early carcinoma have been detected. In these cases invasion of the muscularis mucosae had not yet occurred (Fig. 5) and there were no proven metastases.

Whether the mucosal changes described as 'precancer' really represent a true preneoplastic change of the epithelial cells or not remains to be proved. As far as we know it has not yet been shown that these changes are reversible. Irrespective of what we call this

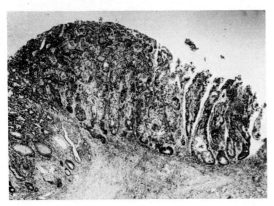

FIG. 5   *'Precancer' of flat mucosa with an early 'microscopic' carcinoma in the centre which has not yet invaded the muscularis mucosa. vanGieson* X *30. Reduced for reproduction 36%.*

mucosal change it is a regularly observed phenomenon in ulcerative colitis with carcinoma and it has not been shown to occur in other forms of colitis. Thus, in practice it has great diagnostic value.

References

Boddington, M. M. and Truelove, S. C. (1956): Brit. med. J., 1, 1318.
Dawson, I. M. P. and Pryse-Davies, J. (1959): Brit. J. Surg., 47, 113.
Filipe, M. I. (1969): Gut, 10, 577.
Gad, A. (1969): Brit. J. Cancer, 23, 52.
Galambos, J. T., Massey, B. W., Klayman, M. I. and Kirsner, J. B. (1956): Cancer (Philad.), 9, 152.
Greco, V., Lauro, G., Fabbriani, A. and Torsoli, A. (1967): Gut, 8, 491.
Hultén, L., Kewenter, J. and Åhrén, Chr. (1972): Scand. J. Gastroent., 7, 663.
Morson, B. C. and Pang, L. S. C. (1967): Gut, 8, 423.

CEA in cancer of the colon*

Norman Zamcheck

Department of Medicine, Harvard Medical School; Mallory GI Research Laboratory, Boston City Hospital; Department of Pathology, Boston University School of Medicine, Boston, Mass., U.S.A.

Gold and Freedman (1965) demonstrated the presence of a glycoprotein antigen in human cancer of the colon and in 1969 Thomson et al. in the Montreal laboratory described a radioimmunoassay for carcinoembryonic antigen (CEA) in serum. The initial series reported 97% positivity in patients with cancer of the colon (Thompson et al., 1969). This finding was promptly confirmed in this laboratory, where 91% positivity was found (Moore et al., 1970), and subsequently by Lo Gerfo in New York City (86%) (Lo Gerfo

TABLE 1   *CEA in colonic cancer: Variations in positivity from series to series*

	Method	No. of cases	'Positivity'* (%)
Montreal (Thomson et al., 1969)	G	36	97
Boston (City Hospital)	G		
Initial series (Moore et al., 1971b) Dec. 1970		35	91
Expanded series (Moore et al., 1971a) May 1971		60	72
Later series (Dhar et al., 1972) July 1972			
Preresection (all stages)		51	59
Postresection with known tumor recurrence		28	96
New York (Lo Gerfo et al., 1970)	H	101	86
Buffalo (Reynoso et al., 1972)	H	33	83
Boston (Lahey Clinic) (Nugent and Hansen, 1971)	G	33	64
London (Chester Beatty) (Laurence et al., 1972)	T	132	67

* See definition of 'positivity' in text

G = Gold's method
H = Hansen's method
T = Todd's method

et al., 1971) and by Reynoso in Buffalo (83%) (Reynoso et al., 1972). An enlarged series from this laboratory later reported a fall in positivity to 72% (Table 1) (Moore et al., 1971a; Dhar et al., 1972). In our initial study we sought patients with 'overt' cases of colonic cancer, many of whom had metastases. Later we sought earlier cases, and the

* The original work reported here was supported by the National Cancer Institute grant (CA-04486) and NIH contract NIH-NCI-E-71-2276; and American Cancer Society grant (CI-19).

This material is an updated modification of articles previously published (see text).

The studies are the work of many collaborators, especially Drs. H. Z. Kupchik, T. L. Moore, P. Dhar, J. J. Sorokin, and R. F. Delwiche, as well as Drs. N. Marcon, A. Keeley, L. S. Gottlieb, and F. Ona.

enlarged series reflects the larger proportion of these. The Gold assay as used in our laboratory and the Hansen (Hansen et al., 1971) and Todd (Egan et al., 1972) assays, as well, are better tests for widespread metastases than for 'early' cancer. A negative assay does not exclude the diagnosis of early cancer although it makes less likely the diagnosis of widespread metastatic cancer; and in patients with known colonic cancer suggests but does not guarantee a favorable prognosis. Of 127 colonic cancer patients, reported later by Dhar from this laboratory (Dhar et al., 1972), tumor was present at the time of assay in 79 (primary in 51, and recurrent or metastatic in 28); serum CEA test results were positive in 57 (72%) of the 79.

Group A. *51 patients with CEA tests done prior to tumor resection*

The incidence of CEA positivity varied from 19% in patients with tumors localized to the bowel wall at operation (Dukes stage A) to 100% in those with distant metastases; those with the more extensive tumors had the higher levels of serum CEA (Table 2). Serum CEA levels, between 2.1 and 2.4 ng/ml in 4 patients became undetectable following resection of the tumors. Tumors were resected in 40 of 51 patients. Of 39 patients who had adenocarcinomas, 18 of 36 with well to moderately well-differentiated tumors and one of 3 with poorly differentiated tumors had positive CEA results. One patient with squamous cell carcinoma of the rectum had a negative CEA result.

TABLE 2   *CEA in colonic cancer: Results on 51 patients tested prior to tumor resection*

Extent of tumor at operation	No.	CEA positive*	CEA 10 ng/ml or greater
1. Localized to bowel wall (Dukes stage A)	16	3 (19%)	1 (6%)
2. Extending to pericolic tissues (Dukes stage B:3; Dukes stage C: 14)	17	9 (53%)	4 (24%)
3. Metastatic to distant tissues	18	18 (100%)	11 (61%)

* CEA level of 2.5 ng/ml or greater in each of duplicate tubes of patients' serum

Group B. *76 patients with CEA tests after tumor resection*

28 of 76 patients had evidence of recurrent or metastatic disease at the time of assay (Fig. 1). Of these, 27 patients (96%) had positive CEA findings. Evidence of hepatic metastases was found in 8 of 19 patients with values greater than 10 ng/ml. 43 (98%) of the 44 patients without evidence of malignancy at the time of assay had negative CEA results. The limitation of these data due (*a*) to the impossibility of ascertaining the exact status of some patients, and (*b*) to the inevitable selection in the study of long-term follow-up patients of 'cured' survivors and the exclusion of patients dying of recurrent cancer, has become apparent on prospective studies.

Lo Gerfo, using the Hansen method, also reported higher occurrence of positivity in patients with more advanced colon cancer: Dukes A (38%); Dukes B (60%); Dukes C (75%); and 'metastatic cancer' (85%) (Lo Gerfo et al., 1972).

Laurence et al. (1972) using a modified Todd assay reported the following correlations of CEA positivity and extent of colorectal tumor: Dukes A (44%); Dukes B (76%); Dukes C (60%); and 'metastasized' (100%).

The diagnostic value of the CEA assay thus varied widely according to the stage of the

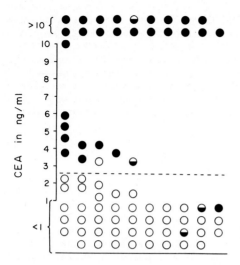

FIG. 1   *Serum CEA in colonic cancer. Results in 76 patients tested only after resection of primary tumors. (o) Patients with no evidence of tumor; (•) Patients with recurrent or metastatic tumor; (◓) Patients with uncertain tumor status.*

tumor. A negative result for preoperative serum CEA determination suggested but did not prove localized tumors, while a strongly positive preoperative serum CEA determination suggested metastases.

Thomson et al. (1969) reported 5 cases in which preoperatively positive assays fell to negative levels after complete resection of colonic cancers. We (Moore et al., 1971a; Dhar et al., 1972) (Fig. 2), Lo Gerfo and his colleagues (Lo Gerfo et al., 1971, 1972), Reynoso and Holyoke at Roswell Park (Reynoso et al., 1972; Holyoke et al., 1972), and Laurence et al. (1972) at Chester Beatty Institute confirmed this finding. Elevated or rising CEA values post-resection were associated with residual or disseminated malignancy and with poor prognosis. Prolonged follow-up observations of many more cases are needed to assess further the use of the assay as an index of completeness of tumor excision.

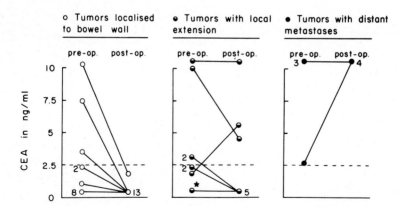

FIG. 2   *Serum CEA in colonic cancer. 26 patients with both pre- and postoperative values. Note: Local extension was accompanied by regional lymph node involvement in all but one patient (*) who had invasion only of the pericolic fat (Dukes stage B).*

26 of our 51 Group A patients had serial pre- and postoperative CEA determinations (Fig. 2) and were observed for 2 to 20 months (average, 8 months) following tumor resection. 14 had tumors limited to the bowel wall and negative CEA test levels following presumed definitive resection of the tumors (Fig. 2, left). Nine of these patients remained well and free from evidence of tumor during the follow-up period; 3 died, apparently of unrelated causes; and 2 others developed metastatic disease secondary to colonic cancer.

Eight patients had local extension of tumors with or without regional lymph node involvement (Fig. 2, center). Three of those with positive CEA determinations following tumor resection included one who subsequently developed local recurrence and 2 who died of suspected (but unproven) metastatic disease. Of the 5 patients with negative postoperative CEA determinations, 4 remained free from evidence of tumor while the fifth eventually developed extensive metastases.

All 4 patients with apparent distant metastases at operation showed positive CEA results following resection of the primary tumors (Fig. 2, right). Three of the 4 died within a year of surgery while the fourth, in the seventh postoperative month at the time of the last follow-up examination, was receiving 5-fluorouracil therapy for peritoneal carcinomatosis.

Positive serum CEA determinations following tumor resection thus showed good correlation with known residual tumor or with the appearance of metastatic disease early in the follow-up period. Negative postoperative CEA levels, however, did not exclude the presence of residual tumor. This was clearly demonstrated by the 3 patients who, despite negative postoperative CEA levels, showed evidence of metastatic disease within 6 to 15 months following surgery. Studies are underway to determine whether serial CEA determinations can detect metastases early enough in the postoperative period to warrant 'second look' surgery.

Potential use of CEA in monitoring chemotherapy   No detailed studies have yet been reported of the use of CEA in monitoring the effect of chemotherapy of digestive tract malignancy, although reports from several laboratories suggest its potential usefulness in this regard (Laurence et al., 1972; Holyoke et al., 1972). Reynoso et al. (1972) observed that the plasma levels of CEA decreased following treatment of 6 children with active neuroblastoma, 2 patients with myeloma and one with Waldenstrom's macroglobulinemia.

Ulcerative colitis   Lo Gerfo et al. (1971) reported that 10 of 31 patients with ulcerative colitis, but without cancer, had positive assays, whereas, using the Gold assay,

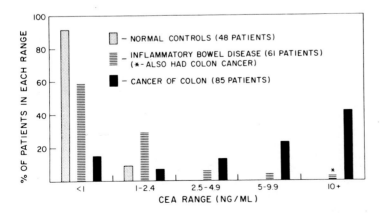

FIG. 3   *Levels of CEA in patients with inflammatory bowel disease or colonic cancer. Number of patients in each range of CEA level is expressed as per cent of the total group.*

we found only one of 61 patients with a persistently elevated positive assay (Moore et al., 1971*a*, 1972); this patient had colonic cancer. Six others had transient CEA elevations without evidence of cancer (Fig. 3). That this difference was due in part to differing selection of patients and in part to differing methodology seems likely (see below). How useful, if at all, the assay will prove to be in helping to select the patients for colectomy who have the greatest risk of cancer of the colon remains to be studied. Other workers have shown higher frequencies of positivity than we have (Laurence et al., 1972; Lebel et al., 1972; Rule et al., 1972).

Benign and malignant polyps   Lo Gerfo et al. (1971) found a positive assay in 1 of 29 patients with benign colonic polyps. The 1 of 15 of our patients with benign polyps who had a positive test (Moore et al., 1971*a*) had cirrhosis of the liver and his assay remained positive after resection of the polyp. Of 5 patients with polyps containing foci of adenocarcinoma in our group only one was positive, and this patient also had cirrhosis. Using immunofluorescence techniques Burtin et al. (1972) identified CEA in all 25 colonic polyps studied with both rabbit anti-CEA antibody and goat anti-CEA antibody. The intensity of fluorescence was variable and, in general, greater in the well-differentiated polyps than in the undifferentiated ones. CEA was always localized on the apical pole of the glandular cells as observed in carcinomas and in fetal intestine. Burtin concluded that 'from an immunological viewpoint polyps behave as cancers'.

Specificity of CEA   Several investigators have indentified CEA or CEA-like antigens in a variety of tumor tissues and normal tissues including normal digestive tract tissues; non-cancerous colonic mucosa (Martin and Martin, 1970; Martin et al., 1972; Von Kleist and Burtin, 1969); polyps, juvenile colonic mucosa and hemorrhoidal mucosa (Burtin et al., 1972*a, b*); in normal lung (Lo Gerfo and Herter, 1972; Pusztaszeri and Mach, 1973); lactating breast (Pusztaszeri and Mach, 1973); normal and cirrhotic liver (Kupchik and Zamcheck, 1972). In each instance, the amount of antigen in the normal or non-malignant tissue was markedly less than that found in the corresponding tumor, especially in the digestive tract.

Each antigen preparation should be assessed chemically, immunochemically and physicochemically before it is called CEA as described by Gold (Gold and Freedman, 1965*a,b*), Krupey et al. (1968), Banjo et al. (1972), and as Terry has done with CEA prepared by Todd (Terry et al., 1972). Martin and Devant (1973) have pointed out that until standards for CEA are universally accepted for clinical laboratory purposes, CEA can only be defined immunologically; i.e., as an antigen giving a reaction of identity with the immunologic system of Gold and co-workers. It is clear that the present assays for CEA are not diagnostically 'specific' for colon cancer.

The methods used for preparation and detection of CEA are highly complex and do not yet lend themselves to 'routine' usage. The Montreal (Gold's) assay (Thomson et al., 1969) analyzes serum and the Hansen and Todd assays (Hansen et al., 1971; Egan et al., 1972) analyze plasma.

A comparative clinical study of both the Hansen and Gold assays, using the respective antisera, performed simultaneously on the same patients' blood specimens was done in this laboratory (Table 3) (Sorokin et al., 1972). Apparent 'differences' between the two assays were primarily quantitative. In the low ranges of antigenemia, values obtained using the Hansen technique were slightly higher than those obtained on the same blood with the Gold technique. The Gold assay tended to read higher than the Hansen assay in the patients with alcoholic liver disease, when values (Gold) were greater than 4 ng/ml. The lowest frequency of agreement between the assays occurred in those groups with low levels of antigen including postoperative colon cancer patients and in ulcerative colitis (Moore et al., 1972) (see Fig. 4). This probably reflects variations inherent in the assays as currently performed.

Variations around the 2.5 ng/ml level accounted for 83% of the apparent non-correlations between 'positive' and 'negative' values. Laurence et al. (1972) found qualitative

TABLE 3   *Comparison of assays for carcinoembryonic antigen: Positive vs. negative*

	Number of comparisons					Agreement*	
Gold (Boston) vs.	+	+	−	−			
Hansen (Boston)	+	−	+	−	Total	Expected	Observed
Malignant - Diseases	50	9	6	47	112	52%	87%
Nonmalignant - Diseases	34	14	6	68	122	54%	84%
Total	84	23	12	115	234	51%	85%
Gold (Boston) vs.	+	+	−	−			
Hansen (Nutley)	+	−	+	−	Total	Expected	Observed
Malignant - Diseases	48	1	13	28	90	53%	83%
Nonmalignant - Diseases	36	7	6	49	98	51%	87%
Total	84	8	19	77	188	50%	86%
Hansen (Boston) vs.	+	+	−	−			
Hansen (Nutley)	+	−	+	−	Total	Expected	Observed
Malignant - Diseases	33	0	15	20	68	55%	78%
Nonmalignant - Diseases	20	1	9	48	78	56%	87%
Total	53	1	24	68	146	50%	83%

* The differences between 'Observed' and 'Expected' agreements are statistically highly significant (p < 0.001) in all categories

agreement in 72% of 272 assays performed on plasma samples by both the Todd and Hansen assays. Further study is needed to define 'positivity'.

Studies of the Gold assay in this laboratory were performed with antigens and antisera provided by the Montreal group. The CEA and resulting antisera used for Gold's initial clinical studies may have been different from those in use today by this and by other laboratories (Kupchik et al., 1972).

Other assays (Lange et al., 1971; MacSween et al., 1972; Go et al., 1972) are presently being studied for possible clinical use. Antigens must be extracted from normal and malignant tissues of all organs and compared. Assay methods must be developed to exploit differences in type or amount of antigen.

Importance of quantitative amounts of CEA   The differences in CEA content between cancerous and noncancerous digestive tissues appear to be quantitative rather than qualitative. 'Malignant' may be differentiated from 'nonmalignant' diseases in part by the *amount* of CEA-like substances found in serum or plasma. The present low serum threshold of positivity (2.5 ng/ml is generally used in the Gold and Hansen assays) misses fewer cancers at the price of reporting more 'false-positive' assays. By setting a higher threshold (for example, greater than 5 ng/ml), greater reliability of a positive diagnosis is achieved at the price of missing some cancers; unfortunately at that threshold many of those missed with the present assays are likely to be 'early' lesions.

At present, with existing assay methods, the use of a high 'threshold of positivity' has some advantages (although there is room for disagreement on this point). Experience has taught pathologists that 'false-positive' diagnoses of cancer may lead to unwarranted surgery. Established diagnostic practices should be followed until more experience with the use of these and newer assays has been gained.

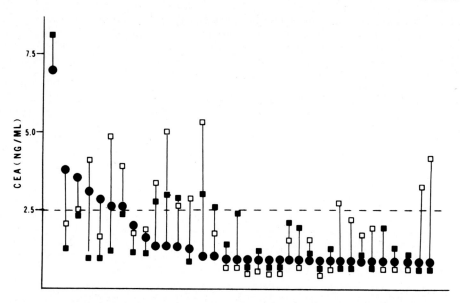

FIG. 4   *Comparison of serum and plasma assays for CEA in patients with inflammatory bowel disease. Serum and plasma samples were drawn at the same time and frozen at -40°C until used. Both assays were considered positive if duplicate tubes of patient's serum contained at least 2.5 ng of CEA/ml. (●) Serum assay (Boston); (■) Plasma assay (Boston); (□) Plasma assay (Nutley, N.J.).*

Conclusion

The CEA studies to date support the promise of clinically useful tests for the detection and diagnosis of colon cancer that may also help assess adequacy of surgical resection and the presence and extent of metastases. The use of this new method may permit better evaluation of premalignant states such as ulcerative colitis (Zamcheck and Moore, 1971).

When the CEA assay or its successor becomes perfected, and reagents are standardized, immunochemical diagnosis will be an important adjunct to (but not a substitute for) experienced clinical judgment and complete X-ray and laboratory study. Whether it will do so early enough to improve prognosis remains to be determined. The performance and interpretation of such assays will require the participation of pathologists, immunologists, and others experienced in the practical diagnosis of malignant tumors and aware of the risks to the patient of misuse of the assays.

Note: Coligan et al. (1972) report that with their method normal serum shows an apparent CEA content of about 0 ng/ml or about 2.5 ng/ml depending on whether the assay is referred to a standard curve obtained with CEA in normal serum or in buffered saline. Using a modification of the Todd assay, Laurence et al. (1972) reported that, in all normal male and female Caucasians studied, the plasma CEA content was less than 12.5 ng/ml.

References

Banjo, C., Gold, P., Freedman, S. O. and Krupey, J. (1972): Nature New Biol., 238, 183.

Burtin, P., Martin, E., Sabine, M. C. and Von Kleist, S. (1972a): J. nat. Cancer Inst., 48, 25.
Burtin, P., Sabine, M. C. and Chavanel, G. (1972b): Int J. Cancer, 10, 72.
Coligan, J. E., Egan, M. L. and Todd, C. W. (1972): Nat. Cancer Inst. Monogr., 427.
Dhar, P., Moore, T. L., Zamcheck, N. and Kupchik, H. Z. (1972): J. Amer. med. Ass., 221, 31.
Egan, M. I., Lautenschleger, J. T., Coligan, J. E. and Todd, C. W. (1972): Immunochemistry, 9, 289.
Go, V. L. W., Schutt, A. J., Moertel, C. G., Summerskill, W. H. J. and Butt, H. R. (1972): Gastroenterology, 62, 754.
Gold, P. and Freedman, S. O. (1965a): J. exp. Med., 121, 439.
Gold, P. and Freedman, S. O. (1965b): J. exp. Med., 122, 467.
Hansen, H. J., Lance, K. P. and Krupey, J. (1971): Clin. Res., 19, 143.
Holyoke, D., Reynoso, G. and Chu, T. M. (1971): Ann. Surg., 176, 559.
Krupey, J., Gold, P. and Freedman, S. O. (1968): J. exp. Med., 128, 387.
Kupchik, H. Z. and Zamcheck, N. (1972): Gastroenterology, 63, 95.
Kupchik, H. Z., Hansen, H. J., Sorokin, J. J. and Zamcheck, N. (1972): In: Monograph on Proceedings Second Conference and Workshop on Embryonic and Fetal Antigens in Cancer, pp. 261-265. Oak Ridge National Laboratory, Oak Ridge, Tenn., 1972.
Lange, R. D., Chernoff, A. I., Jordan, T. A. and Collmann, I. R. (1971): In: Proceedings, First Conference and Workshop on Embryonic and Fetal Antigens in Cancer, pp. 379-388. Oak Ridge National Laboratories, Oak Ridge, Tenn., 1971.
Laurence, D. J. R., Stevens, U., Bettelheim, R., Darcy, D., Leese, C., Turberville, C., Alexander, P., Johns, E. W. and Neville, A. M. (1972): Brit. med. J., 3, 605.
Lebel, J. S., Deodhar, S. D. and Brown , C. H. (1972): Dis. Colon Rect., 15, 111.
Lo Gerfo, P. and Herter, F. (1972): J. Surg. Oncol., 1, 7.
Lo Gerfo, P., Krupey, J. and Hansen, H. (1970): New Engl. J. Med., 285, 138.
Lo Gerfo, P., Krupey, J., Herter, F., Barker, H. G. and Hansen, H. J. (1971): Amer. J. Surg., 123, 127.
MacSween, J. M., Warner, N. L., Bankhurst, A. D. and Mackay, I. R. (1972): Brit. J. Cancer, 26, 356.
Martin, F. and Devant, J. (1973): J. nat. Cancer Inst., 50, 1375.
Martin, F. and Martin, M. S. (1970): Int. J. Cancer, 6, 352.
Martin, F., Martin, M. S., Bordes, M. and Bourgeaux, C. (1972): Europ. J. Cancer, 8, 315.
Moore, T. L., Dhar, P., Zamcheck, N. and Kupchik, H. Z. (1971a): In: Proceedings, First Conference and Workshop on Embryonic and Fetal Antigens in Cancer, pp. 393-400. Oak Ridge National Laboratories, Oak Ridge, Tenn.
Moore, T. L., Kantrowitz, P. A. and Zamcheck, N. (1972): J. Amer. med. Ass., 222, 944.
Moore, T. L., Kupchik, H. Z., Marcon, N. and Zamcheck, N. (1971b): Amer. J. dig. Dis., 16, 1. (Also published as abstract in 1970 in Clin. Res., 18, 680).
Nugent, F. W. and Hansen, E. R. (1971): Lahey Clin. Bull., 20, 85.
Pusztaszeri, G. and Mach, J. P. (1973): Immunochemistry, 10, 197.
Reynoso, G., Chu, T. M., Holyoke, D., Cohen, E., Valensuela, L. A., Nemoto, T., Wang, J. J., Chuang, J., Guinan, P. and Murphy, G. P. (1972): J. Amer. med. Ass., 220, 361.
Rule, A. H., Straus, E., Vandevoorde, J. and Janowitz, H. D. (1972): New Engl. J. Med., 287, 24.
Sorokin, J. J., Kupchik, H. Z., Zamcheck, N. and Dhar, P. (1972): Immunol. Commun., 1, 11.
Terry, W. D., Henkart, P. A., Coligan, J. E. and Todd, C. W. (1972): J. exp. Med., 136, 200.
Thomson, D. M. P., Krupey, J., Freedman, S. O. and Gold, P. (1969): Proc. nat. Acad Sci. (Wash.), 64, 161.
Von Kleist, S. and Burtin, P. (1969): Int. J. Cancer, 8, 874.
Zamcheck, N. and Moore, T. L. (1972): New Engl. J. Med., 287, 43.

Cancer of the colon and rectum: Diagnostic methods

Antonello Franchini

Department of Surgery, St. Orsola University Hospital, Bologna, Italy

The diagnostic methods for cancer of the large intestine can be distinguished in 3 groups: those directed simply towards localizing the tumor, those directed towards establishing its local extension and those for the diagnosis of the advanced stages and recurrences.

Endoscopy and radiology are included in the first group with various techniques which today permit us to discover the tumor even in its initial stages. It is then possible to conduct a precise study of the tumor's anatomical patterns and in particular its extension and diffusion, by means of angiography and lymphography. Finally, many other methods are used by which it is possible to recognize the secondary invasion of other organs and even the recurrences after surgical treatment (Table 1).

It is evident that such numerous methods do not allow us to describe various techniques nor give detailed information of them all; it will be sufficient to mention only their use and give a rapid evaluation of the relative advantages and disadvantages.

The prime importance of *sigmoidoscopy* in the diagnosis of cancer of the large intestine results from the observation, now evidenced by universal experience, that 70% of

TABLE 1   *Detection methods for cancer of the colon and rectum*

Methods for localizing the tumor	Methods for establishing grade of spreading	Methods for diagnosing advanced stages and recurrences
Exfoliative cytology		
Endoscopy:		
rectosigmoidoscopy	Selective angiography	Thoracic X-ray
endoscopy with large tube	Lymphangiography	Paracentesis
fibercolonoscopy	Liver scan	Laparoscopy
operative colonoscopy	Thoracic X-ray	Needle biopsy
Radiology:		Cystoscopy and urography
conventional barium enema		Radiophosphorus
double contrast study		Etc.
hypotonic rectosigmoidography		
bowel parietography		
visualisation with intravenous P.V.P.		
Angiography:		
aortography		
selective angiography		
Silicone foam diagnostic enema		

the cases localize in the rectum and sigmoid — areas within reach of the instruments. The only technical limitation of the method remains in the impossibility to scour the entire tract covered by the length of the tube; this occurs in about 10 — 12% of the cases, because of sharp turns of the intestine or narrowed lumen due to many anatomical and pathological reasons. On the other hand, when favorable conditions recur, the exam can be carried out with a 'big tube' as proposed by Parturier, which is a rectoscope with a proximal diameter of 5 cm and a distal one of 3.5 cm. Its shape permits an excellent endoscopic view with only a frontal mirror without special lighting.

Colonoscopy with optical fiber flexible instruments has acquired popularity in the last few years. The technical progress of this method as compared to traditional sigmoidoscopy does not depend only on the obvious consideration which ensues from the different lengths of the two instruments (i.e. the possibility to explore with the coloscope all of the intestinal tract above the sigmoid colon), but also because of the possibility to explore the sigmoid itself (this to substitute sigmoidoscopy) in the cases mentioned, where traditional endoscopy is not possible.

An opinion on optical fiber colonoscopy cannot be but positive, for in practice, it permits the discovery of all the intestinal tumors, benign and malignant, even the more minute growths of the mucosa vividly evident in the brilliant ocular image. It should not be forgotten, however, that its use in long distances is not at all easy and requires a high degree of training and not mere skill.

Fiber colonoscopy has supplanted *operative colonoscopy* which until now was indicated during tumor operations when there were doubts concerning the extent of removal, or the suspicion of concomitant polyps. Colotomy presents a surgical risk — bound to possible infection — too high for a simple diagnostic method besides encountering technical difficulties related to the not always convenient preparation of the colon.

In spite of the progress in endoscopy the X-ray continues to maintain an irreplaceable position in tumor diagnosis of the large intestine. It is better to admit, however, that the *traditional barium enema* has its limits: difficult cleaning of the feces from certain segments of the colon, over-abundance of folds in other tracts especially sigmoid and flexures, rendering the reading uncertain, overlapping of non-dissociable intestinal loops etc. Therefore, perfect techniques must be used with a meticulously clean colon, the use of liquid barium, the use of high-voltage apparatus, image intensifier, spot camera, film X—ray, and above all *double contrast methods*.

The last are now a part of all modern radiological services in spite of high costs and longer performance, provide maximum details in the morphological study of the mucosa and are above all indicated in the study of polyposis and in the initial stages of malignancy.

During the exam anticholinergic drugs and local anesthetics can be administered, obtaining a transient hypotonic and hypokinetic state of the viscus. This preparation called *hypotonic recto-sigmoidography* (Schiffino et al., 1964) consents a detailed study of the mucosa. Besides a simultaneous gaseous insufflation, intra- and extra-visceral views can be taken obtaining very precise reliefs from the double contrast. This method is called *parietography of the bowel*.

Among the radiological methods, we can recall the visualization of rectal cancer by injection of polyvinylpyrrolidone with bismuth and iron, which impregnates the tumor tissues rendering them opaque (Bodkin, 1967).

Selective angiography of the mesenteric arteries can serve as a 'research' method of an abdominal tumor when there is a strong suspicion and the traditional exams prove negative and can serve as a 'study', when desired, for establishing the benign or malignant nature of an ascertained abdominal tumor and make an exact anatomical inventory of its extension, morphology and vascularization.

Selective arteriography by transcutaneous femoro-aortic catheter represents an indisputable technical progress as compared to traditional aortography. Its main field of study is represented by digestive hemorrhages of any nature whether acute or chronic; the hemorrhage can be viewed outside the vascular bed or the responsible lesion identified. In the case of tumors, these are identified by the presence of 'tumor vessels': increased diameter of the arteries, morphological and structural anarchy of the arterioles, arteriovenous shunts etc. In certain cases a parenchymography of the tumor is obtained.

On the whole, opinion on arteriography is positive and direct experience induces its recommendation as a valuable diagnostic method.

On the other hand, *lymphography* by the Kinmonth method and variants does not enjoy generally favorable opinions. It is applied in the study of the lymphatic spread of tumors of the bowel, being previously known not to visualize the lymph nodes near the colon but only the iliac and lumbar-aortic ones which are only rarely invaded. The findings, moreover, are difficult to interpret and the morphological alterations, whether of the lymphatic vessels or of the lymph nodes (variations of size, number, defects of opacity, irregularity etc.), do not always correspond to the presence of neoplastic invasion. A reliable pattern instead is that of the lymphatic block, that is, of the diminished or missed mono- or bi-lateral injection. This pattern indicates compression or invasion of the corresponding lymphatic territories and characterizes the cases of pelvic carcinosis or of advanced infiltration of the perirectal organs and tissues.

With greater experience, however, lymphography can become a useful instrument whether as a guide in lymph node removal or to avoid useless operations when the tumor has by-passed surgical resources.

Liver scanning is widely justified in the pre-operative study of bowel tumors in search of hepatic metastasis. These are present in 10—15% of the cases and their preliminary identification is very important whether to avoid useless operations or to be ready for eventual hepatic resections.

On the scanning sheet the metastatic liver presents multiple irregular areas more often luke-warm rather than cold, but the descriptions are not always so evident. The limits of scanning are represented by false positivity and false negativity — these last due to the fact that the nodules are smaller than 2—3 cm — or because they lie very deeply or vanish due to respiratory movements or are not visible due to a defect in the instrument.

In spite of these limitations (about 20% of the false results) liver scanning is advantageous as compared to all the other direct methods in predicting hepatic metastasis and in particular the B.S.F. and alkaline phosphatase.

The diagnosis of advanced Ca of the bowel or even of the generalization phase ceases to follow particular rules and depends on the most common methods as suggested by general semeiotics. Recourse is made therefore to the thoracic X-ray to search for the not rare pulmonary mestastasis, to cystoscopy and urography to show the secondary invasion of the ureters and bladder, with eventual colon-bladder fistula, gyn.-exam, abdominal exploration whether with paracentesis if ascites is present, or with laparoscopy, examination of the lymph stations, etc. It is not necessary to dwell on these findings, since they are quite obvious. More important, on the other hand, is the problem of recurrences after surgical treatment. We know that they are revealed by general signs (weight loss) mostly with local signs represented by perineal pain (after abdominal-perineal resection) and rectal bleeding (after resection with anastomosis). In the first case verification is necessary by exploration of the perineal scar whether with palpation or with needle biopsy. In the second case the anastomosis has to be explored with endoscopy and barium enema to search for recurrences on the suture line. This finding is not always easy because the morphological alterations due to surgical anastomosis can be confused with those of the tumor. For this D.D. a Geiger counter can be used, applied to the tip of a probe and introduced into the intestine by means of sigmoidoscopy (Nelson). Injecting radioactive phosphorus which is fixed and remains in the malignant tissues much longer and in higher concentrations than in normal tissues, the G. counter will signal the presence of the tumor even when it is beneath the mucosa or in the midst of a polyposis or pseudopolyposis.

Undoubtedly, an attentive consideration of the recurrence problem will allow discovery of surgically treatable lesions and therefore prolong the life in a certain number of patients.

Not to mention that the systematic control of every patient who has undergone surgery for Ca of the bowel permits us to discover in a certain number of cases an ignored second tumor completely distinct and independent from the very first.

References

Bodkin, L. G. (1967): Dis. Colon Rect., 10, 197.
Schiffino, A., Paolini, F. and Madonia, G. (1964): Minerva gastroent., 10, 208.

Cancer of the colon and rectum

Discussion

Dr. Burdette: Members of the audience are invited to join the discussion or ask members of the panel questions at this time.

Dr. Victor A. Gilbertson: Please clarify the distinction being made between carcinoma of the colon and rectum.

Dr. Wynder: The statistics for each site do not vary sufficiently to suggest that variations in assigning the location of neoplasia introduce a very great error.

Dr. Burdette: The exact point of demarcation between colon and rectum has not been precisely defined. Most surgeons consider that the rectum begins approximately at the sacral promontory where redundancy of the sigmoid terminates. Some clinicians believe that a more logical division on a functional basis is at the midtransverse colon. Although the numbers of neoplasms exhibit a distal increment, studies of the epithelium itself have revealed little to distinguish that derived from the colon from that derived from the rectum.

Dr. Altares: A series of illustrative slides will demonstrate modern radiologic diagnostic techniques for carcinoma of the colon and rectum and carcinoma appearing in cases of ulcerative colitis.

Dr. Chopra: Attention should be directed to the situation in East Africa where there is variation in carcinoma of the large bowel between the different races. It offers an interesting opportunity for studies on etiology.

Dr. Burdette: Dr. Wynder, you suggested that animals had limited usefulness in the study of colorectal carcinoma. Since there are obvious uses for such models, would you clarify your statement?

Dr. Wynder: If one is to conduct metabolic studies relative to carcinogenesis, metabolic pathways in some laboratory animals do not correspond to those in man. Therefore such studies with laboratory animals should take this into consideration. For example, a primate might yield useful information in a given study, whereas a rodent would not be suitable at all.

Dr. Rubel: Please comment on the incidence of colonic and rectal carcinoma in populations that eat a high-fat, low-carbohydrate diet (e.g., the Eskimos).

Dr. Wynder: Unfortunately there are not sufficient numbers of Eskimos accessible for clinical studies. Therefore we are better advised to draw conclusions when there are sufficient numbers with differences in incidence and in which required measurements can be made. For example, the migrants from Japan to Hawaii and California are a very promising group for study. Fortunately there continue to be funds available for such studies from the U.S. Public Health Service. An additional category is the possibility for obtaining support by applying to the Colorectal Cancer Program for which funds have been set aside as a result of the work of the planning committee chaired by Dr. Burdette.

Dr. Makari: Our results with the intradermal test for cancer we have described (Makari, J. G. (1969): The Intradermal Cancer Test (ICT). *J. Amer. Geriatrics Soc. 17*, 755) suggest that it may be useful in diagnosing carcinoma of the colon and rectum.

Dr. Burdette: Is the intradermal test your group uses related in any way to the intradermal test described for detecting CEA by Dr. Herberman and colleagues? Also, would you comment more on the failure of the test to persist when neoplasms of the colon and rectum are completely excised.

Dr. Makari: As far as we know our procedure is different from that for CEA. Reversal after cure is a characteristic of this test, although other hypersensitivity tests are known to persist.

Dr. Martin: We have induced tumors in BD rats with 1,2-dimethyl hydrazine and recently have successfully transplanted several lines in the BD IX strain.

Dr. Burdette: Two years ago we were able to transplant adenocarcinoma induced in BD II rats into animals of the same line. There are 10 of these strains and several have been inbred for over 20 generations. Dr. Martin, have you been able to obtain a carcino-embryonic antigen that cross-reacts with antiserum against human CEA?

Dr. Martin: So far in our studies, which are in the initial stages, there has been no cross-reaction.

Dr. Burdette: The results presented during this segment of the meeting lead to optimism that colorectal carcinoma, a disease associated with a Western life style being assumed by more and more people, may be detected earlier and perhaps even prevented as soon as the approaches discussed are fully explored.

3. Cancer of the lung

Lung cancer

Richard Doll

Department of Medicine, University of Oxford, Oxford, United Kingdom

Few if any cancers can be of so much interest to our conference as cancer of the lung. It is common throughout a large part of the world, highly lethal with normal methods of diagnosis, and very largely preventible — if only we could persuade people to act on the available knowledge. For the academic oncologist, lung cancer has provided a wealth of fascinating data that have already contributed much to knowledge of the causes of cancer and there is reason to suppose that it can still contribute much more.

Subsequent speakers will discuss whether we can use radiology and cytology to diagnose lung cancer at a stage of development when a higher proportion of cases can be cured or even at a pre-invasive stage, when it may be possible to prevent the development of overt disease. Others will discuss the practicability of prevention by changing the character of cigarettes or by reducing exposure to asbestos. Before calling on them, however, it may be helpful to review briefly the principal features of the aetiology of the disease.

Comparison of incidence rates throughout the world, standardised for age within the limits of 35 and 65 years of age so as to avoid falsely low figures due to inadequate case finding in older people (Doll, 1972), shows five notable features. First, lung cancer is the commonest type of cancer in men in a large part of the world, with the possible exception of skin cancer, which is often incompletely recorded. If skin cancer is excluded, lung cancer is the commonest type of cancer in men in half the populations reported in the International Union's collection of registry data (U.I.C.C., 1970) and falls below third place in order of frequency in only 4 out of 55 populations. Secondly, the incidence of the disease varies some 40-fold from Scotland, England, Finland, and Hawaii to Nigeria and Uganda. Thirdly, the disease is much less common in women than in men; among the 55 populations examined in the International Union's book, it is the third commonest in only one, and is relatively less common in all the others. High male rates are accompanied by moderately high female rates only among the Maoris of New Zealand, among whom it is several times commoner in women than in most European countries. High male rates are often accompanied by low female rates and the sex ratio varies from 10:1 in Finland and Latvia to 1:1 in Nigeria. Fourthly, the disease is appreciably less common in men in the U.S.A., Canada, Australia, and South Africa than it is in Britain and much of Europe, despite the fact that the number of cigarettes smoked per person in these countries is as great or greater than it is in Britain. Fifthly, the disease was rare in all countries before the first world war and has become common only in the last 30 years.

The importance of cigarette smoking as a causal factor has been demonstrated frequently, but there are a number of aspects which still need clarifying. I have referred to the relatively low incidence in some countries in comparison with the number of cigarettes smoked; and it is still not clear how far this discrepancy can be accounted for by such factors as age at starting to smoke, the length of butt thrown away, the number of puffs taken per cigarette, the use of filter tips, and perhaps the character of the tobacco as well as the relative extent to which tobacco is smoked in cigarettes, cigars, and pipes. Data from prospective studies in America and from retrospective studies in Britain show

TABLE 1   *Mortality from lung cancer in non-smokers and in women, standardized for age*

Population	Sex	Rate per 100,000
Non-smokers, Britain	M	5.5
,, ,, U.S.A.	M	6.1
,, ,, ,,	F	4.2
All Portugal	F	3.8
,, Norway	F	4.3
,, Switzerland	F	4.9
,, Netherlands	F	5.1
,, France	F	5.5
,, Finland	F	5.9
,, Belgium	F	6.4
,, Sweden	F	6.4
,, Italy	F	6.5
,, Australia	F	6.9
,, Japan	F	7.1
,, German F. R.	F	7.5
,, New Zealand	F	7.7
,, Canada	F	7.8
,, Chile	F	8.2
,, Austria	F	9.1
,, U.S.A. white	F	9.7
,, S. Africa white	F	10.0
,, U.S.A. non-white	F	10.0
,, N. Ireland	F	10.4
,, Denmark	F	10.7
,, Israel	F	11.5
,, Ireland	F	11.6
,, England and Wales	F	15.5
,, Scotland	F	16.9

that the mortality in non-smokers is much the same in each sex, being perhaps 50% higher in men than in women, and is almost identical in men in both countries (Table 1). In these countries the mortality among male non-smokers is near the lower end of the range of mortality rates among all women, irrespective of smoking habits, in the 25 populations throughout the world reported in detail by Segi and Kurihara (1972).

Atmospheric pollution by coal smoke and the fumes of motor exhausts has long been suspected as another cause, mainly on the grounds that the incidence of the disease is greater in the towns than in the country. Direct evidence is, however, weak and considerations like those I have referred to make it unlikely that pollution plays any major role — a conclusion that is borne out by the relatively small increase in risk that has been observed in men who are heavily exposed to the combustion products of coal and oil in the course of their work. It seems probable, however, that it plays some small part, possibly in combination with other factors. Asbestos particles constitute another form of pollution which, like motor fumes, has increased steadily over the last 50 years. The amount present is still relatively small but could be of importance in the future — particularly in the production of pleural mesothelioma.

The effect of ionizing radiations has been known since it was realised that the miners in Schneeberg and Jachymov had been exposed to large amounts of radon in the air of the mines. It has been confirmed in the uranium miners of Colorado, the fluorspar miners of Newfoundland, and the haematite miners of England, as well as in the survivors of the atomic bomb explosions in Hiroshima and Nagasaki and in patients who have been irradiated for the treatment of ankylosing spondylitis. If the carcinogenic effect is proportional to the dose, the small amounts of radon in normal air and the radioactive isotopes in our bodies must contribute some small part to the basic incidence of the

TABLE 2   *Lung cancer: Occupational hazards*

Exposure to high concentrations of radon

    Miners in Schneeberg and Jachymov
    Uranium miners in Colorado
    Fluorspar miners in Newfoundland
    Haematite miners in England

Chromate manufacture

Nickel refining

Manufacture of coal gas

Exposure to arsenic

    In vineyards
    Sheep-dip manufacture

Exposure to asbestos

    Asbestos factories
    Insulation work

Manufacture of mustard gas

* Exposure to di-chlor-di-methyl ether

? Tyre manufacturers (moulders, etc.)

---

  * For animal experiments see Laskin et al. (1971)

disease. Histological studies suggest that ionizing radiations are particularly likely to cause the oat cell variants of the disease.

At least 7 other occupational hazards have been recognised, some of which have been responsible for causing 20 or 30% of deaths in exposed men. These are listed in Table 2. The last two hazards have been described only in the last two years, and I am grateful to Dr. Lloyd Davies, Chief Medical Officer of the Department of Employment in England for permission to refer to the possible hazard among rubber workers, a report of which will be published shortly in the British Journal of Cancer.

From these and other data it has been concluded that some 80 to 90% of cases in men can be prevented in all those countries in which the disease is common. Practical application is difficult, but 3 observations are encouraging. First, the effect of stopping smoking is observed much more quickly than might have been expected, the incidence of the disease being affected appreciably within 5 years (see, for example, Doll, 1971). Secondly, Dr. Wynder has shown that it may be possible to reduce the risk of the disease by changing the method of manufacutring cigarettes (*This Volume*, p. 146). Thirdly, Professor Selikoff has shown that changes in smoking habits may also modify the extent of occupational hazards (*This Volume*, p. 152).

For the rest, our hope lies, as with other cancers, in early diagnosis.

References

Doll, R. (1971): J. roy. stat. Soc. Series A., 134, 133.
Doll, R. (1972): Proc. roy. Soc. Med., 65, 49.

Laskin, S., Kuschner, M., Drew, R. T., Cappiello, V. P. and Nelson, N. (1971): Arch. environ. Hlth, 23, 135.

Segi, M. and Kurihara, M. (1972): Cancer Mortality for Selected Sites in 24 Countries No. 6., 1966-67. Japan Cancer Society Segi Institute of Cancer Epidemiology, Nagoya.

U.I.C.C. (1970): Cancer Incidence in Five Continents, Vol. II. Editors: R. Doll, C. S. Muir and J. A. H. Waterhouse. Springer Verlag, Berlin.

Epidemiological study of lung cancer in the district of Kolín, Czechoslovakia

A. Kubík

Tuberculosis and Respiratory Diseases Research Institute, Prague, Czechoslovakia

The epidemiological study of lung cancer is a prospective investigation of 12,322 males aged 40-64 years each of whom had a normal chest X-ray on entry into the study (Kubík et al., 1970, 1972). The objectives of the study are as follows:
    1. To ascertain basic data on smoking habits and prevalence of respiratory symptoms in the study population.
    2. To study the distribution of the risk of developing lung cancer and its natural history.
    3. To test a simple technique, suitable for large scale investigations, for identifying which groups of persons have a greater risk of developing lung cancer than the average for their age group.

Methods

The study has been carried out since 1966 in the district of Kolín, which lies 50 km east of Prague and is both industrial and agricultural in character. There is a total population of approximately 100,000 inhabitants.
    In the course of the first year of the study (1966), during a mass survey of the population, a photofluorogram of 70 × 70 mm was done and a brief interview was held with each male examinee aged 40-64 years. The interviewers (experienced chest clinic nurses) were trained in the application of the questionnaire in order to standardize the interview technique. The questions concerned smoking habits, the presence of a cough during the past year, the worsening of a cough, expectoration of sputum, blood-spitting and any pneumonic episodes in the past year.
    A 'cigarette-smoker' was defined as a person who was smoking regularly and had smoked not less than 1,000 cigarettes up to the day of the interview. An 'ex-smoker' was defined as a smoker who had stopped regular smoking 6 months ago or earlier. The approximate total number of cigarettes smoked to date was estimated on the basis of the approximate number of smoking years and the average daily consumption of cigarettes; a Table presented as a supplement to Regulation No. 26/1965 of the Czechoslovak Ministry of Health was used. The severity of the symptoms, coughing and the expectoration of sputum, was evaluated according to the answer to a simple question about their presence on most days for as much as 3 months in the past year. The total duration of the interview did not exceed 2 min as a rule.
    During subsequent years lung cancer was diagnosed in patients asking for medical advice on account of their symptoms. In addition, in the year 1969 cases were detected as a result of a mass X-ray survey of the population. Only males in whom lung cancer had been confirmed, by histologial or cytological examination of material obtained from the respiratory system during the patient's life, or by post-mortem examination, were admitted to the present analysis. Data for the patients recorded during the mass survey on entry into the study was then extracted from the file.

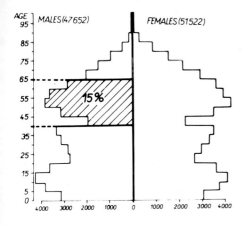

FIG. 1   *Age and sex distribution of popula-*
tion – Kolín district (31/12/1965).

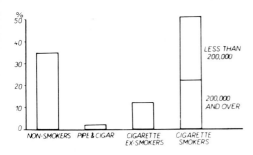

FIG. 2   *Smoking history of 12,322 males*
aged 40-64 years with normal chest
film (Kolín district, 1966).

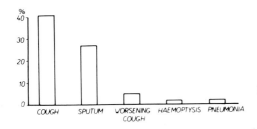

FIG. 3   *Respiratory complaints of 12,322*
males aged 40-64 years with normal
chest film (Kolín district, 1966).

Results

Males aged 40-64 years represented approximately 15% of the total population of the
district of Kolín (Fig. 1). Of these, a group of 12,322 males, aged 40-64 years, with a
normal photofluorogram and a complete interview record obtained during the mass survey in the year 1966, were eligible for the long-term study. In this group there were 35%
non-smokers, 2% cigar or pipe smokers, 12% cigarette ex-smokers, and 51% current
cigarette smokers (Fig. 2). Less than half the number of current cigarette smokers (22%
of all males) have smoked a total of 200,000 or more cigarettes, the remaining fraction of
smokers (29% of all males) have smoked fewer. 41% of the interviewed males had a cough
during the past year of at least 3 months' duration and in 5% the cough had got progress-

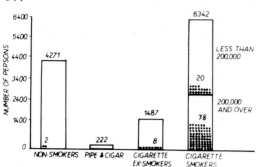

FIG. 4   *Distribution of 108 proved lung cancer cases by smoking history (5.5 year follow-up).*
           (● Confirmed lung cancer)

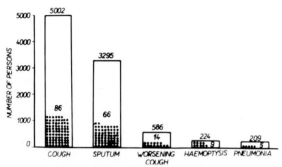

FIG. 5   *Incidence of confirmed lung cancer by respiratory complaints (5.5 year follow-up).*
           (● Confirmed lung cancer)

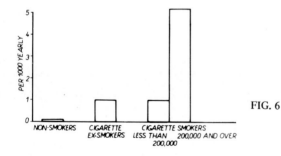

FIG. 6   *Average annual risk of developing*
           confirmed lung cancer – Kolín dis-
           trict (5.5 year follow-up) – in rela-
           tion to the smoking history.

ively worse (Fig. 3). 27% had brought up sputum for 3 months or more. 2% reported
haemoptysis in the past year, and another 2% had had a pneumonic episode.
    In the total group of 12,322 males aged 40-64 with a normal chest photofluorogram in
the year 1966, 108 cases of confirmed lung cancer were diagnosed during the subsequent
5.5 years, that is 1.6 per thousand yearly on average. The incidence of lung cancer was
related to smoking habits, as shown in Figure 4. Out of the 108 confirmed lung cancer
cases, 78 were diagnosed in smokers who had smoked a total of 200,000 or more cigarettes, 20 in smokers who had smoked less than 200,000 cigarettes, 8 in cigarette ex-
smokers and 2 in non-smokers. Further analysis revealed relations between the incidence

of lung cancer and the recorded symptoms (Fig. 5). 86 of the 108 confirmed lung cancer cases were included in the group having a chronic cough. Similarly, in the groups of males with expectoration of sputum, worsening cough, haemoptysis, or a pneumonic episode during the past year, more cases of lung cancer were diagnosed than would have been expected with regard to the number of persons having these symptoms.

The average annual risk of developing confirmed lung cancer was calculated using the figures mentioned so far. It is shown in Figure 6 that for current cigarette-smokers who had smoked a total of 200,000 or more cigarettes the risk of developing lung cancer is 5.2 per thousand yearly. For smokers who had smoked less than 200,000 cigarettes, and cigarette ex-smokers the risk is 1.0 per thousand yearly. The lowest risk of developing confirmed lung cancer was found for non-smokers − less than 0.1 per thousand annually.

Similarly, the risk of developing lung cancer can be related to respiratory symptoms (Fig. 7). A significant increase in the risk of developing confirmed lung cancer was found in groups of males with chronic cough (3.1 per thousand yearly), chronic expectoration (3.6 per thousand yearly), worsening of cough (4.3 per thousand yearly), haemoptysis (7.3 per thousand yearly) and a pneumonic episode (4.3 per thousand yearly) compared with the risk of persons without these symptoms (0.5, 0.8, 1.5, 1.5, and 1.5 per thousand respectively).

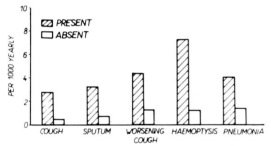

FIG. 7   *Average annual risk of developing confirmed lung cancer − Kolín district (5.5 year follow-up) − as related to respiratory symptoms.*

Conclusions

It is concluded that the risk of developing lung cancer varies not only with age and sex but is associated with heavy cigarette smoking and certain symptoms, namely chronic or worsening cough, chronic expectoration of sputum, haemoptysis and a pneumonic episode during the past year. A simple questionnaire, used in our study during a mass X-ray population survey, was found to be useful in identifying those population groups with a high risk of lung cancer.

If cigarette smokers could be persuaded to discontinue their habit a reduction in the number of new lung cancer cases would be expected in the subsequent period (Doll, 1970). For persons in high-risk groups who continue heavy cigarette smoking, the offer of a periodical X-ray follow-up should be considered, in countries with suitable facilities, as this procedure can contribute to an earlier diagnosis of lung cancer in some cases.

References

Doll, R. (1970): Scot. med. J., 15, 433.
Kubík, A. et al. (1970): Scand. J. resp. Dis., 51, 290.
Kubík, A. et al. (1972): Stud. pneumol. phthiseol. cechoslov., 32, 119. (In Czech)

Some reflections on the epidemiology of lung cancer*

Ernest L. Wynder and Kiyohiko Mabuchi

Naylor Dana Institute for Disease Prevention, American Health Foundation, New York, N.Y., U.S.A.

It has been more than 20 years since the association between tobacco smoking and lung cancer was first reported (Doll and Hill, 1950; Wynder and Graham, 1950). On the basis of the work done since then (U.S. Public Health Service, 1966, 1971, 1973), the following conclusions can be drawn:

1.   The smoking of tobacco, especially cigarette smoking, is related to both histological types (Kreyberg Groups I and II) of lung cancer, although the relationship to smoking is stronger for Kreyberg Group I (squamous/oat cell type) cancer than for Kreyberg Group II (adenocarcinoma/terminal bronchiolar type) cancer.

2.   Kreyberg Group I lung cancer is extremely rare in nonsmokers.

3.   The risk of lung cancer increases with increasing exposure to cigarette smoke, indicating that there is a dose-response relationship.

4.   Smoking intensity factors relating to different exposure levels include age at which smoking was started, duration of smoking, butt length, inhalation practices, and tar yield.

5.   In the United States, the mortality from lung cancer among women which started to rise around 1960 still continues to be lower than among men due to the fact that the exposure to cigarette smoke as measured by these smoking intensity factors are less frequent among women, especially at older ages. Even among younger women, the exposure to cigarette smoke is less frequent than among men for the reason that women more frequently smoke cigarettes with low tar yields than men.

6.   Individuals involved in specific occupations, such as uranium miners, workers in the chromate, nickel and asbestos industries, painters and carpenters have an increased risk of lung cancer. It is of interest to note that the risk is particularly increased if individuals also smoke cigarettes.

7.   It has not been established that, upon standardization for smoking intensity factors, occupational exposure, and the accuracy of case finding and reporting, the lung cancer risk for urban dwellers significantly differs from that of individuals living in rural areas.

8.   The reported relationship between chronic bronchitis and lung cancer (over and above the cigarette effect) remains to be fully established.

The less harmful smoking product

It is clear that when individuals stop smoking there incurs a reduction in lung cancer risk (Fig. 1) (Hammond, 1966; Wynder et al., 1970). How soon this reduction takes place relates to the duration and amount of tobacco consumed before cessation. Among long-term heavy smokers, there is a slight reduction in lung cancer risk 3 to 4 years after

* This review was in part supported by Public Health Service Grant NIH–NCI–E–70–2087 from the National Cancer Institute.

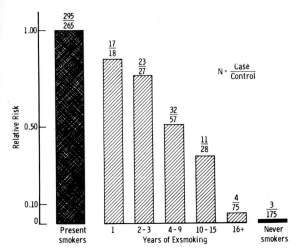

FIG. 1   *Relative risk of lung cancer (Kreyberg Group I) by number of years after cessation of smoking males, New York City, Los Angeles and Houston, 1966–1971. (Data: Memorial Hospital, NYC, Case–210, Control–420, 1966–69; Hospitals in Los Angeles, Houston and NYC (including Memorial), Case–188, Control–376, 1970–71. Controls matched by age and hospital).*

cessation, suggesting that cellular evidence of cancer is present long before clinical signs become evident.

The key epidemiological question in the lung cancer/smoking issue is whether the smoking of certain types of tobacco products results in a reduction of cancer risk. Of great interest in this regard is what has happened to the ordinary type of cigarette in the United States, since cigarettes represent the major tobacco product smoked in the country.

During the past 20 years, there has been a steady decline in the tar and nicotine content of American cigarettes (Fig. 2) (Wynder and Hoffmann, 1972). This has been accomplished through the increased use of low tar-yielding tobaccos, greater utilization of reconstituted tobacco sheets and stems, greater porosity of cigarette paper and effective filters. Experimental studies show that tars obtained from best-selling cigarettes on the U.S. market today are lower in tumorigenicity than cigarettes manufactured 20 years ago (Fig. 3) (Wynder and Hoffmann, 1968). It has been shown that cigarettes made wholly from reconstituted tobacco sheets or stems have a relatively low tumor yield (Fig. 4) (Wynder and Hoffmann, 1965, 1969).

Therefore, it is of interest from an epidemiological standpoint to determine whether the risk of lung cancer among long-term filter (low tar) cigarette smokers is lower than that of nonfilter (high tar) cigarette smokers. Our data, (Wynder et al., 1970), in agreement with Bross and Gibson's (1968) data, do show a reduced risk of lung cancer for long-term filter cigarette smokers (Fig. 5). It should be pointed out, however, that filter cigarette smokers included in these studies started with nonfilter cigarettes and shifted to filter cigarettes. Our future studies will be concerned with the determination of cancer risk among individuals who began their smoking careers with low tar cigarettes.

It is reasonable to assume that in the United States, the effect of the smoking of less harmful cigarettes on the total mortality will be first seen in women. The differences in such smoking intensity factors as daily number of cigarettes consumed, age at which smoking was begun, depth of inhalation and butt length, which existed in the past between men and women are today greatly lessened, particularly among younger smokers (Wynder et al., 1973). However, women generally started their smoking careers with low tar cigarettes since smoking became common among women much later than among men.

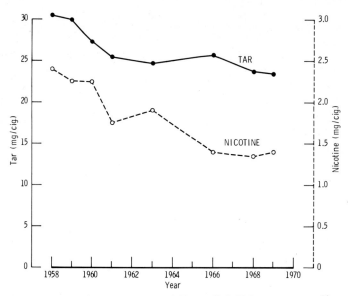

FIG. 2   *Tar and nicotine content of best-selling U.S. cigarettes (80% of total sales: 7-20 brands).*

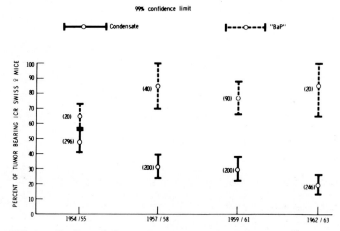

FIG. 3   *Decline of skin tumor response obtained with 50% solutions of smoke condensate over a period of 9 years compared with response obtained with 0.005% BaP over the same period of time. (Figures in parenthesis indicate number of mice per group.)*

It is for this reason that we predict that the lung cancer mortality rate in women will continue to increase in the future but will not achieve the high level reached by men who more often than not started smoking with high tar cigarettes (Wynder et al., 1973).

As far as lung cancer is concerned, included among less harmful tobacco products are pipes and cigars. This is because these products are generally not inhaled. It has, however, been shown that heavy cigar and pipe smokers (e.g., 5+ cigars or 10+ pipes a day) do have an appreciable risk of developing lung cancer even when not inhaling (Abelin and Gsell, 1967; Wynder and Mabuchi, 1972). Epidemiological studies also show that the risk of cancer of the mouth for cigar and pipe smokers is at least as great as for cigarette smokers (Wynder et al., 1957). Animal experiments indicate a greater carcinogenicity of cigar and pipe smoke than cigarette smoke (Croninger et al., 1958; Homburger et al., 1962).

In the United States, the excessive smoking of cigars and pipes has relatively little impact on the statistics because of the small number of cigar and pipe smokers in the general population. However, in Switzerland where cigar smoking is much more widespread, there is a high mortality risk of lung cancer reported (Gsell and Abelin, 1972).

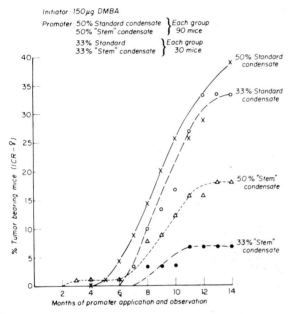

FIG. 4   *Tumor-promoting activity of smoke condensates from cigarettes made with standard tobacco and tobacco stems. DMBA = 7,12-dimethylbenz (a) anthracene.*

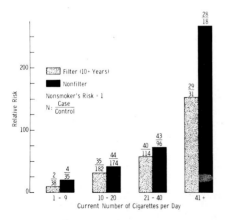

FIG. 5   *Relative risk of lung cancer (Kreyberg Group I) by type and number of cigarettes. Males, New York City, Los Angeles, and Houston, 1966–1971 (408 male lung cancer patients and 2,272 controls).*

There has recently been considerable controversy in the United States with respect to the so-called 'little cigars'. These are manufactured from cigar tobaccos but are the size of regular cigarettes. It can be predicted that, to the extent that certain 'little cigars' are inhalable, they carry a risk for lung cancer similar to that of cigarettes. In a recent paper, we reported on factors that may contribute to the inhalability of tobacco smoke, especially in the form of cigars and little cigars (Hoffmann and Wynder, 1972).

The mortality rate from lung cancer among French males (27.7/100,000) is considerably lower than that of U.S. white males (39.6/100,000) or males in England and Wales (69.7/100,000) (Segi and Kurihara, 1972). As has been suggested by Schwartz, this may be due to the fact that French smokers inhale significantly less smoke than their American or British counterparts (Schwartz et al., 1961), which in turn may be due to the significantly higher nicotine and alkaline content of French cigarettes (Hoffmann, unpublished data).

It would seem that any tobacco product which cannot be readily inhaled should be associated with a decreased risk for lung cancer. This concept obviously does not apply to cancer of the upper alimentary tract.

Conclusions

We favor the attempts of the voluntary health organizations to educate the public (especially younger people) with respect to the health hazards of smoking. It seems, however, that in a social setting where cigarette smoking is accepted and practiced by many adults, such educational programs will fall on deaf ears, especially of the young. It should be emphasized that such programs seem to have had a positive effect on certain adult groups, especially educated males. However, in view of the fact that strong legislation against smoking is not likely in the foreseeable future, much of our educational effort will be diluted. In addition to these mass-education programs, we thus need to concentrate our efforts on making smoking as harmless as possible. Tobacco carcinogenesis is a very specific process related to specific tumor initiators and promoters existing in the tobacco smoke and specific precursors present in the tobacco itself. We have already learned much about the nature of tumorigenic components and their precursors. It is now up to us to put this knowledge to practical application.

While it is unlikely that a completely harmless smoking product will ever be produced, much more progress can be made toward this goal. It appears possible that a smoking product can be developed which, except when used excessively, would carry relatively little risk for developing lung cancer or other tobacco-related malignancies.

One of the things which must be faced, whether we like it or not, is the fact that society, for a variety of reasons, is likely to continue to tolerate tobacco usage. It is because of this realistic assessment that efforts to make smoking products as harmless as possible must be accelerated.

References

Abelin, T. and Gsell, O.R. (1967): Cancer (Philad.), 20, 1288.

Bross, I.D.J. and Gibson, R. (1968): Amer. J. publ. Hlth, 58, 1396.

Croninger, A.B., Graham, E.A. and Wynder, E.L. (1958): Cancer Res., 18, 1263.

Doll, R. and Hill, A.B. (1950): Brit. med. J., 2, 739.

Gsell, O.R. and Abelin, T. (1972): J. nat. Cancer Inst., 48, 1795.

Hammond, E.C. (1966): In: Epidemiological Approaches to the Study of Cancer and Other Diseases. Editor: W. Haenszel. Nat. Cancer Inst. Monogr., 19, 127.

Hoffmann, D. and Wynder, E.L. (1972): Science, 178, 1197.

Homburger, F., Tregier, A. and Baker, J.R. (1962): Fed. Proc., 21, 452.

Schwartz, D., Flamant, R., Lellough, J. and Denoix, P.F. (1961): J. nat. Cancer Inst., 26, 1085.

Segi, M. and Kurihara, M. (1972): Cancer Mortality for Selected Sites in 24 Countries, No. 6 (1966–1967). Japan Cancer Society, Tokyo.

U.S. Public Health Service (1966): Smoking and Health. Report of the Advisory Committee to the Surgeon General of the Public Health Service. Public Health Service Publication, No. 1103, U.S. Department of Health, Education, and Welfare, Washington.

U.S. Public Health Service (1971): The Health Consequences of Smoking. A Report to the Surgeon General: 1971. DHEW Publication No. (HSM) 71-7513, U.S. Department of Health, Education and Welfare, Washington.

U.S. Public Health Service (1973): The Health Consequences of Smoking. DHEW Publication No. (HSM) 73-8704, U.S. Department of Health, Education and Welfare, Washington.

Wynder, E.L., Bross, I.D.J. and Feldman, R.M. (1957): Cancer (Philad.) 10, 1300.

Wynder, E.L., Covey, L. and Mabuchi, K. (1973): J. nat. Cancer Inst., 51, 391.

Wynder, E.L. and Graham, E.A. (1950): J. Amer. med. Ass., 143, 329.

Wynder, E.L. and Hoffmann, D. (1965): J. Amer. med. Ass., 192, 88.

Wynder, E.L. and Hoffmann, D. (1968): Science, 162, 862.

Wynder, E.L. and Hoffmann, D. (1969): Cancer (Philad.), 24, 289.

Wynder, E.L. and Hoffmann, D. (1972): J. nat. Cancer Inst., 48, 1749.

Wynder, E.L. and Mabuchi, K. (1972): Prevent. Med., 2, 529.

Wynder, E.L., Mabuchi, K. and Beattie Jr, E.J. (1970): J. Amer. med. Ass., 213, 2221.

Multiple factor etiology of occupational lung cancer

Irving J. Selikoff and E. Cuyler Hammond

Environmental Cancer Research Project, Mount Sinai School of Medicine of the City University of New York, and the American Cancer Society, New York, N.Y., U.S.A.

The clear identification of the fibrogenic effect of asbestos inhalation (Cooke, 1924) was soon followed by the discovery of 3 important additional characteristics of such exposure: (1) the long-lapsed period between onset of exposure to the dust and the appearance of significant disease (Table 1) (Selikoff et al., 1965) with, generally, 20 years or more required for this disease to be seen; (2) the frequent involvement of the pleura in the disease process (Lynch and Smith, 1935), with a similar time sequence (Table 2), and (3) the potential for neoplastic change in such cases.

TABLE 1   *X–ray changes in asbestos insulation workers**

Years from onset of exposure	No.	Normal %	Abnormal %	Asbestosis (grade)		
				1	2	3
40+	121	5.8	94.2	35	51	28
30 – 39	194	12.9	87.1	102	49	18
20 – 29	77	27.2	72.8	35	17	4
10 – 19	379	55.9	44.1	158	9	0
0 – 9	346	89.6	10.4	36	0	0
	1,117	51.5	48.5	366	126	50

* (From Selikoff et al., 1965)

TABLE 2   *Roentgenographic evidence of pleural abnormality among 1,117 asbestos insulation workers**

Years from onset of exposure	Number examined	Normal pleura	Abnormal pleura	
			Fibrosis	Calcification
40+	121	28	65	70
30 – 39	194	96	62	67
20 – 29	77	47	25	8
10 – 19	379	340	36	5
0 – 9	346	342	4	0

* (From Selikoff, 1965)

TABLE 3   Expected* and observed number of deaths among 625 New York-New Jersey asbestos insulation workers, Jan. 1, 1943–Dec. 31, 1971, twenty or more years after onset of first exposure to asbestos

	1943–1947		1948–1952		1953–1957		1958–1962		1963–1971		Total	
	Expected	Observed	Expected	Observed	Expected	Observed	Expected	Observed	Expected	Observed	Expected	Observed
Total cancer: all sites	5.7	13	8.1	17	13.0	26	9.7	39	15.7	94	52.2	189
Lung cancer	0.8	5	1.4	8	2.0	12	2.4	17	4.8	42	11.4	84
Pleural mesothelioma	**	1	**	0	**	1	**	1	**	5	**	8
Peritoneal mesothelioma	**	0	**	1	**	2	**	1	**	20	**	24
Cancer of stomach, colon, rectum	2.0	4	2.5	4	2.6	7	2.3	14	3.1	12	12.5	41
Cancer all other sites	2.9	3	4.2	4	8.4	4	5.0	6	7.8	15	28.3	32
Asbestosis	**	0	**	1	**	4	**	7	**	21	**	33
All other causes	34.0	15	42.7	36	43.6	55	44.8	42	69.3	53	236.3	201
Total all causes	39.7	28	50.8	54	56.6	85	54.4	88	85.0	168	288.5	423
Person years of observation	1,912.0		2,478.0		2,336.5		2,011.0		2,520.0		11,257.5	

632 members were on the Union's rolls on Jan. 1, 1943. Seven died before reaching 20 years from first employment. All others entered these calculations after reaching the 20-year-from-first-exposure point

* Expected deaths are based upon death rate data reported annually by the U.S. National Office of Vital Statistics. Rates for 1968–1971 were extrapolated from age-specific rates for 1961–1967

** U.S. death rates not available, but these are rare causes of death in the general population

TABLE 4   Expected* and observed deaths among 933** amosite asbestos factory workers first employed 1941–1945, and observed to Dec. 31, 1971

	Before 1952		1952–1961		1962–1971		Total, 1941–1971	
	Expected	Observed	Expected	Observed	Expected	Observed	Expected	Observed
Total deaths	69.98	88	108.27	146	121.24	250	299.49	484
Total cancer: all sites	9.81	15	18.72	44	21.63	84	50.16	143
Lung cancer	1.49	3	3.71	23	6.21	47	11.41	73
Pleural mesothelioma	***	1	***	0	***	2	***	3
Peritoneal mesothelioma	***	0	***	0	***	4	***	4
Cancer of stomach	1.45	3	1.84	4	1.29	4	4.58	11
Cancer of colon, rectum	1.56	2	2.61	5	2.88	8	7.05	15
Cancer of esophagus	0.27	0	0.45	0	0.51	0	1.23	0
All other cancers	5.04	6	10.11	12	10.54	19	25.69	37
Asbestosis	***	3	***	7	***	17	***	27
All other causes	60.17	70	89.55	95	99.61	149	249.33	314

* Expected rates are based upon age-specific death rate data of U.S. National Office of Vital Statistics from 1949–1967. Rates were extrapolated 1941–1948 from rates for 1949–1955 and for 1968–1971 from rates for 1961–1967

** 933 men were employed. In 5 cases, ages were not known and these men have been excluded from these calculations. 877 men were traced to death or to Dec. 31, 1971. 51 men were partly traced and remain in the calculations until being lost to observation

*** U.S. death rates are not available, but these are rare causes of death in the general population

TABLE 5 Expected* and observed deaths among 17,800 asbestos insulation workers in the United States, Jan. 1, 1967–Dec. 31, 1971

| | Total | | Distribution by duration from onset of exposure | | | |
| | | | Less than 20 years | | 20 years and more | |
	Expected	Observed	Expected	Observed	Expected	Observed
Total deaths	805.63	1,092	178.94	211	626.69	881
Cancer: all sites	144.09	459	26.31	51	117.78	408
Lung cancer	44.42	213	7.03	22	37.39	191
Pleural mesothelioma	**	26	**	2	**	24
Peritoneal mesothelioma	**	51	**	3	**	48
Cancer of stomach	6.62	16	0.97	1	5.65	15
Cancer of colon, rectum	17.51	26	2.51	3	15.00	23
Cancer of esophagus	3.21	13	0.44	1	2.77	12
All other cancers	72.33	115	15.36	19	56.97	95
Asbestosis	**	78	**	5	**	73
All other causes	661.54	555	152.63	155	508.91	400
Number of men	17,800		12,681		5,119	
Person-years of observation	86,300		62,673		23,627	

* Expected deaths are based upon age specific death rate data of the U.S. National Office of Vital Statistics. Rates for 1968–1971 were extrapolated from rates for 1961–1967

** U.S. death rates not available, but these are rare causes of death in the general population

Following the initial description of a random case by Lynch and Smith (1935), Doll, in a classic study reported in 1955, demonstrated the lung cancer risk to be an important one, and later observations added mesothelioma (Wagner et al., 1960).

While earlier studies provided data concerning disease resulting from poorly controlled industrial conditions of the 1920's and 1930's, more recent investigations have demonstrated that the lung cancer risk continues to be a major hazard among large groups of asbestos workers. For example, among 632 insulation workers in the New York construction industry, observation to the end of 1962 showed the lung cancer risk to be almost 7 times that expected; 45 deaths occurred of cancer of the lung and pleura (including 3 pleural mesothelioma) while only 6 or 7 had been expected to occur (Selikoff et al., 1964). Observation of the remainder of the group through December 31, 1971, has shown equally unhappy results, with one of every 5 deaths resulting from lung cancer and one in 15 from mesothelioma (Table 3).

Similar experiences among workers in an asbestos textile factory first employed between 1941-1945 and followed through 1971, have been noted. Eleven lung cancer deaths were expected and 73 occurred (Table 4).

Further, current studies of the mortality experiences of a very much larger group of asbestos insulation workers in the United States (all 17,800 members of the Asbestos Workers Union on January 1, 1967) have provided data of equal concern. In this group of men, 44.42 lung cancers were expected between 1967-1971, and 213 occurred. In addition, pleural mesothelioma was again found in very great excess (while this is a rare cause of death in the general population, 26 of the 1,092 deaths in this group were so related) (Table 5). The major increase in lung cancer risk was, as expected, 20 to 40 years from onset of work exposure (Table 6).

Unlike the biological effect which results in asbestosis, however, the lung cancer risk does not have the same strong association with relatively heavy exposure, often for long periods of time. Cases are regularly seen in which there is little or no radiological evidence of asbestosis associated with lung cancer in asbestos workers; this is frequently the case with pleural mesothelioma. Apparently the carcinogenic influence is not necessarily iden-

TABLE 6   *Deaths of lung cancer and pleural mesothelioma among 17,800 asbestos insulation workers in the U.S. and Canada, Jan. 1, 1967–Dec. 31, 1971: relation to elapsed period from onset of work exposure*

Years from on-set of exposure	Lung cancer			Pleural mesothelioma
	Expected deaths*	Observed deaths	Ratio	Observed deaths
< 10	0.48	0	–	0
10–14	1.69	4	2.4	0
15–19	4.68	18	3.8	2
20–24	7.55	25	3.3	4
25–29	8.51	41	4.8	7
30–34	6.24	44	7.1	4
35–39	3.53	23	6.5	1
40–44	4.04	24	5.9	3
45–49	3.72	17	4.6	4
50+	3.81	17	4.5	1
Total	44.42	213	4.8	26

* Expected deaths are based upon age specific death rate data of the U.S. National Office of Vital Statistics. Rates for 1968–1971 were extrapolated from data for 1961–1967

TABLE 7   *Expected and observed deaths of lung cancer among 876 amosite asbestos factory workers, first employed 1941–1945, and observed to Dec. 31, 1971.* Distribution by duration of employment*

Duration of employment	Number of men	Person-years of observation	Deaths of lung cancer		
			Expected**	Observed	Ratio
< 3 months	256	5,869	3.55	13	3.66
3–11 months	294	6,158	3.58	15	4.19
1 + years	326	6,912	4.09	45	11.00′
Total	876	18,939	11.22	73	6.51

*   This table excludes 57 men. 10 died during first year of employment, 39 could not be traced after the first year, 7 had prior occupational exposure to asbestos and 1 had employment of uncertain duration. 17 men of the 876 were partially traced and remained in the calculations only until lost to observation

**   Expected rates are based upon age-specific death rate data of U.S. National Office of Vital Statistics, 1949–1967. Rates were extrapolated 1941–1948 from rates for 1949–1955 and for 1968–1971, from rates for 1961–1967

TABLE 8   *Expected** and observed deaths among 370 New York-New Jersey asbestos insulation workers, Jan. 1, 1963- Dec. 31, 1971*

	Total		No history of cigarette smoking*		History of cigarette smoking	
Number of men Jan. 1, 1963	370		87		283	
Person years of observation	2,520		608		1,912	
	Expected deaths	Observed deaths	Expected deaths	Observed deaths	Expected deaths	Observed deaths
Cancer all sites	15.74	94	4.75	15	10.99	79
Lung cancer	4.57	42	1.26	1	3.31	41
Pleural mesothelioma	***	5	***	–	***	5
Peritoneal mesothelioma	***	20	***	7	***	13
Cancer of stomach	0.94	6	0.30	2	0.64	4
Cancer of colon, rectum	2.15	6	0.69	2	1.46	4
Cancer of esophagus	0.37	–	0.11	–	0.26	–
Asbestosis	***	21	***	5	***	16
All other causes	69.22	53	22.28	15	46.94	38
Total deaths	84.96	168	27.03	35	57.93	133

*   Included 39 men who smoked pipe or cigars

**   Expected deaths based upon age specific U.S. mortality for white males, disregarding smoking habits. Lung cancer estimates based upon U.S. rates for cancer of lung, pleura, bronchus and trachea, categories 162 and 163

***   United States data not available, but these are rare causes of death in the general population

tical with that producing fibrosis. Epidemiological data demonstrating this disassociation are now at hand as a result of the study of the asbestos factory workers; there was significant increase in lung cancer risk even with exposures of less than 3 months, although the risk was still higher among those working for a year or more (Table 7).

There is thus ample evidence of an important lung cancer risk associated with occupational exposure to asbestos. *However, it has now been found that this risk is not a simple one, entirely the result of the asbestos exposure.* Recent experiences have demonstrated that lung cancer among asbestos insulation workers is largely confined to those men with a history of cigarette smoking. Among the 370 New York insulation workers alive on January 1, 1963, 87 men had no history of cigarette smoking and 283 had smoked cigarettes.These men were followed to 1967. Having available expected rates for lung cancer among the general population (Hammond, 1966), it was calculated that fewer than one death should have occurred among the 87 men who had not smoked cigarettes. None occurred. On the other hand, among the 283 smokers, 2.98 such deaths had been expected. 24 died of lung cancer (Selikoff et al., 1968). The cohort has now been traced an additional 56 months. Table 8 shows the findings for the 9 year period, January 1, 1963-December 31, 1971. Of the 283 men who smoked cigarettes regularly, 41 died of lung cancer while of the 87 men who never smoked cigarettes regularly, only one died of lung cancer. This man was a cigar smoker. The expected number of deaths in the table is based upon U.S. mortality data disregarding smoking habits, since death rates related to smoking are not yet available for the period 1967-1971.

We now have data in the far larger study of insulation workers throughout the United States. Among the 17,800 men who were members of this Union on January 1, 1967, 11,656 completed a questionnaire providing, among other details, information concerning their smoking habits. We have followed this cohort through December 31, 1971 (Selikoff et al., 1973).

1,092 deaths occurred, with 213, as noted, due to lung cancer. Among the 9,590 men with a history of regular cigarette smoking (Table 9), there were 596 deaths, 134 of which were due to lung cancer. On the other hand, of the 2,066 non-cigarette smokers, only two deaths due to lung cancer occurred. One of these two men was a cigar and pipe smoker and the other never smoked regularly.

Pleural mesothelioma

In our previous report, we were unable to suggest whether or not pleural mesothelioma was related to cigarette smoking. Only 3 deaths occurred of this disease in our initial report (Selikoff et al., 1964). While all 3 of these men were cigarette smokers, the number was too small for reliable evaluation.

We have now analyzed the deaths in the nation-wide study under way. 26 were due to pleural mesothelioma and of these men, 17 had a history of regular cigarette smoking, 1 was a pipe smoker and 1 never smoked regularly and 7 were unknown as to smoking habits. We still refrain from drawing definite conclusions because of small numbers.

Conclusions

It seems clear, then, that lung cancer is uncommon among asbestos insulation workers who have no history of cigarette smoking and that if the risk is increased, such increase is not great. On the other hand, occupational exposure to asbestos appears to greatly increase the lung cancer risk of cigarette smoking.

Since similar experiences have been reported among uranium miners (Lundin et al., 1969), it appears likely that other occupational lung cancers may be the result of such multiple factor effect. This has important implications for the prevention of this disease (Selikoff et al., 1968).

TABLE 9   Expected and observed deaths among 17,800 U.S. and Canada asbestos insulation workers, Jan. 1, 1967- Dec. 31, 1971*

	Total		No history of cigarette smoking**		History of cigarette smoking		Smoking habits not known	
Number of men Jan. 1, 1967	17,800		2,066		9,590		6,144	
Person-years of observation	86,300		10,163		46,615		29,522	
	Expected deaths	Observed deaths	Expected deaths	Observed deaths	Expected deaths	Observed deaths	Expected deaths	Observed deaths
Cancer all sites	144.09	459	19.92	33	79.58	265	44.59	161
Lung cancer	44.42	213	5.98	2	25.09	134	13.35	77
Pleural mesothelioma	***	26	***	2	***	17	***	7
Peritoneal mesothelioma	***	51	***	9	***	29	***	13
Cancer of stomach	6.62	16	0.95	1	3.60	8	2.07	7
Cancer of colon, rectum	17.51	26	2.52	4	9.53	14	5.46	8
Cancer of esophagus	3.21	13	0.44	0	1.80	7	0.97	6
Asbestosis	***	78	***	4	***	45	***	29
All other causes	661.54	555	92.67	36	356.67	286	212.20	233
Total deaths	805.63	1,092	112.59	73	436.25	596	256.79	423

* Expected deaths based upon age specific U.S. mortality rates for white males, disregarding smoking. Lung cancer estimates based upon U.S. rates for cancer of lung, pleura, bronchus and trachea, categories 162 and 163

** Included 609 men who smoked pipes or cigars

*** United States data not available, but these are rare causes of death in the general population

References

Cooke, W. E. (1924): Brit. med. J., 2, 147.

Doll, R. (1955): Brit. J. Industr. Med., 12,81.

Hammond, E. C. (1966): In: Epidemiological Study of Cancer and Other Chronic Diseases. Nat. Cancer Inst. Monogr., 19, 127.

Lundin Jr, F. E., Lloyd, J. W., Smith, E. M., Archer, V. E. and Holaday, D. A. (1969): Hlth. Phys., 16, 571.

Lynch, K. M. and Smith, W. A. (1935): Amer. J. Cancer, 24, 56.

Selikoff, I. J. (1965): Ann. N.Y. Acad. Sci., 132, 351.

Selikoff, I. J., Churg, J. and Hammond, E. C. (1964): J. Amer. med. Ass., 188, 22.

Selikoff, I. J., Churg, J. and Hammond, E. C. (1965): Ann. N.Y. Acad. Sci., 132, 139.

Selikoff, I. J., Hammond, E. C. and Churg, J. (1968): J. Amer. med. Ass., 204, 104.

Selikoff, I. J., Hammond, E. C. and Seidman, H. (1973): In: Proceedings, Working Group to Assess Biological Effects of Asbestos, I.A.R.C. Scientific Publications, No. 8. I.A.R.C., Lyon (In press).

Wagner, J. C., Sleggs, C. A. and Marchand, P. (1960): Brit. J. industr. Med., 17, 260.

Detection of occult lung cancer by cytological examination

M. R. Melamed

*Memorial Sloan-Kettering Cancer Center, Cytology Service, New York, N.Y.,
U.S.A.*

At the present time there are very limited means at our disposal for the detection and
diagnosis of lung cancers at an early stage while they are potentially curable. This is
reflected in the dismal survival rate for this disease, which is about 8-10% overall, simply
because most lung carcinomas are locally advanced and often metastatic before they are
even suspected.

The chest X-ray which is the most widely used and accepted technique for the detection of lung cancer fails us in the search for very early carcinomas, particularly those that
are centrally located and partially hidden by mediastinal or cardiac shadows.

In very early cancers, even when X-ray abnormalities are present they are frequently
non-specific. To reach a definitive diagnosis then requires an endoscopic biopsy or thora-
cotomy; but too often, unfortunately, there is a deliberate delay until more specific
radiological abnormalities appear and meanwhile the disease progresses.

During the last 15 to 20 years we have devoted considerable attention to the detection
and diagnosis of early lung cancers by cytological examinations of cough specimens of
sputum. It is a basic premise that carcinoma of the lung, like carcinoma of any other
organ, begins with an abnormality of the cells of the surface epithelium. When these
altered cells are dislodged spontaneously or by a vigorous cough and expelled in a specimen of sputum, they provide an epithelial sample of the bronchus — a cytological biopsy
if you will — that enables the skilled examiner to make a diagnosis of carcinoma (and
perhaps of precancerous lesions) with considerable accuracy.

The technique for collecting specimens is simple and not at all uncomfortable. It could
readily be used to survey selected high risk populations.

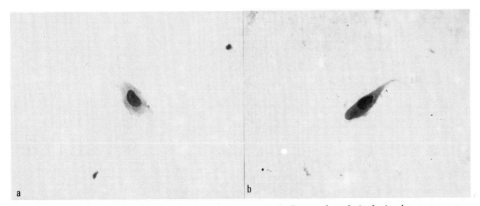

a   b

FIG. 1a, b   *Exfoliated cells of squamous carcinoma usually are found singly in the sputum, or as
loose, small clusters. Nuclei are increased in size, dark staining and often irregular, with
coarsely textured chromatin; cytoplasm is abundant and densely eosinophilic or orango-
philic. Papanicolaou stain. X 560. Reduced for reproduction 46%.*

The sampling of the exfoliated cells in a cough specimen of sputum is random, so that any single specimen may or may not contain diagnostic cells. But if we arbitrarily examine three or more specimens, then it is possible to make a definite diagnosis of carcinoma in nearly 80% of patients with the disease, and a probable diagnosis in 10% more, making a total of 90%. If we include patients who have only a single specimen examined, rather than three or more, then the probability of such a diagnosis is reduced to a little over 60%, but even this is at present three times better than that obtained with a bronchial biopsy and certainly much easier for the patient.

The value of cytological diagnosis is also reflected in the accuracy with which the histological type of the carcinoma present can be predicted from the expelled cancer cells

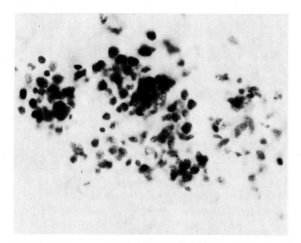

FIG. 2   *Oat cell carcinoma. Exfoliated tumor cells are small, non-uniform, usually loosely clustered and often only slightly larger than lymphocytes. Nuclei are hyperchromatic but some contain visible nucleoli. Cytoplasm is typically scanty or totally inapparent. Papanicolaou stain. X 560. Reduced for reproduction 35%.*

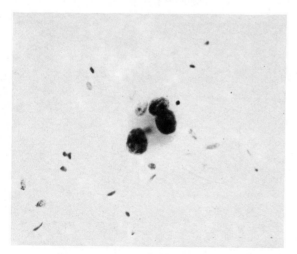

FIG. 3   *Glandular cancer cells in sputum from a patient with bronchiolar lung carcinoma. Nuclei are large, rounded, with delicate or coarse nuclear chromatin and sometimes very prominent nucleoli. Cytoplasm is abundant, but lighter staining and less eosinophilic than for squamous carcinoma. Clusters are common, as are multinucleated tumor cells. Papanicolaou stain. X 560. Reduced for reproduction 35%.*

in the sputum; for instance, Figure 1 shows a classical example of squamous carcinoma in the sputum. This can be compared with oat cell carcinoma, which is quite different as illustrated in Figure 2 and both differ from bronchiolar or adenocarcinoma which is shown in Figure 3. All of these three major forms of lung carcinoma have different clinical behavior and may require diffent therapeutic approaches. Thus, proper classification of cell type is essential.

Some years ago, Dr. Jorgen Hastrup who was then working in our laboratory, compared the accuracy of cytological and histological classifications of lung cancers. In more than three-quarters of the cases studied by him, he was able to make a precisely accurate prediction of histology. In occasional cases, actual fragments of tumor are expelled in the sputum, resembling microbiopsies as seen from Figure 4.

One of the major potential advantages of cytology may be its use as a supplement to the chest X-ray in lung cancer detection. The X-ray will identify small peripheral carcinomas most easily, while cytology can best be used to detect the central carcinomas of the large bronchi that are difficult to see at an early stage on an X-ray.

In a publication some years ago by Drs. Koss, Goodner and myself, we summarized the initial X-ray diagnoses of over 1,000 consecutive patients with lung carcinoma seen at the Memorial Hospital. There were 130 cases or about 13% that had either no definite diagnosis or the diagnosis of a benign lesion was favored. In 102 of these patients without a radiological diagnosis of carcinoma, a cytological examination was also carried out and 65% then had a positive cytological diagnosis of cancer while 10% more were suspicious.

The following is one example of the cases in that group (Fig. 5). The subject, a doctor's father, had a large thin-walled cyst in the left lower lobe. It was thought to be a benign cyst. He was operated on and the involved lobe was resected only because of the finding of squamous carcinoma in the sputum. The cyst proved to be a large cavitating carcinoma. Today, more than 5 years later, this man is alive and well. In another case, a patient with symptoms and X-ray evidence of pneumonia in the right upper lobe underwent lobectomy because of cancer cells in the sputum. He did indeed have pneumonia, but we also found a very well developed carcinoma in situ involving the lobar bronchus proximal to it — probably the reason for his developing pneumonia in that lung.

Even more interesting are a number of cases of very early lung carcinoma discovered by sputum cytology in patients with normal chest X-rays. In one case the man was a cigarette smoker, but otherwise well when we received a sputum specimen from him. His sputum unexpectedly showed evidence of epidermoid carcinoma. There was considerable

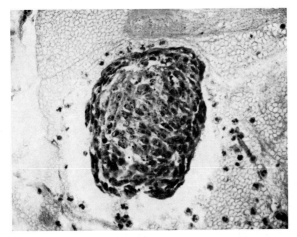

FIG. 4   *A fragment of epidermoid carcinoma expelled in the sputum by deep, spontaneous cough. This is a microtome section of fixed and paraffin embedded sputum. Hematoxylin and Eosin. X 350. Reduced for reproduction 35%.*

difficulty in localizing the source of these cancer cells, a problem that I think Dr. Frost will be discussing later. I will only note that in this particular case the patient had multiple chest X-rays, 2 bronchograms and 3 different bronchoscopies before one of several biopsies of major bronchi revealed a carcinoma in situ within the right intermediate bronchus. A right middle- and lower-lobe bi-lobectomy was performed (Fig. 6). If you look carefully at the bronchus on the left of the figure, you will see that the mucosa

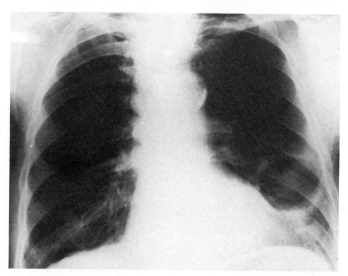

FIG. 5   *Chest X-ray of an elderly man, interpreted as showing a benign cyst of the left lower lobe with some secondary pneumonitis. Surgery was not planned initially, but after cancer cells were found in the sputum a left lower lobectomy was performed. The thin-walled cyst proved to be cavitating carcinoma and this patient is alive and well more than 5 years later.*

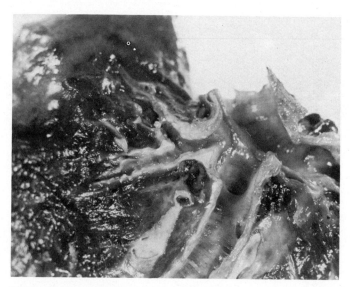

FIG. 6   *Gross specimen of resected lung showing thickened, opaque mucosa of bronchus on the left, due to carcinoma in situ. The other bronchi are normal, with delicate transverse mucosal rugae. No tumor mass is present.*

is thickened and opaque compared with the normal bronchi present. This represents an area of carcinoma in situ, which you can see in a histological section from this site illustrated in Figure 7.

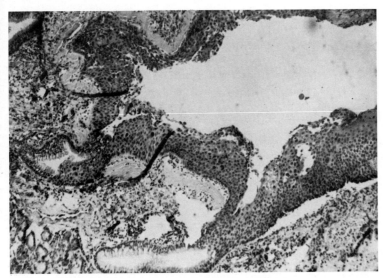

FIG. 7   *Histologic section of bronchus showing carcinoma in situ. Compare with Figure 6. Else-where there was superficially invasive carcinoma, still confined to the bronchial wall. Hema-toxylin and Eosin X 280. Reduced for reproduction 39%.*

In yet another case detected by examination of the sputum, again an illustration of carcinoma in situ, in this instance in a segmental bronchus, there was a single focus of superficial invasion that was confined to the level of the bronchial cartilage, and did not penetrate through the bronchial wall. This patient also had a normal chest X-ray.

Dr. Nael Martini, of the Thoracic Service at Memorial Hospital with Dr. Edward Beattie, Dr. Eugene Clifton and myself have recently reviewed a series of 26 lung cancer patients presenting with essentially normal chest X-rays at the time that their sputum showed carcinoma. I have summarized the results in a preliminary fashion.

16 of the 26 patients were treated by surgical resection and 12 (75%) were apparently cured. One other patient died as a result of surgery. This was an early case and the surgical complications resulted from difficulty localizing the source of the cancer cells. If this patient had survived, and I think today he would, the survival rate would be 80%.

There were 8 patients who for one reason or another were treated by radiation without resection. Of those, one is surviving for 39 months with metastases; all the others died in shorter periods of time. One other patient refused all therapy and died.

Similar figures have been given by two other institutions which have had a relatively large experience with these early lung cancers: In reports by Dr. Woolner and his associates from the Mayo clinic the survival rates of patients treated by surgery for early and occult lung cancers are approximately the same as ours. Drs. Pearson and Thompson from Toronto had a series of 19 cases, showing excellent survival rates in those whose disease was promptly localized and properly treated.

It is not known how long lung carcinoma remains in a clinically and radiologically occult phase while being detectable by exfoliated cancer cells in the sputum, or whether all histological types of lung cancer behave in the same way. Efforts to answer these and other questions are under way at present, particularly those concerning the practical usefulness of sputum cytology in screening an asymptomatic population. Perhaps when we meet again in a few years time, we will have some answers to these questions.

166

The use of the mass radiography for the detection of lung cancer

P. Veeze

Overijsselse Vereniging tot Bestrijding der Tuberculose, Enschede, The Netherlands

The best possibility as yet of controlling lung cancer lies in prevention rather than cure. However, prevention has failed to yield impressive results so far and we may be sure that for many years to come we shall have to cope with a continuous stream of new patients, whose only hope lies in sufficiently early diagnosis and treatment. It is the task of the medical profession to provide these for all patients who appear to have any chance at all.

Many of us have had exaggerated expectations of periodic mass radiography as a means of improving the outlook for lung cancer patients. So far, it has not caused a very dramatic rise in the proportion permanently cured. However, in view of the depressingly low survival rate in this common disease (below 10%), even a modest improvement would be worth making great efforts to achieve.

There has been some confusion about the real value in this respect of mass miniature radiography. The first question which must be answered, is: 'Will periodic radiography, when repeated at suitable intervals, result in an improved overall cure rate for lung cancer?'

To be sure, such an assumption is perfectly logical, for we know that this disease when untreated generally runs a fatal course, whereas some patients, even when suffering from very malignant varieties of lung cancer, may be cured if treated in time. Moreover we know that diagnosis and treatment may be considerably accelerated in a large proportion of cases by radiographic detection. But statistical evidence, to prove the influence of early detection upon survival, is remarkably meagre and inadequate.

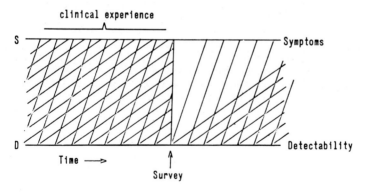

FIG. 1   *Selection of slowly developing tumours by screening.*

Let us first recall one of the principles of screening for cancer. In Figure 1, which is a modification of a graph by Saxén and Hakama (1964), the sloping lines at different angles symbolize a hypothetical mixed population of two types of cancer, supposed to have the same incidence but exhibiting different rates of progression. The steeply rising lines represent fast growing, centrally located tumours, soon giving rise to serious symptoms.

The more oblique lines stand for less malignant peripheral cancers, which tend to go unnoticed for a long period of time after having reached a size which renders them radiologically detectable. In clinical experience, both types will be encountered equally often, but it can easily be seen that a screening examination will reveal proportionally far more tumours of the slowly progressing variety.

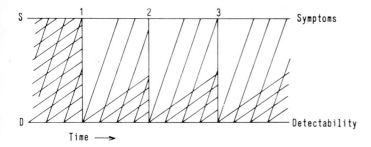

FIG. 2   *Effect of repeated screenings.*

With repeated screenings (Fig. 2) all tumours will be classifiable into two categories, the survey-cancers and the so-called clinical fall-out cancers, the latter coming to light between surveys. Both subgroups are quite different from each other biologically and prognostically.

As a consequence, the fact that in a given population those patients with survey-cancers generally fare better than do those with clinical fall-out cancers (as many authors have demonstrated) is no proof that early detection will improve the prognosis. In order to arrive at a valid conclusion one has to include all of the tumours (survey-cancers *and* clinical fall-out cancers) arising in a frequently screened population within a given period. Few authors have done so. Their long-term results are shown in Table 1.

Unfortunately the test population used by Boucot and co-workers in Philadelphia (Weiss, 1971) included a large proportion of older men with pre-existing respiratory disease preventing surgical treatment. The South London study by Nash et al. (1968) has been criticized by Weiss (1971) for the fact that the test population was not very clearly defined, which under the circumstances implied that the case material was more or less restricted to co-operative patients.

The only investigator to have used a proper control group is Brett (1969). He actually found an overall cure rate 2.5 times better for the frequently screened population than

TABLE 1   *Overall results (survey + clinical fall-out cancers). 6-monthly radiographic screening for lung cancer in men*

		Population	Cases	Cured	Cure rate
Philadelphia (Weiss, 1971)		6,137	121	7	6% (5 years)
45 years and over		(many with pre-existing pathology)			
South London (Nash et al., 1968)		67,400	197	35	18% (4 years)
45 years and over		(group not clearly defined)			
N.W. London (Brett, 1969)	Study	29,723	101	15	15% (5 years)
40 years and over	Control	25,311	77	5	6% (5 years)

for the controls, but unfortunately the numbers are rather small. The difference is suggestive, but not quite significant at the 5% level.

I am afraid this is all we have in the way of statistical evidence. To summarize, the assumption that early detection may improve the overall survival rate for lung cancer is well-founded logically, but so far it has been insufficiently tested. The available evidence supports the assumption, but is not conclusive. Clearly more well-designed large-scale studies are needed.

An equally important question is: 'What chance of cure have we to offer to survey-detected cancer patients, justifying their being prematurely disturbed? '

As a matter of fact, those patients not eligible for curative treatment need not be uselessly disquieted by early detection. Those obviously inoperable need hardly be disturbed at all, some of the incurable ones may benefit from well-planned anticipatory palliative care, and the illusion of well-being of the majority would not have lasted very much longer anyway.

TABLE 2   *Survey cancer, 5-year survival*

	Cases	Cured	Cure rate (%)
Leipzig (Baudrexl et al., 1970)	217	26	12
Berlin (Berndt, 1970)	462	58	12.5
Magdeburg (Kirsch, 1968)	634		14
Finland (Riska, 1971)	54	12	22
Philadelphia (Weiss, 1971)	80	5	6
Harwell (England) (Duncan et al., 1968)	90	15	17
S. London (Nash et al., 1968)	147	40	27 (4 years)
N.W. London (Brett, 1969)	65	15	23

Table 2 shows a rather wide variation in the cure rates for survey-cancer, which is no doubt due mainly to differences in age distribution, general health etc. between the populations concerned. However, other factors, notably divergences in the screening routine and patient management, may play a significant role as well. For, as we all know, the radiographic detection of small and inconspicuous lesions may be extremely difficult and in such cases making a prompt diagnosis of lung cancer may at times require not only the utmost skill and determination but also, of course, the patient's full cooperation. The fact that those being screened are asymptomatic or nearly so only contributes to the difficulty.

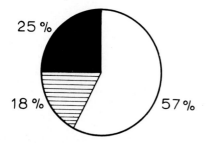

FIG. 3   *239 persons with radiologically visible lesions due to lung cancer: effectiveness of detection by mass radiography. (White area = cancer diagnosed within 3 months; shaded area = lesion overlooked; hatched area = diagnosis unduly delayed).*

TABLE 3   *Malignant tumours detected by mass miniature radiography in males aged 40 years and over*

	40 – 49	50 – 59	60 – 69	70 – 79	> 80	Total
4 towns* Overijssel '69 – '70						
Examined	6,319	5,258	5,769	3,627	911	21,884
Malignant tumours	3	18	31	30	6	88
Malignant tumours per 10,000	4.7	34.2	53.7	82.7	65.9	
4 cities West Holland '68 – '69**						
Examined	59,873	59,491	57,933	35,793	8,290	221,380
Malignant tumours	18	91	198	166	31	504
Malignant tumours per 10,000	3.0	15.3	34.2	46.4	37.4	
Netherlands '68 – '69 (excluding 4 cites)**						
Examined	182,989	150,727	135,415	81,982	22,914	574,027
Malignant tumours	48	192	385	285	85	695
Malignant tumours per 10,000	2.6	12.7	28.4	34.8	37.1	

* Deventer, Enschede, Hengelo, Zwolle

** Amsterdam, The Hague, Rotterdam, Utrecht

The difference between the yields in the Overijssel towns on the one hand and the Western cities on the other is highly significant (T=4.98, P≤0.001)

Our personal experience may illustrate this point (Fig. 3). In the course of a retrospective study (Veeze, 1972) it was discovered that 239 persons had (mostly in the years 1959 to '64) participated in one of our radiographic surveys while harbouring a radiologically visible lesion which ultimately proved to be lung cancer, albeit some of those lesions were very small at the time. Only 75% had been detected by the survey. Worse still, only 3/4 of the cancers detected were correctly diagnosed at once. Thus, no more than 57% of all visible lung cancers were actually recognized as such within 3 months of the survey. It appeared that the diagnosis of *early* lung cancer posed special problems with which many clinicians were unfamiliar.

We realized that small, inconspicuous cancers, which are so easily overlooked or misdiagnosed, are precisely the ones likely to offer the best chance of cure if diagnosed at that stage. So an attempt was made to improve the effectiveness of mass miniature radiographic surveys, in 3 ways, viz.:

(1) by paying special attention to those inconspicuous abnormalities which experience had shown to be suggestive of early cancer;

(2) by carefully comparing any abnormality, however slight, with previous films; and

(3) by cultivating the closest possible cooperation with those responsible for further clinical studies (which is not always as easy as it sounds).

Two phenomena already seem to reflect the partial success of these endeavours. Firstly, an improved detection rate in our province has been demonstrated (Table 3): far more cases have been diagnosed in the medium-sized towns of Overijssel than in the large Dutch cities, which in turn generally have higher detection rates than elsewhere in The Netherlands. As you may notice, this applies to all age groups.

Secondly, most encouraging long-term results have been obtained. We have been reviewing 99 consecutive cases of primary lung cancer, detected in patients of up to 70 years of age during the 3 years 1966 to 1968, which allows for a follow-up period of at least 5 years. The age and sex distributions are shown in Table 4, and the distribution

TABLE 4   *Age and sex distribution of 99 consecutive patients with survey-cancer*

	35 – 39	40 – 44	45 – 49	50 – 54	55 – 59	60 – 64	65 – 69	All ages
Males	1	2	9	12	18	20	28	90
Females			1		2	2	4	9
Total	1	2	10	12	20	22	32	99

TABLE 5   *Distribution according to cell type of 99 consecutive survey-cancers*

Squamous cell cancer	47
Adenocarcinoma	15
Bronchiolo-alveolar cancer	4
Large-cell undifferentiated cancer	11
Small-cell carcinoma	9
Mixed type carcinoma	2
Carcinoid tumour with regional lymphogenic spread	1
Cylindroma (histologically malignant)	1
Not typed (all deceased within 2 years)	9
Total	99

TABLE 6   *Survey-cancer, long-term results – Overijssel, patients under 70 years*

		At risk	Cured
Detected 1966	(7 years follow-up)	36	10
Detected 1967	(6 years follow-up)	36	13
Detected 1968	(5 years follow-up)	27	11
Total 1966–'68	(at least 5 years follow-up)	99	34 (34%)

TABLE 7   *Survey-cancer, presenting as a solitary nodule – Overijssel, patients under 70 years*

Number of patients	45 (100%)
Resections	38 (84%)
Postoperative deaths	3
Surviving resection	35 (78%)
5 - year survival	23 (51%)

TABLE 8   *Survey-cancer presenting as solitary nodule: Long-term survival following resection*

		Surviving resection	Cured
Detected 1966	(7 years follow-up)	10	6
Detected 1967	(6 years follow-up)	11	8
Detected 1968	(5 years follow-up)	14	9
Total 1966–'68	(at least 5 years follow-up)	35	23 (66%)

according to cell type in Table 5. Of these 99 patients, 59 underwent a resection and 34 (34%) are still alive, 5 years following treatment (Table 6).

We may conclude from this that when special attention is paid to accurate screening and proper management of suspected cases the outlook for survey-detected lung cancer is far from hopeless. An active diagnostic and therapeutic approach is fully justified.

Those survey-cancers which present as solitary pulmonary nodules deserve a separate discussion. At a rough estimate, 30% of all lung cancers will pass through this stage, which often covers many months. With tumours of this variety, virtually the only possibility of diagnosis at a curable stage lies in detection by radiography and then the prospects are comparatively favourable. Of 45 patients with such cancers, 23 (51%) have survived for at least 5 years following resection (Table 7). Of those successfully operated on the long-term survival rate even amounts to 66% (Table 8).

In our opinion, these results alone provide ample justification for a carefully designed radiographic detection programme.

References

Baudrexl, L. a. A., Rothe, G. and Kurpat, D. (1970): Z. Erkr. Atmungsorgane, 132, 111.
Berndt, H. (1970): Germ. med. Mth., 15, 103.

Brett, G. Z. (1969): Brit. med. J., 4, 260.
Duncan, K. P. and Howell, R. W. (1968): Brit. J. prev. soc. Med., 22, 110.
Kirsch, M. (1968): Z. Tuberk, 129, 251.
Nash, F. A., Morgan, J. M. and Tomkins, J. G. (1968): Brit. med. J., 2, 715.
Riska, N. (1971): Geriatrics, 26, 172.
Saxén, E. and Hakama, M. (1964): Ann. Med. exp. Biol., 42 (Suppl. 2), 5.
Veeze, P. (1972): In: Proceedings, Second Congress of the European Association of Radiology, Amsterdam, 1972, pp. 73 – 78. Editors: J. R. Blickman, W. H. A. M. Penn, E. H. Burrows, A. Somerwil, K. H. Ephraim and P. Thomas. Excerpta Medica, Amsterdam.
Weiss, W. (1971): Arch. environm. Hlth, 22, 168.

4.   Cancer of the urinary tract

Environmental and occupational factors in urinary bladder cancer

Johannes Clemmesen

Cancer Registry, Institute for Cancer Epidemiology, The Danish Anticancer League, Copenhagen, Denmark

It is well known that while cigarette smoking plays the major part in the aetiology of lung cancer, its share in the aetiology of bladder tumours is more limited, and it is assumed that occupational and industrial factors play a larger part in the aetiology of bladder tumours. It is the purpose of the present paper to compare the incidence of lung cancer with that of bladder tumours to gain information about the factors influencing their aetiology.

Lung cancer and neoplasms of the urinary bladder − in the following the so-called papillomas have been included − have been increasing for some time in most western countries. In Denmark, this trend has been most pronounced in the capital, but closely followed in other towns and, to a lesser extent, in rural areas. For either neoplasm therefore, the incidence for a particular cohort will be higher the later that cohort was born. At the national level, or for the population of a city like Copenhagen, there will therefore be a peak in the overall age distribution and this peak will appear later in life, as the exposed groups go on in age. Hence the age distribution will change in shape over the years, until all cohorts have experienced the same exposure.

An individual cohort, however, will show a smooth age dependence curve typical of malignant neoplasms and the shape will be the same for all cohorts, but the curve will be displaced upwards the later the cohort was born. Therefore, if we want to know the true age distribution for such temporarily increasing neoplasms we can combine observations on several cohorts, provided that we have accurate data for a long period of time as in Copenhagen, where such data exist for the years 1943 to 1967.

Data from the Danish Cancer Registry were fed into a computer programmed for the best approximation of an arbitrary number of observations to the simple exponential function $y = ab^x$, by means of the method of least squares. Since we found the correlation coefficient (Spearman's R) at 0.97 for the lung and the same for the bladder, the approximation for the points observed and the i., curve is as close as may reasonably be expected from clinical data.

Figure 1 gives data covering men diagnosed in Copenhagen from 1943 to 1967 and born later than 1895. The diagram shows the following:

1. approximate formulae fitting the two curves of age dependence;
2. that these formulae are identical for all practical purposes; and
3. that the average curve of age dependence for bladder neoplasms is displaced by about 10 years relative to the curve for lung cancer.

The usual estimate of the average time necessary for the induction of lung cancer is 20 years, so for bladder cancer we would assume 30 years, which is consistent with practical experience.

Figure 2 shows the age-adjusted mortality rates for lung cancer in various countries plotted against cigarette consumption 20 years earlier. It should be noted that Denmark, Norway and Sweden are at the lower end of the regression line and Finland followed by the United Kingdom at the upper end.

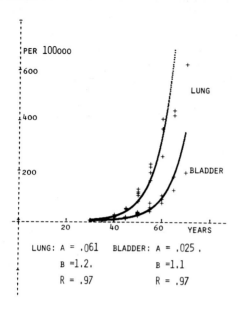

LUNG: A = .061   BLADDER: A = .025 ,
      B =1.2,   B =1.1
      R = .97   R = .97

FIG. 1   *Lung cancer and urinary bladder neo-*
          plasms by age, men born later than
          1895, Copenhagen 1943–1967.
          (Morbidity rates per 100,000; least
          square fit-exponential $y = ab^x$*).*

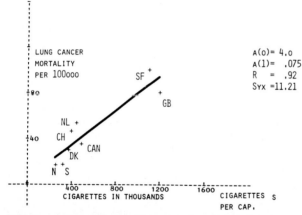

A(o)= 4.0
A(1)= .075
R = .92
Syx =11.21

FIG. 2   *Lung cancer mortality, Europe and Canada, 1950, per 100,000. Age-adjusted for European*
          standard, plotted against national cigarette consumption per capita, 1930. (Linear regression
          $y = a(o) + a(1)x$*).*

It was demonstrated by Lockwood in 1961 that for men living in Copenhagen there is an association between bladder tumours and the smoking of tobacco, although less pronounced than the association found elsewhere for lung cancer. This is in accordance with the findings in prospective studies in the United States by Hammond, Dorn and others. They found that the risk of lung cancer for smokers was 10 times the risk for non-smokers, whereas the risk of death from bladder cancer for smokers was twice the risk for non-smokers, which gives an approximate ratio among smokers of 5 lung cancers to 1 bladder cancer.

We next tried plotting bladder cancer mortality against cigarette consumption 30 years earlier as we had done previously for lung cancer (though against cigarette consumption 20 years earlier), but we found no correlation, except for Denmark, Norway and Sweden where a possible correlation was found. This is, of course, not conclusive evidence but it made us examine whether there was a constant ratio between lung and bladder neoplasms. So, we plotted data collected during 25 years for men from 20 different 5-year birth groups, living in Copenhagen, other towns, suburbs, and rural areas, and included Norwegian and Swedish data covering three and two periods respectively.

The number of lung cancer cases were plotted on a scale reduced by 3:1 compared with that for the bladder cancer cases (Fig. 3). A close correlation is found in Spearman's R again amounting to 0.97, which suggests a high comparability of the data for these countries.

However, the ratio found in Denmark, Norway and Sweden does not apply to other countries. In Finland and the United Kingdom there are far more cases of lung cancer per bladder cancer case and as indicated tobacco consumption in these two countries has for a long time been higher than for the three other Scandinavian countries (Fig. 4). In England where occupationally associated tumours have often been demonstrated and where the rate of smoking is greater than in these other countries, bladder tumours are no more frequent than in Denmark, even though occupationally associated bladder tumours are so far not known to occur in Denmark.

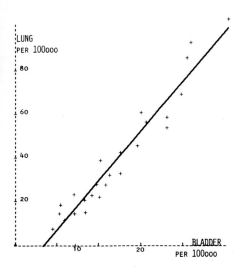

FIG. 3   *Lung cancer plotted 3:1 against urinary bladder neoplasms, morbidity per 100,000 men, age-adjusted to European standards. Denmark, 1943–1967, urban/rural, 20 OBS; Norway, 1953–1966, 3 OBS; Sweden, 1959–1965, 2 OBS. Linear regression analysis: (y = a(o) + a(1)x), a(o) = −16.0, a(1) = 1.1, R = 0.97, S(xy) = 6.7.*

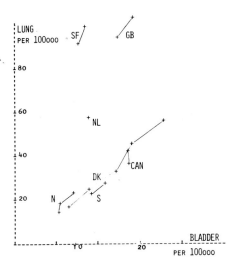

FIG. 4   *Lung cancer plotted 3:1 against urinary bladder neoplasms. Morbidity rates per 100,000 for men, age-adjusted to European standard. European and Canadian Registries CA, 1960.*

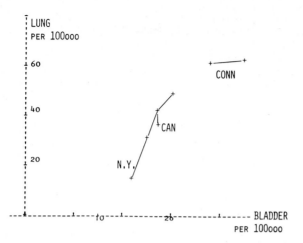

FIG. 5   *Lung cancer plotted 3:1 against urinary bladder neoplasms. Morbidity per 100,000 men, age-adjusted to European standard. 3 North American Registries.*

It may be objected that prospective studies in the United States have suggested that the number of deaths from lung cancer and bladder cancer are in the ratio of 5:1 among smokers. This is not, however, a direct contradiction of our findings which are not limited to smokers nor to deaths. The situation in North America is different from that in Europe: Figure 5 shows, for Connecticut, an increase in bladder tumours but not for lung tumours, whereas almost the opposite trend is shown for New York and the direct opposite trend for Canada.

It seems then that sufficiently well established data are available for Denmark, Norway and Sweden to form the basis for detailed studies concerning the effect of factors other than smoking and the conditions which modify the oncogenic effect of tobacco on the bladder.

References

Clemmesen, J. (1965a): Acta path. microbiol. scand., Suppl. 174.
Clemmesen, J. (1965b): Acta path. microbiol. scand., Suppl. 174.
Clemmesen, J. (1969): Acta path. microbiol. scand., Suppl. 209.
Clemmesen, J. and Bremerskov, V. (1973): Biomedicine, 19, 198.
Clemmesen, J. and Nielsen, A. (1973): Acta path. microbiol. scand., 81, 95.

Histological changes in pre-malignant lesions of the urinary tract

C. K. Anderson

Departments of Pathology and Urology, University of Leeds, Leeds, United Kingdom

Table 1 shows the general mortality figures for England and Wales for the year 1971, the last year for which complete records are available. The trends shown there are mirrored in all industrial societies. Consideration of these figures shows that approximately 20% of all deaths, male and female, are due to neoplastic disease, but that carcinoma of the urinary bladder does not appear to be one of the prime causes of death in this group. Consequently, it would seem that, excepting those persons engaged in employment thought to be associated with an increased incidence of bladder tumours, the routine screening of populations to detect pre-symptomatic bladder cancer cannot be justified. But the mere stating of bald mortality statistics gives no indication of the clinical importance of bladder cancer in urological practice. Bladder carcinoma exhibits a wide range of clinical behaviour. On the one hand we have patients with tumours so malignant and aggressive that they prove lethal within a short period of time; at the other extreme we see patients who survive for many years with multiple, recurrent tumours and who require repeated treatments to control the disease (Anderson, 1973). Table 2 shows the survival from initial attendance in 162 cases of patients with bladder cancer coming to post-mortem examination in the General Infirmary, Leeds, over the 10 year period 1963–1972. This series is obviously biased as to selection, but it does indicate that there is a substantial group of patients whose disease is untreatable when first seen. Most of the deaths occurring within 2 years of presentation were caused by the original tumour which first drove the patient to seek treatment. At 3 years and over it was usually a subsequent tumour arising after successful treatment of the first lesion which caused the death of the patient.

Most patients who present with the symptoms of bladder cancer are found to have cystoscopic evidence of tumour at the time of presentation. There is, however, a small group of patients who seek advice for lower urinary tract symptoms (pain, frequency and haematuria, singly, or in combination) in whom no cystoscopic evidence of tumour is found. These patients subsequently develop bladder cancer, but until a tumour has ap-

TABLE 1   *General mortality figures for England and Wales for the year 1971*

	Male	Female
Total deaths	288,359	278,903
Deaths from:		
1. Neoplastic disease	63,649	54,567
2. Carcinoma of bronchus and lung	25,113	5,588
3. Carcinoma of prostate	4,027	
4. Carcinoma of breast	80	11,182
5. Carcinoma of urinary bladder	2,763	1,107

TABLE 2   *Survival from initial attendance. Patients with bladder carcinoma. Post-mortem series (Leeds) 1963–1972*

| Survival period | No. of cases | | Total |
	Males	Females	
Less than 6 months	28	9	37
Up to 1 year	40	20	60
Up to 2 years	21	7	28
Up to 3 years	16	5	21
Over 5 years	10	6	16
Total	115	47	162

peared the tendency is to diagnose them as having 'cystitis' or 'prostatitis'. If the urologist suspects such a patient is at risk of developing a bladder tumour then the most useful investigation that can be performed is repeated, carefully-done exfoliative cytology with further cystoscopy at intervals, or whenever abnormal cellular forms are detected in the urine deposit. In a small number of these patients areas of abnormal-looking bladder mucosa will be seen at cystoscopy at some stage before the development of a true tumour. We need to know, or to attempt to discover, the common histological appearances of such abnormal areas and what these appearances mean in terms of the subsequent production of bladder cancer. How likely is a given histological abnormality in the bladder mucosa to be associated with tumour formation and what length of latent period may there be before a tumour emerges?

The epithelial lining of the bladder may be subjected to a series of environmental changes or assaults of differing degrees of severity and over varying periods of time (Kerr, 1970). Among the physical agents may be listed inflammatory change, particularly when associated with infection or stasis, friction due to calculi or foreign bodies, and friction with surface drying in ectopia vesicae. More important are the various carcinogenic agents, whether exogenous from the environment or the patient's employment, or endogenous due to dietary habits or smoking. In some instances these stimuli will affect the bladder epithelium simply through the process of normal replacement, only at enhanced rate. But if the stimulus is long continued, or of an extreme type, the epithelium may respond by the production of abnormal growth forms. Both normal replacement and abnormal growth forms may progress to clinical cancer.

The first of the abnormal growth forms are those that mirror normal transitional epithelium. Under this heading may be grouped simple hyperplasia where there is an excess of growth over cell loss so that the epithelium is thickened. This process is seldom uncomplicated and is frequently associated with the appearance of abnormal cell forms so that atypical hyperplasia is produced. The process continues with cell nest formation and increasing cellular atypicism until the grossest form of dysplasia, carcinoma in situ, is reached. Any of these abnormal growth forms may move by progression into the succeeding form and at any stage in this pathway transformation to carcinoma may occur. Secondly, there are the metaplastic forms of abnormal growth — squamous and glandular metaplasia, both of which may progress to carcinoma which may either resemble the metaplastic epithelium of origin, or be undifferentiated. Any cellular abnormality produced by abnormal growth may persist over a long period of time, or may under favourable circumstances undergo resolution to normality, or progress to carcinoma.

The histological appearance of abnormal growth forms are sometimes very clear cut and obvious and occasionally difficult as to recognition and interpretation. This makes any uniformity in histological reporting between one centre and another hard to achieve. For instance, an area of epithelial irregularity may be passed as 'abnormal hyperplasia' by one pathologist and called 'carcinoma in situ' by another. Only improved standards of recognition and data recording with free exchange of information between centres can help iron out these difficulties.

The histological terms and criteria for diagnosis may be stated briefly as follows.

Simple hyperplasia there is increased cellularity of the epithelial layer, but the growth arrangement is regular throughout.

Atypical hyperplasia here the growth pattern is more disorderly and bizarre cells are seen within the epithelial cell mass and these changes may be coupled with the genesis of small cell nests growing into the submucosa. Where small papillary projections are seen the lesion is termed *papillary hyperplasia* and is an obvious forerunner of papillary transitional cell carcinoma.

Carcinoma in situ this is morphological cancer without invasion. There is increased cellularity, marked irregularity of growth pattern, cellular pleomorphism, nuclear pyknosis and frequent mitoses, many of which are irregular. The underlying stroma is frequently vascular, oedematous and infiltrated by inflammatory cells. In some instances the diagnostic partition between gross atypical hyperplasia and carcinoma in situ is very difficult to make.

Any consideration of the significance of abnormal growth forms in the genesis of bladder cancer is difficult because the statistics at our disposal are frequently inadequate and inconclusive. Nevertheless, certain conclusions may tentatively be drawn. Table 3 shows the incidence of epithelial hyperplasia in Leeds over the 10-year period 1962–1971. All the patients presented with symptoms. Out of a total of 99 there were 76 males and 23 females in whom no previous tumour had been detected. Although 22% are seen to be tumour free for periods ranging up to 11 years no less than 40% have developed a bladder tumour during the period under review, and so there is a significant association between epithelial hyperplasia and the development of bladder tumours.

Table 4 shows the incidence of squamous metaplasia over a 10-year period in Leeds. None of these patients had had a previous tumour, and all presented with symptoms. There were 5 males and 8 females. Of these, 1 male and 4 females are living without any evidence of bladder tumour, but 3 males and 1 female developed rapidly invasive, poorly differentiated squamous carcinoma from which they died. It is obvious that there is a

TABLE 3 *Epithelial hyperplasia (Leeds) 1962–1971. No previous tumour (76 males, 23 females)*

Tumour free	Alive	10
	Dead	12
Tumour developed	Alive	18
	Dead	22
Lost to follow-up		37

TABLE 4 *Squamous metaplasia (Leeds) 1962–1971. No previous tumour*

	Males	Females
Alive tumour free	1	4
Dead tumour free	1	3
Died of tumour	3	1
Total	5	8

significant risk of the development of invasive squamous carcinoma with squamous meta-plasia, particularly in the male, and particularly when this is associated with stricture, infection, stone formation and repeated instrumentation. In the female the position is much less obvious. Squamous metaplasia in most female patients appears as a very orderly process with dense surface keratinisation (leukoplakia), but when there is marked, irregu-lar acanthosis of the squamous cell area the risk of developing carcinoma is probably as great as in the male.

TABLE 5   *Carcinoma in situ (Leeds) 1962–1973). No previous tumour (14 males, 3 females)*

	No. of cases
Invasive carcinoma within 6 months	7
Invasive carcinoma within 1 year	2
Invasive carcinoma 1 – 2 years	2
Invasive carcinoma 2 – 3 years	1
Invasive carcinoma 3 – 5 years	2
No tumour 11 months and 27 months	2
'Resolution' at 5 years	1

Table 5 shows the incidence of carcinoma in situ over an 11-year period to date in Leeds. There are 14 males and 3 females. All but 3 of these patients have developed invasive carcinoma within periods of 6 months to 5 years following diagnosis. In 2 of the patients, no tumour has been observed at 11 months and 27 months and one patient has undergone resolution 5 years after the original diagnosis.

One should note that all abnormal growth forms, with the exception of squamous metaplasia, are significantly more common in males than in females.

Conclusions

1. Proliferative lesions

The facts and figures are both hard to come by and extremely difficult to correlate. Nevertheless, such lesions, including all forms of hyperplasia, atypical hyperplasia and cell nest formation, show a significantly increased incidence of bladder tumour formation after a very variable latent period.

2. Carcinoma in situ

This carries a very high incidence of invasive carcinoma after a variable latent period of time, which is usually shorter rather than longer (Anderson, 1973; Utz et al., 1970).

3. Metaplasia

The position here is the most difficult of all. Cystitis cystica has not been observed transforming into cystitis glandularis, although the two conditions may co-exist (Bell and Wendel, 1968). A patient with extensive cystitis glandularis which cannot be controlled by endoscopic resection is probably at risk of developing a glandular carcinoma (Kitter-edge et al., 1964).

Irregular squamous metaplasia carries a definite risk of carcinoma and even the most inert and regular type of leukoplakia may ultimately undergo malignant change (Holley and Mellinger, 1961).

Whenever one reviews the literature on these topics, one must be at pains to differentiate those cases in which epithelial hyperplasia, metaplasia or carcinoma in situ were discovered before the incidence of the tumour, rather than those cases which occurred coincidentally or concurrently with a bladder tumour. This distinction is often not drawn (Melamed et al., 1964). The general conclusion is that any abnormal growth form of bladder epithelium must be viewed with considerable suspicion in a patient in the cancer age group presenting with urinary tract symptoms, when these cannot be adequately explained on the grounds of infection or obstruction. Any suspicions aroused by the histological appearances will be further enhanced by discovering that the patient is particularly at risk either because he is a heavy smoker or because his occupation is known to be associated with an increased incidence of bladder tumours.

References

Anderson, C.K. (1973): Proc. roy. Soc. Med., 66, 283.
Bell, T.E. and Wendel, R.G. (1968): J. Urol., 100, 462.
Holley, P.S. and Mellinger, G.T. (1961): J. Urol., 86, 235.
Kerr, W.K. (1970): Modern Trends in Urology, 3. Editor: Sir E. Riches. Butterworth, London.
Kittredge, W.E., Collett, A.J. and Morgan Jr., C. (1964): J. Urol., 91, 145.
Melamed, M.R., Voutsa, N.G. and Grabstald, H. (1964): Cancer (Philad.), 17, 1533.
Utz, D.C., Hanash, K.A. and Farrow, G.M. (1970): J. Urol., 103, 160.

Identification of the malignant potential of bladder tumours and detection methods

E. H. Cooper

Department of Experimental Pathology and Cancer Research, University of Leeds, Leeds, United Kingdom

In considering the problem of how to identify the malignant potential of bladder tumours one must first be fully conversant with their natural history and how treatment may modify the evolution of the disease. The accompanying paper by C. K. Anderson (*This Volume,* p. 177) succinctly summarizes the natural history of bladder tumours. It is evident that there is a wide range of behaviour. The very aggressive tumour that soon invades through the bladder and produces distant metastases is one end of the scale. Whilst the other end is represented by the very well differentiated non-invasive tumours, that are often a source of controversy as to whether they are truly malignant, although it is wiser to assume all tumours are malignant so that the patient will have the benefit of an adequate follow up.

The second factor is that treatment is frequently by local endoscopic resection of the tumour with or without radiotherapy which retains the bulk of bladder mucosa. Consequently, as many of these tumours are recurrent, the antecedent history of urothelial cancer and the site of the tumour will influence the prognosis.

The surgeon and pathologist between them, from a consideration of the history, physical signs, pyelograms, endoscopic appearances and histology, can make a reasonable estimate as to the likely behaviour of the tumour. Indeed, this is the basis for all decision making in the management of urothelial cancer, but though an experienced team will have a fair idea of the average behaviour of a tumour of a particular stage and grade, it is evident that there is a considerable variation in the eventual evolution of the tumour from one patient to another. The problem lies in knowing how to select the best therapy for a TII or TIII (UICC Classification) tumour. It is known some of these tumours will rapidly become worse and others of apparently the same type show a good response to endoscopic resection and radiotherapy. The surgeon often faces the dilemma of deciding, on slim scientific evidence, whether to perform a total cystectomy or the more conservative measures. Furthermore, there is the added morbidity and mortality that is associated with coincidental events such as haemorrhage and renal failure which are dependent on vagaries of tumour vascular construction and tumour site that are not simply correlated with tumour grade.

Examining this problem in more detail in the light of the experience of the Urology Department at Leeds, it is essentially the invasive tumours that keep their fronded structure with some evidence of dedifferentiation that are the most difficult to predict in their likely behaviour. The well differentiated tumours usually have a good prognosis and the anaplastic solid tumours usually have a poor prognosis, though even in these tumours occasional unexpected tumour progression in the former and long survival in the latter may occur.

It is a simple matter to say that it would be an advantage to be able to make a more precise prognosis in bladder cancer, but in practice it is proving to be a very complex task. Our group in Leeds has been involved with this problem during the past 5 years and it may be useful to outline our previous experience and indicate our current thoughts.

Examination of the biopsy specimens

We began by trying to find out whether a more detailed study of the tumour tissue can reveal additional information that can be used in predicting tumour behaviour. Measurement of the DNA content of the tumour cells (Levi et al., 1969) confirmed the rise in DNA content associated with anaplasia and indicated small populations of aneuploid cells may occur in well differentiated tumours. This approach was extended by a detailed analysis of the chromosome constitution of 65 tumours (Spooner and Cooper, 1972). We confirmed the diploid origin of bladder tumours; it must be remembered that they arise from a polyploid epithelium, and their tendency to increase their chromosome number to about twice normal in their more anaplastic forms. There is nothing remarkable about the chromosome constitution of bladder tumours to distinguish them from any other solid tumours. The patterns of gain and loss of chromosomes was varied both within a tumour and between tumours of the same type of pathology.

Three points emerged that are of interest to the histopathologist. First, in recurrent well differentiated tumours there was often a marked chromosome stability and marker chromosomes could be identified in specimens taken with intervals of up to 21 months apart. Secondly, most tumours had modal chromosome numbers in the diploid range (44-49, normal diploid = 46). Whilst all the well differentiated tumours were in this diploid range, about half the tumours considered to be de-differentiated were also in this range, the remainder had higher chromosome numbers. In practical terms this means that chromosome analysis is unlikely to be able to distinguish high and low risk groups within the papillary tumours, as there is considerable overlap of the chromosome constitution of histological types found at the 2c mode. In all cases in which high chromosome numbers were encountered there is no doubt about the anaplastic nature of the tumour.

Finally, this provides confirmatory evidence that within the individual fronds of papillary tumours which have a modal chromosome number in the diploid range, clones of malignant cells with higher chromosome numbers may be found, this focal change taking place in a well differentiated tumour. Hence, it has been our practice to regard these areas as being an indication of instability in the tumour and may have increased its malignant potential. However, it is not clear whether these focal areas of tumour progression can be the source of invasive cells or whether they behave more like carcinoma in situ (Melamed, 1972).

Cell proliferation and tumour grade are generally taken to be related. A more detailed study of this parameter suggested that this is a general rule in bladder tumours but occasionally well differentiated fronded tumours have a high rate of cell proliferation and some conversely anaplastic tumours may be fairly quiescent. Once again, the unexpectedly high proliferation in an apparently well differentiated tumour should always be regarded with suspicion. In our view, studies of ^{3}H-TdR labelling are prone to inaccuracy and offer little value to the histopathologist.

Detailed ultrastructural examination has revealed several points of interest about tumour organisation (Fulker et al., 1971), but it is unsuited for any routine procedure. Histochemistry has failed to reveal any major differences of cell organisation within tumours, but may help to distinguish between tumour and non-malignant areas (Burghele et al., 1965).

The prognostic significance of lymphoid and plasma cell infiltration that may be present in bladder tumours is uncertain. In our series of more than 1000 biopsies (Tanaka et al., 1970), there was a significantly higher association of lymphoid infiltration with bladder cancer compared to benign diseases of the bladder mucosa when considered as a whole. However, there was a variation within a tumour grade and it was intermittent in several recurrent tumours. We did not consider lymphoid infiltration had any significance on the 3 year survival, although Sarma (1970) reported it was a favourable sign. Pommerance (1972), examining total cystectomy specimens, suggested plasma cell infiltration was a good sign of prognosis, but its absence did not necessarily mean the prognosis was unfavourable. There is growing evidence that bladder tumours are antigenic and the host may have cytotoxic lymphocytes that are capable of killing bladder tumour cells in vitro

(Bubenik et al., 1970). However, patients with advanced disease have blocking factors in their serum that tend to interfere with this cytotoxic action of the lymphocytes. It is tempting to think that the presence of the lymphocytes and plasma cells may in some way have something to do within the patient's immunological response against his tumour. But, it is premature to jump to this conclusion; more evidence is needed before the significance of such infiltration can be evaluated. This can only be done by careful grading and recording the amount and type of infiltration and patiently waiting a sufficient number of years to see if it is an important factor.

At present, study of the immunology of bladder cancer is still in an experimental stage. The tests for cellular immunity and blocking factors are too complex for routine use and preliminary results do not suggest that they will be able to provide evidence that can readily be incorporated into the scheme for making prognostic assessment. The patients with extensive disease have limited responses and their sera contains blocking factor. Possibly the alteration of the characteristics of the serum after therapy may help to predict survival (O'Toole et al., 1972). On the other hand, other tests of immunity may be helpful. There is evidence that skin delayed hypersensitivity reactions to tuberculin and dinitrochlorobenzene (DNCB) (Cooper et al., 1973) are decreased in bladder cancer. The extent of the depression is correlated with invasion of the tumour. This type of immunological response is seen in many tumours. It is to be hoped that the very considerable effort being made in devising suitable tests for studying immunological reactions to tumours in vitro (Bloom et al., 1973) will result in development of a set of tests that can be used routinely in surgical practice.

Studies of the urine of bladder cancer-bearing patients may be helpful in surveillance. Cytology is one of the mainstays of follow up and in competent hands is an invaluable method of screening for recurrence, although carcinoma in situ may give a positive cytology in the absence of a tumour detectable by cystoscopy. It has been found that the muramidase (Kovanyi and Letanski, 1971) and β-glucuronidase (Hradec et al., 1965) content of the urine rises in bladder cancer. If urine content in these two enzymes is measured, and its concentration corrected for the urine creatinine content, this is able to provide the basis of a useful test to discriminate highly active invasive tumours from well differentiated non-invasive tumours (Cooper et al., 1973).

Progress in the management of urothelial cancer is slow, in part due to the long period of time required to see the effect of any change and in part due to the multiple factors that may influence the outcome. Ultimately, success or failure can only be expressed in terms of survival. However, the quality of life up to survival is important but more difficult to assess objectively.

The future requires meticulous data collection and use of modern data analytical methods to try to resolve precisely what is happening to the patients and to improve the criteria for selection of the mode of therapy that is best suited to the needs of the individual patient. The recent review by Williams and Smith (1973) on the achievements of therapy in urothelial cancer shows there is little reason for, and we are a long way from, the solution of knowing what is the best way to treat a patient with urothelial cancer.

References

Bloom, B. R., Landy, M., Lawrence, H. S. (1973): Cellular Immunol., 6, 331.
Bubenik, J., Perlmann, P., Helmstein, K. and Moberger, G. (1970): Int. J. Cancer, 5, 39.
Burghele, T., Mases, V., Ulad, C. and Vulcan, R. (1965): Urol. int., 20, 42.
Cooper, E. H., Anderson, C. K., Steele, L. and O'Boyle, P. J. (1973): Cancer, (in press).
Fulker, M. J., Cooper, E. H. and Tanaka, T. (1971): Cancer, 27, 71.
Hradec, E., Petrik, R. and Pezlardva, J. (1965): J. Urol., 94, 430.
Kovanyi, G. and Letansky, K. (1971): Europ. J. Cancer, 7, 25.
Levi, P. E., Cooper, E. H., Anderson, C. K. and Williams, R. E. (1969): Cancer, 23, 1074.
Melamed, M. R. (1972): Europ. J. Cancer, 8, 287.

O'Toole, C., Perlmann, P., Unsgaard, B., Almgard, L. E., Johansson, B., Moberger, G. and Edsmyr, F. (1972): Int. J. Cancer, 10, 92.
Pomerance, A. (1972): Brit. J. Urol., 44, 451.
Sama, K. P. (1970): J. Urol., 104, 843.
Spooner, M. and Cooper, E. H. (1972): Cancer, 29, 1401.
Tanaka, T., Cooper, E. H. and Anderson, C. K. (1970): Europ. J. clin. biol. Res., 15, 1084.
Williams, R. E. and Smith, P. (1973): Brit. J. Urol., 45, 310.

Mass or selective screening for bladder cancer

H. G. Parkes

*Health Research Unit, British Rubber Manufacturers' Association Ltd., Birmingham,
United Kingdom*

My intention in this short paper is to discuss one or two points in order to illustrate some of the problems associated with the introduction of a cytodiagnostic screening programme in an exposed to risk population. I propose to state very briefly what we are doing and why we are doing it. I hope also to discuss some of the problems and some of the lessons we hope we have learned during our 15 years' experience in this field.

In Great Britain we have a large population of chemical and rubber workers at risk as a result of their exposure to carcinogenic aromatic amines between 1927 and 1949. Undoubtedly, the most important of these amines was β-naphthylamine, the use and manufacture of which was abandoned in Great Britain in 1949. The withdrawal of these chemicals was followed shortly after by the implementation of early diagnostic screening procedures, and the first of these was a simple urine test for the presence of red blood cells. This was carried out routinely in the chemical industry, but was in practice found to be an effective diagnostic tool in only 50% of cases.

The cytodiagnostic technique was introduced into the chemical industry on a trial basis in 1951, and 6 years later a report was published by Geoffrey Crabbe et al. evaluating their experience and showing quite conclusively that the cytodiagnostic method was much to be preferred. On the appearance of this report a programme of cytodiagnostic screening was started in the British rubber industry, and in both these two industries the technique has been used continuously ever since. Insofar as the British rubber industry is concerned, and this is my personal area of interest, we have had to contend with a number of problems. For a start it was necessary for us to attempt to define the high risk areas of exposure and this was particularly difficult due to the size and the complexity of our industry. In this context we have since come to realise the enormous value of reliable epidemiological data in establishing the high risk occupations, and by using such information we have gradually accumulated within the rubber industry an exposed to risk study population of approximately 20,000. These 20,000 individuals do of course include not only current employees but also those who have retired or left for other occupations. Inevitably as time moves on it becomes more and more of an ageing population. To carry out our task we have had to evaluate the various techniques available to us and we have also had to determine from actual experience the optimum frequency of testing. We now consider that cytodiagnostic tests should ideally be carried out not less frequently than 3 times a year. This frequency is particularly desirable in view of the possibility that occasional false negative results may be obtained on the basis of a single test. In order to provide the required facilities we now maintain in Birmingham a cytodiagnostic laboratory with 4 full time technicians, and we are aware that similar facilities are independently provided for the chemical industry and that a small amount of testing is also done by National Health Service laboratories.

Use of the cytodiagnostic technique in the manner just described has thus far resulted in the diagnostic detection of some 200 cases of bladder cancer within the chemical and rubber industries. It should however be appreciated that this can only be regarded as a small proportion of the total of occupational tumours which have arisen. Understandably, there is no compulsion about participation in the screening arrangements, and there are inevitably a considerable number of cases of bladder cancer amongst men who, for one reason or another, do not participate in the cytodiagnostic programme. Because of this, it has been an important part of our work to compile an independent register of all known cases of bladder cancer arising in our industry whether or not these have been detected on cytodiagnostic screening.

There are 3 principal reasons which may be advanced as a justification for the implementation of a mass screening programme.

1. We are concerned with a population for which there is epidemiological evidence of an enhanced risk of bladder cancer.

2. It is a reasonable presumption that early diagnosis will facilitate treatment and may improve prognosis.

3. A recent High Court case has established for the employer the need to protect himself against legal liability.

1. Enhanced risk of bladder cancer

Each year in Great Britain there are some 4,000 deaths attributable to bladder cancer and it is estimated that between 1 and 10% of this total may be occupational in origin. It must surely be evident from this that no case can really be made out for a mass screening programme which is not clearly related to a population in which there exists a defineable risk. Such a programme could not be justified in cost benefit terms and might well be considered a waste of both money and medical manpower.

2. Benefits of early diagnosis

It is unfortunately clear that amongst cytologists, epidemiologists and statisticians involved in diagnostic screening programmes today there is no real agreement about the long term evaluation of their work. The debate will no doubt continue with conflicting claims and opinions being advanced by the protagonists in the columns of the medical journals. We ourselves feel that we can contribute little to this because our own experience suggests that the lead time which may be gained by cytodiagnosis is so variable that it makes the calculation of comparative survival times highly unreliable. I believe however, that we should start from the simple premise that early diagnosis does indeed offer the patient a brighter prospect, and I see no justification for abandoning that assumption unless and until we have conclusive evidence to the contrary. One reason why it is especially difficult to evaluate a cytodiagnostic urine screening programme is that results may sometimes be vitiated by delay in treatment. For this, one cannot blame the surgeon, he cannot act unless he has a positive finding on cystoscopy and, unlike the situation which obtains in cervical cancer, he is not free to carry out a cone biopsy.

3. Employer's liability

It has to be appreciated that this consideration does have a special importance in all cases of industrial cancer. Under British Law it is held that an employer has a duty to take all reasonable care to protect the health of his employees. There is of course much room for argument about what constitutes such reasonable care, but in so far as our screening programme is concerned the position has recently been clarified by a very important High Court Judgment, in which the Dunlop and I.C.I. companies were joint Defendants in an action brought by two Plaintiffs suffering from industrial bladder cancer. In this case the Court held that there was a duty on the part of the employer, having once become aware of the hazard to which his employees were exposed, to provide for them satisfactory cytodiagnostic screening arrangements or, alternatively, and at least, to ensure that they were properly advised of the need to secure such facilities. For the present time therefore, and for the forseeable future, it is evident that cytological screening of men at risk from industrial bladder cancer will have to continue.

Criteria

If the points which I have thus far made are valid, then I suggest that it is possible and reasonable to propose 4 criteria which might reasonably be adopted and applied in a selective screening programme for occupational bladder cancer: (1) Significant exposure to known or strongly suspected carcinogens should be firmly established before any screening programme is considered. (2) There should be available clear epidemiological evidence of an enhanced risk of cancer resulting from such exposure. (3) It should be demonstrable that the diagnostic techniques to be applied will have a high degree of efficiency. (4) There should be an upper age limit for entry into the screening programme (this is a more controversial proposal, but I personally can see little justification for descending upon ex rubber workers, and others who may already have spent several years in retirement who are aged perhaps 65 to 70, and who are going to be seriously alarmed if they are suddenly told that for the rest of their lives they should be subjected to regular urine tests because they may get bladder cancer).

In conclusion I would offer just one or two thoughts for the future.

Hopefully, our present screening programme will cease to have a useful purpose when the exposed to risk population which it now serves has disappeared from the scene.

What is needed for the remainder of this term is improved diagnostic efficiency matched with similar advances in treatment. At present we can claim diagnostic success in about 80% of our cases and we should certainly try to improve upon that. We have in the past year been looking hopefully for alternative or additional diagnostic procedures including for example the test for carcinoembryonic antigen. Unfortunately, present indications are that this, at least at the present time, is unlikely to be able to offer us much help. We are however also exploring the possibility of collaborating with Professor Field and others at Newcastle working on lymphocyte sensitisation, but it is too early yet to report on the results of this work and there are special difficulties particularly with regard to the collection of samples that have yet to be overcome. In summary therefore, I would say that our own experience of industrial screening argues strongly for a selective approach. What is needed surely is quality rather than quantity.

Perspectives in the treatment of cancer of the prostate*

A. Coune and H.J. Tagnon

*Service de Médecine et d'Investigation Clinique de l'Institut Jules Bordet,
Centre des Tumeurs de l'Université Libre de Bruxelles, Bruxelles, Belgium*

In the different fields of modern medicine, prospective comparative studies are now widely used to determine the efficiency of new drugs and various therapeutic methods. Usually, these clinical trials require a large number of patients, randomly assigned to the several therapeutic groups. The only way of gathering a large number of patients in a short period of time is the establishment of a cooperative group. The important role of such a group in medicine can no longer be questioned, as it allows the collection of a homogenous group of patients, from whom the response rate as well as the frequency of the side effects of the tested therapy can be determined. The recent development of new concepts in the treatment of human prostatic cancer provides a striking example not only of the usefulness but indeed of the necessity of the cooperative clinical trials. Prior to 1967, when the unexpected results of the Veterans Administration Cooperative Urological Research Group (VACURG) study were reported, high doses of diethylstilboestrol had been given to an amazingly high number of patients with prostatic cancer, without the lethal cardiovascular side effects of this drug being suspected (VACURG, 1967a). This clearly indicates how important a cooperative clinical trial may be since the widespread use of a drug is no guarantee of its harmlessness.

According to the VACURG clinical classification, stage I prostatic cancer is defined as an unsuspected carcinoma detected in a few areas of benign hyperplastic tissue resected because of symptoms of prostatism; at the present time the generally held opinion is that no further therapy is needed. A VACURG study, comparing placebo with radical prostatectomy followed by placebo has been in progress for 48 months. For stage II carcinoma, a palpable prostatic carcinomatous nodule without extraprostatic extension of the cancer, several therapeutic methods are available: radical prostatectomy, cryosurgery, supervoltage radiation therapy, and endocrine therapy, both pharmaceutical and surgical. Despite several clinical studies, most of them without adequate control series, nobody knows the best therapeutic procedure. In the United States of America, radical prostatectomy seems the favourite procedure for men under 70 years of age (Jewett, 1970). Nevertheless, as a high percentage of prostatic cancer develops in older men and grows at a relatively slow rate, it is not certain that all stage II patients need treatment. Relevant information will be available in the future as a result of the VACURG study number 2.

Stage III prostatic cancer exists when there is extraprostatic extension of the tumour without involvement beyond the pelvis. Stage IV is the disseminated stage of the disease. Both these stages are usually treated either by endocrine surgery or oestrogens.

Although the first favourable response to the endocrine modification of the host was observed in a case of prostatic carcinoma, the effect of hormonal treatment has been assessed with much greater accuracy in the treatment of disseminated breast carcinoma in the human being, because of the presence of multiple accessible and accurately measurable metastatic lesions. Experience has repeatedly shown the small number of direct

*This work was supported by the Fonds Cancérologique de la Caisse d'Epargne.

specific objective criteria available for evaluating the response of prostatic carcinoma to therapy; usually evaluation is based on indirect objective criteria and even on subjective criteria. To avoid this drawback, the duration of survival from the start of treatment is used as the criterion for evaluating the response to a drug. As a matter of fact, the objective improvement induced by the endocrine treatment of patients with advanced prostatic carcinoma is not known; the VACURG study indicates that 40% of patients with progressive cancer show definite clinical improvement; however, the criteria used for the evaluation are not described (VACURG, 1967*b*). It is very important for further clinical trials on prostatic cancer to try to define precise objective criteria for evaluation. These criteria may be direct ones, like the size of the prostatic tumour or its metastases, or indirect ones, like the determination of, kidney function. Refinement of methods of measurement used today are urgently needed. The size of the prostatic tumour will probably be more accurately determined by the use of ultrasonic scans or scintigrams, following uptake by the prostatic tissue of radio-iodinated sex hormones. Methods for quantifying bone metastases are being studied and may result in a more precise evaluation of lytic as well as plastic lesions. The EORTC Genito-Urinary Tract Cancer Cooperative Group B has launched a clinical trial using only objective criteria for the evaluation of prostatic cancer cases. As a matter of fact a very important conclusion emerged from the VACURG study: evaluation of a drug using survival as a major criterion may be biased by the lethal side effects of oestrogenic compounds. This is confirmed by the recent results of this study on a 10-year follow-up basis. For stages III and IV, treatments without oestrogen are significantly better than treatments including oestrogen. A new clinical study has been started by the VACURG for determining if a smaller dose of diethylstilboestrol would be as effective while being much less toxic than the usual 5 mg a day dose (Bailar III et al., 1970). After 54 months follow-up it appears that there is nothing to indicate that the 1.0 mg dose is less effective than the 5.0 mg dose in controlling cancer of the prostate, while there is a significantly greater risk of death from cardiovascular diseases when the 5.0 mg dose is used. Definition of the parameters which would indicate the patients most susceptible to these side effects is a very important task for the near future. Diethylstilboestrol induces major modifications in several blood components like plasminogen, fibrinogen and other proteins. Possible relations between these modifications and the appearance of the cardiovascular and thrombo-embolic side effects are being studied. It is possible that the oestrogens may act on one of the 3 different proteolytic systems contained in the human prostate (Nijs et al., 1971). The VACURG has also started a clinical study using a natural conjugated oestrogen instead of diethylstilboestrol. Finally it will be very interesting to determine the action and the side effects of anti-oestrogenic compounds endowed with weak oestrogenic properties.

Using electron microscopic autoradiographic studies, Sinha et al. (1973) have shown that ^{3}H-oestradiol is incorporated in vitro in the basal and invasive cells, but rarely in the differentiated cells, of human prostatic carcinoma. This suggests that oestrogens may act directly on some of the prostatic cancer cells. Further development in this field may perhaps allow oestrogen sensitive cancer cells and oestrogen insensitive cancer cells to be distinguished. On the other hand, determination of the sex hormone steroid receptors in the prostatic cancer cells may perhaps provide additional understanding of the therapeutic effect as has been suggested in the field of human breast cancer (Mainwaring and Milroy, 1973).

Another class of compounds studied in relation to prostatic cancer is the progestational one. In the latest VACURG clinical trial one group of patients is receiving medroxyprogesterone. Another progestational drug, endowed with potent anti-androgenic properties, is under current investigation. Although no results of a comparative randomized trial versus diethylstilboestrol are available, the preliminary results suggest that cyproterone acetate may be a valuable drug for the treatment of human prostatic cancer (Wein and Murphy, 1973). Unfortunately its side effects are not as yet well known. A non-steroidal anti-androgen is also available and is being tested on animal tumours.

Experimental work indicates that prolactin and testosterone stimulate the growth of the lateral lobe of the prostate in hypophysectomized and orchiectomized rats. In vitro, sheep prolactin, at a concentration of 1.5 μg per ml, stimulates adenylate cyclase activity in rat prostatic tissue homogenate (Golder et al., 1972). Evidence that the growth of the prostate can be affected by prolactin has prompted the EORTC Genito-Urinary Cancer Cooperative Group B to launch a clinical trial using an ergocryptine derivative to reduce pituitary prolactin secretion. This study is now in progress.

In cases of failure of the initial endocrine treatment or in cases of reactivation of the disease after a first regression, radioactive pituitary implantation has been advocated; nevertheless no case of long lasting objectively-assessed regression has been reported after such a procedure (Fergusson and Hendry, 1971). A recently published series of 22 patients treated by bilateral adrenalectomy indicates an objective response rate of 36% and a median survival of 9 months; it must be stressed that the response criteria are not described and that this trial is not a comparative one (Mahoney and Hartwell Harrison, 1972). Further investigation is needed to determine the real value of major ablative endocrine therapy in human prostatic cancer.

As far as cytotoxic chemotherapy is concerned, only a few reports are available in the literature. The frequent involvement of numerous bones in disseminated prostatic cancer may necessitate dose adjustment because of severe marrow toxicity; nevertheless further study of chemotherapy, alone or in combination, may be rewarding.

It is a paradox that throughout the 25 years since Huggins's publication the availability of a reliable and innocuous treatment for cancer of the prostate has been taken for granted (Huggins and Hodges, 1941). Only in the last few years have we become aware of the necessity of investigating more deeply the difficult field of prostatic cancer in order to develop a harmless and efficient therapy.

References

Bailar III, J.C., Byar, D.P. and Veterans Administration Cooperative Urological Research Group (1970): Cancer (Philad.), 26, 257.
Fergusson, J.D. and Hendry, W.F. (1971): Brit. J. Urol., 43, 514.
Golder, M.P., Boyns, A.R., Harper, M.E. and Griffiths, K. (1972): Biochem. J., 128, 725.
Huggins, C. and Hodges, C.V. (1941): Cancer Res., 1, 292.
Jewett, H.J. (1970): J. Urol. (Baltimore), 103, 195.
Mahoney, E.M. and Hartwell Harrison, J. (1972): J. Urol. (Baltimore), 108, 936.
Mainwaring, W.I.P. and Milroy, E.J.G. (1973): J. Endocr., 57, 371.
Nijs, M., Brassinne, Ch., Coune, A. and Tagnon, H.J. (1971): Thrombos. Diathes. haemorrh. (Stuttg.), 25, 481.
Sinha, A.A., Blackard, C.E., Doe, R.P. and Seal, U.S. (1973): Cancer (Philad.), 31, 682.
Veterans Administration Cooperative Urological Research Group (1967a): J. Urol. (Baltimore), 98, 516.
Veterans Administration Cooperative Urological Research Group (1967b): Surg. Gynec. Obstet., 124, 1011.
Wein, A.J. and Murphy, J.J. (1973): J. Urol. (Baltimore), 109, 68.

5. *Uterine cervix carcinoma*

Follow-up studies of untreated cervical dysplasia

Magnus Nasiell, Karen Nasiell, Vlasta Vaclavinkova and Vivi Roger

Departments of Cytology, and Obstetrics and Gynecology, Sabbatsberg Hospital, Stockholm, Sweden

Dysplasia of the uterine cervix has been studied in the Departments of Cytology and Obstetrics and Gynecology of Sabbatsberg Hospital, Stockholm, for approximately 10 years with a long term follow-up of about 1,700 women including vaginal-cervical smears, colposcopy, punch biopsy in a selected part of the series, etc. The intention was to study the development of mild, moderate, and severe cervical dysplasia in relation to various parameters such as biopsy, age, pregnancy/deliveries, and inflammation.

In order to check the diagnostic accuracy of cytology, a special experimental study was designed to correlate the cytological diagnosis with the final histological diagnosis. This study showed that out of all the cases diagnosed cytologically as moderate dysplasia, no case had a histological diagnosis of carcinoma in situ or invasive carcinoma and only one case had a normal histology. Out of the patients having a cytological diagnosis of severe dysplasia 26% showed carcinoma in situ, but no case showed invasive carcinoma at the histological examination.

The patients in the follow-up study have been grouped according to whether or not a biopsy had been performed. Thus, the patients in this study do not include cases treated with cone biopsy, cautery, radiation, or cryosurgery. The follow-up time varies from 1-12 years, with average times of 1.8 years for mild dysplasia, 4.1 for moderate dysplasia, and 3.5 years for severe dysplasia.

Out of 550 patients with mild dysplasia 3/5 showed regression and 1/5 persistence of the dysplasia. The remaining cases showed progression to moderate or severe dysplasia or carcinoma in situ. 8% of the patients with mild dysplasia had a final diagnosis of severe dysplasia or carcinoma in situ.

There were 3 patients, all from the retrospective part of the material, who showed progression to invasive carcinoma. Otherwise a cone biopsy was always performed when the cytological examination indicated progression to in situ carcinoma.

Out of the 850 patients with moderate dysplasia, slightly more than 50% showed regression of the abnormality, about 25% showed persistence and the remainder showed progression. There was no statistically significant difference between the biopsy group and the non-biopsy group with respect to regression, persistence, and progression.

Out of the 265 patients with severe dysplasia somewhat more than 1/3 showed complete regression. Out of these patients only 12 had not had a biopsy. Somewhat more than 1/3 showed progression to carcinoma in situ and the remaining patients showed persistence of dysplasia, i.e. mild, moderate, or severe dysplasia. In the severe dysplasia group with complete regression it was found that the performance of a biopsy significantly influenced the tendency to complete regression.

It is possible to conclude that certain patients with dysplastic lesions will develop more advanced lesions including carcinoma in situ, that some will regress to normal and that the highest frequency of progression is seen in patients with severe dysplasia. However, biopsies are frequently performed on the patients in this particular group, a fact which makes the evaluation of the biological development difficult.

The most interesting findings of this study concern the more easily defined changes, i.e. mild and moderate dysplasia. According to the results obtained the diagnosis of mild or moderate dysplasia indicates that a careful follow-up of the patient is necessary.

The effects of mass screening on morbidity and mortality from cervix cancer*

William M. Christopherson

Department of Pathology, University of Louisville School of Medicine, Louisville, Ky., U.S.A.

The incidence of carcinoma of the cervix in the United States is exceeded only by breast and colon-rectum cancer in women. This is also true for other western countries. Cervix cancer, however, is the major cancer problem in the developing, highly populated countries of the world. Unlike other sites, cervical cancer is a controllable disease. The method of control is accurate, painless, and economical. It requires organization and an extraordinary amount of hard work and perseverence. Many health authorities have been slow to recommend, and even slower to establish, effective cervix cancer control programs, often citing the writings of a minority who cast doubt on the indisputable evidence that cancer of the cervix, like other sites, must of necessity arise from carcinoma in situ.

Another major reason for the slow development of cervix cancer control programs is a misunderstanding of cost factors. The ability of trained paramedical personnel (cytotechnologists) to screen a large number of slides each day has been well demonstrated in our laboratory and many others in various areas of the world. Effective screening is not directly related to a minimal workload. Quite the contrary, those who do the best job of screening can often cover up to 100 patients a day. The cost-benefit ratio for any screening program should be large. In the United States it has been calculated by our Public Health Service to be 1:9. In other words, $9 accrue for every $1 spent on cervix cancer screening.

The following is a brief outline documenting the fact that: (1) It is possible to reach almost the entire female population in a mass screening program; (2) in such a program invasive cancer will be detected at a much earlier stage (usually the asymptomatic stage) and, therefore, produce higher cure rates; (3) the incidence of invasive cancer will decrease due to the elimination of carcinoma in situ from the population; (4) death rates will eventually show a significant decrease due to the combination of earlier diagnosis and lower incidence; and (5) the average age of deaths in the failures will increase by several years.

Louisville, Jefferson County, Kentucky has a population of slightly over 800,000. There are approximately 220,000 women at risk. Currently 140,000 women are examined each year. The smears are obtained by direct visualization by private physicians in their offices. A clinic is maintained in the University Hospital for the screening of clinic patients who do not have a private physician. In the latter clinic the examination is free and is recommended to all women attending out-patient clinics. I would like to stress that the important thing is to screen asymptomatic out-patients rather than women who are hospitalized. It is also just as important to screen women attending dental clinics, eye clinics, etc., as those attending obstetric and gynecologic clinics. In point of fact, our highest yield has come from women attending ear, nose and throat clinics; followed by those attending dental clinics. This is largely due to the age group involved. Another important facet of mass population screening is to be sure to reach the older women. For example, women 30 years of age and younger are easily screened since they are

* This work was supported by a grant from the American Cancer Society, Inc. and by the Kentucky Division of the American Cancer Society.

receiving obstetrical care, postpartum care, contraceptive advice etc. This group produces less than 4% of all invasive uterine cancers. On the other hand, women 50 years old and older (usually postmenopausal) produce the majority of invasive cervix cancers and contribute highly towards death rates. These women normally do not attend gynecologic clinics.

With such a screening program, approximately 94% of the population has been screened at least once. A high percentage of these have been screened on multiple occasions. The small percentage that has not been reached consists mainly of women 60 years old and older.

Of equal importance to identifying the women with positive cytology, is obtaining a biopsy diagnosis, providing treatment and maintaining a follow-up. In recent years 99.6% of all cervix cancers have been histologically proved.

Results

The percentage of patients diagnosed as having Stage I disease showed an increase of 78% over the precytology control years of 1953 to 1955. The most remarkable improvement of diagnosing the cancer at Stage I was in women under 50 years of age. Stage I disease decreased with each decade and reached a low of 15% for those 70 years old and older. These older women with cancer rarely had prior screening and they contributed heavily to death rates.

Carcinoma in situ increased proportionately with screening activities. After reaching a peak in 1967, carcinoma in situ has steadily decreased.

The age adjusted incidence rates for invasive squamous carcinoma of the cervix has decreased by over 50%.

The ultimate test of the effectiveness of a cancer control program is a demonstrable decrease in death rates attributable to that program. One would logically assume that with a decrease in incidence rates and with earlier diagnosis, death rates must of necessity come down. However, the rationale for screening is still being questioned because of delay in documenting a decrease in death rates.

Since Jefferson County was the only county in Kentucky where a mass effort at cytologic screening was undertaken, we used the rest of the state outside of Jefferson County as a control population. The death rates in Jefferson County changed from 23.7 per 100,000 in 1953 to 10.8 per 100,000 in 1970, whereas there was no significant change in the rest of the state.

It could be argued that physicians in Jefferson County had improved in delineating cervix cancer from other uterine cancers during the last several years of the study, while the physicians in the rest of the state had not shown this improvement. To test this, total deaths from uterine cancer were computed and showed a similar change in Jefferson County, whereas there was no statistically significant change in the rest of the state.

An additional dividend attributable to the screening program was a remarkable increase of 7.6 years for residents of the County in the average age at time of death from cervix cancer.

Conclusions

Morbidity and mortality from cervix cancer is highly controllable through mass population screening — statements to the contrary notwithstanding. While sporadic, limited screening is of great benefit to the individual in whom an early lesion is detected, it will not show appreciable effects either on incidence or death trends.

Since the method is not only economical, but has a high cost-benefit ratio, and since the uterine cervix has proved to be the only cancer site that can be effectively controlled, it is to be hoped that this method which has been applied now for over a quarter of a century will finally receive more attention from health authorities and the medical profession in general.

6.   Cancer of the breast

Assessment of etiological factors in human breast cancer relevant to prevention

F. De Waard

Department of Epidemiology, University of Utrecht and The Cancer Registry, Amsterdam, The Netherlands

In preventive medicine there is a distinction between primary and secondary prevention. Theoretically, only primary prevention is true prevention, viz: reducing the incidence of the disease by eliminating one or more causal factors. No causal factors have come to light so far which warrant investigation aimed at the primary prevention of breast cancer.

Paraphrasing from Roman history: *Senatu deliberante periit Saguntum*   It may be pertinent to ask whether epidemiologists have not been wasting valuable time while the enemy (cancer) has been gaining ground. The answer is, that for a strategy to be successful, time is needed in order to choose the right direction in which to strike. The cancer enemy has provided a number of traps which may lead the research worker into a swamp from which he will not be able to rescue himself. These traps are called: 'Spurious associations and correlations'. An illustration of this kind of trap, which is sufficiently obvious to be easily identifiable as such, is the inverse relationship between the incidence of breast cancer and mean annual outdoor temperature in the countries studied so far. Few among the members of this audience will suggest a mass migration to tropical regions to prevent breast cancer! Nevertheless, less obvious traps have seriously hampered progress in the field of prevention. Up to 1970 many statistics showed an inverse relationship between breast cancer risk and the number of children delivered. These findings resulted in a widespread belief that some event related to childbearing, e.g. lactation, afforded protection in an unknown manner against human breast cancer.

Due to the work of an international group under the leadership of MacMahon it is now being recognised that lactation offers no protection against mammary cancer, and that the inverse relation between parity and breast cancer was a trap indeed. The relationship disappears if the data are standardised for age at *first* pregnancy, and this variable seems to be an important one with regard to the risk of breast cancer. Cole and MacMahon have postulated that certain risk-associated hormonal patterns existing during young adulthood may be modified by pregnancy. Thus, an early first pregnancy means an early intervention in the hormonal actions upon the reproductive organs, including the breast. Without speculating on the nature of hormonal risk factors – e.g. the estrogen ratio as Cole and MacMahon believe, or abnormal androgen production as Bulbrook, Hayward and Spicer have shown – the potential consequences of the age-at-first-pregnancy issue seem to be of importance when family planning is practiced.

In contrast to the situation with respect to primary prevention, in secondary prevention programmes (population screening) it is not of vital importance to know whether a statistically established risk factor is a causal factor or not. E.g., in screening programmes for cervical cancer it is well known that the prevalence will be highest in the lower socio-economic groups although socio-economic status as such is not considered by most scientists to be a causal factor of this kind of malignancy.

When high-risk groups can be identified, ways of increasing the yield of screening are both feasible and desirable. However, for particular high-risk factors, there are practical limitations. Very often it will be difficult to find an acceptable 'threshold' below which a group will not be offered screening opportunities.

We strongly advise against regarding parity as a risk factor in breast cancer screening. This is because the statistical relationship between age at first pregnancy and number of children may gradually disappear. In The Netherlands at least, there is a tendency to marry earlier and to have smaller families. Thus, in the not too far distant future the factor, parity, may lose its statistical relationship with breast cancer altogether.

Up to now, cancer screening programmes have been largely exercises in good organization, health education, technology and statistics; only few attemps have been made to use these studies as a means of learning more about the natural history of breast cancer. Even less has been published about the applications of biological insight to cancer control programmes.

Recently our group has developed a theory about biological aspects of population screening for mammary cancer. These ideas were stimulated by findings in the breast cancer study of the Health Insurance Plan of greater New York. That study revealed that the benefits of screening in bringing down the case fatality rate were limited to the postmenopausal group.

We suggest that the difference in outcome between pre- and postmenopausal women may be explained biologically. It is a fundamental rule in cancer screening that slow-growing tumors have a greater chance of being picked up in a curable stage than fast-growing tumors. It is well known that the growth rate of existing breast cancers can be accelerated by estrogens if the tumor cells contain the specific receptor sites for these hormones. Since estrogenic stimulation is markedly reduced at the menopause, a decrease in tumor growth rates is quite natural. In fact, such a decrease has been described by those who were able to follow a number of untreated patients.

The question remains whether estrogenic stimulation continues in some women after the cessation of menses. Our cytological studies in 7000 normal postmenopausal women have shown that there is an almost linear relation between the frequency of estrogenic smears and the degree of overweight of these women. It may be of interest also that obesity is more common in postmenopausal breast cancer patients than in the general population of the same age.

These findings have been put into perspective by recent biochemical studies which have shown that estrogen production in postmenopausal women takes place in peripheral tissues (notably in adipose tissue) from adrenocortical androstenedione.

In preliminary studies in obese postmenopausal women we have obtained evidence both cytologically and biochemically that even moderate weight reduction is accompanied by a further drop in the estrogen level. Under these conditions estrogen-responsive tumors will grow very slowly indeed.

Based on this idea we have designed a study which combines breast cancer screening with nutritional intervention, viz: weight reduction.

Of course, many problems of a practical nature will have to be dealt with. Still, we think the basic concept is solid enough to go ahead with in 1974.

Some reflections on the etiology of the cancer of the breast*

Ernest L. Wynder, Rebecca C. Gantt and Peter Hill

Divisions of Epidemiology and Nutrition, Naylor Dana Institute for Disease Prevention, American Health Foundation, New York, N.Y., U.S.A.

When examining the role of the environment in the development of various cancers, logical reasoning led to the suspicion that an inhalant such as cigarette smoke could result in the development of lung cancer and that nutritional factors could play a role in the carcinogenesis of large bowel cancer. A great many studies thus far on breast cancer have been mainly concerned with functions of the breast and environmental factors most readily related to these functions such as marriage, parity and lactation. While these have been contributory toward descriptive epidemiology, not all prominent factors have been consistently supported on a widespread basis. Therefore, it is less readily apparent which environmental factors really lead to cancer of the breast. Since breast development and maturation are dependent upon hormones, and breast tissue and function are maintained by hormones, it would seem logical that any environmental factor which alters hormone production or action could be of etiological significance. It would thus seem evident that epidemiological studies dealing with oral contraceptives and long-term hormonal therapy should be done as well as laboratory studies which assess the hormonal milieu.

Demographic leads

The major leads on the etiology of breast cancer come from its demographic distribution. The major clues are: (1) the difference in mortality rates among Japanese and American populations, especially for post-menopausal breast cancer (Fig. 1) (WHO, 1970); (2) the breast cancer mortality increases (although less rapidly than colon cancer) among Japanese immigrants to the United States (Fig. 2) (Haenszel and Kurihara, 1968); (3) the incidence seems to be increasing especially among age groups 34—44 in America (Fig. 3) (Conn. State Dept. Health, 1966, 1964 *a*, *b*, 1965, 1971); (4) there is a positive correlation between breast cancer and prostatic cancer mortality (Fig. 4) (Segi et al., 1972); (5) there is a positive association between fat consumption and the mortality of breast cancer (Fig. 5) (Segi et al., 1972; FAO, 1970); (6) in New York City, cancer of the breast is relatively more common among Jewish women (Fig. 6) (Newill, 1961; Seidman, 1970). It is possible that the general factor underlying all these observations appears to be nutrition, especially in terms of fat and/or cholesterol.

Case control studies

A number of investigators have carried out case control studies in which they have compared various factors (DeWaard et al., 1960; Lilienfeld, 1963; Shapiro et al., 1968;

---

* This work was supported in part by Public Health Service grant CA 012376-03 and in part by grant ET 33-0 from American Cancer Society, Inc.

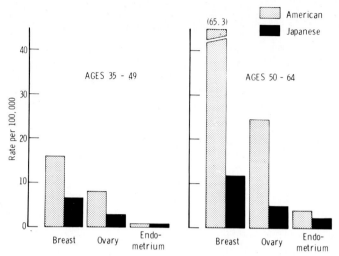

FIG. 1   *Mortality rate from hormone-related cancers in American and Japanese women by age, 1964–65.*

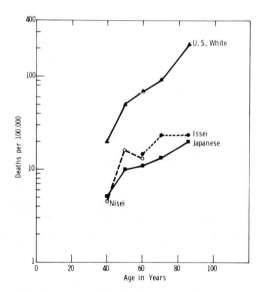

FIG. 2   *Age-specific death rates for breast cancer in women. Issei (1959–62), Nisei (1959–62) and U.S. Whites (1959–61). (From: Haenszel and Kurihara, 1968).*

Staszewski, 1971; Trichopoulos et al., 1972; Wynder, 1969; Wynder et al., 1960; Zippin and Petrakis, 1971). Among these factors which have been shown to be positively related to cancer of the breast are: (1) older age at first pregnancy; (2) early age of menarche; (3) late menopause; (4) a family history of breast cancer; (5) a history of fibrocystic disease of the breast; (6) size of the breast; and (7) obesity. It should be pointed out, however, that none of the differences in these factors are large enough, even though repeated in various studies, to account for the major difference, which is approximately 5-fold, in rates existing between American and Japanese populations.

The high frequency of breast cancer in obese Dutch women as observed in The Netherlands has not been confirmed in this country (DeWaard, 1969). It should be stressed that if obesity does play a major role in the American rate of breast cancer, then the rate should be especially high in Negro women since obesity is far more common among them than among Caucasians. Also, data standardized for socio-economic status indicate that in Memorial Hospital, N.Y.C., the higher the status, the less frequent is obesity, and yet breast cancer is more prevalent in the more affluent and better educated groups (Wynder, 1969). Obviously, potential as well as overt obesity should be examined as well as the differences, if any, in obesities induced by carbohydrate or fat intake.

Our own data did not show a difference in age of first pregnancy between study and control groups (Wynder et al., 1960). It remains to be shown whether this difference is related to differences in matching for socio-economic status, a factor known to influence age of first pregnancy (Cole and MacMahon, 1969).

Early reports do not indicate that the rate of breast cancer is affected by birth control medication, though admittedly the number of cases — particularly in terms of long-term usage — on which these results are based are quite small (Fechner, 1970; Vessey et al., 1971; 1972). Our own studies dealing with birth control medication are currently in progress. Recent evaluation of the data indicates that socio-economic variables such as age, education, race, religion, and other epidemiological factors; age at first marriage, age at first intercourse, age at first pregnancy and number of pregnancies are important determinants of oral contraceptive usage. All these variables must be considered in the deter-

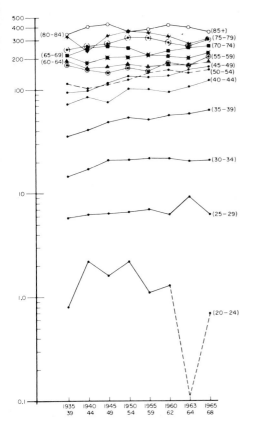

FIG. 3   *Age specific breast cancer incidence rates per 100,000 population. Connecticut (1935–68). (From: the Connecticut State Department of Health).*

mination of the carcinogenicity of hormones. In recent data analyzed, the percentage of long term oral contraceptive users (5 or more years) amounts to only 5.3% for age groups 30–49. It is important, therefore, to emphasize the limited size of the current sample and the fact that this percentage is controlled only for age.

Rough preliminary evaluation of data thus far within these stated limitations supports the concept that use of 'The Pill' does not increase the risk of developing cancer of the breast. In fact, there is some indication that it may reduce the risk.

A number of studies have suggested that women on long-term hormonal therapy may

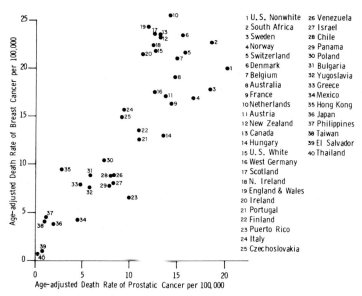

FIG. 4   *Correlation between breast cancer in women and prostatic cancer in men (1964–1965).*
(From: Segi et al., 1969).

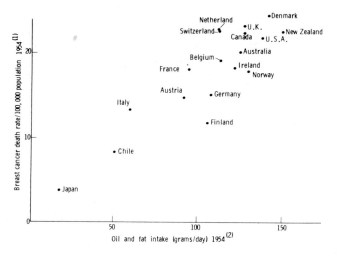

FIG. 5   *Correlation between oil and fat intake and breast cancer. ((1) From: Segi, 1964; (2) From:*
U.N. Food and Agricultural Organization, 1960).

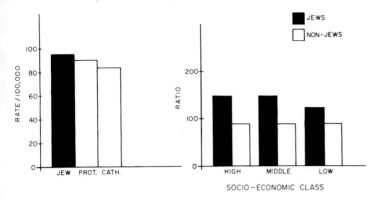

FIG. 6   *(Left) Estimate average annual death rates from breast cancer in Caucasians, age 45 or over*
(N.Y.C., 1953–58) (From: Newill, 1961); (Right) Age adjusted breast cancer death rates in
N.Y.C. Caucasians, ratios in Jews and non-Jews by socio-economic status (1949–51).
(From: Seidman, 1970).

have a reduced risk of developing breast cancer (Table 1) (Burch and Byrd, 1971; Geist et
al., 1941; Henneman and Wallach, 1957; Leis, 1966; Mustacchi and Gordan, 1958;
Schezler-Saunders, 1960; Wilson, 1962). Studies of this nature need to be conducted in
further detail (J. nat. Cancer Inst., Editorial, 1973). This also is a difficult epidemiological
undertaking because of the highly selective nature, as well as the relatively small number
of women who are on long-term hormonal medication.

Metabolic epidemiological studies

A number of investigations have suggested that different hormonal patterns may be
related to a woman's risk of developing breast cancer.

It has been postulated that the ratio of estriol to estradiol and estrone decreases in
breast cancer patients (MacMahon et al., 1971; Briggs, 1972). A higher ratio has been
reported in Japanese or Indian women who have a low incidence of breast cancer. The
ratio in healthy Caucasians compared to those with breast cancer overlap and may even
increase in premenopausal breast cancer patients (Table 2) (Briggs, 1972; Lemon et al.,
1966; Arguelles et al., 1973). The interpretation of the urinary levels of estrogens is
ambiguous since estriol arises as a breakdown product of estradiol and estrone or by
peripheral conversion of androgens. If the urinary level of estradiol in Caucasians is higher
than in Japanese, one may assume that this may also be the case in the peripheral
circulation. Without knowledge of the ovarian production rate (Lloyd et al., 1971) or
metabolic clearance of estradiol in the two populations though, no valid judgement can
be made. No difference in the plasma estrogen has been reported in pre-menopausal
patients (Bulbrook, 1972), and it is unproven that either estradiol or estriol is carcinogenic in women.

Comparative studies of British and Japanese women indicate a lower secretion of
androgens in young women, and a significant alteration in the urinary excretion of
androsterone to aetiocholanolone (5a/5b ratio) in older Japanese women (Bulbrook and
Thomas, 1964; Bulbrook et al., 1967). However, in early breast cancer cases, no difference has been found in the plasma 17-oxosteroid or 11-deoxy-17-oxosteroid levels
(Deshpande et al., 1965). Also, the urinary level of 11-deoxy-17-ketosteroids has been
reported to be the same in Japanese and American patients (Kumaoka et al., 1968).

Furthermore, no difference has been found in the aeticholanolone excretion in breast
cancer patients in general (Gleave et al., 1969). A change in this excretion was found only

TABLE 1   Incidence of breast and gynecological cancer subsequent to long-term administration of estrogens

Authors (years)	No. of patients	Age (years)	Reasons for estrogen administration	Methods and duration of administration	Years of follow-up	Cancer incidence site obs./exp.
Geist et al., 1941	206	25–80	Menopausal syndrome, functional amenorrhea, senile vaginitis, kraurosis vulvae	Estrogens only 6 mth – 5.5 years	1–5	Breast/gyn 0/12
Henneman et al., 1957	292	15–83 (avg. 51)	Menopausal syndrome, postmenopausal, osteoporosis	Cyclic estrogens > 1 yr (average 5.1 years)	1–25	Gyn 7/22 (Cervix 1, ovary 2, endometrium 4)
Mustacchi et al., 1958	120	15–84 (avg. 62)	Osteoporosis	Estrogens 3–8 years alone, androgens, or estrogens + androgens	> 1	Breast/gyn 0/5–6*
Wilson, 1962	304	40–70 (avg. 51)	Estrogens deficient women according to Pap smear tests	Cyclic estrogens 1–27 years	1–27	Breast/gyn 0/18
Schleyer-Saunders, 1960	300	30–60	Artificial menopause, osteoporosis, senile vaginitis etc.	Estrogen/androgen and DOCA. Combination pellet Several years	Several	Breast 3 gyn 4 (Cervix 1, ovary 2, endometrium 1)
Leis, 1966	158	36–54 (avg. 46)	Menopausal syndrome, incl. some cases art. menop.	Cyclic estrogens 8 years Progesterone 10–14 years	8–14	Breast/gyn 0/Unknown
Burch et al., 1971	511	27–72 (avg. 54)	Hysterectomy	Estrogens only long-term	29	Breast 9/39

* Expected number for all malignant tumors

TABLE 2   Urinary estrogen in premenopausal women ($\mu g/24$ hr)

Authors	No. of women	Race	Breast cancer	Age	Estrone	Estradiol	Estriol	Estriol (estradiol and estrone)
Lemon et al. (1966)	16	White	No	28	5.6 ± 1.1	5.3 ± 1.5	10.0 ± 0.3	1.5 ± 0.3
	6	White	Yes	34	1.3 – 8.0	1.3 – 4.8	1.0 – 8.6	0.6 ± 0.4
MacMahon et al. (1971)	29	Asians	No	39	5.3 – 7.7*	2.5 – 3.6	8.2 – 15.1	1.27 – 1.64
	30	North Americans	No	39	7.0 – 13.3*	3.4 – 7.6	8.3 – 14.3	0.83 – 0.89
Argüelles et al. (1973)	8	Argentine	No	Unknown	16.2 ± 4.7	4.5 ± 1.7	20.8 ± 4.0	1.02 ± 0.14
	47	Argentine	Yes	Unknown	10.1 ± 4	3.6 ± 2.0	17.2 ± 8.3	1.28 ± 0.25

* Follicular and luteal mean values

in advanced breast cancer patients (Forrest, 1971), so the use of altered androgen excretion, 5a/5b ratio in the early diagnosis of breast cancer or in the identification of high breast cancer risk individuals, remains unproven. This ratio of 5a/5b appears to be determined by puberty and is specific for the individual (Tanner and Gupta, 1968). Whether the hormonal conditions initiating benign (Brennan et al., 1973) or malignant breast disease are the same is unclear.

We feel, however, that whatever hormonal pattern has been established so far — perhaps because the techniques used were based on urinary analysis or perhaps because the differences were related to other variables — cannot account for large-scale geographical differences in the incidence of breast cancer. It is possible that what is related to the development of breast cancer may be 'initiating' exposure which could well be hormonal in nature, whose onset is early in life, perhaps around puberty. This is then followed by a promoting factor which we hypothesize might be dietary in nature and which has its effect later in life.

Chan and Cohen (1974) in confirmation of earlier studies (Carroll and Khor, 1970, 1971) have shown that a diet high in fat enhances mammary tumor incidence in DMBA treated rats. Explorations are currently being made on the possible role of mechanisms in the endocrine system underlying this phenomenon. Data thus far appear to indicate that high dietary fat intake, in an as yet unexplained manner, raises the serum prolactin in rats, and this elevation in turn stimulates the growth of mammary tumors. Extrapolating these rat model findings to human breast cancer, which can only be done with the greatest of caution suggests that high dietary fat intake stimulates, via the pituitary prolactin, in situ mammary lesions to grow into overt tumors.

Conclusion

We conclude that some of the promising leads in the etiology of breast cancer which need to be explored now relate to birth control medication in early life, long-term hormonal therapy in later life, and to the apparent interrelationship between nutrition and cancer of the breast.

References

Argüelles, A.E. et al. (1973): Lancet, 1, 165–8.
Brennan, M.J. et al. (1973): Lancet, 1, 1076–9.
Briggs, M. (1972): Lancet, 2, 324.
Bulbrook, R.D. (1972): J. Nat. Cancer Inst., 48, 1039.
Bulbrook, R.D. and Thomas, B.S. (1964): Nature (Lond.), 201, 189.
Bulbrook, R.D. et al. (1967): J. Endocr., 38, 401.
Burch, J.C. and Byrd, B.F. (1971): Ann. Surg., 174, 414.
Carroll, K.K. and Khor, H.T. (1970): Cancer Res., 30, 2260.
Carroll, K.K. and Khor, H.T. (1971): Lipids, 6, 415.
Chan, P.C. and Cohen, L. (1974): J. nat. Cancer Inst., 52, 25.
Cole, P. and MacMahon, B. (1969): Lancet, 1, 604.
Connecticut State Department of Health (1964a): Cancer in Connecticut, Incidence and Rates, 1963.
Connecticut State Department of Health (1964b): Cancer in Connecticut, Incidence and Rates, 1964.
Connecticut State Department of Health (1965): Cancer in Connecticut, Incidence and Rates, 1965.
Connecticut State Department of Health (1966): Cancer in Connecticut, Incidence and Rates, 1935–62.
Connecticut State Department of Health (1971): Cancer in Connecticut, Incidence and Rates, 1966–68.
Deshpande, N. et al. (1965): J. Endocr., 32, 167.
DeWaard, F. (1969): Int. J. Cancer, 4, 577.
DeWaard, F., DeLaive, J.W.J., Baanders and Van Halewijin, E.A. (1960): Brit. J. Cancer, 14, 437.

FAO (1970): Production Yearbook, Vol. 23. Food and Agricultural Organization of the United Nations, Rome, 1970.

Fechner, R.E. (1970): Cancer, 26, 1204.

Forrest, A.P.M. (1971): Proc. roy. Soc. Med., 64, 509.

Geist, S.H., Walter, R.I. and Salmon, U.J. (1941): Amer. J. Obstet. Gynec., 42, 242.

Gleave, E.N. et al. (1969): Brit. J. Surg., 56, 627.

Haenszel, W. and Kurihara, M. (1968): J. nat. Cancer Inst., 40, 43.

Henneman, P.H. and Wallach, S., (1957): Arch. int. Med., 100, 715.

Journal of the National Cancer Institute (1973): Exogenous Hormones – Boon or Culprit? (Editorial) 51, 729.

Kumaoka, S. et al. (1968): J. clin. Endocr., 28, 667.

Leis, H.P. (1966): Int. J. Surg., 45, 496.

Lemon, H.M. et al. (1966): J. Amer. med. Ass., 196, 13, 112–20.

Lilienfeld, A.M. (1963): Cancer Res., 23, 1503.

Lloyd, C.W. et al. (1971): J. clin. Endocr., 32, 155.

MacMahon, B. et al. (1971): Lancet, 2, 900.

Mustacchi, P. and Gordan, G.S. (1958): In: Proceedings, Second Biennial Louisiana Cancer Conference, pp. 163–169, New Orleans, January, 1958. Editor: A. Segaloff. C. V. Mosby Co., St. Louis, Mo.

Newill, V.A. (1961): J. nat. Cancer Inst., 26, 405.

Schezler-Saunders, E., (1960): Med. Press, 244, 337.

Segi, M. et al. (1972): Cancer Mortality for Selected Sites in 24 Countries, No. 6 (1966–67). Japan Cancer Society, Tokyo.

Seidman, H. (1970): Environ Res., 3, 234.

Shapiro, S., Strax, P., Venet, L. and Fink, R. (1968): Amer. J. Publ. Hlth., 58, 820.

Staszewski, J.L. (1971): Cancer, 47, 935.

Tanner, J.M. and Gupta, D. (1968): J. Endocr., 41, 139.

Trichopoulos, D., MacMahon, B. and Cole, P. (1972): J. nat. Cancer Inst., 48, 605.

Vessey, M.P., Doll, R. and Sutton, P.M. (1971): Cancer (Philad.), 28, 1395.

Vessey, M.P., Doll, R. and Sutton, P.M. (1972): Brit. med. J., 3, 719.

Wilson, R.S. (1962): J. Amer. med. Ass., 182, 327.

World Health Organization (1970): Mortality from Malignant Neoplasms, 1955–65. W.H.O., Geneva.

Wynder, E.L. (1969): Cancer (Philad.), 24, 1235.

Wynder, E.L., Bross, I.J. and Hirayama, T. (1960): Cancer, 13, 559.

Zippin, C. and Petrakis, N.L. (1971): Cancer (Philad.), 28, 1318.

Histological parameters defining minimal breast cancer

Robert W. McDivitt

Division of Surgical Pathology, The University of Utah College of Medicine, Salt Lake City, Utah, U.S.A.

Minimal breast cancer can be interpreted to mean many different things. For some it describes in situ carcinoma; for others, atypias or so-called precancerous lesions; and yet for others, invasive cancers that have not yet metastasized. Regardless of which definition we prefer, we still are concerned with the histological parameters identifying breast cancer at some early point in its evolutionary course.

In situ carcinoma

Perhaps we should defer consideration of atypias and so-called precancerous lesions for the moment, and begin on somewhat surer footing by discussing in situ carcinoma. In situ carcinoma of the breast arises both within the terminal ducts comprising lobules and within larger, more central ramifications of the duct system. In the former, the designation, in situ lobular carcinoma is applied; for the latter, in situ duct carcinoma or more simply, intraductal carcinoma. In situ carcinoma of breast lobules was first described in 1947 by Foote and Stewart (1947). They observed the frequent association of this lesion, seen in Figure 1, with certain types of infiltrating carcinoma. However, their suggestion that this was an in situ form of carcinoma was based, at that time, primarily on circum-

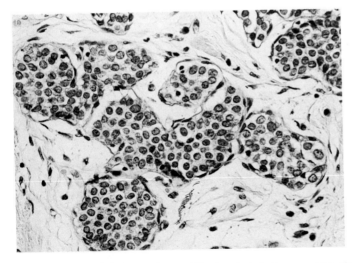

FIG. 1   *In situ lobular carcinoma. The terminal ducts comprising this lobule are distended with loosely cohesive tumor cells. H&E 400X. Reduced for reproduction 46%.*

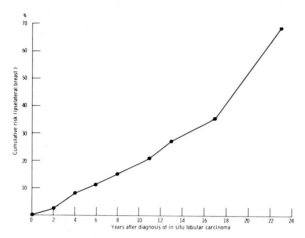

FIG. 2   *Cumulative risk of ipsilateral invasive breast carcinoma following excision of in situ lobular carcinoma.*

stantial evidence; therefore, the concept did not receive unqualified acceptance. This permitted subsequent prospective follow-up of women who had had this lesion excised from their breast, but no additional therapy. By doing so the clinical significance of this histological marker was more precisely defined. The following chart (Fig. 2), subsequently compiled, shows the cumulative risk of ipsilateral invasive breast cancer in a group of such women followed at Memorial Hospital in New York (McDivitt et al., 1967). Note that the cumulative risk of later invasive cancer is dependent on time at risk, being approximately 15% at 10 years, but rising further to 30% at 20 years. Note alternately that many

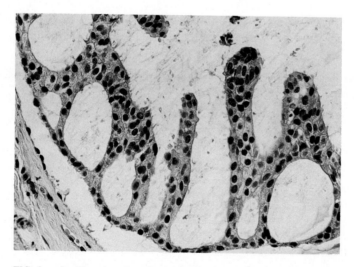

FIG. 3   *Papillary intraductal carcinoma. The margin of the duct wall is seen in the lower left corner. No fibrovascular stalk suspends fronds of tumor cells extending out from the duct wall. These cellular fronds bridge to form microtubular structures sometimes referred to as a cartwheel pattern. H&E 400X. Reduced for reproduction 46%.*

patients did not develop invasive cancer during the prolonged period of follow-up. Data of this sort permit a rather precise, if arbitrary, histopathological definition of in situ lobular carcinoma because they give an explanation of what is meant by this pathological diagnosis.

No comparable data are available to define the meaning of in situ carcinoma of the larger ramifications of the breast duct system, intraductal carcinoma. Figures 3 and 4 show the histology of the most common, generally accepted varieties of in situ duct carcinoma; the papillary and comedo types. Most pathologists in the United States agree with these visual definitions; even though they cannot say precisely what is meant by this pathological diagnosis, in terms of subsequent invasive cancer risk, or time factors concerned with subsequent risk. In the United States, breasts containing intraductal carcinoma are usually removed because of concern that the risk of subsequent invasive cancer, although unknown, is sufficient to render inappropriate prospective follow-up studies, such as have been conducted for in situ lobular carcinoma.

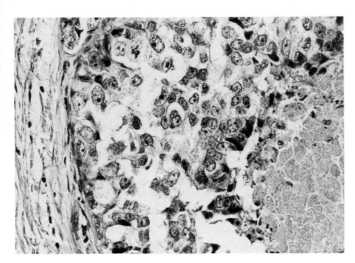

FIG. 4   *Intraductal carcinoma, comedo type. The margin of the duct wall is on the left. Except for the central necrotic detritis, tumor cells almost completely fill the duct lumen. H&E 400X. Reduced for reproduction 46%.*

Atypical epithelial hyperplasia

Assaying the risk of less advanced epithelial proliferations within breast ducts and lobules, proliferations which histologically seem less atypical than in situ carcinoma becomes even more difficult. For example, do we know the meaning of an epithelial proliferation within a lobule, such as is seen in Figure 5? We might suspect that lobular lesions of this type would incur some of the risk of in situ lobular carcinoma since they somewhat resemble in situ lobular carcinoma histologically. However, this is difficult to prove, since a large number of cases and prolonged follow-up are required. Atypical epithelial proliferations within breast ducts, such as seen in Figure 6, pose similar problems. In reviewing records of patients who had had mastectomy for infiltrating papillary carcinoma, Holleb and I found disappointingly few who had had benign papillomas previously excised; however, Jensen and Wellings have found histologically benign papillomas in direct continuity with intraductal or infiltrating duct carcinomas in more than a third of cases studied by whole organ breast sections (Jensen and Wellings, personal communication).

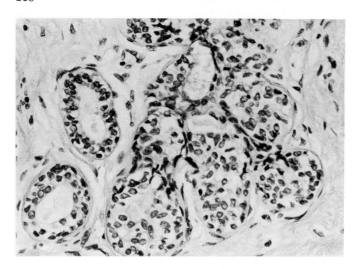

FIG. 5   *Lobular atypia. In contrast to Figure 1, proliferating epithelium less completely fills and distends the terminal duct lumens. In addition, there is more cellular cohesion and less nuclear symmetry. H&E 400X. Reduced for reproduction 46%.*

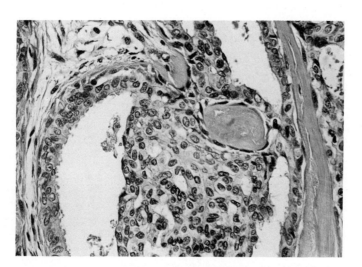

FIG. 6   *Duct papilloma. In contrast to intraductal carcinoma, neither the cartwheel pattern or detritis formation are present here. H&E 400X. Reduced for reproduction 46%.*

As an alternate approach to the problem, a follow-up clinic has been started at Memorial Hospital for patients who have had atypical epithelial proliferations removed from their breasts. Results so far are tentative because of short follow-up; but there is some indication that lobular atypias at least may prove to increase subsequent cancer risk, although to a lesser degree than that demonstrated for in situ lobular carcinoma (Ashikari et al., 1974; McDivitt et al., 1969).

Benign dysplastic lesions

Aside from the proliferative lesions mentioned above, I know of no benign dysplastic lesion of the breast that has been proved precancerous by means of statistically valid prospective follow-up studies. Of course, there have been numerous articles, most of them retrospective, purporting to show that one lesion or another increases the subsequent cancer risk; but all suffer from complex assumptions and manipulations of data which weaken their conclusions (Ashikari et al., 1974; Berg and Robbins, 1966; Davis et al., 1964; Warren, 1940). Most concern themselves with fibrocystic disease and in doing so fail at the outset to make allowance for the fact that pathologists use the term, fibro-cystic disease, as a wastebasket category, applying the diagnosis to many diverse histo-pathological entities; even charitably at times when no specific histopathology is found.

Sclerosing adenosis is perhaps second to cystic disease in frequency of being miscon-strued as precancerous. In reviewing consultations from the 1940's and 50's one finds that it was not unusual for pathologists in the United States to misinterpret the distinct histopathology of adenosis as a variant of infiltrating carcinoma (Fig. 7). Although this is less of a problem today, as judged by consultations; adenosis has again become falsely linked with carcinoma through different circumstances. With the expansion of mammo-graphy during the past few decades, some radiologists have been slow to realize that a micropunctate pattern of intramammary calcification as seen on these films is not specific for carcinoma but seen almost as frequently with adenosis. Because of this, many mam-mographic 'positives' prove histologically to be adenosis rather than carcinoma. For some, this has again raised suspicion concerning the relationship between adenosis and carci-noma.

Minimal invasive carcinoma

As mentioned before, some physicians do not accept in situ carcinomas as true cancers of the breast, restricting their use of the term, minimal, to describe those infiltrative breast

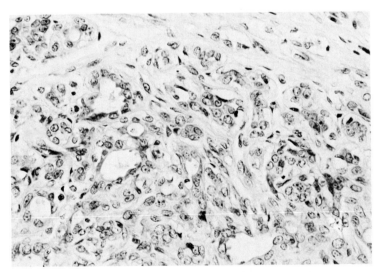

FIG. 7   *Sclerosing adenosis. Epithelium is trapped and compressed by myoepithelial hyperplasia. Produces an overall whirled, concentric pattern which is more apparent at lower magnifica-tion. H&E 400X. Reduced for reproduction 46%.*

cancers, which for one reason or another they believe early in their evolutionary course (Kreyberg, 1941). Frequently by convention the word early is used to describe breast cancers which have not yet produced regional lymph node metastases; a stance which has some merit, since long term survival can be correlated with the presence or absence of axillary metastases and with the extent of axillary lymph node metastases as well. In studying a group of several thousand breast cancer patients at Memorial Hospital in New York, Berg and Robbins found that those who had no axillary metastases had approximately a 70% chance of surviving 20 years postmastectomy; those with only proximal axillary lymph node metastases, a 40% chance of surviving for the same period; but among those who had metastases in distal axillary lymph nodes, the chance of survival for 20 years was only 10% (Berg, 1967; Berg and Robbins, 1966). Since, as was shown by Fisher et al. (1969), there is a direct statistical relationship between primary tumor size and propensity for axillary metastases, it becomes reasonable to equate minimal with small, when speaking of infiltrating carcinomas. In comparing primary tumor size with chance of postmastectomy 20 year survival, we found that those patients whose primary tumor was less than 1 cm in diameter had approximately a 75% chance of long term survival following radical mastectomy; those whose primary tumor was between 1 and 2 cm, a 60% chance; and that beyond this, chance of long term survival fell off progressively in proportion to increase in primary tumor size, producing less than a 20% chance of survival when tumor size exceeded 6 cm in diameter (Berg and Robbins, 1966; McDivitt et al., 1969).

Microcalcification and minimal cancer

Of course, the smaller the infiltrating cancer, the less chance of its being detected by physical examination of the breast. Because of this, ancillary procedures such as mammography have been used with increased frequency in our country in an attempt to discover small or minimal cancers. This has posed special problems for the pathologist who must attempt to correlate his histological findings with the radiological findings in the clinical mammograms. To facilitate this correlation we have found it useful to keep a small industrial X-ray machine within our pathology department, which we use to X-ray biopsy specimens of all patients who have had suspicious clinical mammograms. We have found this procedure an aid in localizing calcifications within the specimen, thus telling us where to take blocks for histologic study. It is particularly useful when searching for small or minimal infiltrating carcinomas and in situ carcinomas that may not be obvious on gross examination of the biopsy specimen (Owen et al., 1954; Westbrook and Gallager, 1971).

These then are some of the parameters which I, as a pathologist, have found useful in defining minimal breast cancer, as well as some which I have not. In some areas, the implications of our terminology are rather clear, whereas in others, they are much less so. One thing is certain; that is, with increased clinical emphasis on the identification and treatment of these so called minimal cancers, it behooves us to critically dissect areas of pathological certainty from those of speculation.

References

Antonious, J. I. and Jones, H. W. (1963): Bull. Mason Clin., 17, 17.
Ashikari, R., Huvos, A. G., Snyder, R. E., Lucas, J. C., Hutter, R. V. P., McDivitt, R. W. and Schotten-
    feld, D. (1974): Cancer (Philad.), 33, 310.
Bauer, W. (1967): Zbl. Chir., 92, 2322.
Berg, J. W. (1955): Cancer (Philad.), 8, 776.
Berg, J. W. and Robbins, G. F. (1966): Surg. Gynec. Obstet., 122, 1311.
Davis, H. H., Simons, M. and Davis, J. B. (1964): Cancer (Philad.), 17, 957.
Devitt, J. E. (1972): Surg. Gynec. Obstet., 134, 803.

Fisher, B., Slack, N. H. and Bross, I. D. J. (1969): Cancer (Philad.), 24, 1071.
Foote Jr, F. W. and Stewart, F. W. (1947): Amer. J. Path., 17, 491.
Kreyberg, L. (1941): Brit. J. Cancer, 7, 491.
McDivitt, R. W., Holleb, A. I. and Foote Jr, F. W. (1968): Arch. Path., 85, 117.
McDivitt, R. W., Hutter, R. B., Foote Jr, F. W. and Stewart, F. W. (1967): J. Amer. med. Ass., 201, 82.
McDivitt, R. W., Stewart, F. W. and Berg, J. W. (1969): AFIP Atlas of Tumor Pathology: Tumors of the Breast, Second series. Institute of Pathology, Armed Forces Fascicle 2, 1969, Washington, D. C.
Owen, H. W., Dockerty, M. B. and Gray, H. K. (1954): Surg. Gynec. Obstet., 98, 302.
Warren, S. (1940): Surg. Gynec. Obstet., 71, 257.
Westbrook, K. C. and Gallager, H. S. (1971): Amer. J. Surg., 122, 607.

Correlation between mammographic and histological diagnosis

Gianfranco Coopmans De Yoldi

Institute of Radiological Sciences, University of Milan, and Radiological Department, National Cancer Institute, Milan, Italy

At the Institute of Radiological Sciences of the University of Milan, and the Radiological Department of the National Cancer Institute, mammographic examination was carried out for the first time, in 1958, by modified traditional equipment. Since 1965 special equipment has been used: at present we have at our disposal two Senograph CGR and a Siemens Mammomat. From 1958 to the present day about 40,000 women, of whom 6,000 had undergone surgery, have been examined. In the majority of cases they were sent for the examination by surgeons of our Institute in order to remove a clinical doubt; therefore, I am speaking here of clinical mammography and not mass screening.

The cases selected were in general premenopausal women with cancers at an early stage (T_1 and some T_2) or with extended dysplasia which are difficult to diagnose clinically. What I have discovered has great importance concerning the accuracy of diagnosis by mammography: the different reliabilities quoted by certain authors, from 65 to 95%, may result from qualitative differences in the cases examined.

TABLE 1   *Patients examined with lesions whose nature had been established histologically*

Total no. of patients	No. with benign lesions	No. with malignant lesions	Accuracy of diagnosis by mammography
817	363	454	685 (84%)

From the Institute of Radiology, University of Milan and National Cancer Institute, Milan

This report concerns the results of a study of 817 patients, in whom the precise nature of the disease had been established by the histology found at a biopsy: 363 patients out of the 817 had a limited or extended dysplasia and 454 had cancer (Table 1). Among the dysplasias we have included the so-called benign tumours (adeno-fibromas, philloid-adenomas, papillomatosis etc.) and also steatonecrosis and specific and aspecific inflammatory lesions.

454 patients had early epithelial cancers, generally invasive scirrhous carcinomas, but also a lymphosarcoma and a carcinosarcoma.

TABLE 2   *Accuracy of mammography in diagnosis*

Benign lesions	Malignant lesions
319 (88%)	366 (81%)

From the Institute of Radiology, University of Milan and National Cancer Institute, Milan

The radiological and clinical diagnosis was correct in 685 cases out of 817 (84%). I want to emphasize that this diagnosis was based on both the results of clinical examination and the study of radiograms. It is important that the two methods should always be carried out in combination. Analysis of the relevant literature shows that greater diagnostic precision is achieved for dysplasias than for cancers (Table 2): in fact the radiological diagnosis was correct in 319 of the 363 dysplastic cases (88%), while of the 454 cancer cases the diagnosis was confirmed histologically in only 366 (81%). The above is supported by other authors, in particular Friedman et al. (1966) (Table 3) and Clark et al. (1965) (Table 4). In 94 patients out of 817 our radiological diagnosis was wrong; more precisely, in 35 we made a wrong diagnosis of malignant tumour (false positive cases) and in 59 the opposite (false negative cases).

TABLE 3   *Accuracy of mammography in diagnosis*

Benign lesions	253	(75%)
Malignant lesions	233	(68%)

Most of the patients were 45 years of age, 60%, and premenopausal (From Friedmann et al., 1966)

TABLE 4   *Effect of age on diagnostic accuracy*

Age (years)	Non-malignant pathology	Malignant pathology	Diagnostic accuracy: benign lesion	Diagnostic accuracy: malignant lesion
Under 30	243	8	97.2%	50.0%
30–44	463	63	94.9%	55.6%
45–59	280	191	84.5%	77.0%
60 and over	109	207	67.9%	90.3%
Total	1095	469	90.3%	79.5%

(From Clark et al., 1965)

In the other 26 cases it was impossible to make a radiological diagnosis owing to the deep and uniform opacity of the breast due to physiological or pathological causes: at present the problem of deep and uniform opacity of the breast is insoluble. Moreover in 12 cases our diagnosis was doubtful because at the X-ray examination no changes were apparent.

The causes of error are shown at Table 5 for the false negative and the false positive cases. In 36 false negative cases the heart of the tumour was partially or totally hidden by a concomitant dysplastic process. An epicritic analysis shows that in at least 20 out of the 36 cases a correct diagnosis might have been obtained if many detailed radiograms in different projections had been carried out, instead of a few.

It follows that the care necessary in carrying out mammography is particularly important in cases of dysplasia associated with cancer. In the other 23 false negative cases the primary lesion was clearly evident in the various radiograms but was incorrectly diagnosed owing to the absence of pathognomonic and indirect signs of malignity.

The histology of the lesions present in the 35 false positive cases is detailed in Table 5. 15 patients had cysts with aspecific inflammatory reaction of the wall: the differential diagnosis of a cyst and a tumour is possible on the basis of the changes which appear in

TABLE 5   *Diagnostic errors and failures in mammography*

Deep and uniform radio-opacity in the breast:		

Impossible to diagnose	26	
Diagnosis doubtful	12	

Errors in diagnosis	94	(11.5%)

False negative cases	59	
(a) Malignant lesions hidden by concomitant benign lesions		36
(b) Malignant lesions with non-pathognomonic X-ray aspects		23

False positive cases	35	
(a) Cyst with inflammation in the wall	15	
(b) Fibrocystic disease (gross cystic disease)	12	
(c) Sclerosing adenosis	3	
(d) Steatonecrosis	2	
(e) Cystosarcoma phylloides	2	
(f) Tuberculosis of the breast	1	

From the Institute of Radiology, University of Milan and National Cancer Institute, Milan

the course of X-ray examinations repeated 2 or 3 months later, biopsy and aspiration or insufflation; 12 had cystic disease or complex mastopathy which our pathologists consider a precancerous condition, therefore our diagnosis should not be considered wrong. Also among the false positive cases were 3 adenoscleroses, 2 steatonecroses and a mammary tuberculosis. These are uncommon diseases, difficult to diagnose differentially from cancer on a clinical basis. Consequently the radiological diagnosis may be the definitive one.

In order to complete the study and emphasize the necessity of combining radiological and clinical methods, I will remind you that diagnosis based only on palpation by a surgeon were correct in 610 cases (75%) out of 817, while in 207 (25%) they were wrong (120 cancers and 87 dysplasias).

The deficiencies of either a radiological or a physical examination are compensated by the other, so that when performed together by a surgical oncologist the possibility of error is reduced to 7-9%. Concerning the false positive cases, it should be noted that there is frequent disagreement between the clinical and radiological diagnoses.

Concerning the patients with deep and uniform opacity of the breast, the diagnosis was correct in 10 out of the 26 cases studied and it was possible to show that 6 patients had cancer.

References

Clark, R.L., Copeland, M.M., Egan, R.L., Gallager, H.S., Geller, H., Lindsay, J.P., Robbins, L.C. and White, E.C. (1965): Amer. J. Surg., 509, 127.

Friedmann, A.K., Askovitz, S.I., Beiger, S.M., Dodd, G.D., Fisher, M.S., Lapayowker, M.S., Moore, J.P., Parlee, D.E., Stein, G.N. and Pendergrass, E.P. (1966): Radiology, 86, 886.

What are the potentialities of thermography for detection of breast cancer in a preclinical stage ?

N.J.M. Aarts and G. Vermey

Department of Radiodiagnostics, St. Elizabeth Hospital, Tilburg, The Netherlands

By the time a cancer has reached the clinical phase (Fig. 1), i.e. become detectable by clinical examination, it is already between a half and two thirds of the way along its life-span. A tumour 1 cm in size is already middle aged. In comparison, the size of a tumour (Table 1) seems to be less important than is generally accepted. The statistics from Fisher and co-workers show that some carcinomas can be as big as 6 cm and more without metastasising. The 5-year survival rate of patients with these tumours is only slightly less than that of patients with small tumours, 1 cm in size, also without lymph node involvement. The statistics show 75 to 85% survival. On the other hand cancers, approximately 1 cm in diameter, are not uncommonly accompanied by several involved lymph nodes. The survival rate here is worse, only 65%.

We may presume the existence of two types of carcinomas, fast-spreading and slow-spreading. Professor De Waard also mentioned this in his communication (De Waard, This Volume, p. 195). Both the 5-year survival rate and the life history of the tumour indicate the necessity for diagnosis in the preclinical stage. Roentgenology has its limits and it is very difficult to detect the small tumours we are looking for by roentgenological examination. For clinical examination these carcinomas also present a problem. Although from the first, thermography has been used to diagnose a breast cancer, its usefulness is still under discussion. It is even denied.

Indeed, it is reported in the literature that even big carcinomas have been missed thermographically. This seems to be an inherent disadvantage of the method. Several theories to explain this phenomenon have been put forward. The most plausible in our

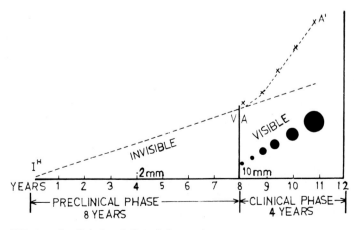

FIG. 1   *Preclinical and clinical phases of cancer.*

TABLE 1   *Effect of primary tumour size and nodal status on 5-year survival rates*

Tumour size	Nodal status									
	Negative nodes		Positive nodes		1-3 positive nodes		4+ positive nodes	
	No. of patients	Survival (%)	No. of patients	Survival (%)	No. of patients	Survival (%)	No. of patients	Survival (%)
0.1–0.9	17	76	5	100	4	100	1	100
1.0–1.9	85	85	58	67	38	68	20	65
2.0–2.9	146	80	101	59	60	65	41	51
3.0–3.9	107	69	131	44	65	63	66	26
4.0–4.9	78	72	79	43	40	60	39	26
5.0–5.9	43	74	85	42	41	54	44	32
6.0+	63	75	107	27	33	55	74	15
Total	539	76	566	46	281	62	285	31

opinion is that heat production and transfer decrease as both the immune reaction and the metabolism and vascularity of the tumour decrease during its development. Small but increasing carcinomas face a strong reaction and many new and pathological vessels are being formed. This favours an increase in heat production and transport. So it seems more likely that small tumours will be detected by their thermal output than big ones. In order to compare readings, standardization of thermograms is necessary. Criteria for their evaluation must be laid down and if appropriately formulated a computer might be used in the initial evaluation. It is expected however that the computer would merely select 'normals' from 'non-normals'. However, this is for the future. Several years ago we listed some criteria for systematic evaluation. The scheme was based upon our own experience in analysing several hundreds of thermograms and was also intended to instruct other workers. Soon however, we added to our list the 'edge-sign' as described by Isard. A review of our material supplied ample justification for this addition.

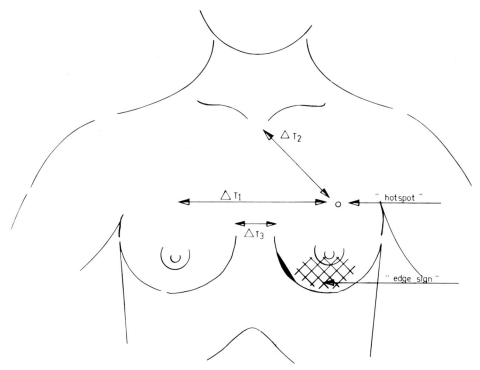

FIG. 2   *Criteria for the evaluation of thermograms.*

Our criteria are listed as follows (Fig. 2):
1. a 'hot spot' on the affected side
2. a $\Delta T_1 \geqslant 1.5°C$. ($\Delta T_1$ is the temperature difference between the 'hot spot' and the other side)
3. a $\Delta T_2 \geqslant 1.0°C$ (ΔT_2 is the temperature difference between the 'hot spot' and the suprasternal fossa)
4. a $\Delta T_3 \geqslant 1.0°C$. ($\Delta T_3$ is the temperature difference between average temperatures of both sides)
5. a diffuse and increased heat pattern of the affected side; a normal pattern on the other side
6. the 'edge-sign'
7. a 'hot spot' coinciding with clinical/mammographic findings.

The more criteria fulfilled, the more likely it is that malignancy is present. It is obvious that basing the decision on a single parameter, e.g. comparing only the temperature difference between the hot spot or affected side and the symmetrical part on the other side, is insufficient. As the number of subclinical carcinomas we may have found is very small, we have given no statistics.

In our material we found 20% false positives. In the literature a false positive rate between 20 and 30% can be found. We are almost convinced that some of these 'false positives' are due to subclinical carcinomas. In the first instance biopsy and mammography failed to confirm them. But our theory is supported by our own experience as well as that of others in that confirmed cancers appeared in this group a few months to just over a year after the first false-positive thermogram. Of course not all false-positive cases did develop carcinoma. Thus we became more and more convinced of the need for more objective testing of the possibilities of thermography. In other words we wanted to know if thermography could contribute to the detection of subclinical breast cancers. The question was formulated as follows: 'would it be possible to detect occult cancers, in the sub- or pre-clinical stage, by means of the thermographic equipment available at the moment'. This question was put to Mr. Vermey, engineer of the Department of Electronics of the Technological Institute of the University of Twente.

We knew that a computer model, which would be developed by Mr. Vermey, might possibly supply an answer. For reasons concerning the computer 'soft-ware' he started with a 'cancer' of 1 mm in size and at a temperature of 37°C. Our first attempt, formulated by Mr. Vermey, is now described. A model of the heat transfer in the skin was formulated for either rectangular or spherical volumes. The skin was assumed to consist of two different layers, one of wet tissue and the other of fatty tissue. The differential equations describing the physical system were solved using an iterative method, by a digital computer. Temperature sources, which serve to represent the clinical picture, were introduced into the model. From the computed temperature distribution, the necessary resolution of the thermograph can be deduced. To illustrate the differences in the resolution required, a 1 mm source at 37°C, located at a variable depth under the skin surface, will be considered. To detect this source when it is at a depth of 5-6 mm, a thermograph is required with a temperature resolution of better than 0.1°C and a spatial resolution of at least 1 mm. This conclusion holds both for rectangular and spherical volumes of skin. The environmental temperature was chosen to be 18°C as a compromise between a degree of vasoconstriction and the comfort of the patient. This environmental temperature was assumed in all the computer simulations.

As this study is continuing with sources of different sizes and temperatures, only a preliminary conclusion can be given. Prospects seem to be good for detecting breast cancers of 5 to 10 mm in size at a subclinical stage by thermography. With more sensitive machines even smaller ones might be detectable if they were located rather superficially. But the problem of the speed of the machine versus the resolution remains to be solved. Already however, it seems possible to use thermography for screening purposes. In this computer model neither vascularity nor better heat transport by blood flow have been considered. We must not forget however, that all the different diagnostic methods available should be used to obtain the correct diagnosis in time. On the basis of 'heat' alone malignancy can never be diagnosed.

Practical mass screening for breast cancer

Philip Strax

The Stella and Charles Guttman Breast Diagnostic Institute, New York, N.Y., U.S.A.

Mass screening for breast cancer is emerging as a practical means for earlier detection of this disease with the potential for lowering the mortality.

The basis for such screening procedures is the data from the large breast cancer screening program conducted by the Health Insurance Plan of Greater New York under contract with the National Institutes of Health. In a 5-year follow-up, a one-third reduction in mortality was achieved in a study group of 31,000 women compared to a matched control group (Shapiro et al., 1971). Although perhaps an additional 5 years are needed for definitive long range follow-up, the findings are sufficiently encouraging to warrant study of practical methods for mass screening for earlier detection of breast cancer.

The H.I.P. study also made it apparent that improvements in techniques and methodology were needed for a realistic practical method for the following reasons:

1. The Egan method used in the H.I.P. study carried with it a comparatively high cost in manpower and equipment. Much technical skill was needed with great attention to detail. Wear and tear on equipment was substantial. Time of examination was too high for practical mass screening. Although radiation dosage was kept to acceptable levels, improved techniques that would permit lower radiation dose in periodic examinations were desirable. In other words, for large-scale mass screening of the general population, improvements in equipment and technique that could result in increased speed, lower cost, less wear on equipment and greater efficiency were indicated.

2. 'Interval' cancers – or cancers detected between examinations – which amounted to 15% of the total, presented a challenge. Improved techniques or new modalities that might enhance cancer detection appeared desirable.

3. The case fatality rate applied to the H.I.P. study revealed that the reduction in mortality was concentrated in women over the age of 50. Those under 50 showed no such improvement. In these younger women, breasts tend to be more glandular and dense on the mammogram, making cancer detection more difficult. It was felt that improved techniques in mammography might enhance the detection of cancers by the radiologist in this more difficult group of women.

These considerations led to the development in 1968 of the Guttman Breast Diagnostic Institute in New York City with the basic objective of developing a mass screening approach that would be feasible and could reach the general population of women. The two major problems to be solved were: how to develop a practical, economical and efficient method that could produce a satisfactory yield of earlier cancers and how to motivate women to accept such a procedure (Strax, 1971).

A tandem approach to breast cancer detection has been developed that has offered the best opportunity for greatest yield. Two types of screening are done. A fixed facility has been developed where an increasing number of women are examined. Mobile screening is also carried out in communities. Such mobile programs maintain an umbilical cord to the fixed facility where definitive treatment is advised and follow-up is carried out. Modalities used in both types of screening are as follows:

At the central location, examination is made available through the New York City Division of the American Cancer Society which uses the press, radio and television to make women aware of the problem and offers to provide them further information including an opportunity for free examination at the Guttman Institute.

All examinations are done independently so that the contribution of each modality may be assessed. Data are collected on special cards for easy compilation and retrieval. A complete examination consists of the following:

1. *Interview*   Demographic data, including ethnic background, education, menstrual, parity, breast and family history, are obtained, usually by volunteers specially trained for this task.

2. *Clinical examination*   This phase is under the supervision of a physician well versed in this procedure. General breast characteristics are recorded. Impression of non-malignant no mass, non-malignant mass or suspicious of malignancy is noted. Recommendation is made for 1 year recall, early recall or biopsy or aspiration.

3. *Mammography*   Soft tissue X-ray examination of the breast is performed with the Senograph – a special apparatus developed for breast study which produces mammograms of a high technical excellence rapidly (about 10 women per hr) with low radiation dose (2-2.5 rads per exposure), by using non-screen film. Two views (cranio-caudal and medio-lateral) are made.

Data are recorded on special cards. Breast type is noted. Summary of findings such as non-malignant no mass, non-malignant mass or suspicious of malignancy is recorded. Recommendation for routine 1 year recall, earlier recall because of minimal suspicion, immediate recall for technical reasons or biopsy or aspiration is made.

4. *Thermography*   A graphic representation of the infrared emanation from the breast is made with an AGA Thermovision. This device produces an instantaneous photographic image on Polaroid film or on 70 mm photographic film. Impression of normal venous pattern, increased heat pattern or localized area of increased heat is recorded. Recommendations for 1 year recall, earlier recall on suspicious findings, or immediate recall for technical reasons are made. Since areas of increased heat do no necessarily correspond to the location of a cancer, thermographic findings are used to alert the clinician to findings on the other modalities.

Since clinical examination, mammography and thermography detect different facets of breast cancer and since these methods are complementary, all 3 are used on all patients over 35. Under 35, the X-ray is omitted. Additional modalities will be added when proved effective.

Training of paramedical personnel, supported in part by the New York City Division of the American Cancer Society, is directed to several areas. Several of the Institute's personnel have been trained as pre-screeners in clinical examination of the breast. Several non-technicians have been trained to do thermography. Three of the X-ray technicians have developed considerable skill in reading mammograms as pre-screeners. Non-technical personnel have been trained as health aides to canvass the community, spreading knowledge of the presence and value of the screening procedure.

With efficient logistics and concentration of examinations in one room so that all are done under cooling conditions, the entire examination can be done in under 15 min. With 10,000 women examined per year, the cost for the complete examination can be brought to under $ 20.00.

In mobile screening, the same 4-part technique is used as above. However, mammography is performed with a 70 mm device which uses ordinary house current, is transportable and is capable of examining up to 20 women per hr with a radiation dose of 1-1.5 rads per exposure. Another unit for mammography is also transportable and has a stationary molybdenum anode tube. It uses ordinary current and produces mammograms on 8 x 10 film.

A most recent development is a 26 foot mobile unit which incorporates the tandem techniques in entirety (Strax, 1972). This makes the entire screening process completely mobile. Even more, it stimulates widespread acceptance of the procedures on a community level.

Non-health facilities such as community centers or churches are used as sites for screening for better acceptance by the women. Neighborhood personnel are involved in the actual screening process, if possible. Health aides are used to canvass the community with flyers and door-to-door solicitation for 2 weeks prior to a screening. Informational material is written in the languages used in the community.

Results

(January 1, 1971 to December 31, 1971)

1. Number of women examined (at fixed facility) 11,668
   Initial exam 5997
   Subsequent exam 5671

   Age distribution:
   Under 35 . . . . 16%
   35-39 . . . . 15%
   40-49 . . . . 31%
   50-59 . . . . 24%
   60 and over 14%

2. Number of biopsies (or aspirations) recommended 462

3. Number of biopsies (or aspirations) performed 287

4. 80 cancers found for detection rate of 6.9/1000
   Initial exam . . . . 66 Ca – 11.0/1000
   Subsequent exam . . 14 Ca – 2.5/1000

5. In these cancers:
   (a) 38 had neg. axillary nodes 48%
       Initial exam . . 30 of 66 Ca – 45% (14 nodes unk.)
       Subsequent exam 8 of 14 Ca – 57% (2 nodes unk.)

   (b) 10 were 'interval' Ca – not detected at screening
       All were found after initial exam.
       8 were under 49 years of age.
       6 with neg. nodes, 3 with pos. nodes, 1 node unk.

   (c) Of 70 Ca 19 (27%) were found on mammography only.
       13 (19%) were found on clinical only.
       39 (54%) were found on both.

   (d) If clinical and thermography were used without mammography
       9 Ca or 13% would have been missed.
       (4 were 49 or under)
       (5 had neg. nodes, 3 unk. nodes)

   (e) Age distribution:
       Under 35 . . . . 1%
       35-39 . . . . 2%
       40-49 . . . . 29%
       50-59 . . . . 34%
       60 and over 34%

Conclusions

1. Mass screening for breast cancer is a practical procedure.
2. A complete examination should include clinical evaluation, X-ray study and thermography. All 3 contribute to the yield. An interview for demographic data and

history is useful to help delineate high risk groups. Breast self-examination must be encouraged for 'interval' pick-up.

3. Paramedical personnel can be trained for pre-screening clinical examination and mammography reading. They can also be trained to do thermography and act as health aides.

References

Shapiro, S., Strax, P. and Venet, L. (1971): J. Amer. med. Ass., 215, 1777.
Strax, P. (1971): Cancer (Philad.), 28, 1563.
Strax, P. (1972): Prevent. Med., 1, 422.

7. Recent advances on tumours with particular racial and geographical distribution

Oesophageal cancer

G. P. Warwick

Chester Beatty Cancer Research Institute, London, United Kingdom

The problem has recently been extensively reviewed by Warwick and Harington (1973).

The distribution of oesophageal cancer throughout the world presents features of interest for studies of cancer epidemiology and environmental carcinogenesis. Thus the incidence of oesophageal cancer varies more than that of any other type of alimentary tract cancer, areas of very high and very low incidence often occurring in close proximity.

This is probably nowhere more vividly portrayed than in Southern Africa where on the one hand the incidence is very high among the Xhosa people of the Transkei area of Cape Province, and very low in neighbouring Mozambique. Again in Western Kenya there appears to be an area of relatively high incidence while across the border in Uganda the incidence is low. The highest incidence in the world occurs among the people of the Guriev region of Kazakhstan where there has been reported to be an annual rate of 547 per 100,000 aged 35-64 years, standardised for age (Doll, 1969). As stressed by Doll, studies of the geographical distribution of cancer are an important way of obtaining clues as to causation. It is most instructive to study the world distribution not only of one type of cancer but of as many as possible simultaneously. Such studies are of course often fraught with difficulties (Keen, 1970), particularly in developing countries where cancer registration may be far from complete. Studies of possible aetiology should of course only be carried out where adequate epidemiological surveys have been done.

The interesting geographical distribution of oesophageal cancer suggests that some environmental factor or factors could contribute to causation. On this basis studies of aetiology, however complex, should be undertaken. One useful method of approach is to carry out prospective and retrospective questionnaire surveys based on customs and habits in areas of high and low incidence. Again such surveys are often most difficult to conduct in the very areas in which the populations are at high risk, which is certainly the case for oesophageal cancer. There is thus a need for a systematic and co-ordinated study of the aetiology of oesophageal cancer on an international basis. Such surveys as have already been carried out have pointed to various possible contributing factors which may be more or less important depending on the population under study. The most important of these include smoking, the consumption of alcoholic drinks, a combination of both, and chewing various mixtures.

There is some suggestion that a background of certain types of malnutrition might contribute to the development of oesophageal cancer. In almost all studies which have been made of the aetiology of oesophageal cancer a relationship has been found with alcohol and/or tobacco consumption, whether incidence has been low, moderate, or high. This comment is at best an oversimplification partly because both entities vary not only in composition, but also in the manner of their consumption throughout the world. In the case of tobacco there are differences not only of the type and method of smoking but also in methods of curing. Thus air-dried and flue-cured tobaccos differ in chemical composition – the latter having a much higher residual sugar content – which is reflected in the chemical composition of the smoke and other products of combustion (Elson et al.,

1972). It was suggested by Warwick and Harington (1973) that the chronic smoking of tobacco which produces an alkaline smoke (air dried tobacco) could result in the oesophagus, and other parts of the alimentary tract, being chronically exposed to an alkaline irrigation. The authors drew attention to the chewing of *Nass* (a mixture of tobacco and wood ash, and therefore also alkaline) in some areas where carcinoma of the oesophagus is common. The importance of alkali in the genesis of oesophageal cancer in man has often been stressed (reviewed by Warwick and Harington, 1973). Further studies along these lines could be informative.

Unless alcohol is an oesophageal carcinogen per se, for which there is no particular evidence, then the other components of alcoholic drinks should receive particular study since variation in the nature of these could be responsible for variations in the relative importance of alcoholic drinks apparently to influence the process of oesophageal carcinogenesis from one place to another. Obvious candidates for analysis include nitrosamines, metals and tannins (Warwick and Harington, 1973), although only the former class have been shown unequivocally to produce oesophageal cancer in experimental animals. Cook (1971) has produced suggestive evidence that a correlation exists between the development of oesophageal cancer and the consumption of beer made from maize. This matter is being further investigated, and it is of interest that in at least two areas where the incidence of oesophageal cancer is high or moderate (the Transkei and parts of Western Kenya) there is evidence for an increased use of maize for general consumption and for brewing home-made and (in the former area) commercial beer during recent decades. Morton (1968, 1970) suggests an interesting correlation between oesophageal cancer and the consumption of tannins present in a variety of products such as sorghum and certain wines. This suggestion deserves a detailed follow-up.

Regarding smoking, much more valuable information could be made available if the variety of tobacco, the manner in which it has been treated after picking, and the way it is smoked are noted in future surveys. Similarly for alcoholic drinks it would be instructive as a basis for aetiological studies to know the nature of the crude constituents, details of brewing procedures, methods of distillation, and whether or not other foreign materials ('concoctions') are added at any stage during these processes.

As mentioned earlier there is some suggestion that certain types of malnutrition, e.g. vitamin and mineral could be involved in a synergistic manner in the development of oesophageal cancer, at least in some areas, particularly where people grow their own food. The Transkei (Cape Province) and Curaçao represent 2 areas where there has been drastic impoverishment of the soil during recent decades (Warwick and Harington, 1973) and in parts of Iran where the incidence of oesophageal cancer is high, the quality of the soil is traditionally poor (Kmet and Mahboubi, 1972). Poor soil is reflected in these areas often by poor crop yields associated with low quality protein, overstocking of grazing land, and diets deficient in fruits, vegetables, milk, eggs and meat. Diets deficient in riboflavin, nicotinic acid, vitamin A or zinc have been shown to produce oesophageal damage in experimental systems, and there is some evidence to suggest that the same could be true for man (Warwick and Harington, 1973). There is evidence that cell proliferation is a potentiator of carcinogenesis and it is in the production of abnormally high levels of proliferation of the epithelial cells of the oesophageal that certain dietary deficiencies could be influencing the carcinogenic process (Warwick and Harington, 1973).

It is not suggested that malnutrition per se can produce cancer of the oesophagus, but rather that it might 'condition' the oesophagus, possibly in at least some cases by producing hyperplasia of the epithelial cells making the oesophagus more vulnerable to exogenous carcinogens.

The Conference concerns both cancer prevention and detection. What has been said so far concerns areas of research aimed at producing suggestions for prevention. Unfortunately there are no tests for the early diagnosis of oesephageal cancer, and outlook following current methods of treatment is poor. Thus, every effort should be made to prevent this form of cancer, and already some tantalizing clues have emerged.

References

Cook, P. J. (1971): Brit. J. Cancer., 25, 853.
Doll, R. (1969): Brit. J. Cancer, 23, 1.
Elson, L. A., Betts, T.E. and Passey, R.D. (1972): Int. J. Cancer, 9, 666.
Keen, P. (1970): S. Afr. med. J., 44, 1143.
Kmet, J. and Mahboubi, E. (1972): Science, 175, 845.
Morton, J. F. (1968): Cancer Res., 28, 2268.
Morton, J.F. (1970): Econ. Botany, 24, 217.
Warwick, G. P. and Harington, J. S. (1973): Advanc. Cancer Res., 17, 81.

Oral cancer and precancerous conditions amongst 50,915 villagers in four states of India

Fali S. Mehta and J. J. Pindborg

Basic Dental Research Unit, Tata Institute of Fundamental Research, Bombay, India

The aim of this study was to establish a registry of oral cancer and precancerous conditions amongst 50,915 villagers in 5 districts of India, and to note the prevalence of oral cancer and precancerous conditions from this registry, which was to form a basis for a follow up study of the same individuals in order to know the incidence of these lesions, and to establish how rapidly, with what regularity and with what chances of interruptions, remission or disappearance these precancerous conditions progress.

Material and methods

Selection of study population

We knew, during the planning stage of this study, that chewing and smoking habits vary within India. Therefore, 4 states were selected in which different types of habits prevailed. The state of Gujarat was chosen because of the widespread tobacco smoking habit, Andhra Pradesh for the reverse smoking habit, Kerala for placing the tobacco-containing quid in the lower buccal groove, and Bihar for keeping the tobacco-containing quid in the lower labial groove behind the lower lip. In India, the states are divided into districts, which comprise a group of villages or towns.

Villages in the district were selected by employing the random sampling technique. Only those villages where population figures were between 500 and 3000 were selected for survey. The smallest population unit in the District Census Handbook of the respective districts was taken as the sampling unit. All such sampling units, where population figures were between 500 and 3000, were numbered and listed. Also the number of units that would give an adult population of approximately 10,000 was calculated. The required number of units was selected using the random numbers given in Fisher and Yates Statistical Tables. In each family, all members 15 years old and over were examined.

Definition of clinical conditions

Leukoplakia is a white patch of the oral mucosa measuring 5 mm or more which cannot be scraped off and which cannot be attributed to any other diagnosable disease. The definition carries no histologic connotation.

In the evaluation of clinical features of leukoplakia, the following 3 types were taken into consideration: (1) the homogeneous type; (2) the ulcerated type; and (3) the speckled type. The homogeneous type is characterized by raised plaque formation consisting of plaques or groups of plaques varying in size and with irregular edges. These lesions are predominantly white, but may have areas of a grayish-yellow color. The ulcerated type of leukoplakia gives the impression that ulceration has been caused by trauma either of chewing or of burning in cases of reverse smoking. The affected area is usually uniformly red, but yellowish areas of fibrin may be present. The speckled leukoplakia has the characteristics of white patches on an erythematous base.

Chewing and smoking habits

Although various types of chewing and smoking habits are practised in India, only the most common ones will be described here.

The habit of chewing betel nut ('areca' nut) is usually practised in the form of chewing a 'Pan'. 'Pan' is a preparation of betel leaf, areca (betel) nut (raw or cured), slaked lime, and catechu. It may or may not be combined with tobacco. The bolus formed by chewing the preparation is either spat out, swallowed, or kept in the mouth for hours, sometimes even during sleep. Usually, the bolus is kept in the lower buccal sulcus. In some areas, tobacco may be chewed alone or with lime, and the bolus is kept in the lower labial or buccal sulcus (this preparation is called 'khaini').

A 'bidi' is an Indian form of cheap cigarette, made by rolling between the fingers a rectangular dried piece of 'temburni' (Diospyros melanoxylon), also called 'tendu' leaf, with 0.30-0.36 g of tobacco and securing the roll with a thread. The length of a 'bidi' varies from 4 cm to 7.5 cm.

'Chutta'. The name cheroot is derived from Tamil 'curuttu', which means roll (of tobacco). 'Chutta' is a more coarsely prepared cheroot and is often smoked with the burning end inside the mouth.

'Hookli' is a clay pipe with a rather short stem, varying in length from 7 to 10 cm and used in Gujarat.

Methods of clinical examination

The examinations in the field were done by 9 dentists, divided into 4 teams. The dentists had been trained by the authors, who had conducted similar studies among urban Indians in other parts of India.

A history form was completed for each person before the clinical examination. Information for the history was obtained by a trained interviewer and the forms were completed in the absence of the dental examiner to reduce examiner bias. Identifying information, such as name, age, sex and information on chewing and smoking habits was recorded.

The examination took place in natural light using two mouth mirrors. All lesions were registered on diagrams designed for this study, where the oral mucosa was divided into 41 topographic areas. The lesions were photographed in color by a Polaroid camera, and all the lesions were biopsied.

Standardization of clinical methods

Two pilot surveys were conducted with the following objectives: (1) to note the comparability among examiners; (2) to note the accuracy and reliability of recording habits and ages; and (3) to test the design of the examination form.

Results

Clinical findings

The percentage of men and women examined within each group was nearly equal in all districts. About 50% of the persons examined were within the age group of 15 to 34 years. Thereafter, the number of persons examined within each group decreased rapidly. This particular pattern of age and sex distribution of the examined samples conforms to the age and sex distribution of the entire population in each district. This result was achieved by random selection of the population.

Looking at the sex, average age, and geographic distribution of habits, some wide differences could be observed. In all states, women outnumbered men in the 'no habits' group. The difference was highest in Bihar (Singhbhum) (9.1% men, 35.2% women) and lowest in Andhra Pradesh (10.2% men, 15.6% women). The average age of men and women in the 'no habits' group was considerably lower than the average age of men and women in all states, except for Bihar (Singhbhum). Within the 'no habits' group, the average age of men was lower than the average age of women.

Among the various habit groups different patterns could be observed in the different states. Except for Bihar (Darbhanga) and Andhra Pradesh, more women were practising chewing habits alone than men in the other areas studied. The highest number of persons with chewing habits alone was in Kerala (26.2%) and the lowest in Andhra Pradesh (3.3%). Average age of men and women in this habit group was higher than the average age of men and women in the entire sample, except for the women of Andhra Pradesh and Bihar (Singhbhum).

Ordinary smoking habits were rarely practised by women in all districts, except Bihar (Darbhanga), where women smokers outnumbered men smokers. The average age of women smokers was higher than the average age of all women examined in each of the 5 districts.

The reverse smoking (of chutta) was found in Andhra Pradesh only. The percentage of women reverse smokers alone was 26.9 compared with 16.9 men who smoked in the reverse way. Their average ages were higher than the average age of the population.

Prevalence figures

26 oral cancer cases were found in this house-to-house survey, with almost half the cases in South India (Kerala). 17 of the cancer cases were diagnosed clinically. The remaining 9 cases were diagnosed as leukoplakia (5 cases), submucous fibrosis + leukoplakia (1 case), or ulcer (1 case). A biopsy from these cases revealed the true nature of the lesion.

The prevalence of leukoplakia ranged from 0.2% in Bihar (Singhbhum) to 4.9% in Andhra Pradesh.

All the oral cancer patients had one or several chewing or smoking habits. With regard to location of the cancer, it is interesting to note that 5 of the 12 cases from Kerala were connected to the tongue, and they had chewing habits. Nine of the 10 cases from Andhra Pradesh were found in the palate and all 9 had the habit of reverse smoking. 13 patients had simultaneous leukoplakia, 3 submucous fibrosis and one lichen planus.

It is striking that 30 patients with leukoplakias were observed in the 15 to 24 year age group and 124 in the 25 to 34 year age group. The highest number of leukoplakias was found in the 35- to 44-year age group. There was an overwhelming predominance of men with leukoplakia, except in Andhra Pradesh, where women comprised 58.1% of the leukoplakias.

Interesting differences were brought out when comparing the results from the 4 states. The labial mucosa was the seat of one-fifth of the leukoplakias in Gujarat and Bihar (Darbhanga), whereas Kerala and Andhra Pradesh showed very low figures. In Gujarat, the commissures were more often affected than in Kerala. In both states, a predilection for the right side seemed to exist. The buccal mucosa was most frequently affected in Kerala, where this location made up 64.8% of all leukoplakias. An impressive finding was the occurrence of 71.3% of keratotic lesions of the palate in Andhra Pradesh.

Low figures were found for leukoplakias on the gingiva, tongue (except Bihar Singhbhum), floor of the mouth, and alveolar ridge.

Correlation of leukoplakia with smoking and chewing habits

The highest percentage of leukoplakia (8.7%) is found among the reverse smokers in Andhra Pradesh. Next in association with leukoplakia are the smoking habits in Gujarat and Kerala. In Gujarat, Kerala, and Andhra Pradesh, mixed habits (except reverse smoking) are associated with quite high figures for leukoplakia.

Recent research on naso-pharyngeal cancer: Clinical implications

Arthur G. Levin

Nairobi Research Centre, International Agency for Research on Cancer, Nairobi, Kenya

Introduction

Naso-pharyngeal cancer (NPC) is a tumour of strikingly variable incidence with important epidemiological, virological, genetic and immunological implications. More than that, it is a serious clinical problem (Shanmugaratnam, 1971; Ho, 1972; Muir, 1972). Although it is rare in Europe and North America it is fairly common in some parts of Africa, such as East Africa, Tunisia and the Sudan. It is quite common in many places in the Far East such as Indonesia, Malaysia, Hong Kong and Singapore, and approaches the dimensions of a major public health problem in Southern China where it is, for example, the commonest tumour seen in Kangchow.

I will comment on recent research on this tumour not only from the point of view of laboratory and theoretical aspects but also ongoing clinical research determining how patients respond to current methods of treatment.

Aspects of the natural history of NPC

There are many neoplasms which can arise in the naso-pharynx but NPC as dealt with in this report is a well-defined clinical entity. Because it is so rare in Europe and North America it may not be fully appreciated that the natural history of this tumour is such that in areas in Africa and the Far East where it is seen frequently, there is no question of its being a discrete clinical entity with characteristic pathological and clinical features.

Table 1 lists in general form various aspects of this disease.

Certain additional comment is called for. A very high *incidence* seems clearly to be in areas where people of Southern Chinese origin live. It appears to be fairly common in other areas of China, such as North China, and fairly common among people of Mon-

TABLE 1   *Aspects of naso-pharyngeal cancer (NPC)*

Incidence	Very high:	S. China and Chinese immigrants
	High:	Other Mongoloid peoples
	Raised:	Parts of Africa (Kenya, Tunisia)
Pathology	Epidermoid, undifferentiated	
	Often lymphoid infiltration	
Clinical	Spread to neck nodes, skull	
Treatment	Radiation therapy: Chemotherapy	
	Long term results unsatisfactory	

goloid origin such as Malaysians and Indonesians. The question of its incidence in developing countries such as those in Africa is bedevilled by inadequate medical facilities, short life expectancy, and inadequate collation of health statistics. Further, the frequency with which a tumour is seen is often a function of the interest of medical personnel in seeking out and studying patients with that tumour. In these countries, the safest statement is that this tumour is seen frequently. These clinical impressions are not to be discounted.

The *pathological picture* of undifferentiated and/or epidermoid carcinoma is characterized by lymphoid infiltration. The belief that this was a lympho-epithelioma is now discredited: the lymphoid cells are host cells. It is clearly not easy to quantitate the extent of this host cell infiltration but the lymphoid cell response has been reported in a varying percentage of patients up to 90%. Less frequently commented on is the fact that plasma cells are very often seen in great abundance. Many eosinophils may also be seen but these may be secondary to parasitic infestation. Such a host cell reaction in patients with other tumours has been taken to suggest host resistance to the tumour based on a correlation between the extent of lymphoid infiltration and the patients' clinical course. Such a correlation is being investigated with regard to NPC but no clearcut evidence is, as yet, forthcoming.

Clinically the tumour may be confined to the naso-pharynx but characteristically spreads either to the base of the skull causing CNS problems or to lymph nodes in the neck. In Kenya, patients will usually have much larger neck nodes than in, for example, Singapore. This is probably due to the less well developed medical services in the former country so that patients present with more advanced disease. Nevertheless, it cannot be ruled out that a faster growing tumour is seen in Kenya.

Treatment. The common modalities, radiation therapy and to a lesser extent chemotherapy, frequently render the patient free of disease but it is generally agreed that the long term results are not good.

The points noted above underline different factors which may be associated with the natural history of NPC.

Genetic factors

The disease shows a striking predilection for those of Southern Chinese origin and newer methods have recently been utilized to study genetic factors in this population. This involves studies of the HL-A system which is felt to be the major human histocompatibility locus. With the use of specific antisera, and immunological tests utilising peripheral leucocytes, it is possible to determine the presence or absence of many of the HL-A antigens. In the mouse, where the H2 system is analagous to HL-A in the human, there is a relationship between some forms of mouse leukaemia and antigens of the H2 system (McDevitt and Bodmer, 1972). Recently, evidence has been presented by Simons and his colleagues suggesting that NPC patients in Singapore show particular HL-A patterns (Simons et al., 1973). The HL-A system is by no means completely understood and additional data will be forthcoming when techniques and antisera are further refined. The possible relationship between certain genetic types and a particular cancer has important implications for understanding the natural history of that cancer but also may have clinical significance in pinpointing groups or individuals at high risk.

There is little evidence for an association between ethnic groups of non-Mongoloid origin and susceptibility to NPC. For instance, in Kenya most NPC patients belong to the Kalenjin group of tribes. However, this is very likely because of the peculiar geographic distribution of the tumour, to be noted below. Nevertheless, HL-A studies of NPC patients in areas of high incidence outside of the Far East are clearly indicated.

Environmental factors

These have been investigated extensively in studies such as those concerning inhalants and ingestants which might affect those racial groups known to be at high risk. There is, however, little evidence that any of these are significant in that they are associated with NPC patients as opposed to those of the same background who do not have the tumour. Now under investigation are such factors as the possibility that food additives or preservatives used in South East Asia may lead to the formation of carcinogenic nitrosamines.

Mention should be made of a recent finding suggesting that Caucasians born and raised in the Far East where NPC is very frequently seen, are at greater risk than Caucasians in general (Buell, 1973). This may implicate some environmental factor in the broadest sense (including a virus).

In Kenya one environmental factor seems of interest. NPC appears to be largely confined to high areas above 5,000 or 6,000 feet. The significance of this is unclear as environmental factors stemming from this, such as increased exposure to carcinogens in fires inside dwellings, have not been implicated (Shanmugaratnam, 1971). It is of note that NPC in South China is seen mainly in the low coastal areas (Wu Shan, personal communication).

Viral factors

Research has concentrated in this area on the Epstein-Barr virus (EBV). This member of the herpes group was first shown to be associated with Burkitt's lymphoma. In this children's tumour, common in some parts of Africa, patients have high levels of antibody to one or more of the antigens associated with this virus. In the case of NPC it has also been shown that many patients have high levels of antibody (Lin et al., 1972; De Schryver et al., 1969), and there is recent evidence that there is some correlation between antibody level and clinical condition (Lin et al., 1973).

It is striking that in Kenya, which is one of the rare places where both Burkitt's lymphoma and NPC are frequently seen, they appear to be geographically mutually exclusive. Burkitt lymphoma patients come from lower altitudes than NPC patients and it is extremely rare to see an NPC patient in a Burkitt lymphoma endemic area. Biochemical studies have contributed toward elucidation of this viral problem. EBV DNA has been isolated from NPC biopsies (Zur Hausen et al., 1970). Since there is very often lymphoid cell infiltration in the tumour the question arises as to whether or not the anti-EBV antibody levels stem from the presence of EBV simply as a lymphotropic virus. Recent studies have indicated that the virus has been identified through presence of its nucleic acid in epidermoid cells derived from NPC (Zur Hausen et al., 1973). This may be of considerable interest in elucidating the role of this virus in NPC. It must be emphasised that EBV has *not* been shown to be the cause of any human tumour and analysis of its role in the natural history of human tumours is still far from complete.

Hormonal factors

Although there is a striking sex ratio in the tumour, in that men are far more often affected than women, there is little evidence as yet indicating any relationship between hormonal factors and predisposition to the tumour.

The complexity of factors perhaps associated with the natural history of this tumour may be illustrated in a comparison of the above factors as they affect patients in 2 widely separated parts of the world, Kenya and Singapore (Table 2). The same pathological entity is affected by factors which are both common to the areas and distinctive to each of them. This type of comparison may point the way to future work that can give possible clues which will further our knowledge of this tumour.

TABLE 2   *Naso-pharyngeal cancer in Kenya and Singapore*

Incidence	Singapore much greater
Genetic factors	Probably different
Environmental factors	Probably different
Viral (EBV) antibody	Probably similar
Clinical picture	Probably similar
Response to treatment	Probably similar

Clinical response

To illustrate this most important aspect of the problem, one may cite clinical experience in Kenya. Characteristically patients present with very large neck nodes, or erosion of the base of the skull, or both. Patients with disease in neck nodes only are treated by radiation therapy. Disease elsewhere is treated with chemotherapy. (Table 3 summarises the clinical picture.) Of patients treated with radiation therapy, many are clinically free of disease after completion of treatment. Many of these patients remain free of disease for lengthy periods of 2, 3 or 4 years. However, after this disease-free interval there is a very high rate of recurrence. These general statements represent a strong clinical impression. Preliminary analysis of patient data supports this but is still under way (Clifford et al., 1968; Singh and Larsson, personal communication). The response to treatment of these patients suggests that at the period of clinical 'remission' after radiation therapy, there are a few cancer cells remaining which are kept in check by host defences until these are overcome and the tumour recurs. The possibility of a host reaction against the tumour is indirectly supported by histological evidence (lymphoid infiltration) and by anti-EBV antibody if indeed this virus is associated with the tumour in any fundamental way.

This situation, suggestive of a few cancer cells held in check for a period, but later causing recurrence, is very much a case in which immunotherapy may be considered. From both animal data and preliminary clinical trials there is a suggestion that host defences against cancer can be exploited in conditions where there are relatively few cells to combat (Klein, 1968). The term 'minimal residual disease' has been employed to describe this. A corollary to this in any consideration of immunotherapy is that there should be, as there is in NPC, a high recurrence rate. Further, to permit an adequate clinical trial there must be a large enough number of patients fitting the clinical criteria as suitable for immunotherapy. It is not the purpose of this report to discuss approaches to immunotherapy but merely to state that a possible approach would be to attempt either specific tumour associated immune stimulation (e.g. from irradiated NPC cells) or non-specific immune stimulation (e.g. BCG) to be administered after radiation therapy during the period of minimal residual disease. It is noteworthy that the clinical response of

TABLE 3   *Clinical aspects of naso-pharyngeal cancer in Kenya*

Disease site	Treatment	Results
Base of skull	Chemotherapy	Poor
Neck nodes	Radiation therapy	Many 'remissions' but disease often recurs

Natural history of patients in 'remission'

'Remission'	Minimal residual disease	Most recur, usually after more than 2 years

NPC patients in Singapore (Kim Boon and Ewe Hong, personal communication) based on discussion with clinicians involved, appears to be very much the same as in Kenya. The general pattern or response to treatment seems to be the same in that radiation therapy results in a high percentage of patients being rendered free of disease and many of these patients show recurrences often after a long interval. From discussions with clinicians elsewhere, including those in Tunisia (Mourali and Tabbane, personal communication) and the People's Republic of China (Wu Shan, personal communication) there is evidence that similar clinical responses to NPC are seen in those countries.

One must mention, however, that there are other possible explanations for the clinical picture described above and seen in NPC patients in many parts of the world. It may be that one is dealing with a cancer cell which proliferates very slowly and recurrence only becomes apparent after a long period of time. Thus, the disease-free interval after radiation therapy might not be due to host factors but to a slow build up to tumour cells. Even if this were so it would not militate against the use of immunotherapy to destroy those cells.

Clearly, host factors in NPC must be investigated, and if possible quantitated, to serve as a method of monitoring the success of any immunotherapy. While serological tests may be of use, and as mentioned above, anti-EBV antibodies may play a part, it is generally felt that cell-mediated reactions are the best index for an anti-tumour response. Though these are hard to measure, an approach is being undertaken through the use of preserved immunologically stimulatable lymphocytes which can be tested in vitro. In this way, serial specimens from the same patient or cells from different patients may be tested under similar experimental conditions. Such cells are available and relevant studies are being carried out at the Nairobi Research Centre of the International Agency for Research on Cancer.

Conclusion

Two main conclusions may be drawn. First, analysis of the factors known or suspected to be involved in the causation of NPC would suggest that study of these in various parts of the world might not only be an appropriate way of investigating NPC but might also be a model for analyses of a multifactorial aetiology of cancer. Second, it seems possible that NPC is a very suitable tumour target for immunotherapy and discussion of the possibilities of this should be undertaken.

Acknowledgment

I am grateful to the various clinicians who are concerned with the diagnosis and treatment of NPC and who are cited in the bibliograpy. Special thanks are due to Drs. L.G. Larsson, C.A. Linsell and K. Shanmugaratnam for valuable discussions.

References

Buell, P. (1973): Int. J. Cancer, 11, 268.
Clifford, P., Sternsward, J. and Singh, S. (1968): In: Cancer in Africa, p. 365. Editors: P. Clifford, C.A. Linsell and G.L. Timms. East African Publishing House, Nairobi.
De Schryver, A., Freiberg Jr, S., Klein, G., Henle, W., Henle, G., De Thé, G., Clifford, P. and Ho, H.C. (1969): Clin. exp. Immunol., 5, 443.
Ho, H. C. (1972): In: Oncogenesis and Herpes Viruses p. 357. Editors: P. M. Biggs, G. De Thé and L. N. Payne. International Agency for Research on Cancer, Lyon.
Klein, G. (1968): Cancer Res., 28, 625.
Lin, T. M. et al. (in press)

Lin, T. M., Yang, C. S., Ho, S. W., Chiou, J. F., Liu, Tu, S. M., Chen, K. P., Ito, Y. H., Kawamura, A. and Hirayama, T. (1972): Cancer, 29, 603.

Linsell, C. A. and Martyn, R. (1962): East Afr. med. J., 39, 642.

McDevitt, H. O. and Bodmer, W. F. (1972): Amer. J. Med., 52, 1.

Muir, C. S. (1972): In: Ontogenesis and Herpes Viruses, p. 367. Editors: P. M. Biggs, G. De Thé and L. N. Payne. International Agency for Research on Cancer, Lyon.

Shanmugaratnam, K. (1971): Int. Rev. exp. Path., 10, 361.

Simons, M. et al. (in press)

Zur Hausen, H. et al. (in press)

Zur Hausen, H., Schulte-Holthausen, H., Kelin, G., Henle, W., Henle, G., Clifford, P. and Santesson, L. (1970): Nature (Lond.), 228, 1056.

Recent advances in hepatocellular cancer

C. A. Linsell and G. Warwick

International Agency for Research on Cancer, Research Centre and Medical School, Nairobi, Kenya

The interest in hepatocellular cancer (HCC) has many facets. There is the marked geographical variation in incidence of the tumour, which is relatively rare in Europe and North America, but the most commonly occurring tumour in males in some parts of Africa and the Far East. As the treatment of HCC remains so depressing, the evaluation of aetiological factors, a necessary prerequisite for possible prevention, has attracted much attention. This cancer is associated with cirrhosis, almost invariably in North America and Europe and commonly in other areas of the world. The exact relationship between the two diseases is not yet clear but the occurrence of a tumour in the course of a disease, characterized by marked regeneration of the cells eventually incriminated in the neoplasm, is thought-provoking.

Attempts to relate the disease to many of the hazards, both parasitic and bacteriological, to which populations in the areas of higher incidence are exposed, have not been fruitful. In animal experiments, tumours of this type are a frequent expression of the carcinogenicity of a wide range of agents.

The diagnosis of HCC, although its occurrence is always to be suspected in patients with cirrhosis who show marked clinical deterioration, is not easy as the biochemical parameters of liver function are of little diagnostic value. A surgical biopsy, although presenting many problems even in countries with well-developed health services, was considered until recently the only certain method of diagnosis. However, the demonstration of alpha-feto-protein in the serum of many patients with this tumour offers an advance in diagnostic methods, particularly relevant in developing countries with their increased HCC incidence. Approximately 70% of HCC patients in Africa have diagnostic levels of this onco-feto-protein when simple immuno-diffusion techniques are used. The subject has been reviewed recently by Abelev (1971) and in another series of publications Purves et al. (1973) have discussed the limitations of alpha-feto-protein as a diagnostic tool and the possibility of its use in epidemiological surveys.

The readiness with which liver cells in animals respond to laboratory carcinogenic agents has fostered the theory that a chemical agent might be an important factor in the aetiology of the human disease. The demonstration that the aflatoxins produced by some fungi were powerful liver carcinogens brought this facet of the problem out of the laboratory and as these fungi commonly contaminate poorly stored cereals, their geographical association with human liver cancer was suspected. A number of studies have indeed supported this hypothesis of association between the opportunity for aflatoxin contamination of foodstuffs and liver cancer. A recent population-based study (Peers and Linsell, 1973) showed a significant association, but urged caution in assuming that aflatoxin was causally related to human cancer until further evidence had been evaluated.

The discovery of the hepatitis B antigens, previously known as the Australia or hepatitis-associated antigens, has greatly advanced our knowledge of one type of viral hepatitis and the geographical incidence of this type of hepatitis may be an important factor in the aetiology of HCC.

Chronic antigenaemia is significantly more frequent in the general population of most developing countries and in some cirrhotic patients, particularly where the aetiology is associated with infection rather than alcohol. The number of HCC patients with the antigens is even higher, in some series as high as 80%.

Although a causal relationship between the antigens and hepatitis must now be seriously considered, it is still far from clear what their role is in cirrhosis and liver tumours. The association may be related to the suggested sequence of hepatitis- cirrhosis-cancer but much more knowledge is needed, particularly in view of the attractive hypothesis of Dudley et al. (1972) that the chronicity of antigenaemia may depend on a defect of cell-mediated immunity, so often suggested as a factor in carcinogenesis.

Recent knowledge therefore offers some possibilities for control of HCC. We may be able to consider vaccine prophylaxis for hepatitis type B and the provision of improved storage of foodstuffs may decrease the opportunities for fungal contamination. We may now be justified in tempering the pessimism associated with the treatment of these tumours with some hope of prevention.

References

Abelev, G.I. (1971): Advanc. Cancer Res., 14, 295.
Dudley, F.J., Fox, R.A. and Sherlock, S. (1972): Lancet, 1, 723.
Peers, F.G. and Linsell, C.A. (1973):Brit. J. Cancer, 27, 473.
Purves, L.R., Branch, W.R., Geddes, E.W., Manso, C. and Portugal, M. (1973): Cancer (Philad.), 31, 578.

238

8. Public health aspects of cancer control

Socio-economic factors in cancer prevention

Ivan Vodopija

Institute for Health Protection, Zagreb, Yugoslavia

'Knowledge of the incidence of different types of cancer in different communities living under different conditions has provided many clues to the aetiology of the disease and pointed to ways in which the disease can be prevented in practice' (Doll, 1970).

The mortality pattern differs greatly from country to country, but also shows striking similarities. In both sexes the death rates for neoplasms increase with age. Excess male mortality, increasing with age, has profound demographic and social implications (De Haas, 1967). A decrease of only a fraction of a percent in the existing trends of some types of cancer could bring enormous benefits.

TABLE 1   *Age groups and deaths from neoplasms in Zagreb, 1971*

Age	Deaths from neoplasms	Total No. of deaths	Deaths from cancer as % of all deaths	Deaths from neoplasms per 10,000 inhabitants
0–4	2	224	0.89	0.5
5–9	1	8	12.50	0.3
10–14	–	4	0.00	–
15–19	6	32	18.80	1.8
20–29	12	91	13.19	1.1
30–39	28	163	17.18	2.7
40–49	80	368	21.74	8.7
50–59	154	618	24.92	26.5
60–69	346	1154	29.98	63.7
70 and more	444	2367	18.76	173.9
Total	1073	5029	21.34	17.8

To demonstrate the scale of the problem of cancer in a single area, figures from our registry in the City of Zagreb are presented in Table 1. Certification of the cause of death in Zagreb is quite accurate and there is a significant correlation between clinical and post-mortem diagnoses. The relative mortality statistics for the total number of deaths and for cancer deaths (period 1963-1971) show similar trends.

$y = 3880.78 + 142.85 \ x$

$y = 823.49 + 27.7 \ x$

The proportion of cancer deaths in the total number of deaths is more or less constant to within 20%. These data show clearly that from the socio-economic point of view intensive

TABLE 2   *Deaths from neoplasms in Zagreb, 1971*

Rank	ICD code	Location	No. of deaths	Per 10,000
I	151	Stomach	197	3.3
II	162	Lung	170	2.8
III	174	Breast	69	1.1
IV	155	Liver	63	1.1
V	153	Colon	56	0.9
VI	154	Rectum	49	0.8
VII	182	Corpus uteri	39	0.7
VIII–IX	185	Prostate	31	0.5
VIII–IX	157	Pancreas	31	0.5
X–XI	183	Ovaries	26	0.4
X–XI	180	Cervix uteri	26	0.4
XII–XIII	156	Gall bladder	22	0.4
XII–XIII	188	Urinary bladder	22	0.4
XIV	200	Lymphosarcoma	14	0.2
XV	170	Bones	10	0.2

measures in the age group under 40 are not necessary. The age of 40 appears to be a border line from where the rates of cancer deaths significantly increase.

However, on the other hand, it takes decades of prolonged and continuous exposure to a carcinogenic agent for the disease to develop. Since the causes of cancer are multifactorial, viz, environmental, hormonal, immunological, nutritional, viral, etc., emphasis on public education can only partially improve the situation.

Table 2 shows the significance of neoplasias as the cause of death in Zagreb in 1971. These figures clearly indicate that the greatest challenge is the control of common tumours, such as those of the stomach, lung, breast, liver, and colon. Although there are many 'cures' for cancer patients it is better to use the term normal life expectancy (Zubrod, 1972).

It is interesting to note the average age of patients who died from cancer in Zagreb, as seen in Table 3. When we take into consideration that the normal life expectancy in Zagreb is about 68.5 years, the following question immediately arises: what types of cancer should be dealt with first? Cancer of the cervix uteri is at the top of the list because of the early average age of death in the female population from this cause. This is followed by breast cancer and then cancer of the corpus uteri. But when we observe their rank (as seen in Table 2) it appears that only breast cancer deserves full attention.

From such data it appears to be impossible for any one country, let alone any single institution, to mount a prospective study which could lead to valid conclusions regarding prevention, within a reasonable length of time (Zubrod, 1972). However, individual attempts could improve cancer detection. It is intended that the onset of cancer should be prevented in the entire population. Just as the evolution of neoplasia is a long-developing process so are the appropriate preventive measures. In fact, legislation is required to provide the opportunity for a substantial improvement in cancer prevention. What Denoix (1970) said is 'Le dépistage est efficace s'il a une influence sur la mortalité globale par cancer dans la région considérée'. If it is a *sine qua non* for detection campaigns, is it not so *a fortiori* for prevention?

Our knowledge about the prevention of cancer is still regrettably incomplete, but we know enough about the high risk factors to start or intensify preventative measures. 'Health education, based on explanation and aimed at primary prevention, must start in adolescence in order to get lasting results.' (De Haas, 1967). If we want to improve the

TABLE 3   *Average age at death of patients dying from cancer in Zagreb*

ICD code	Location of cancer	Male	Female	For both sexes
151	Stomach	66.5	70.6	68.3
153	Colon	65.9	69.4	67.9
154	Rectum	67.8	62.8	65.9
155	Liver	65.3	71.9	68.5
156	Gall bladder	74.5	70.1	71.1
157	Pancreas	63.2	66.9	65.2
162	Lung	65.1	67.8	65.6
174	Breast		59.2	
180	Cervix uteri		58.5	
182	Corpus uteri		63.3	
185	Prostate	71.2		
188	Urinary bladder	70.4	73.8	71.6

health of mankind in developed countries, we have to embark on a whole series of resourceful innovations and systematic improvements. Basic research in the prevention of cancer is the most important. Prevention not only relieves human misery, but can also save enormous amounts of money, which can then be reinvested in improving human life.

Thus, from what has been stated, the following means of furthering cancer prevention are suggested.

1. We are witnessing today the rapid growth of the realisation of the interreactions between environmental protection and cancer prevention.

2. We know a lot about the relation between smoking habits and lung cancer, such as the incidence of lung cancer in smokers, the fate of heavy smokers, and the prospects for individuals if they give up smoking. The increase of life expectancy for those who give up smoking is considerable.

3. Similarly a movement to clean the air is taking place in many areas with some visible results. However, the components which really spoil the air in large cities (CO_2, aromatic hydrocarbons, metals such as lead) are still there and thus basically the situation has not improved as much as we would like. Reports from megalopoles, such as Tokyo, clearly indicate that air pollution is continuously increasing. This is due to the increase in the number of cars on the streets and fumes in the atmosphere of our cities.

4. It is well know that for high agricultural production, a significant amount of such active substances as fertilizers, herbicides, pesticides, mercury containing crop protection products and others are required. There is a demonstrable increase of mercury in many fish, not only in fresh water fish but also in sea fish. How does this mercury enter the flesh of so many animal species? Research studies have shown the pathways and the possible breakdowns of many substances, but a lot of this is not yet known. Much discussion is being carried on regarding the role of DDT as a possible carcinogen. Can mankind at this point refrain from using all this agricultural armoury for the sake of cancer prevention, especially since there is an ever-increasing need for food throughout the world?

5. We are witnessing the increased pollution of the seas but who has the power to stop the transport of oil to those areas where this energy is so badly needed?

6. Man has added considerably to the pollution of his own environment in his efforts to preserve life and to benefit his family. Now he must find new ideas and approaches to combat this pollution, if he is going to embark on the road towards proper cancer prevention.

The socio-economic aspects of such an endeavour can only be contemplated at present, because looking at the practical side three questions appear (a) who, (b) what, and (c) when.

(a) Regarding the question of *who* has to do the job, we feel the answer is simple: governments must undertake the responsibility of making proper arrangements and agreements for controlling the many carcinogenic substances. Such legislation could influence not only social, but also economic changes in many existing organizations.

Is this impossible? In the present world of so many rivalries, one can only hope to realise such an aim. Many of the more developed countries have taken the initiative in prohibiting the use of certain products by the public, but stocks of these products are still available in many of the developing countries. This means that people there are exposed to new dangers.

Another example of what is happening is that many of the developed countries, under the pretext of wanting to help developing countries, are now transferring 'dirty' industry which processes very toxic substances to Africa and Asia. The workers and the people in the developed countries are basically protected, but what about the people in those areas where these poisons are just being introduced – no answer is forthcoming.

(b) The most difficult question is *what* has to be done? We have to begin in the light of present-day knowledge and with realistic possibilities, such as reducing smoking and air pollution. This is a great challenge since thousands are earning their daily living from the industries involved.

(c) Finally, *when* can these problems be tackled? The time is ripe and everyone knows that we must begin now. Something has to done if we want to see results in the future. Socio-economic aspects of cancer prevention are quite different from cancer detection activities. The approach is different. The legislation required is also different. The methods used for achieving results are not medical, but rather of a technical nature. This means that a whole group of additional co-workers may be needed. It is normal for the expected results or the yield from invested money to be rather slow in appearing in the early decades of this work.

In conclusion, we ask from where the money might come? Firstly, governments in many countries earn quite a lot from the taxation of tobacco, oil, and the car industry. Secondly, it is our opinion that man, who now has a life expectancy of more than 70 years must contribute something if he wants to add a few more years to his life span. A fraction of his pension or earnings could be diverted into a so-called *Cancer Prevention Fund*. From such a fund future research and possible compensation for redundancy in affected industries could be financed in part. Thirdly, the initiation of long term studies (which would last at least 20 years) leading to cancer prevention might be another answer. This suggestion is never welcomed because very few wish to start a programme they may not see finished.

Obviously there are no quick answers – we have only the bare facts about the experience of many countries with various types of cancer and the possible socio-economic consequences of cancer prevention.

References

De Haas, J. H. (1967): In: Health of Mankind, pp. 79-102. Editors: G. Wolstenholme and M. O'Conner. J and A. Churchill Ltd., London.
Denoix, P. (1970): Cancer Bull., 8, 13.
Doll, R. (1970): Cancer Bull., 8, 15.
Zubrod, C. G. (1972): Cancer, 30, 1474.

Socio-economic factors in cancer detection

G. Riotton

Centre de Cytology et de Dépistage du Cancer, Geneva, Switzerland

When prevention is not feasible, we must rely on detection, sometimes called secondary prevention. I will only outline and introduce, the discussion on the socio-economic factors in cancer detection since some of these are being treated by other speakers.

This subject may be approached from two quite different directions: a purely cost/benefit assessment of disease control, taking account of the priorities of public health, or consideration of the relevance of the apparent differences in socio-economic level of communities or populations, to the implementation of cancer control procedures. It may be useful to stress the basic elements required to make cost-benefit assessments and how to evaluate their reliability.

Some of these basic elements include: the natural history of the disease; the age-adjusted incidence and prevalence of the cancer being studied; the cure rate, disablement and the cost of treatment at different stages of the disease; the economic value of human life during illness or at the time of death versus the overall cost of the programme. These are only some elements of the equation: some are evidently difficult to assess with reasonable accuracy or even approximately.

It is most important to assess the reliability of the data collected. For example, data collected in Cancer Registries such as clinical or pathological diagnosis and patient identification are not nearly as reliable as is usually supposed and may be misleading. When cost-benefit analysis is not feasible a different calculation may be done if a gross evaluation makes it evident, or at least sufficiently probable, that a programme is really needed. In such a situation *cost-effectiveness* is used instead of cost-benefit analysis. Cost-effectiveness does not evaluate benefits, but permits the identification of the least expensive of the alternative courses of action.

We will not discuss the many types of screening for cancer, which have been suggested at one time or another, nor the appropriate techniques, e.g. mass screening, selective screening for high risk groups, multiple screening combining the search for two or more cancers in the same individual etc. The main criteria for the choice of a screening procedure are, as for any other disease: *validity* which comprises *sensitivity* (few false negatives) and *specificity* (few false positives) (sensitivity and specificity can be varied reciprocally according to the threshold chosen) and *reliability*. If a test is valid, that is to say if it is a good index of the disease sought, two factors are involved in the efficiency of the method: reproducibility and observer-variations.

In addition, the *yield* must be considered. This is primarily related to the prevalence of the given cancer in the population under study and also to the efficiency of the method, which must be high. The cost must be bearable and, finally, the test must be acceptable to the individual tested. For example, in our region the most easily detected cancers are those of the uterus (cervix and corpus) and the breast. Much has been said about these cancers. For the uterus the quality of the cytological technique is of crucial importance and the entire efficiency of the programme depends on it. There are too many ambitious programmes for the detection of cervical cancer which are meaningless and very costly due to the lack of decent quality control at the laboratory level.

There are many techniques available for screening for breast cancer, e.g. mammography, thermography and xerography, but none of them are suitable for mass screening, at this point in time. Another alternative, using public health education, is to train women to make a simple, regularly repeated self-examination of their breasts. Inherent in this programme is the prior education of doctors in the necessity of promoting self-examination among their patients. The planning of any programme of detection which deals with a large number of individuals must be included in a national, or regional, public health programme. It would be very unwise to organize the programme as an individual, isolated activity although this is often done. Remember that the costs must be related to the benefits that would have been derived from spending the same sums on other forms of medical care.

The aims, as well as the priorities, will be different depending on the level of development of the region, the medical facilities and, in particular, the treatment facilities. The priorities are decided, not only by the frequency, mortality, age at onset etc. of the disease, but by its specific social impact in the region, or in the population group under study. Included in the calculation are the purely financial aspects. It seems self evident that a Ministry of Finance cannot spend more money than is available and it has other budgets than the Public Health one. The Ministry of Health also has many priorities which may vary widely depending on the region. This is why the final decision must be as unemotional, technical and realistic as possible. Prestige and politics should play no part in the decision: it is the final benefit for the community which must be the deciding factor.

This is especially true for countries where cancer may not be a major public health problem for some time. In such a situation only small, restricted projects and laboratories need be set up to prepare an infrastructure of technically able people and to provide training for them. However, these small units must work according to strict scientific principles. The units may be easily expanded when the situation demands. They will permit the accumulation of limited, but pertinent, data.

Education of the public

Gisela Gästrin*

Cancer Society of Finland (1962-1973), Helsinki, Finland

When I speak about *Education of the public* I include the following two items:
1. *Medical education* using popular terms and language.
2. *Information* on cancer control programs including social counselling and practical advice on prevention, early detection, treatment, check-ups and so on.

I think Finland presents an example of how cancer education can be organized in a small country. There are 4.6 million inhabitants in Finland. There is one cancer organization, the Cancer Society of Finland, which is a voluntary organization, established in 1936. It has a nationwide coverage with 10 regional *Chapters*. The Cancer Society has 60,000 members. They represent the general public, but there are also doctors, nurses, health workers, teachers etc. – and cancer patients.

According to the by-laws of the Society, education takes first place in its program of action. Education is planned by the Chief of Education who has to be a physician. The plans are submitted for approval to the board of the Cancer Society which represents the highest medical authorities in the fields of oncology, pathology and gynecology. Funds for education are raised through campaigns, donations, wills, a congratulation and condolence address service and through membership fees. Since the implementation of the National Health Act in 1972 municipalities pay the Cancer Society for the material received.

The recommendations of the WHO and UICC and the plans of the Scandinavian Cancer Union are of central significance in the selection of target groups for cancer education. The UICC, IARC, IUHE and the Finnish Cancer Registry are the most important scientific sources in the preparation of educational material. National health legislation and the program of on-going school reform are essential in the preparation of material to suit the current conditions.

Six leaflets, the exhibitions and *a teaching kit* are the present educational material financed by the Cancer Society.

The six leaflets are for the public. Some of them refer to specific kinds of cancer; some of them are aimed at young people – others are directed towards adults. In each case the reader is advised what to do on observing any of the cancer symptoms.

Exhibitions, complete with movable stands and supports, are used. The exhibition material gives the same type of information as the leaflets.

The teaching kit consists of slides as well as printed and experimental material. It is used by doctors, nurses, teachers and medical students in the education of the public and in schools etc. Posters and films are also used in the education of the public.

The services provided for particular target groups will now be described (Fig.1):

A Chief of Information is employed half-time as the managing editor of a magazine delivered to the members of the Cancer Society. The editor-in-chief is the leading physician of the Helsinki University Clinic of Radiotherapy. The magazine contains articles on different cancerous diseases as well as a great deal of social counselling and advice. It is published 8 times a year.

The Chief of Education is in charge of the direct counselling of the public, lectures, radio, TV and press comments – and of the production of leaflets, posters, teaching kits and exhibition materials.

* Present address: P.B. 21, Helsinki 57, Finland

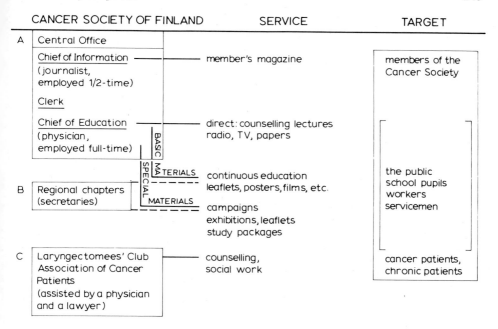

FIG. 1   *Services of the Cancer Society to target groups (1962-1973).*

The regional Chapters have secretaries, employed either full-time or half-time, for administrating the 11 cytological laboratories of the cervical cancer mass-screening network and the 7 detection centers. They also distribute material, arrange campaigns, exhibitions and lectures as well as produce articles for the local press.

The Association of Laryngectomees and the Association of Cancer Patients make use of specialists in their efforts to promote various social and medical improvements for patients.

The public is thus being served in a multitude of ways. It is divided into several target groups such as the members of the Cancer Society, school pupils, workers, the military, women participating in mass-screening, patients in different hospitals, patients in cancer detection centers, cancer patients and chronic cancer patients.

In the continuous process of education and during campaigns, the following groups, in addition to the regional Chapters of the Cancer Society, contribute:

Continuous education

regular subscribers
municipalities, maternity welfare stations
mass screening offices
various public health organizations
out-patients
clinics of various hospitals
schools and institutes
temperance organizations
industry
private subscribers

Campaigns

assisting organizations
National Board of Health
medical faculties of universities
National Board of Schools
medical interns
labor unions
the armed forces
trade fairs

The determination of priorities in cancer detection programmes

R.J. Wrighton

Department of Health and Social Security, Alexander Fleming House, London, United Kingdom

The principles of early disease detection were stated by Wilson and Jungner in their monograph on the Principles and Practice of Screening for Disease published in 1968. They listed 10 main points which they suggested should be regarded as guidelines to the planning of case finding schemes. These principles were intended to apply to the planning of screening schemes for all types of disease including screening for all types of cancer and the development and launching of any scheme must start from a consideration of the factors covered by these principles.

One aspect of the determination of priorities in the implementation of schemes depends in effect on how well or otherwise a particular scheme measures up to the principles. It is not necessary to enumerate these principles at this point but I should like to discuss their application to different cancer detection schemes later.

The determination of priorities in cancer detection programmes can however be considered both from the viewpoint of priorities between competing programmes and the degree of priority of cancer detection programmes individually or as a whole over health care programmes in other fields.

In general the determination of priorities *between* cancer detection programmes has not so far proved a big problem because the number of types of cancer which can be successfully screened for with present techniques is strictly limited. It is not so much a question, at least in the United Kingdom, of weighing the desirability of screening for one type of cancer against screening for another type, when satisfactory techniques are available for both and the returns in terms of lives saved or usefully prolonged are roughly similar. Rather it has been a question of looking for any practical opportunity for effective screening and applying it in the most appropriate way. Reaching the decision to launch a cancer detection programme, whether on a national basis or on a more limited basis, involves the consideration of the factors already mentioned.

Determining the priority of screening for cancer in comparison with other desired developments in health care is a more difficult exercise and as yet we do not really know how to do it in any scientific way. The nearest we can get at present is to draw up an economic equation which attempts to balance the cost of a screening programme against the likely gains to be expected from the prolongation of productive life as a result of early detection and treatment of the disease. It is perhaps not too difficult to arrive at a reasonably accurate estimate of the cost of the actual screening procedure in terms of staff, materials and overhead costs and in the case of cervical smears, for instance, a cost per unit test can readily be arrived at. What is more difficult is the estimation of the cost of further procedures and treatment generated by the screening scheme against which has to be offset the cost of treatment that would have become necessary at a later date for those positive cases discovered.

The calculation of the other side of the equation, the gain produced, is perhaps even more difficult and undoubtedly the immediate and purely economic aspect is of relatively minor importance.

We can perhaps start with the idea that in the absence of effective prevention (which is of course the ideal solution) it would probably be desirable to be able to detect all types of cancer at the earliest possible stage in their development. In the present state of the art we are largely limited to the finding of gross morphological change in a tissue or in some cases the recognition of abnormal cells derived from an epithelial surface. The stage in the history of the cancer at which these changes can be found may in fact be quite late and the effect on the prognosis of instituting treatment at that stage, assuming an effective treatment is available, may not be all that great. It is however not unlikely, that there will be developed over the next few years tests depending on chemical and/or immunological reactions which will detect cancers very much earlier. One which has already become established is urinary chorionic gonadotrophin assay in screening for and monitoring cases of choriocarcinoma. I shall say more of this in a moment. Tumour-associated antigens are at present of limited usefulness in diagnosis and because of their poor specificity are of no value as screening tests but it is at least possible that more specific tests will emerge along these or similar lines which will enable the existence of cancerous change to be detected before there is any morphological evidence of its presence, and long before any symptoms appear. If at the same time there are available chemotherapeutic or immunotherapeutic techniques which are effective at this early stage (and again it is certainly possible and in time probable that there will be such) then the possibility of real control over cancer through early detection will have been brought much nearer. With existing treatment techniques of course, we need to know where the cancer is before it can be treated and unless one knows this, early detection is of no value. Thus, a high carcino-embryonic antigen level, if it is shown to be a reliable indicator of the presence of cancer, cannot be acted on unless other signs to enable localisation are present. Sputum cytology for early lung cancer has proved to be of no value as a screening test for this reason.

If and when we have developed the screening techniques and effective chemo- or immuno-therapy a number of the problems which colour our present thinking about the establishment of screening programmes will have been overcome but there will remain complex social and economic considerations which will become progressively more difficult of solution. But that is for the future. I would like now to say something of the current cancer detection programme in the United Kingdom which I hope may serve to illustrate some of the general points I have made.

Choriocarcinoma

The Department of Health and Social Security for England and Wales, together with the Scottish Home and Health Department, has recently launched a national screening scheme for women who have had a hydatidiform mole pregnancy. About 800 mole pregnancies occur annually in the United Kingdom and about 1 in 40 of these patients will develop a malignant trophoblastic tumour over the ensuing 1 to 2 years. These 20 cases constitute roughly half of the expected annual number of cases of malignant trophoblastic tumour in the country.

The characteristics of choriocarcinoma are that once established it is frequently rapidly fatal but in its early stage it is highly susceptible to chemotherapy and if adequately treated within 6 months of the evacuation of the mole a cure rate of 95% can be expected; delay of treatment beyond 6 months progressively reduces this. Therefore even with such a small annual number of cases the degree of improvement in prognosis that can be attained by early detection makes a good prima facie case for a screening scheme. Furthermore the group to be screened is small, readily identified and readily accessible in that the vast majority will be under the care of a gynaecologist at the time of the diagnosis of hydatidiform mole pregnancy.

The third major factor is the availability of a specific screening test, a radioimmunoassay procedure for urinary chorionic gonadotrophin. The test is non-invasive merely requiring the patient to provide at given intervals a small specimen of urine which is sent in a container provided, direct to the laboratory. The laboratory reminds the patient when the next specimen is due and ensures as far as is possible that the specimen is actually produced. There are therefore very few problems with patient acceptability of procedure or with defaulting.

The principal costs with this scheme are laboratory costs and the costs of special treatment facilities. In fact treatment costs are reduced overall since the time required to treat these cases early is considerably less than is required later in the course of the disease. Three laboratories and at present one special treatment centre (later two) provide the required resources for this scheme for the whole country.

This example provides a picture of the ideal screening situation, albeit in miniature; the only one of Wilson and Jungner's criteria that it may be questioned whether it satisfies, is that the condition should be an important health problem. But the weight to be attached to any one criterion is modified by the strength of the others and in this instance the obvious prognostic gains, the readily identifiable and accessible high-risk group and the availability of an acceptable, specific and relatively inexpensive test easily justified the establishment of this scheme.

It is unfortunately not always so straightforward.

Breast cancer

The importance of this as a major health problem in many countries is indisputable. In the United Kingdom it is the commonest cause of death from cancer in women and accounts for approximately 4% of all female deaths. In 1971 there were 10,600 deaths attributed to carcinoma of the breast; 16,000 new cases were registered. The social and economic cost of breast cancer to the nation, even if it cannot be exactly quantified, must clearly be very high and on these grounds alone breast cancer must be considered to have high priority as a subject for general screening facilities.

But in looking at the other criteria for screening as they apply to this case the situation becomes complicated. There is little clear evidence that the treatments currently available for the disease are effective though there is some evidence to suggest that about 40% of women with Stage I and Stage II cancers enjoy a similar expectation of life after surgery as women of comparable age without breast cancer. And whilst there has been no appreciable change in mortality rates from breast cancer in any country there is evidence from North American cancer registry data which suggests that 5-year survival rates have shown some improvement over the last 20 years. This may be partly attributable to improved treatment. But there is little agreement on the form treatment should take and we are only just beginning to get evidence from controlled trials.

There are several tests available, none being clearly superior to the other, and the combination of tests with which to achieve the highest degree of validity has yet to be demonstrated. Clinical examination and thermography are non-invasive and as such preferable to mammography and xerography, but the first is expensive of professional time and is not capable of detecting cancers as early as one would like, and the second is not yet technically adequate. Studies have been set up in a number of centres in the United Kingdom in an attempt to clarify some of the problems related to validation of the various tests – we need to know the degree of sensitivity and specificity of the tests individually, the degree of observer variation to be expected and the relative contributions of each test to diagnosis. Breast cancer, more than some other forms, is an emotive subject and it is likely that there would be a high demand for the screening service. With the shortage of professional staff available it would be necessary to employ trained non-medical staff, for example nurses and radiographers, to carry out palpation and initial screening of radiographs, using medically qualified staff for second-stage screening only. Also we need to know more about the population to be screened, particularly whether it is possible to define high-risk groups.

The early results from the HIP study in New York suggest that a significant reduction in mortality may be achieved in the over-50 age group by means of annual screening using clinical examination and mammography. My department will be closely observing the later results of this excellent study which, with the results of the studies now begun in the United Kingdom, will help us to decide the case for instituting what would be a massive programme on a national scale and one which would necessarily have to be considered in competition with other health care needs for the allocation of limited resources.

Bladder cancer

The success of treatment of cancer of the bladder is markedly affected by delay in application. The 3-year survival rate for patients treated within one month of development of symptoms is about 70% but declines to 35% after 6 months delay. Accurate diagnosis at the time of the first symptom or before is therefore likely to have an appreciable effect on prognosis. Pre-symptomatic detection in a high-risk population is likely to be even more effective. The overall incidence of carcinoma of the bladder is not high – in the United Kingdom approximately 6,000 new cases occur annually and in 1971 there were 3,800 deaths attributed to bladder cancer. Urinary exfoliative cytology is not a simple procedure – it requires careful attention to specimen collection, preservation and speed of handling to minimize the appreciable false negative rate as well as highly skilled processing and interpretation. It is therefore unsuitable for mass screening. It is, however, suitable for use in the screening of high-risk groups, particularly in certain industries where the risk of development of bladder cancer is increased. In the United Kingdom the rubber industry has provided a screening service for employees since 1957 based on urinary cytology and my Department is about to offer a similar service to some 19,000 employees who were in the industry during the time that benzidine and naphthylamine derivatives were in use but who had left before the screening scheme was established. We have been able to trace the majority of those people whose names were obtained from the records kept by the industry through our National Health Service Central Registry where named records of all NHS patients are kept up-to-date.

Improvement of tests for bladder cancer could improve the efficiency of screening but the techniques available, cytology of fresh bladder washings and endoscopy, do not lend themselves to large scale application. These techniques are however being assessed in the early diagnosis of another high-risk group, those presenting with haematuria, between 10 and 20% of whom may be expected to have early bladder cancer. The use of urinary carcino-embryonic antigen in early diagnosis is also being investigated in this group.

Other cancers

Apart from cancer of uterine cervix for which a national screening programme has been established in the United Kingdom since 1967, there is at present little further scope for screening for cancers except within certain well-defined groups or under certain circumstances, for example, rectal examination and endoscopy during routine medical examination, especially in the elderly, for the early detection of colo-rectal cancers. In a number of cases it is not because the problem is not a major one that it does not justify high priority for screening – rather it is the absence of widely acceptable and economically feasible tests or, as in the case of lung and probably stomach cancers, it is the intractability of the disease which makes early diagnosis of little practical value to the individual. However, the increasing sophistication of techniques for examination of the stomach may perhaps lead to some reappraisal of the case for early diagnosis of stomach cancer.

There is another factor however in cancer detection which should perhaps receive high priority in its own right and this is public (and professional) education in the recognition of early symptoms. Instruction in self-palpation of the breast is an established part of the function of Well-Women clinics and whilst its efficacy is hardly capable of proof it is probable that a few cancers will as a result present in Stage I rather than later. Recognition of the early symptoms of bladder or rectal cancer, particularly in the latter, may materially affect the prognosis; alertness on the part of the patient and the physician or dentist to non-healing lesions of the mouth and tongue might lessen the delay in these notoriously late-diagnosed cancers and improve the results of treatment. Cancers of the skin similarly could be recognized earlier.

Health education must therefore form an essential part of any cancer detection programme and it should be closely linked with research to determine the nature of the population one is trying to reach and the most appropriate means of so doing, an approach which has been pursued in depth by workers in Manchester with particular relevance to the cervical cytology screening service. In the United Kingdom the general practioner with his health care team (nurse, health visitor, social worker) forms one of the main sources of health education and health surveillance and in the recent proposals for the establishment of regional oncological services the general practitioner will play an important part in cancer education as well as in the other aspects of cancer care. In the last analysis all early detection activities, mass screening, selective screening of high-risk groups, early diagnosis clinics, cancer education, must be an integral part of the overall health care programme if they are to be maximally effective and plans for the organization of cancer services in a number of countries now recognize this.

Public health structures for control

Leila M. Watson

City of Edinburgh Health Department, Edinburgh, United Kingdom

Introduction

There is evidence from many countries where cancer is a major cause of morbidity and mortality that cancer control programmes vary greatly. For example, diagnostic and treatment facilities may or may not be centralised, cancer registries vary from hospital based to total population based, education of the public may be highly organised to cover the whole population or merely concerned with segments of it, and departments of public health play roles of lesser or greater importance. Why has cancer control grown in a fashion as disorganised as cancer itself? I suggest we have worked in isolation in a diversity of specialities, but failed to co-ordinate and thus reinforce our efforts.

Levels of control

Diseases can be controlled by effective prevention, by earlier detection, and by improved treatment. Wherever possible, we must promote the control of cancers simultaneously at these 3 levels. The primary level is true prevention, including removal of carcinogenic hazards as well as education in avoiding them. Secondary control depends upon early detection and diagnosis, and more importantly, the identification and protection of the vulnerable and high-risk. These basic oncological approaches have been examined throughout this symposium. Tertiary control must ensure the holistic fulfilment of patients' needs for active treatment, follow-up, rehabilitation, and terminal care – that is, physical, mental, social, environmental, vocational and economic aspects which demand an interdisciplinary team approach.

In this short paper I refer to separate measures, or 'microstructures' of control; indicate the role and aims of one local public health department and how it contributes at each level of control to provide what might be called a 'mesostructure'; and, finally, outline a nationally organised 'macrostructure' which I suggest is essential for more effective community control.

Present public health structures

The National Health Service (Scotland) Act (1947) included the prevention of illness, care and aftercare in the powers and duties conferred upon local health authorities. As community health workers our role is to service and to co-ordinate the medical, remedial and social care services, using our skills and resources to detect and fulfil the health needs and to solve the medico-social problems of our community.

In Edinburgh, with its population of 453,000, over 2,000 neoplasms are diagnosed every year and the annual death rate from malignant diseases is 2.9 per 1,000 population. Resources for cancer control are allocated in competition with the valid claims of over 6,000 neonates, 32,000 pre-school and 78,000 school children, 65,000 elderly citizens, a wide range of infectious, degenerative, chronic and handicapping diseases, and many environmental problems. Support for the cancer programme is not increased by doubts in decision-makers about the effectiveness of control measures; and some services are held at low pitch lest false expectations and too heavy demands result.

All evidence emphasises the multiple causality of cancers and the importance of augmenting and contributing factors; but when they cannot be modified, a major public health effort must be to prevent exposure to carcinogens resulting from personal behaviour, occupation or other elements of our total environment. As information from clinicians, radiologists, epidemiologists, and research workers composes the natural history of each cancer the optimum level for intervention can be more exactly selected.

Public health policy is shaped by these competing facts. Our aim is to promote public and personal co-operation in the prevention of cancers, the proper utilisation of screening procedures, and timely self-referral for treatment. Our present control measures can be summarised under the headings: total care, education, information, and legislation.

Total care   Our contribution to prevention and detection includes the provision of cytotest and breast examination facilities and smokers' clinics. We have 114 health visitors who are nurses trained in prevention and working in the community. Every one of these in her daily work with individuals and groups fosters preventive action, early self-referral and acceptance of screening, treatment and rehabilitation. They have proved themselves invaluable field workers in several research studies. The City has 132 district nurses who provide complete nursing services and support in every stage of home after-care.

Often it is these community nurses who alert the family doctor to the need of patients and their families for social services and ancillary help. As primary care teams develop, the skills of these public health workers are increasingly enlisted in all aspects of care because they are accepted by people in their homes. Thus at every stage they help allay the fear and stress which are part of the burden and problem of cancer, and encourage patients and their relatives to come to terms with the illness and the aftermath of treatment. In the event of death, two post-bereavement visits are made by home nurse, then health visitor to give support and advice. This is all of very real importance in changing the image of cancer for affected families and in modifying beliefs and attitudes in the community.

With such a team approach the public health sector contributes to treatment and care.

Education   We have a prevention-detection-treatment education programme designed for the whole community. Repetition reinforces awareness of action, which is further consolidated through community participation. The programme is appraised at different stages and accordingly improved.

It was a simple evalution which revealed a great need for education in health workers. Briefly, assessment of the knowledge, attitudes and practice of 196 of our female professional staff (a 70% response) revealed that 1 in 10 did not believe that earlier treatment improves the prognosis of mammary cancer, or felt that the anxiety engendered outweighed the value of self-examination or mass screening. In discussion, many revealed similar feelings resulting from unforgettable personal memories despite their professional knowledge of successful treatment. 78 (39.8%) of the responders did not perform breast self-examination; and 125 (64.8%) had never had a cytotest, the majority arguing that '*only* sexually active and promiscuous women of lower social classes develop carcinoma of the cervix . . . . . .'. How often we defend ourselves by denying or misinterpreting facts! This study led to in-service training sessions and discussions which have greatly improved our understanding and work-performance. The importance of personal example set by health workers cannot be over-estimated and it is especially important in cigarette smoking. Surely we should practice what we preach.

Convinced that cancer control demands community action, we are developing deeper involvement of people in many ways, though not yet to the extent achieved in several countries represented here. We have a promising participation project where local housewives are trained as health aides to help change attitudes to cancer in the hitherto unreachable. Their own beliefs and actions have changed radically — all have had the cytotest, the majority have already stopped smoking, and their message has become hopeful ('it may not be cancer . . . . . . and if it is they can do a lot for you nowadays . . . . . .

so see your doctor NOW'). One aide, still in training, has finally convinced 3 women to consult their doctors with conditions they had feared for months to be cancer yet had approached no professional worker.

The very foundation for cancer control is extensive education of the public and the profession: all clinical advances are diminished without it.

Information and communication   Our own data, central department reports, and medical literature provide cancer incidence information and a profile of our population structure from which to make epidemiological decisions. Alert to note unusual local incidence, we monitor area morbidity and mortality, and are continually improving information, the better to establish then communicate priorities for action (e.g. cancer-site selection, target-group identification, appropriate objective). A public health department is uniquely placed to collect 'soft' as well as 'hard' data about its population.

Our own staff of over 300 (including doctors, health visitors, nurses, midwives and sanitary inspectors) are the epidemiology fieldworkers in daily contact with the community at professional and public levels, and are invaluable in identifying those most at risk. We have established strong lines of communication with all health workers and opinion leaders in our society, and have enlisted the help of voluntary organisations, the mass media and other local authority departments. (For example social work and housing departments assist in reaching lower socio-economic groups; and a cohort of mothers has been contacted for the cytotest through the education department).

Legislation   Comprehensive national legislation exists for environmental health measures controlling recognised carcinogens and co-carcinogens in industry, and pollutants in air, water, food, drugs and other substances. Several central departments, boards and other bodies are involved in implementation and also in the investigation of possible new hazards. Local powers vary and would benefit from standardisation, however, our public health environmentalists, the sanitary inspectors, now have duties in checking food, food additives and drugs, the working conditions in non-mechanical factories, and the safe disposal of radioactive waste. They report the law is honoured best where the danger is immediate or the hazard can be eliminated, but less so when risks are not so apparent and personal action and integrity are required. We believe that appropriate education can make legislation more acceptable.

Conclusions and recommendations

Thus the services and staff of a public health department are involved in a variety of ways in the control and management of this group of diseases. The extent of such services varies greatly in different areas. Critics may question their value but planners see their potential. I believe that presently, with these daily and necessary services, we provide the bonds which link essential microstructures into a mesostructure. A small growth, entirely benign! It must progress from 'Public Health' with capital letters into a macrostructure of community care which incorporates the following:

1. *Personal Care Systems*   Appropriate prevention, detection and treatment services must be developed and maintained. Closer liaison with primary care teams is urged to avoid omissions in care and to achieve co-ordination.

2. *Information Systems*   Accurate data about the cancer diseases and the population must be collected and analysed; then organised communication between all health workers and the community. Unless clinicians are convinced of the usefulness of information, they will not supply it. Existing and new information must be usefully applied, for instance to select priorities, improve services and allocate resources.

3. *Research and Monitoring Facilities*   These are necessary for the whole range from cell to community, from psyche to environment. Collaboration and exchange between workers is vital.

4. *Legislation*   The necessary statutory powers to control industrial and environmental carcinogens should be swiftly enacted and reinforced by international and national standardisation.

5. *Education*   Extensive education of the public and profession is the very foundation for cancer control. From it come understanding and conviction which can make the previous measures effective and the control of hazards possible. Education will secure professional commitment for the control programme and it must be extended to all students and colleagues in nursing, paramedical and medical disciplines.

6. *Evaluation*   Auditing and monitoring are not always welcome, yet only critical assessment of the effectiveness of the foregoing components can return information necessary for continuing progress.

7. *Co-ordination*   At present there are excellent systems for diagnosis, treatment and research. It is essential to extend the community health structures which can add new dimensions to clinical services and facilitate their effectiveness. Separate specialist achievements require development through the services of medical co-ordinators with responsibility at every stage of the total scheme. Wherever they are based, these specialists should not be divorced from the community lest both perspective and opportunities are lost.

Since local and national policy-makers must allocate precious resources according to the total needs and priorities of that society, and to the proven merit of services, perhaps we must all do more to dispel doubts about the value of measures for cancer control.

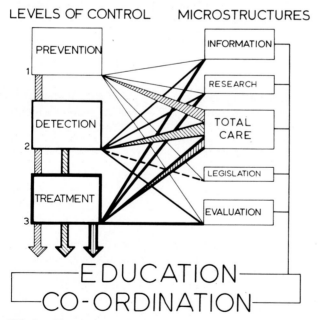

FIG. 1   *Macrostructure for cancer control.*

When epidemiological facts demonstrate that specific cancers occur in certain socio-economic groups then community action is required too.

Only by involving all clinical and research workers, public and central departments, and society itself in a comprehensive dynamic plan shall we so interfere with the ecology of the cancers as to control them.

Summary

Cancer control is seen to consist of essential units (microstructures) of individual care and research which have developed in too great isolation.

A public health system is examined and shown to provide a mesostructure at the 3 levels of prevention, detection and treatment. But public health services vary greatly and an integrated community approach is considered essential.

Management of this group of diseases is seen to demand a team effort — a multidisciplinary collaboration by all cancer workers — and a catalytic role is suggested for a community-based medical co-ordinator.

Society itself must also be involved in such a scheme, to combine total care services, comprehensive education, information systems, legislation, and evaluation into a macrostructure for control.

Public health aspects of cancer control

Discussion

The discussion, stimulated by the 5 panel speakers, covered a variety of aspects of cancer control with a substantial amount of personal experience. There was great interest in the concept that cancer was a community problem requiring a community approach for its solution. It was suggested, therefore, that the detection of the disease required trained members of the community to assume the technical duties and gather the data which accumulated from the programme. There was some concern expressed over the community approach in terms of the confidence of the community in cancer control activities. It was generally agreed that such confidence is directly proportional to the involvement of the medical members of the community − especially in terms of the follow-up of suspicious cases. The suggestion was offered that professional participation determined the success of any cancer control activity and far exceeded the effect of economic factors. Nevertheless, the economic factors did enter the discussion and comparisons of costs between annual examinations, after age 40, and treatment of malignant disease were cited. In general, treatment costs were 5 times greater although it was admitted that screening costs were easily derived, whereas the cost of subsequent treatment was difficult to estimate.

Some good points were made in the discussion of screening programmes as part of the cancer control programme. It was suggested that, in cancer of the breast, the high risk group was relatively well identified but the actual screening method had not been so clearly described. There was agreement that a broad approach to cancer screening pays dividends, that priorities are not difficult to ascertain in view of the limited number of sites. However, it was admitted that new screening techniques may affect the determination of priorities. The need for more trained paramedical personnel was stressed although the question of variation in their status of acceptability remained unresolved.

A.J. Phillips,
Chairman

Symposia

Contents

1. Endoscopic diagnosis of gastrointestinal tract neoplasms

Value of aimed endoscopic cytology as diagnostic confirmation in esophageal cancer

A. Bigotti, N. Campioni, S. Di Matteo and M. Crespi

Cancer Detection Center, Regina Elena Institute for Cancer Research, Rome, Italy

The diagnosis of esophageal cancer by radiological and endoscopic procedures is in a majority of cases rather easy. In some instances however, it may be difficult to reach a clear cut diagnosis: that is in cases where hard stenosis is present or the cancer is developing in diverticula. Also very early cases and some inflammatory lesions may pose rather serious problems of differential diagnosis.

According to our experience, the answer to most of these problems could be in endoscopic examinations completed with aimed biopsies and cytological abrasive smears. In fact, in our Institute, aimed cytology is a matter of routine. This procedure is performed by a rotating brush which scratches the superficial layers of the mucosa. Cytological sampling could also be obtained by washing, but with quite less satisfactory results.

Results

In order to evaluate the accuracy of the methods available for obtaining a morphological diagnosis, we have compared aimed bioptic and cytologic samplings in 28 cases of esophageal cancer (Table 1). As can be seen, in 3 cases in which the biopsy was negative, cytology allowed us the obtain a morphological proof of malignancy. In one case out of 8 of adenocarcinoma of the terminal esophagus, biopsy as well as cytology were negative.

TABLE 1   *Results of aimed endoscopic cytology in 28 cases of esophageal cancer (histologically confirmed at surgery)*

Histologic type	No. of cases	Accuracy of different procedures			
		Aimed cytology		Aimed biopsy	
		+	−	+	−
Adenocarcinoma	9	8	1	8	1
Squamous cell carcinoma	18	18		16	2
Indifferentiated carcinoma	1	1		1	
Total	28	27	1	25	3

In Figures 1 to 6, different cytological aspects of malignant esophageal tumors are shown. The highly keratinized abnormal cells, with either completely pyknotic, hyperchromatic nuclei, or with nuclear shadows, represent a common pattern. Besides, smaller

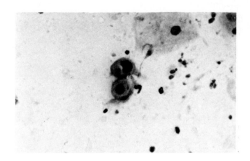

FIG. 1   *'Cell-in-cell' pattern: a small cancer cell is completely surrounded by the cytoplasm of a larger cell.*

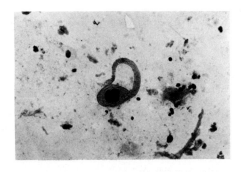

FIG. 2   *Tadpole cell with round, hyperchromatic nucleus eccentrically located within the larger area of the cytoplasm.*

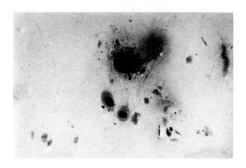

FIG. 3   *Squamous cancer cells: note the club-shaped cell with fully keratinized cytoplasm and faint outlines of the nucleus.*

and less differentiated cells are present, some of which are with very scanty basophilic cytoplasm. Fairly typical cancer cells of glandular type are also present. The 3 main cytotypes of esophageal cancer (adenocarcinoma, squamous cell and indifferentiated carcinomas) may be clearly identified.

Comment

The reason for the discrepancy between bioptic and cytological samplings is of technical origin, i.e. that the bioptic forceps slide on the mucosal surface owing to the tangential direction of the approach. Instead, the cytological brush leans against the esophageal wall and is therefore in a better position to withdraw a satisfactory sample. This is especially worthwhile in esophageal strictures due to malignant or scarring processes, in which a

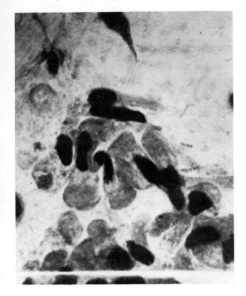

FIG. 4 *Poorly differentiated carcinoma: small cell variety.*

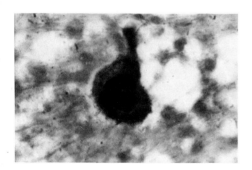

FIG. 5 *Poorly differentiated carcinoma: large cell variety.*

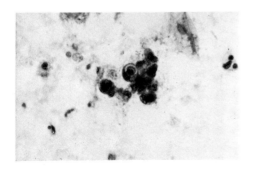

FIG. 6 *Adenocarcinoma: cluster of cancer cells. Note the irregular nuclear outline and the large irregular nucleoli.*

satisfactory sample may be obtained very frequently by abrasive cytology performed through the stricture.

We want to stress that in experienced hands the cytological examination per se is sufficient in achieving a morphological diagnosis of malignancy when radiological and endoscopic data have already aroused a strong suspicion. A possibility of misinterpretation is only in the case of post-radiation cellular changes, but the personal history is always instrumental.

The data presented seem to us a further confirmation of the importance of aimed cytology as a routine diagnostic tool, to be used in close association with aimed biopsy. Its accuracy permits us also to rely on it in excluding malignancy, because a repeatedly negative cytology may rule out a malignant process also if suspicious clinical and radiological data are present.

Reference

Crespi, M. et al. (1971): Minerva Gastroent., 17, 142.

Endoscopic diagnosis of ulcerated gastric cancer (Type III) in the early stages

F. Faggioli, R. Corinaldesi, G. Di Febo, A. Romano and G. Biasco

Istituto di I Patologia Speciale Medica e Metodologia Clinica dell'Università di Bologna, Bologna, Italy

The development of modern endoscopic instruments using fibre optics has facilitated the early diagnosis of gastric cancer. The use of gastroscopy together with direct vision biopsy, washing cytology and brushing cytology has helped to raise the percentage of accurate diagnoses in Italy too. The aim of this communication is to present our data on the early diagnosis of ulcerated gastric cancer Type III according to the classification established by the Japanese Endoscopy Society in 1962.

The data has been gathered over a period of 10 years. The patients observed during this period were sent to us either with abnormal radiological findings or with disorders of the alimentary tract showing negative radiological findings.

From a total of 8,500 endoscopic examinations, we found 320 cases of benign ulcer and 158 cases of ulcerated cancer. From this last group, all of whom underwent surgical intervention, we selected 62 patients with cancer in the early stages (affecting the mucosa and submucosa), and in whom it was possible to carry out direct vision biopsy and washing cytology in addition to endoscopy.

From the analysis of the results it can be seen that when an accurate endoscopic diagnosis is made, biopsy and cytology confirm the diagnosis in fewer cases, but when the endoscopic diagnosis is inaccurate or doubtful, biopsy and cytology are of great help (Table 1). Comparing the results obtained by biopsy and cytology, it may be noted that

TABLE 1   *Diagnostic accuracy by endoscopy, gastric biopsy under direct vision and gastric lavage cytology in 62 cases of early ulcerated gastric cancer*

Endoscopy		Biopsy		Cytology		
		Positive	Negative	Positive	Negative	Technically uncertain
Accurate diagnosis	53	48	5	47	8	2
Inaccurate diagnosis	3	2	1	1	–	1
Doubtful diagnosis	6	4	2	2	1	–
Total		54	8	50	9	3

TABLE 2   *Comparison of results of biopsy under direct vision and gastric lavage cytology in 62 cases of early ulcerated cancer*

Biopsy positive Cytology positive	Biopsy positive Cytology negative	Biopsy negative Cytology positive	Biopsy negative Cytology negative
46	8	4	4

there are more cases showing positive biopsy and negative cytology than those showing negative biopsy and positive cytology. In 4 cases it was impossible to reach a diagnosis either by biopsy or cytology (Table 2). Table 3 summarizes the data about the diagnostic accuracy obtained in the 62 cases. It can be seen that in 3 cases it was not possible to reach a conclusive diagnosis with any of the 3 methods used.

It is evident that whichever method is used, either alone or in conjuction with the others, there is always a percentage of ulcers left which cannot be diagnosed with certainty. Even using brushing cytology under direct vision (which was not carried out on our patients), it does not seem possible to attain a 100% accurate diagnosis. This means that these particular cases present a problem until the end of the therapy. The percentage of accurate diagnoses can vary between fairly wide limits in different cases, depending on various factors. It is clear that the experience of the endoscopist and of the cytologist plays a fundamental role. The correct endoscopic evaluation of an ulcerative lesion requires considerable experience and depends on a subjective interpretation which it is difficult to quantify. The possibility of obtaining direct vision samples for biopsy depends on various factors, the principal being the position of the lesion. It is common knowledge that some ulcers can be easily identified but not so easily reached with forceps and brush. Not forgetting the difficulty, even with accessible lesions, of performing all the manipulations necessary to ensure the accuracy of the diagnosis, many authors recommend that between 6 and 10 biopsies and at least 3 brushings under direct vision be. taken.

TABLE 3   _Diagnostic accuracy in 62 cases of early ulcerated gastric cancer_

Accurate diagnosis by endoscopy	53
Accurate diagnosis by biopsy	54
Accurate diagnosis by cytology	50
Cases in which it was impossible to make a diagnosis using all three methods	3

As to the success rate in obtaining numerous samples for biopsy, Table 4 shows the number of biopsy samples we were able to obtain in 492 ulcerative lesions. It clearly shows that in most cases we were not able to take more than 3 samples, while in 35 cases the lesions were not accessible. At times, it is only possible to see the neoplasm tangentially and this presents a serious disadvantage. If it is not possible to obtain a sample either for biopsy or brushing cytology under direct vision, the results of the cytological examination following gastric lavage can, in particular cases, be the determining factor. However, there are several differing opinions regarding the validity of this last technique. In particular in the case of ulcerated gastric cancer, from 1−19% of false positives have been reported, depending on the case study in question. We do not agree on this point, as up till now we have only found false negatives. The importance of this statement is evident since it implies that if the technique is carried out correctly there should be no risk of mistaking a benign lesion for a malignant lesion. Unfortunately, there still remains a high

TABLE 4   _Possibility of obtaining biopsies under direct vision in 492 ulcerative lesion patients_

1 − 3 biopsies	4 − 6 biopsies	7 − 10 biopsies ·	Impossible to obtain
305	110	42	35

percentage of false negatives. In some cases the diagnosis may be further helped by brushing cytology under direct vision, as previously mentioned.

Considering the difficulty of reaching an accurate diagnosis it is obvious that all the methods at our disposal must be employed, gastroscopy, multiple direct vision biopsy and both washing and brushing cytology, which may in particular patients remove any doubts. Even so, there are still some cases in which it is not possible to reach a conclusion. It is therefore advisable to follow the evolution of the lesion with care over a long period, even when it appears to be healing under treatment. In fact, it has been noted that malignant ulcers often show an improvement. We ourselves have found 12 such cases, and it may be noted that a complete temporary healing may occur following a life cycle, that may be repeated several times over a period of years. These rather disconcerting factors indicate that all ulcerative lesions should be approached with extreme caution.

We would like to make one final point. The early stages of a pure Type III cancer are rarely observed, as it is generally associated with other types, particulary Type II-C. At present we are not sure if the characteristics of the excavation depend on the aggressive chloride-peptic factors which make the endoscopic appearance similar to that of a benign ulcer, but it is certain that this similarity occurs more often in cases with hyper- or normal chlorhydria than in cases with hypo- or achlorhydria.

The results of a study of the gastric acid secretion, carried out on our patients, can be seen in Figures 1 and 2. The patients were divided into two groups based on the endoscopic morphology of the lesion. In the first group of 49 patients with ulcerative lesions (Fig. 1) shown to be neoplastic by endoscopy, the secretion values were variable but

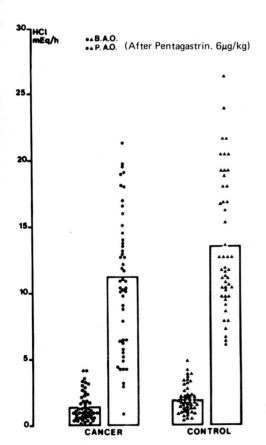

FIG. 1   *A group of 49 patients with ulcerative lesions shown to be neoplastic by endoscopy.*

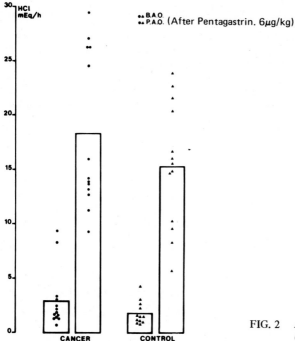

FIG. 2 *A group of 13 patients with early cancer resembling benign ulcer.*

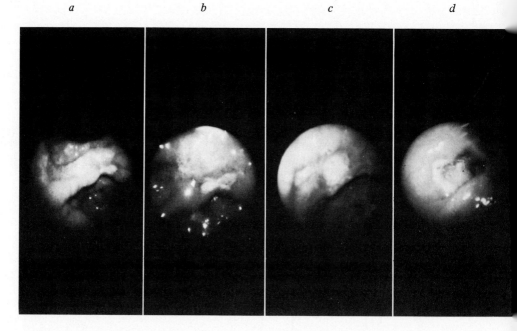

FIG. 3 *Endoscopic features of cancer in early stage. (a), (b): Neoplastic ulcer designed as Type III and II − C. (c), (d): Ulcerated cancer designed as Type III. These aspects clearly demonstrate that the differential diagnosis with benign lesion is difficult and uncertain.*

tending towards hyposecretion. In the second group of 13 patients (Fig . 2) with early cancer resembling benign ulcer, the secretion values were practically identical to the controls.

These results have no statistical significance, but we feel that the evidence tends to confirm the theory of peptic digestion of the tumor already suggested by various authors to reject the theory of neoplastic degeneration at the edges of a benign ulcer. This could explain the partial healing of the cancer following peptic ulcer therapy occurring in some cases, and the relative ease with which an attentive endoscopist can make an early diagnosis of a malignant ulcer, a diagnosis which paradoxically, is more difficult to make in a slightly more advanced stage.

The endoscopic aspect of ulcerated cancer in the early stages is notably different from those of benign ulcer permitting easy diagnosis in the majority of cases by noting the depression, the irregular edges and the crater-like form. These characteristics, so distinctive especially in older patients with hypochlorhydria, may not be present however, if the lesion strikes the hyperchlorhydric stomach of a younger patient.

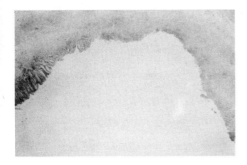

FIG. 4   *The histological specimen after surgical removal showing ulcerative cancer in the early stages. On the right you can see the neoplastic cells and on the left the same type of cells partly destroyed by ulceration. In the central area of ulceration the characteristics of the peptic ulcer can be recognised: necrosis, fibrin, exudation and sclerosis.*

In the cases in which Type III is associated with Type II—C, the diagnosis may be made on the basis of the examination of the surrounding area, where it is preferable to take specimens in order to obtain reliable results. In some rare cases, undoubtedly Type III, it is extremely difficult to differentiate this neoplasm from a benign form (Fig. 3), even with the aid of a biopsy (Fig. 4) and exfoliative cytology.

References

Kuru, M. (1967): Atlas of Early Carcinoma of the Stomach. Nakajama − Shoten Co., Tokyo, 1967.
Prolla, J. C. (1972): Gastroenterology, 1, 33.
Sakita, T. and Oguro, Y. (1971): Gastroenterology, 60, 835.
Debray, C. (1972): In: Advances in Gastrointestinal Endoscopy, p. 355. Piccin Ed., 1972.
Flood, C. A., Lattes, R. and Bachner, P. (1967): In: 3rd World Congress of Gastroenterology, p. 542. Nankodo Co., Tokyo, 1967.
Palmer, E. D. (1969): Gastrointestinal Endoscopy, 117.

268

Gastric mass survey with the gastrocamera: Performance and results*

W. Bergmann, W. Rösner, H.U. Rehs, H. Reiner, T. Székessy, H. Mahmud and H. Oshima

Department of Medicine and Surgery, Stomach Research Group, Klinikum Steglitz, Free University Berlin, Berlin

Introduction

In countries with a high incidence of gastric carcinoma, like Germany, an early diagnosis of cancer is desirable (Bergmann et al., 1970, 1973; Oshima, 1971, 1972; Oshima et al., 1973; Schäfer et al., 1970). The present diagnostic procedures often start too late. For the detection of cancer cases in curative stages, medical check-ups are necessary. Basically, diagnostic methods should be simple and quick, with low-risk and useful results (Bergmann et al., 1973; Oshima, 1972). Mass surveys with special radiological and endophotographic procedures are suitable (Oshima, 1972; Sakita and Fukutomi, 1972). Ex-

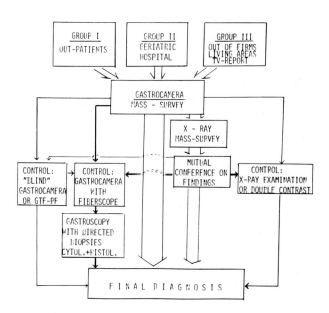

FIG. 1   *Stomach mass survey programme: Course of our mass survey programme since 1968 on persons aged over 45 years.*

---

* The examinations were partly conducted with support of the Deutsche Forschungsgemeinschaft as well as from funds of our own hospital. They contain partial results from studies (Inaugural-Dissertationen) of W. Rösner and T. Székessy.

perience and results from Japan demonstrated the possibilities: more than 2 million persons per year have been examined and more than 40% early carcinomas were detected among the total number of operated gastric carcinomas (Kano et al., 1972; Oshima, 1972; Oshima et al., 1973; Sakita and Fukutomi, 1972). A gastric check-up system, adapted to the present facilities of Germany, should therefore be tested. Because X-ray-mass surveys have been considered ineffective and unpracticable, we started, 5 years ago in Berlin, with gastrocamera mass surveys only. Financial difficulties, such as payment for technicians and equipment, have created special problems.

Material and methods

In 1968 we started to examine, by a stepwise program (Oshima, 1972), out-patients of our clinic who had non-characteristic epigastric complaints (Group I) (Fig. 1).

Beginning in 1969, check-ups were offered to patients who consulted doctors with other diseases and who usually had no epigastric complaints. In particular, we examined persons of higher age from geriatric hospitals, as well as in-patients (Group II). In 1970, we began to examine groups of persons over 45 years of age. They came from firms, residential areas, and in response to a medical television report (Group III A – C).

Persons from Groups I and II who suffered from a chronic-atrophic gastritis were candidates for re-examination some years later (Group IV).

The examinations were performed with so-called 'blind' gastrocameras, at present with model GT-PA. To clarify a suspected finding, the necessary additional tests were conducted in the normal endoscopical, or radiological, manner (Fig. 1). Since May 1972, the radiologists of our stomach research group performed stomach mass surveys with 70 mm fluorography, as in Japan (Treichel et al., 1972). This was usually done a day after the gastrocamera examination. The data were fed into a computer*.

Results

Willingness for gastrocamera check-up   This was found in 7.9% of persons from firms (Group III A).

Fear of examination   83.2% of 955 examined persons of Group III were not afraid, 17.2% were slightly and 1.8% very much afraid. In 3.4% (out of 1000), the examination could not be conducted generally for psychological reasons.

Simplicity of examination   The gastrocamera examination can be easily learned. After 50-100 gastrocamera films performed by a beginner, the diagnostic evaluation was sufficient. Two thirds of the examinations were performed by medical students under supervision of a resident.

Speed of examination   In 966 cases, the average examination period was 4.05 min, and less in women and older persons. The frequency of examinations depended on facilities such as examination places, dressing cabins, and number of assistants. Today, 25 persons can be examined in the morning, and the case history compiled.

Low risk   There was no evidence of risk in more than 3000 examinations.

Diagnostic capacity   Out of 960 films, most of them taken with GT-PA, only 2.4% were inadequate for diagnosis. 55.2% were good, 42.4% were adequate: thus 97.6%

* We wish to express our acknowledgement to Prof. Dr. P. Koeppe and Mr. K.-H. Lehmann, Department of Radiology and Nuclear Medicine (Body Counter), Klinikum Steglitz, Free University Berlin.

were suitable for diagnosis. The important stomach sections were represented in more than 90 up to 100%. The proportion of films for which additional tests were needed for clarification was 9.1% in 966 examinations.

Number of examined persons, most frequent age group, sex distribution, epigastric complaints   A total of 3039 persons has been examined up to December 1973 in 3 different groups (Table 1). Among the employees (Group III A) there were more men, but in the other groups, women predominated. The highest average age was seen, not surprisingly, in patients from the geriatric hospital. Many of the patients had epigastric complaints.

TABLE 1   *Gastrocamera mass survey: Number of examined persons, most frequent age groups, sex distribution, and percentage of epigastric complaints*

	Group					Total
	I	II	III A	III B	III C	
Most frequent age group (yr)	51 – 60	71 – 80	51 – 60	51 – 70	41 – 60	–
Sex	> 50% female	> 75% female	∿ 66% male	∿ 50% male	> 50% female	–
Epigastric complaints	> 90%	∿ 20%	> 60%	> 80%	> 85%	–
No. of examined persons	1037	576	639	312	475	3039

TABLE 2   *Pathological findings of gastrocamera screening tests on 3 different groups of persons aged over 45 years (Feb. 1968 – Dec. 1972)*

Diagnosis	Group			Total
	I	II	III	
Advanced cancer	9 (0.9%)	6 (1.0%)	6 (0.4%)	21 (0.69%)
Early cancer	1 (0.1%)	3 (0.5%)	1 (0.1%)	5 (0.16%)
Ulcer and scar	34 (3.3%)	25 (4.3%)	53 (3.7%)	112 (3.69%)
Polyp	18 (1.7%)	37 (6.4%)	29 (2.0%)	84 (2.77%)
No. of examined persons	1037 (100%)	576 (100%)	1426 (100%)	3039 (100%)

TABLE 3   *Pathological findings of gastrocamera screening tests on persons aged over 45 years from firms, residential areas and responding to a TV - report*

Diagnosis	Group			Total
	III A From firms	III B From residential areas	III C Through TV - report	
Advanced cancer	0	0	6 (1.3%)	6 (0.4%)
Early cancer	1 (0.2%)	0	0	1 (0.1%)
Ulcer and scar	14 (2.2%)	27 (8.7%)	12 (2.5%)	53 (3.7%)
Polyp	13 (2.0%)	10 (3.2%)	6 (1.3%)	29 (2.0%)
No. of examined persons	639 (100%)	312 (100%)	475 (100%)	1426 (100%)

Specific pathological findings Table 2 shows the number of specific findings detected in the various groups. In each of the 3 groups we found early carcinomas, amounting to 0.16% overall. Advanced carcinomas, of which some had not reached the serosa, were detected in a total of 21 patients, i.e. in 0.69%. The highest proportion was in Group II (1.0%). Gastric ulcers, including scars, were detected in 3.7%, and polyps in 2.8%. In Group III (Table 3) we see that all 6 advanced carcinomas were detected in persons responding to the television report. The early carcinoma type III + II C was diagnosed in a doctor of a firm from Group III A.

Follow-up examinations (Group IV) We have not yet detected a carcinoma in patients with chronic-atrophic gastritis (Table 4). The average time between the first, and the follow-up examination was 37 months for the 81 persons examined in 1971/72; 49 months for 56 persons examined in 1972/73 from Group I; and 27 months for 32 patients from Group II. The frequency of ulcers was as high as in Group III B.

TABLE 4   *Follow-up screening test with gastrocamera from out-patients (Group I) and patients from geriatric hospitals (Group II) with chronic-atrophic gastritis. Average time between first and control examinations was 37 months (81 persons) and 49 months (56 persons) from Group I and 27 months (32 patients) from Group II*

Diagnosis	Follow-up screening tests from Groups I and II
Advanced cancer	0
Early cancer	0
Ulcer and scar	14 (8.3%)
Polyp	6 (3.5%)
No. of examined persons	169 (100%)

Discussion and conclusions

The frequency of specific, especially malignant, findings differs from group to group. The percentage of early carcinomas (0.16%) is similar to that found in Japanese statistics (Sakita: 0.22%) (Kano et al., 1972; Oshima, 1972; Sakita and Fukutomi, 1972). The incidence of detected advanced carcinomas (0.69%) is higher in our series than in those from Japan: Ariga obtained 0.27% in over 333,000 examined persons; Sakita found 0.29% in 8,161 examined persons (Bergemann et al., 1970, 1973; Oshima, 1971, 1972; Oshima et al., 1973; Sakita and Fukutomi, 1972); Yamagata found 0.175% in 67,134 examined persons. These differences can be explained in terms of the advanced age of person, frequency of epigastric symptoms and high cancer incidence (Bergemann et al., 1973; Oshima et al., 1973). In addition to the diagnosis of the malignant conditions, the benign lesions detected confirm the value of the gastrocamera method.

The follow-up studies of persons with chronic-atrophic gastritis are still of too short a duration to evaluate the problem of the high risk groups (Székessy and Bergemann, 1973). To detect such groups, the previously mentioned check-ups should be far simpler and more effective than elaborate acid-analyses or bioptical examinations (Oshima, 1971).

By combining our examinations with X-ray mass surveys, the number of diagnostic findings can be increased (Oshima, 1972; Oshima et al., 1973; Sakita and Fukutomi, 1972). The number of persons examined by us with both methods is still too small to obtain a reliable comparison. Public relation, funds for the examinations described, and the creation of additional examination centres should be the next steps in the early detection of gastric carcinomas.

Summary

Because of the high mortality from gastric cancer in Germany, we began gastrocamera mass surveys in 1968 to detect gastric cancer at a curable stage. Three different groups of people were examined: (I) out-patients; (II) patients from geriatric hospitals; and (III) in-patients, persons from industrial firms, residential areas, and those responding to a TV-report. The examinations were simple and easy to learn; they could be conducted quickly and with low risk. The diagnostic capacity, resulting from the use of gastrocamera films, was very high. In 0.69% of 3,039 examined persons, we detected advanced carcinomas; and in 0.16%, early carcinomas. Gastric ulcers were detected in 3.7%; and polyps in 2.8% of all examined persons. The high frequency of carcinoma can be explained partly by the high average age, and partly by the high frequency of epigastric complaints among the persons examined. The results show the high effectiveness of stomach mass surveys when gastrocamera and 70 mm fluoroscopy are combined.

References

Bergemann, W., Schäfer, P. K., Knöchelmann, R. and Oshima, H. (1970): In: Advance Abstracts, 4th World Congress of Gastroenterology, p. 276. Copenhagen, 1970.

Bergemann, W., Rösner, W., Heidinger, F. P., Rehs, H. U., Reiner, H., Assheuer, J. and Oshima, H. (1973): In: Fortschritte der Gastroenterologischen Endoskopie, Vol. 4, pp. 61-69. Editor: H. Lindner. Witzstrock-Verlag Baden-Baden – Brüssel.

Kano, A. et al. (1972): In: Advances in Gastrointestinal Endoscopy, p. 49 and 653. Editors: G. Marcozzi, and M. Crespi. Piccin Medical Books, Padova.

Oshima, H. (1971): In: Gastrokamera-Untersuchung, Grundlagen, p. 129. Editor: H. Oshima. De Gruyter-Verlag, Berlin – New York.

Oshima, H. (1972): Dtsch. Z. Verdau.-Stoffwechselkr., 32, 139.

Oshima, H., Treichel, J., Rösner, W. Heitzberg, H., Rehs, H. U., Behrendt, Ch., Bergemann, W., Friedrich, E. and Mahmud, H. (1973): Aktuelle Gastrologie, in press.

Sakita, T. and Fukutomi, H. (1972): Arch. franc. Mal. Appar. dig. (Suppl.), 61, 422.

Schäfer, P.K., Mikat, B., Knöchelmann, R., Bergemann, W. and Oshima, H. (1970): Dtsch. med. Wschr., 21, 966.

Szekessy, T. and Bergemann, W. (1973): Aktuelle gastrologie, 3, 139.

Treichel, J. et al. (1972): Aktuelle Gastrologie, 2, 53.

Gastric mass survey with 70 mm fluorography: Methods and first results

J. Treichel, H. Heitzeberg, Ch. Behrendt and E. Friedrich

Klinik für Radiologie und Nuklearmedizin, Klinikum Steglitz, Freie Universität Berlin, Berlin

At the present time the results of the treatment of gastric cancer can only be improved by early diagnosis. If a carcinoma is already suspected, the detection of the tumor, even at an early stage, is no longer insurmountable if modern examination methods — especially radiology, endoscopy, biopsy, and cytology — are applied. As the symptoms experienced usually arouse the suspicion of gastric cancer in a relatively late stage, most early carcinomas can only be detected by mass surveys. Thus, the problem of early detection leads to the question of whether mass surveys are practicable.

Methods

The radiological method (Treichel et al., 1973) of stomach mass-surveys developed by us, is based on the well-known technique of photofluorography. Our 70 mm films are recorded from a 9-inch-image-intensifier. The radiographs of the stomach are taken in 6 defined body positions (Table 1) under fluoroscopic control. In each of these positions, a particular stomach section is to be recorded in a particular state of filling. The sequence of the body positions was chosen to allow rapid examination so that, on the double contrast radiographs, an adequate coating of the contrast medium to the stomach wall can be expected. Brief fluoroscopy is used for the observation of the esophageal passage, for the determination of the image section, and for an appropriate distribution of air and barium sulphate in the stomach ('patient-adapted standardization').

TABLE 1   *The sequence of body positions in the standardized radiography of the stomach*

Position	Visualized region	Predominant image
I Prone	Anterior wall	Mucosal study
II Supine: frontal	Lower corpus Gastric angle Antrum	Double contrast
III Supine: right anterior oblique	Prepyloric region Antrum Lower corpus	Double contrast
IV Supine: semirecumbent left anterior oblique	Fornix-Upper corpus	Double contrast
V Prone: right anterior oblique	Esophagogastric region Region of the cardia Fornix	Barium filled — double contrast
VI Upright: right anterior oblique	A) Fornix: Region of the cardia (Upper corpus)	Double contrast
	B) Antrum: Lower corpus	Barium filled

Soon after beginning our mass surveys, we improved the quality of the double contrast pictures by administering effervescent granules to increase the volume of gas in the stomach. These granules contain, in addition to sodium bicarbonate and tartaric acid, a substance which reduces the formation of bubbles. For a better visualization of the anterior wall, which may be difficult to view radiologically, we now supplement our standard radiographs with a mucosal study in the prone position. The evaluation of the 70 mm films was always carried out by two doctors, either simultaneously, or successively.

Up to now, 707 persons over 45 years of age have been examined. Part of this group came from Berlin firms, others had expressed their interest as a result of a televised program on our gastric surveys. It must be concluded that a somewhat select group of persons was examined, because it seemed unreasonable to exclude those with more severe complaints. This selection needs to be considered in the light of the relatively high incidence of pathological findings in our series. With few exceptions, all patients were also examined with the gastrocamera. At present, it is not yet possible to compare in detail the radiological results with those of the endoscopic mass survey.

Results

Before conducting large-scale mass surveys, experience of the organizational prerequisites is necessary, especially the quality of the examination method. For this purpose, the diagnostic value of the radiographs, the visualization of the various stomach sections, the duration of fluoroscopy, and the diagnosis reached were recorded for electronic data processing.

The duration of fluoroscopy was measured in 610 cases and averaged 1.8 min per examination. The overall examination lasted approximately 4 min. The percentage of examinations viewing the entire stomach sufficient to establish a diagnosis is shown in Table 2. Approximately 10% of the examinations performed were technically inadequate. This percentage was expected from the results of previous tests (Treichel et al., 1973). It may be assumed that it can be further reduced by a better technique and an improved image-intensifier. A particular area of the stomach was regarded as sufficiently diagnosable by X-rays when it had been viewed as a double contrast, or mucosal study, or had at least been filled with barium in several projections. We endeavour, however, to visualize each stomach section in at least one 'transparent image' (mucosal study or double contrast). Figure 1 demonstrates how often, in 63 unsatisfactory examinations, the various stomach regions were not diagnosable. Taking into account that with our anatomical division the regions 'cardia', 'angulus', and 'prepyloric antrum' have a lesser extension than the remaining stomach sections ('antrum', 'upper corpus', etc.), it can be concluded that our examination technique does not significantly neglect any part of the stomach. The differences in viewing the anterior and posterior wall, however, must be assumed and are not considered in this scheme.

When planning mass surveys, it is important to know how many re-examinations will be necessary. Naturally, all patients with technically insufficient examinations have to be re-examined, in addition to those patients in whom pathological findings were detected or suspected. Normally, we only recalled persons with the following diagnoses or tentative

TABLE 2   *Diagnostic value of the photofluorographic studies*

Diagnostic value	No. of examinations
Sufficient	632 (89.4%)
Insufficient	75 (10.6%)
Total	707 (100 %)

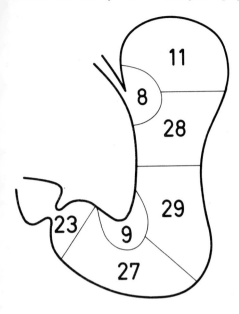

FIG. 1 *Frequency of insufficient visualization of the different regions of the stomach in 63 unsatisfactory examinations.*

diagnoses: tumor, gastric ulcer, ulcer scar. We had to recommend a check-up in 123 cases, i.e. in about 17% (Table 3).

The diseases of the esophagus, the stomach, and the duodenum detected radiologically in our 707 patients are shown in Table 4. In 10% of all first examinations, pathological findings were detected. The same percentage showed questionable pathological or suspected findings. Apart from other diseases, we detected 3 cases of advanced carcinoma of the stomach, 2 of which had been diagnosed radiologically (Fig. 2). In the 3rd case an ulcer was suspected, but the radiographs had been stated as technically inadequate and re-examination has been recommended. In all 3 cases, the carcinoma was operable and still limited to the muscularis propria. Up to now, 1 early carcinoma (Fig. 3) has been detected in a 52-year-old man who had been almost free of complaints. The tentative diagnosis of the radiological mass-survey in this case was determined 'early carcinoma, type IIc'; it was confirmed histologically after the operation (IIc + III). The total number of lesions detected so far justify the continuation of the mass-surveys which we had started to conduct in 1972.

TABLE 3 *Persons recalled for re-examination*

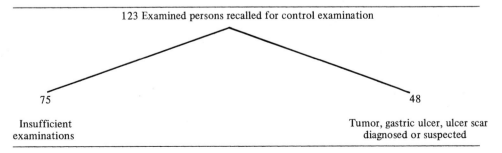

123 Examined persons recalled for control examination

75
Insufficient
examinations

48
Tumor, gastric ulcer, ulcer scar
diagnosed or suspected

TABLE 4   *Findings in 707 screened persons*

Disease	I Diagnosis	II Tentative diagnosis	Findings of groups I + II confirmed by control
Advanced carcinoma	2 (0.3%)	14 (2.0%)	2 (3) (0.3-0.4%)
Early carcinoma		2 (0.3%)	1 (0.14%)
Gastric ulcer	5 (0.7%)	8 (1.1%)	7 (1.0%)
Ulcer scar	2 (0.3%)	1 (0.14%)	2 (0.3%)
Tumors of esophagus	2 (0.3%)		2 (0.3%)
Duodenal ulcer	6 (0.8%)	15 (2.1%)	Not recalled
Hiatal hernia	45 (6.4%)	30 (4.2%)	for control
Other	11 (1.6%)	5 (0.7%)	
Total	73 (10.3%)	75 (10.6%)	

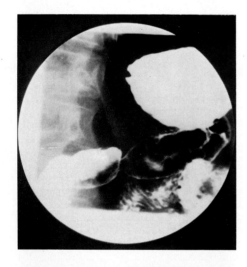

FIG. 2   *Advanced carcinoma of the stomach involving the antrum and the lower part of the corpus. 70 mm film of the mass screening examination.*

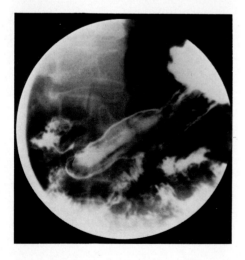

FIG. 3   *Early carcinoma of the type IIc + III in the middle of the corpus, clearly visualized in the position III of the screening examination: Converging folds broken off near the border of a slightly depressed area.*

Conclusions

Nowadays it is possible to conduct radiological mass surveys of the stomach with the aid of 70 mm photofluorography. Our method, the patient-adapted standardized fluorography, combining mucosal study, double contrast and barium filling technique, enables us to evaluate all parts of the stomach in almost 90% of the examined persons. Statistical statements and comparisons with Japanese findings, however, are not yet possible due to the relatively small number of examined persons.

Summary

707 patients have been mass-surveyed with patient-adapted standardized radiography of the stomach. The 70 mm radiographs taken in 6 defined body positions permit an adequate evalution of the entire stomach in approximately 90% of examined persons. Apart from other diseases, 2 advanced carcinomas and 1 early carcinoma of the stomach have so far been detected radiologically.

References

Treichel, J., Heitzeberg, H. and Friedrich, E. (1972): Aktuelle Gastrologie, 1/2, 53.
Treichel, J., Heitzeberg, H. and Friedrich, E. (1973): In: Proceedings, Deutscher Röntgenkongreß, pp. 109-110. Editor: F. Heuck. Thieme, Stuttgart.

Contribution to gastrointestinal tract cancer diagnosis by endoscopic aimed radioisotope scanning

S. Di Matteo, A. Bigotti, V. Casale and M. Crespi

Gastroenterology Unit, Cancer Detection Center, Regina Elena Institute for Cancer Research, Rome, Italy

The use of radioactive phosphorus has proved of considerable value in locating malignant processes of the gastrointestinal tract, owing to its selective uptake by cancer cells. After the first attempts in connecting a Geiger counter to an endoscope (Gregor et al., 1965), the situation was fully reviewed some years ago and the theory and practice of the method were fully assessed (Nelson, 1967).

Today, however, with flexible fiberendoscopes and new scanning devices, the potential value of this diagnostic procedure must be entirely reconsidered. The method is of particular interest in those non-specific mucosal patterns which often represent the first visual mark of a malignant process in its earliest phases, in the cases in which the process has a submucosal spreading. In fact, in early phases of malignancy the lesions may be multifocal, it is often impossible to submit every suspected site to aimed biopsy and, moreover, biopsy may be sometimes inconclusive.

Of special interest is the assessment of the exact spread of the tumor in esophageal neoplasms, in which the therapeutical planning is strictly related to the extension of the process. It is well known that in esophageal pathology the endoscopist is very often unable to reach the suspected site for the presence of strictures. The limited diameter of the probe (5 mm) often permits instead the precise assessment of the extension of the involvement by a step by step scanning through the restricted area.

Methods

A close contact between the probe and the lesion under investigation is in fact essential for obtaining an accurate result, thereby reducing the number of 'false positive' and 'false negative' cases. This is made possible by closely connecting the scanning device itself to

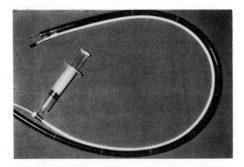

FIG. 1   *Esophago-gastro-duodenoscope connected with the probe carrying tube.*

modern endoscopes, so as to permit direct visual control of the scanning, as may be seen in Figure 1, which shows a terminal view esophago-gastro-duodenoscope connected to the probe carrying tube. Figure 2 shows the detail of the probe extruding from the tube.

The probe consists of a miniaturized solid state detector, which has several advantages over the conventional Geiger counter, particularly, a 150 x greater sensitivity. Continuous washing of the probe to remove mucus and blood is achieved by external flushing with saline.

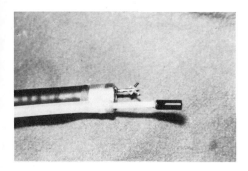

FIG. 2   *Detailed view of the probe extruding from the tube.*

By intravenous administration of 500 μC of ^{32}P 24 hours before the examination, it is possible to obtain fairly acceptable differential counts (30 to 40%) in normal versus neoplastic mucosal areas.

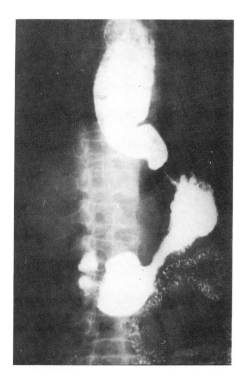

FIG. 3   *X-rays showing suggestive evidence of esophageal acalasia.*

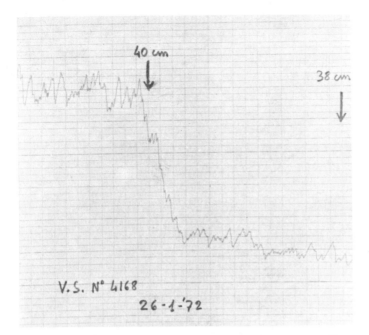

FIG. 4   *Recording of radioactive levels showing a step increase at 40 cm.*

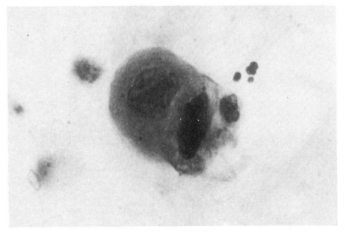

FIG. 5   *Malignant cells at the cytological examination.*

Results

Two cases reported here in detail provide a practical demonstration of the value of this procedure. In the first case, with a long history of esophageal acalasia once more confirmed by X-rays taken a few days before our examination (Fig. 3), endoscopy was not conclusive for the inability of passing the restricted point. The scanning performed subsequently under direct vision by passing the probe through the restricted point revealed a higher count (Fig. 4); an aimed abrasive cytological sampling into the stricture was positive for malignant cells (Fig. 5). In the second case, X-rays showed an infiltration of the esophageal walls in the lower third (Fig. 6). By endoscopy the point of the lesion was clearly identified. The scanning of the esophagus showed very high counts at this level (38 cm) but higher than normal counts were also found at 30 and 20 cm (Fig. 7). The bioptic and cytological samplings at those levels was positive for malignant cells and at surgical intervention a partly submucosal spreading malignant process was found in the medium and lower third of the esophagus, in accordance with previous findings.

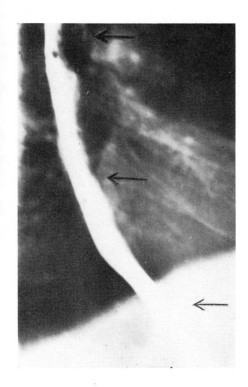

FIG. 6   *X-rays showing infiltration of the lower third of the esophagus. The arrows mark the points in which higher counts were found.*

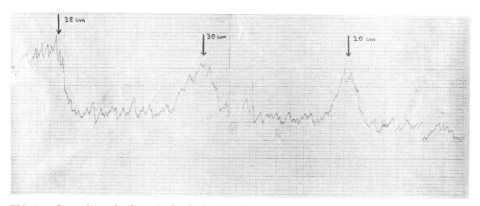

FIG. 7   *Recording of radioactive levels showing the points in which higher counts were found.*

Conclusions

In conclusion, we believe that scanning of the gastrointestinal tract under direct visual control through endoscopes increases the probability of detection of early and often overlooked malignant changes, by providing a precise target for bioptic and cytological sampling. Another interesting application of the method is an accurate definition of the limits of neoplastic infiltration in cases of esophageal and colonic cancer, thus enabling the surgeon in better planning the management schedules. A third application is the control and early detection of local recurrences after major surgery in cancer cases.

The biological problem not fully clarified up to now consists in the real cause of the increased uptake by neoplastic tissues, i.e. if it is caused by the vascular component of the malignant process or by the increase of the mitotic activity.

From a technical point of view we are moving now in two main directions: We try to further reduce the diameter of the probe, so as to fit it into the biopsy channel of endoscopes and we are developing an endoscope with a bigger internal channel, so as to be able to pass the probe without the additional external unit. All this with the aim of having this method operational as routine diagnostic tool in all major endoscopic centers.

References

Gregor, O. et al. (1965): Gut, 6, 234.
Nelson, R. S. (1967): In: Recent Results in Cancer Research. Springer-Verlag, New York, N.Y.

The diagnostic value of X-rays, endoscopy, endoscopy brush cytology and biopsy in a consecutive series of 377 patients with gastric disease

A. Serck-Hanssen, J. Marcussen and I. Liavåg

Department of Pathology, Ullevål Hospital and The Deaconess Hospital, Oslo, Norway

The flexible gastroscope with movable tip has made it possible not only to examine practically every region of the stomach, but also to take biopsies and cytological samples from any suspicious area. Cytological material can be obtained either by lavage after selective water jet washing (Shida et al., 1967), or by selective brushing (Williams et al., 1968; Prolla et al., 1970; Kobayashi et al., 1970; Witte, 1970; Liavåg et al., 1971. By these methods, a diagnostic accuracy for malignancy of from 80-100% has been reported. Few series, however, deal with the relative merits of cytology and biopsy on the same material and compare the results of these refined diagnostic tools with the results of X-ray and gross endoscopic evaluation.

We aim in this publication to present the diagnostic value of X-rays, gross endoscopic evaluation, endoscopic brush cytology and biopsy in a consecutive series of patients.

Material and methods

The series comprises 377 patients referred to the gastro-enterological unit of the Diakonissehuset Hospital in Oslo (Table 1). All patients had a radiographic examination of the upper gastrointestinal tract prior to gastroscopy and they had either radiological evidence of gastric disease or clinical symptoms of gastric disease.

Among the total of 377 patients, 309 had benign diseases of the stomach (Table 2). In 129 of these, the diagnosis was confirmed histologically by operation, or at autopsy (Table 3). In the remaining 180 cases, the benign nature of the disease is based on repeat radiography, gastroscopy with repeated biopsies and cytological examination with clinical observations for a period of from 6 months to 4 years.

There were 68 patients with malignant gastric disease (Table 4). In all of them the diagnosis has been confirmed histologically by operation, or at autopsy.

Gastroscopy is performed in the morning after a 12 hr fasting overnight, using either

TABLE 1   *Total material*

Diagnosis	Men	Women	Total
Benign gastric lesions, unoperated	108	72	180
Benign gastric lesions, operated	79	50	129
Malignant gastric lesions	47	21	68
Total	234	143	377

TABLE 2   *Results of selective brush cytology in benign gastric diseases*

Diagnosis	No. of cases	Cytology Negative	Suspicious	Positive
Gastric/pyloric ulcer	179	173	4	2
Stomal ulcer	10	10		
Gastritis	74	67	6	1
Gastritis in resected stomach	39	39		
Menetrier's disease	2	1	1	
Polyposis	2	2		
Lipoma	1	1		
Leiomyoma	1	1		
Amyloidosis	1	1		
Total	309	295	11	3

the Olympus GFB or the ACMI Mark '87' fibregastroscope.

Premedication is given in the form of an antihistamine ('Phenergan' 25—50 mg) intra-muscularly 1 hr prior to the gastroscopy. At the same time, a surface-tension reducing substance ('Antifoam' 2 tab.) is swallowed with a sip of water. One half hour prior to gastroscopy, atropine 0.5—0.6 mg is given subcutaneously. Prior to insertion of the gas-troscope the throat is sprayed with a surface anesthetic ('lidocaine-spray') and diazepam 5—10 mg is given by slow intravenous injection.

During the gastroscopy a methodical survey is made of the whole stomach and biop-sies are taken from any lesion seen. In the initial half of this series, 2—3 biopsies only were taken, in the latter, 8—10. The brush for cytological sampling is then introduced and the lesion is abraded several times under visual control. In cases of ulcerating lesions, care is taken to brush the floor of the ulcer as well as the adjoining mucous membrane for a distance of up to 2—3 cm from the edge of the ulcer. The brush containing the cells is then withdrawn just inside the distal part of the gastroscope, the opening closed and the gastroscope withdrawn. The brush is then pushed out of the gastroscope and 4 smears are made by rubbing the brush directly against the slides. Care is taken that the smears are fixed immediately with a spray fixative (Pro-Fixx, Scandialab). The fixed smears are stained by the Papanicolaou method.

In certain cases with large lesions or multiple lesions, the brush has been withdrawn through the channel and re-introduced to take a second sample.

The smears have been examined by a cytologist experienced in gastric cytology, and after a full description of the cellular contents and quality of the smears, a cytological conclusion is given in the form of one of the following diagnoses:

Negative for malignancy (Pap. grade I and II).
Suspicious of malignancy (Pap. grade III).
Positive for malignancy (Pap. grade IV and V).

The results of the other investigations are grouped similarly, allowing conclusions as 'probably malignant', or 'almost certainly malignant', to be recorded in the group of malignant diagnosis.

Results

Among the 309 patients with benign gastric disease (Table 2) the cytological diagnosis was correctly negative for malignancy in 295 (95.5%), false positive in 3 (0.9%) and suspicious of malignancy in 11 (3.6%)

Among the 129 patients with benign conditions where the diagnosis was verified histo-

TABLE 3 *Results of various investigations in benign diseases, histologically verified*

Histological diagnosis	No. of cases	X-ray			Endoscopy			Cytology			Biopsy		
		−	?	+	−	?	+	−	?	+	−	?	+
Gastric/pyloric ulcers	105	85	18	2	82	17	6	101	3	1	100		
Stomal ulcers	5	2	2	1	5			5			4		
Extra gastric malignancy	12	8	2	2	7		5	11		1	11		
Menetrier's disease	2		1	1			2	1	1		2		
Polyposis	2	1		1		1	1	2			2		
Lipoma	1		1			1		1			1		
Leiomyoma	1		1		1			1			1		
Amyloidosis	1		1		1			1			1		
Total	129	96	26	7	96	19	14	123	4	2	122		
		Negative 74%			Negative 74%			Negative 95%			Negative 95%		

− = Negative for malignancy; ? = Inconclusive; + = Positive for malignancy

TABLE 4 *Results of various investigations in gastric malignancy*

Histological diagnosis	No. of cases	X-ray			Endoscopy			Cytology			Biopsy		
		−	?	+	−	?	+	−	?	+	−	?	+
Carcinoma in situ	5	5			2	2	1	1		4	2	1	
Early inf. carcinoma	6	1	1	4			6	1*	1	4	4		2
Advanced carcinoma	47	8	10	29	3	3	41		2	45	12	3	26
Advanced carcinoma in resected stomach	8	2	4	2	1	1	6	1	1	6	4		3
Leiomyosarcoma	1	1			1			1			1		
Malignant lymphoma	1			1			1			1			1
Total	68	17	15	36	7	6	55	4	4	60	23	4	32
		Positive 53%			Positive 81%			Positive 88%			Positive 47%		

− = Negative for malignancy; ? = Inconclusive; + = Positive for malignancy   * Malignant cells found in gastric washing

logically on resected specimens, or at autopsy (Table 3), the cytology gave a conclusive diagnosis of no malignancy in 123 (95%), whereas X-ray and gross endoscopic evaluation gave a conclusive non-malignant diagnosis in only 74%. Bioptic material was obtained from only 122 patients, all negative for malignancy.

On the 68 patients with gastric malignancy (Table 4), brush cytology was correctly positive in 60 (88%), false negative in 4, and in 4 patients only a suspicion of malignancy was diagnosed. This compares favourably with the X-ray diagnosis that was positive in only 36 (53%), and the biopsies that were positive in only 32 (47%).

Compared to the other methods of investigation, cytology gave a definite diagnosis of malignancy in the greatest number of histologically verified cases and was the only method that revealed with certainty the early malignant changes occurring in 4 of 5 patients with *carcinoma in situ* (borderline lesions) at the edge of chronic peptic ulcers. It was also the only method that gave microscopic proof of the malignant nature of a lesion believed by endoscopy to be cancer, and that proved by histological examination to be a very small intramucosal carcinoma developing in an area of *carcinoma in situ* (Figs. 1*a,b*).

Comments

In this series endoscopic brush cytology was the most reliable method, both in differentiating between malignant and benign conditions, and also in the diagnosis of gastric malignancy, including very early lesions.

Cases of false positive cytological diagnosis, or unwarranted suspicion of malignancy,

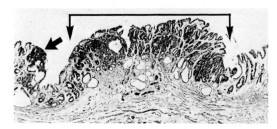

FIG. 1a   *Small elevated area close to chronic peptic ulcer. Area marked with bracket shows carcinoma in situ. Area marked with fat arrow shows, in Fig. 1b, a small intramucosal carcinoma. H & E x 20. Reduced for reproduction 36%.*

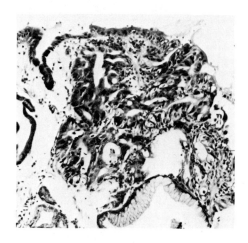

FIG. 1b   *Area marked with fat arrow in Fig. 1a, shows small intramucosal carcinoma. H & E x 160. Reduced for reproduction 33%.*

have all been obtained on material from patients with gastric ulcers or severe gastritis. The diagnosis was made during the early stages of the series before we fully realised that a considerable degree of morphological deviation from the normal, including mitosis in the surface epithelium, may accompany these conditions (Figs. 2–4).

With regard to false positive or unwarranted suspicion of malignancy, cytology compares, however, very favourably with radiological and endoscopic evaluation, where 26% of the diagnoses were inconclusive, or false positive (Table 3).

The high rate of correct negative biopsies must be seen in relation to its high failure rate in cases with malignant disease, and consequently, cannot be relied upon to the same extent as a negative cytological report. It should be stressed, however, that it was only through the latter half of the series that we fully realised the necessity of taking a large number of biopsies in order to secure representative material. Thus, for the last 27 malignant cases, the biopsies have been positive in 74%, but among these there is only one early carcinoma.

The false negative cytological diagnosis has been due partly to non-representative material (2 cases), and partly to the highly differentiated nature of the tumour from

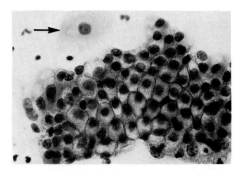

FIG. 2   *Sheath of normal surface gastric epithelium. Note regular pattern, distinct cellular borders and no nuclear pleomorphism. Arrow points to a sq. cell. Pap. stain, X 650. Reduced for reproduction 40%.*

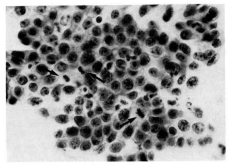

FIG. 3   *Surface gastric epithelium obtained by brushing close to edge of chronic benign ulcer. Note the marked reactive nuclear changes, including mitosis (arrows), indistinct cellular borders and some degree of nuclear variation. Pap. stain, X 650. Reduced for reproduction 40%.*

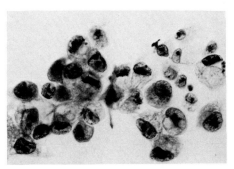

FIG. 4   *Group of malignant cells obtained by brushing. Note good preservation and marked nuclear atypism with generally enlarged nuclei, pleomorphism and very large nucleoli. Pap. stain, X 650. Reduced for reproduction 40%.*

which the cells have originated with resulting lack of marked cellular atypism (4 cases).

Non-representative material is most likely to be submitted in cases with large necrotic tumours, or in ulcerating lesions where the ulcer floor is covered with fibrin, although this tendency is probably less than when using gastric washing (Serck-Hanssen, 1967). It also tends to occur in some cases of diffusely infiltrating carcinomas because these tumours tend to grow under an intact surface epithelium and frequently exhibit only moderate cellular atypism (Bach-Nielsen, 1966; Brandborg and Wenger, 1968; Serck-Hanssen, 1967).

From the diagnostic point of view, the most interesting cases in the present series are the 11 with early carcinoma. These include 5 cases with *carcinoma in situ*, 2 with intramucosal carcinomas and 4 with infiltration in the submucosa (Fig. 5). Brush cytology was positive or suspicious in 9 (82%), whilst in one, malignant cells were found only after blind gastric washing. Kawashima (1966), using different techniques for cytological sampling, reported 78% positive tests in 40 cases with early carcinoma, whereas Shida et al. (1967) reported positive cytology in all of 20 cases using the water-jet method.

Of the cases designated *carcinoma in situ*, 4 were found in the mucous membrane adjoining chronic benign peptic ulcers, and one was found in the gastric stump left after a resection for a bleeding ulcer 10 years earlier.

In none of these cases did biopsies secure the diagnosis, nor did biopsies give the diagnosis in 2 cases with intramucosal carcinomas that also developed in relation to chronic peptic ulcers, and were very limited in their extent.

These small lesions, although to some extent found to be suspicious by the gastroscopist, are certainly too small to be diagnosed with certainty by other than bioptic or cytologic means, and in our experience brush cytology appears better than biopsies, probably because the cellular sampling can be done from a larger area than can be covered even by a large number of biopsies.

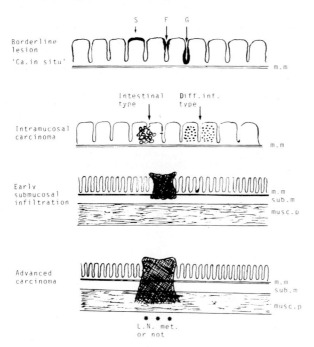

FIG. 5   *Diagram illustrates stages in development of gastric cancer (simplified) with carcinoma in situ developing in either surface, foveolar, or glandular epithelium. Intramucosal carcinoma of the two main types: glandular and diffusely infiltrating; early infiltration in the submucosa and advanced gastric carcinoma with infiltration in muscularis proper.*

Although too little is known of the natural history of *carcinoma in situ* in the stomach, one of the cases in this series demonstrates the transition from *in situ* to intramucosal infiltration (Figs. 1*a,b*).

Conclusion

When properly done by a trained gastroenterologist to collect the material and an experienced cytologist to evaluate the smears, brush cytology is an accurate and reliable method for the diagnosis of gastric malignancy, including the very early lesions. In this series, brush cytology was the most accurate single method for differentiating between malignant and benign conditions.

Although this series was not conducted to compare the results of blind gastric washing and selective brush cytology, 10 years' experience with the blind gastric washing has made it clear to us that brush cytology has the following three main advantages:

1. Brush samples contain far more and much better preserved cellular material.
2. There is little contamination with cells from the respiratory and proximal alimentary tract, making screening more rapid and reliable.
3. Smears have a locating value that makes possible correlation with endoscopic findings and histology on bioptic and surgical specimens.

Summary

The report describes a consecutive series of 377 patients and compares the diagnostic value of X-ray, gross endoscopic evaluation, endoscopic brush cytology and biopsies, in the ability to diagnose and differentiate between benign and malignant conditions.

In 129 patients with benign conditions where the diagnosis was verified by histology on resected specimens, or at autopsy, X-ray and gross endoscopic evaluation gave an inconclusive or false positive diagnosis of malignancy in 26%, whereas the cytological and bioptic diagnosis were inconclusive or false positive in 5%.

In 68 patients with gastric malignancy the X-ray diagnosis was positive for malignancy in 53%, and the gross endoscopic diagnosis in 81%. Brush cytology was positive in 88%, including 8 of the very smallest lesions, whereas the endoscopic biopsies were positive in only 47%, missing 9 of the 11 early carcinomas.

In the present series, endoscopic brush cytology was the most reliable single diagnostic method, both in differentiating between malignant and benign conditions, and also in the diagnosis of gastric malignancy, including the very early lesions.

The advantage of brush cytology compared to blind gastric washing is stressed.

References

Bach-Nielsen, P. (1966): Nord. Med., 75, 239.
Brandborg, L.L. and Wenger, J. (1968): Med. Clin. N. Amer., 52, 1315.
Kobayashi, S., Prolla, J.C., and Kirsner, J.B. (1970): Acta cytol. (Philad.), 14, 219.
Kawashima, S. (1966): Scand. J. Gastroent., 1, 248.
Liavåg, I., Marcussen, J. and Serck-Hanssen, A. (1971): Acta. chir. scand, 137, 682.
Prolla, J.C., Kobayashi, S., Yoshii, Y. and Kasugai, T. (1970): In: Proceedings, 10th International Cancer Congress Houston, Tex., 1970, p. 565. Editors: R. Lee Clark et al. Year Book Medical Publ., Chicago, Ill.
Serck-Hanssen, A. (1967): J. Oslo Cy Hosp., 17, 221.
Shida, S., Sawada, Y., Takamura, S., Kondo, T., Takomoto, T. and Tsuneoka, K. (1967): Gastroent. Jap., 2, 101.
Williams, D.G., Truelove, S.C., Gear, M.W.L., Massarella, G.R. and Fitzgerald, N.W. (1968): Brit. med. J., 1, 535.
Witte, S. (1970): Endoscopy, 2, 86.

Duodenoscopy in the early diagnosis of tumoral lesions of the Vater papilla

M. Banche, L. Bonardi and F. P. Rossini

Ospedale Maggiore S. Giovanni Battista e della Città di Torino, Divisione di Gastroenterologia, Torino, Italy

At the end of February 1973 we had performed 607 endoscopic examinations of the duodenum using Olympus instruments, either the front view type, GIF-D, or the side view type, JF-B. Our experience is summarized in Table 1.

We have observed the duodenum of 463 patients with the GIF-D instrument and 143 with the side view type: the ratio between the two instruments is therefore about 3 to 1. Although we have been using the JF-B since 1971 and the GIF-D only since 1972, at present we prefer the latter in routine practice because of its superior handiness. The first instrument is being used now in a limited number of investigations of patients with suspected disease of the duodenal papilla or of the biliary tree.

It follows that the percentage distribution of the various duodenal diseases differs according to the type of instrument employed. It emerged, for instance, that the number of normal cases was higher with the GIF-D, when compared to the JF-B: a similar result

TABLE 1   *Results of 620 endoscopic examinations of the duodenum using Olympus instruments*

Findings	GIF-D		JF-B		Total	
	Cases	%	Cases	%	Cases	%
Normal	176	37.7	53	34.6	229	37
Duodenitis	77	16.5	31	20.3	108	17.4
Ulcers	108	23.1	24	15.7	132	21.3
Scars	37	7.9	16	10.5	53	8.6
Polyposis	10	2.1	2	1.3	12	1.9
Diverticula	11	2.3	1	0.6	13	2
Others	44	9.4	12	7.8	56	8.9
Vater neoplasm	0	0	4	2.6	4	0.7
Total	463	75.3	143	24.7	607	100

TABLE 2   *Factors determining the preference of the side view instrument to the GIF-D type*

Findings	GIF-D		JF-B	
	Cases	%	Cases	%
Papilla	24	5.2	47	30.7
Jaundice	3	0.6	36	23.5

was found in the diagnosis of duodenal ulcer. This may depend upon the absence of selection of patients sent to our service.

Quite different are the percentage values of duodenitis and duodenal scars detected by the side view instrument. The most interesting data concern, however, the endoscopic incidence of the cancer of the Vater papilla. It was detected in 4 patients out of 153 examined with the side view instrument, while none was observed with the GIF-D type. This is due, in our experience, to two factors (Table 2):

(1) The front view duodenoscope is unsuited to the routine examination of the papilla. (2) The side view duodenoscope is used only for a certain kind of patient. For instance, only 3 subjects examined with the GIF-D were suffering from jaundice, while the JF-B was used in 36 patients with obstructive jaundice in order to detect some kind of papillar disease and for making an attempt at cannulation.

Of the 4 patients with cancer of the papilla, 2 were male and 2 female, ranging from 31 to 82 years of age.

In three the tumor was excised and 6 months later 2 patients were still free from local and general metastases, while the third showed a duodenal spread of the neoplasm. In the fourth patient, the surgeon was only able to perform a simple coledochojejunostomy. In all cases, the tumor was an adenocarcinoma.

We can draw some brief conclusions:

1. The early endoscopic diagnosis of the cancer of duodenal papilla is now possible in many cases.

2. Patients with obstructive jaundice or a defect in the duodenal radiologic pattern should be submitted to duodenoscopic examination.

3. In patients with a suspected papillar disease, the side view duodenoscope should be used. The front view type must be reserved for routine examination of the oesophagus, stomach and duodenum.

Duodenoscopic wirsungography in cancer of the pancreas

B. Watrin, P. Gaucher, R. Jeanpierre, J. Laurent, G. Mauuary and F. Vicari

Groupe de Recherches et de Physiopathologie Digestive et Nutritionelle, et du Service de Médecine 'C', Professeur F. Heully Hôpital Saint-Julien, Nancy, France

Introduction

The pancreas often escapes the various conventional clinico-biological and radiological examinations. Pancreatic arteriography and scintigraphy certainly constitute advances, but they have not transformed the diagnostic problem in diseases of the pancreas, especially in cancer of the pancreas. The introduction of the direct exploration of the pancreas should allow further progress. The ductal and parenchymatous structure can now be investigated by retrograde opacification of the pancreatic passages during transpapillary endoscopic catheterization. From the strictly technical point of view, this method does not pose any practical problems for an experienced endoscopist.

Study material and results

Thirteen cases are available: 11 exocrine tumors and 2 endocrine tumors. Six of the 11 exocrine cancers were localized in the head: the topography of one was corporeo-caudal.

Unfortunately, the presence of a jaundice, giving evidence of a previous carcinomatous stage, considerably limited the value of the catheterization, which often only confirms a diagnosis already strongly suspected by the current clinical and para-clinical examinations. However, based on these observations, we have been able to segregate the most characteristic pancreatographic signs.

Results

There were 3 failures on 13 catheterizations, i.e. about 23% of the cases; this percentage is much higher than the failure rate observed in chronic pancreatitis, which is to the order of 6%. However, in view of the small number of observations, this figure is not very significant. It should be noted that 3 recurrences of a cancer of the head were involved, with stenosis and invasion into the duodenum.

The 2 cases of endocrine tumor were: one patient suffering from a glucagonoma with invasion into the duodenum which entirely prohibited catheterization; in the other case, there was a suspicion of an insular tumor of the caudal region, where normal pancreatography conflicted with the arteriographic findings. In this patient, the clinical development seemed to go into the opposite direction indicated by the arteriography.

A. Analyses of the pancreatographic abnormalities (Table 1)

1. Ductal abnormalities   The presence of a tumoral mass in a duct is rather distinct. The following changes observed are evident most of the time:

TABLE 1   *Analyses of the pancreatographic abnormalities*

	No.	N.P.	A.P.	Failures	Verified operatively
Exocrine cancers					
Head	10	1	7	2	10
Body-tail	1	–	1	–	1
Endocrine tumors	2	1	0	1	1

N.P. = normal pancreatogram; A.P. = abnormal pancreatogram

Definite obstruction of Wirsung's canal (Figs. 1 and 2).

This obstruction may assume a dome-like aspect (Fig. 1), the significance of which is highly disputable, for it may be caused by an air bubble, a false cyst, or a reflux filling starting from the retrograde cholangiography. The combination of a choledochal stenosis due to neoplastic invasion with a dilatation of the higher lying biliary passages (Figs. 1 and 2), certainly constitutes an argument in favor of a neoplastic etiology.

Ductal obstruction is much more characteristic, because it takes the form of an insurmountable 'radish-tail' stenosis (Fig. 2).

A longer or shorter filiform constriction of the main ducts, with, next to this stenosis, a lacunary pancreatographic zone expressing the absent opacification of the secondary canals (Fig. 3).

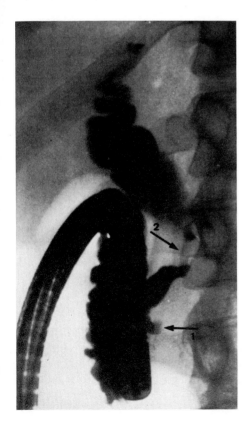

FIG. 1   *(1) Solid dome-shaped obstruction of the canal of Wirsung after 1 cm opacification. (2) Neoplastic stenosis of the bile duct with dilatation of the higher biliary passages.*

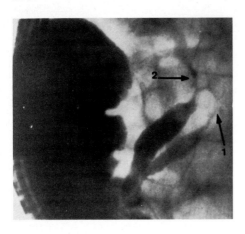

FIG. 2   (1) Insurmountable 'radish-tail' neoplastic stenosis of the canal of Wirsung. (2) Concomitant stenosis of
the choledochus in its retro-pancreatic part.

An aspect of localized stenosis with, next to it, a breakthrough of the contrast
medium, giving a 'pool' image (Fig. 4).

A moniliform aspect of the main canal (photo 5) and of the collateral ductal system.

Finally, a disorganization and a forcing-back of the ductal system associated with
these manifestations (Fig. 5).

2. Parenchymatous abnormalities   Unfortunately, parenchymatography was not

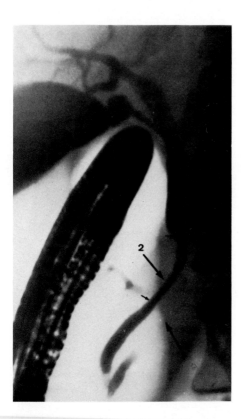

FIG. 3   (2) Filiform constriction of the canal
of Wirsung, disorganized and forced
back. Absence of opacification of the
secondary canals next to this stenos-
ed area. Constriction of the choledochus in its retro-pancreatic part due
to neoplastic invasion (small arrows).

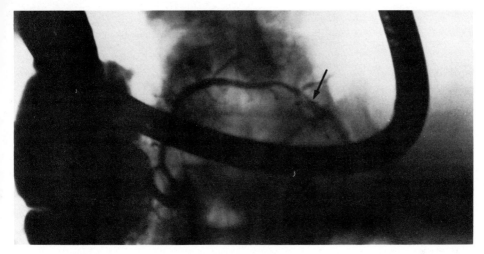

FIG. 4   *Localised stenosis of the canal of Wirsung at the level of the corporeo-caudal junction with, next to it, breakthrough of the contrast medium.*

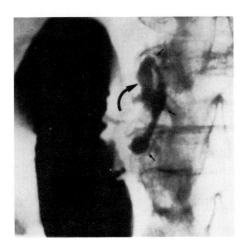

FIG. 5   *Moniliform canal of Wirsung, forced back (small arrows), ending in a 'pool' owing to a localized breakthrough of the contrast medium.*

systematically carried out in all examinations. We wish to say that in none of the cases did we observe any characteristic parenchymatous abnormality. In particular, in the patient in whom we suspected an insular tumor in the caudal region, parenchymatography yielded a strictly-normal result.

B. *Significance of the pancreatographic abnormalities*

The anomalies described above being in general morphologically evident, their specificity and especially their importance with regard to cancer of the pancreas, should be discussed.

With respect to their specificity, we have already called attention to the several pitfalls in the interpretation of a massive ductal obstruction. We wish to remark that certain blockings of injections or certain complicated opacifications of the canal of Wirsung are sometimes difficult to interpret: in these cases, the possibility of an anatomical disposition of embryonic type with an accessory canal of Wirsung, independent of the duct of Santorini, should not be overlooked.

The essential problem is the differential diagnosis between chronic pancreatitis and cancer. According to traditional surgical opinion, preoperative pancreatography afforded an exellent diagnostic distinction. If, as happens in many cases, the pancreatographic manifestations are unusual, judgement becomes difficult. Certain differential criteria are of very great importance, and these are listed in Tables 2 and 3.

Remember that a serrated or filiform constriction of the canals of Wirsung and Santorini, or of one of the principal accessory canals, combined with a localized ductal rarefaction, is by far the most suggestive sign of cancer (Fig. 6).

On the other hand, a non-homogeneous parenchymogram with one or several localized lacunae, might suggest a neoplastic etiology or, more often, an artefact due to bad filling conditions (Fig. 7).

However, ambiguity of diagnosis persists rather frequently, as shown by the following case report of a patient with a corporeo-caudal tumor.

    Mr. F. . . ., age 43 years (first admission, October 1971)
        Clinical aspects: alcoholism
                                  unexplained abdominal pains
                                  normal biology
        Radiological aspects: abdomen, without preparation: calcified ganglion at the
                                  level of $L_1 - L_2$
                                  radiography of the stomach: normal
                                  combined duodenocholangiography: normal
        Duodenoscopy: opacification of the excretory pancreatic passages

There were no apparent abnormalities of the main canal and the secondary canals.
    Tentative diagnosis: alcoholic gastritis

The second admission took place in May 1972.
    Persistence of the painful abdomen
    Radiological and clinical aspects: nothing in particular
    Anti-ulcerative treatment

Third admission, September 1972.
    Spectacular deterioration of the general condition with weight loss of 25 kg
    Biological aspects: important inflammatory syndrome
    Radiological aspects: not very demonstrative
    Gastric endoscopy: spasms of the pyloro-bulbar region

No renewed duodenoscopic catheterization.

Surgical intervention by Professor Grosdidier. Operative and anatomo-pathological report:
    Chronic cholecystitis with cholesterosis without signs of malignancy
    Chronic pancreatic lesions in 2 removed fragments
    A third fragment with a tumoral aspect: an excretory-pancreatic adenocarcinoma. The three fragments originated from the corporeo-caudal region, which was the only macroscopically affected region.

Such a case is interesting from several points of view:
    1. The anatomo-pathological examination revealed the combination of manifestations of chronic pancreatitis with an excretory-pancreatic carcinoma. This combination occurs frequently, and explains why it is often difficult to determine an anatomo-pancreatographic correlation. In this particular case, the pancreatographic aspect rather suggested a neoplastic affection.

TABLE 2   *Differential criteria: Chronic pancreatitis*

Main duct	
Dilatations + stenoses	C.P.
Tortuous constriction	C.P. probable
Enormous dilatation	C.P.
Obstruction	C.P. if dilatation downstream of main duct and secondary ducts
Cystic dilatations	C.P.
Calculi	C.P.
Localized stenoses Indentations Disintegration Segmentary moniliform aspect	In favor of C.P. if the abnormalities are associated with an evocatory bio-clinical context
Collateral ductal system	
Moniliform aspect Cyst-shaped dilatations Cylindrical dilatations Calculi	Signs of great value for C.P. Most often associated with changes of the main duct
Irregular distribution	Very disputable significance Isolated sign: no certainty
Parenchymatous tissue	
Polymacular aspect	Suggestive of C.P.
Homogeneous parenchymatogram	No significance at all
Lacuna	In the center of the opacification: cancer rather than C.P.

C.P. = chronic pancreatitis

TABLE 3   *Differential criteria: Cancers*

Main duct	
Stenosis	Isolated: little significance Associated with breakthrough of contrast medium: great significance
Filiform constriction	Cancer very probable Pathognomonic in case of adjoining lacumary pancreatographic zone
Massive obstruction	Little value
Pressing-back Disorganization	Great value
Isolated moniliform aspect	No value at all
Collateral ductal system	
Dilatations	Against the Δ of cancer
Absence of localized opacification	Pathognomonic, associated with a ductal constriction adjoining it
Parenchymatous tissue	
Lacunary aspect	In the center of the opacification: cancer rather than C.P. Most often artefact

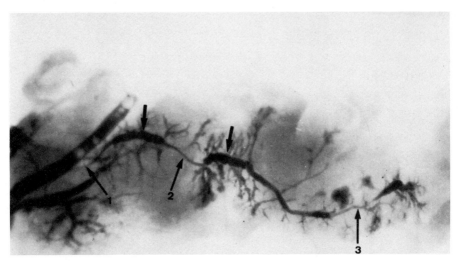

FIG. 6   *Post-mortem opacification of a very extensive cancer of the pancreas. Characteristic aspect:*
Stepwise filiform constrictions (1, 2, 3) with lacunary pancreatographic zones next to them.
Dilatation of the segments situated between these stenoses (non-numbered arrows).

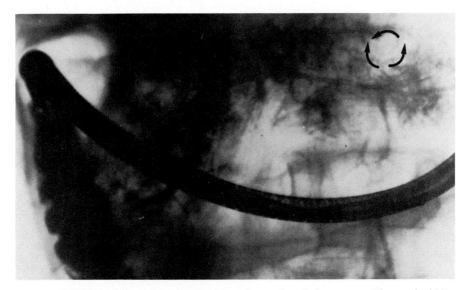

FIG. 7   *Diffusion of the contrast medium spread over the whole pancreas. The canal of Wirsung is*
entirely normal. This parenchymatogram is not homogeneous and shows lacunary zones
(round arrows) without pathological change, but which arise from technical artefacts due to
bad filling.

2.   Admitting that the pancreatographic aspect accorded well with a cancer of the
pancreas, the lesion was seen at an early carcinomatous stage, but the diagnosis was not
accepted until several months later.

3.   Granted that with our experience of pancreatography the wirsungographic aspect
seemed suspect to us, could an indication to operate have been based on the combination
of unexplained abdominal pains and a change in the pancreatogram?

Conclusion

The conclusions to be drawn from such a study are of course fragmentary. It seems that duodenoscopic pancreatography would not appear to be a method of early diagnosis of cancer of the pancreas; such a diagnosis can only be a chance diagnosis. On the other hand, there is unfortunately no strict correlation between the importance of the pancreatographic manifestations and the degree of the neoplastic lesions.

The value of this examination can be increased by combining it with a cytological analysis after endoscopic aspiration of the pancreatic juice.

References

Watrin, B. (1973a): L'opacification perduodénoscopique des voies pancréatiques normales et pathologiques. Academical Thesis, Nancy (mimeographed), pp. 198.
Watrin, B. (1973b): Acta Endoscopica, Vol. 3, No. 6.

Colonoscopy in the diagnosis of neoplastic diseases: Limits and possibilities

L. Gennari, P. Spinelli and G. Fariselli

Istituto Nazionale dei Tumori, Milan, Italy

We believe that colonoscopy is no substitute for radiography. It should always come after an X-ray examination and, most important of all, the position of the instrument must be easily and rapidly controlled. Endoscopic patterns are fairly easy to interpret: only in a few cases is diagnosis doubtful. But the investigation is not always easy to carry out, because particularly sharp intestinal loops can be very awkward to negotiate. However, the X-ray pattern will have told us where we are likely to encounter difficulty and the degree of difficulty.

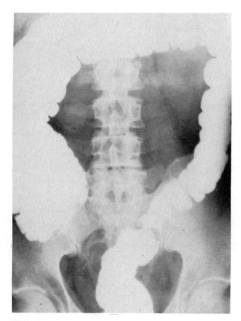

FIG. 1

Figures 1 and 2 illustrate two typical cases. In the first, the intestinal morphology is such that, unless any pathologic processes are present, the instrument should be able to get as far as the cecum without difficulty. The second shows a combination of many possible difficulties: an abnormally long large bowel, and multiple tortuosity or marked kinking, as at the sigmoid and the two flexures. In this latter case, it is easy to get a full view of the whole colon. However, although the angle of the tip of the colonoscope is controllable, it cannot be bent beyond a certain limit.

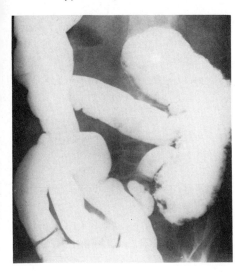

FIG. 2

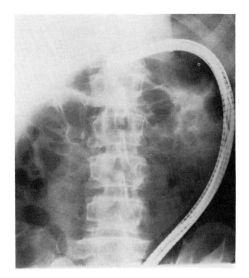

FIG. 3

Figure 3 refers to the first case and shows the instrument in the transverse colon. The instrument is a short one, 86 cm long, but had it been 1 meter 80 long it would have reached the cecum without much difficulty. Forward viewing allows us to see a few centimeters further as long as the intestinal lumen is perfectly straight.

Figure 4 shows the instrument at the level of the sigmoid in the second case. Here the length of the sigmoid loop, its mobility and a kink even before we get to the sigmoid-colon junction, constitute an almost insurmountable obstacle.

Failure to advance is explained by the physical law of the resolution of a force. According to this law, the force imparted to the instrument longitudinally is resolved, at the point at which it encounters a non-rigid obstacle, into two components. Hence part of

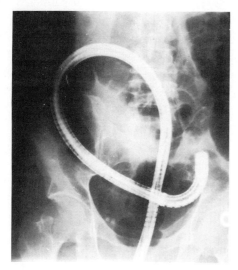

FIG. 4

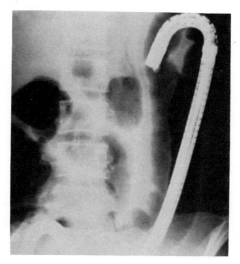

FIG. 5

the force is dispersed against the obstacle, thereby causing, when the intestinal segment is fairly mobile, a displacement and distension of the intestine; and the greater the length of the mobile loop and the ampler the peritoneal fold, the more marked will be the displacement and distension. The second component of the force allows the instrument to advance. The same principle applies at every bend and so, because part of the applied force is lost, when we want to get past a curve it is necessary to apply a force directly related to the number of curves already negotiated. Because the colonoscope has a movable, angling tip, the amount of force needed and the difficulty of getting past the curves are reduced. Lastly, the possibility of advancing the instrument will depend on the angle formed by the intestinal loop. In Figure 5 we see that the tip of the instrument has got past the splenic flexure, but any attempt to push the instrument further fails because of the acute angle formed by the colon.

To overcome the most frequent obstacle, namely the various folds encountered in the splenic flexure and at the junction of the sigmoid with the colon, several suggestions have been made; the most useful seems to be a derotation of the sigmoid flexure so that it forms a Greek alpha. These maneuvers are often feasible and not dangerous if they are carried out under radiologic control.

We draw attention to these points to show how essential X-ray examination is both before endoscopy and during the later investigation.

To date, we have performed 155 colonoscope investigations in 136 patients (76 females and 60 males). The investigation was repeated in 14 cases, either to check the efficacy of subsequent treatment, or to re-examine the site of an operation for recurrences. In the other 5 cases, colonoscopy was repeated for various reasons, such as an imperfect intestinal toilet through intolerance to the investigation (one case) as a result of which it had to be done under general anesthesia.

The sigmoid was observed 140 times (Fig. 6), the descending colon 61, the splenic flexure 22, the transverse colon 9 times and the cecum twice. It is worth noting that in a large number of cases the instrument used was 85 cm long and had one-way tip angulation. With this instrument, the difficulties are greater and the maximum limit of viewing is the splenic flexure. Indeed, in the cases in which we got as far as the cecum, and in at least three-quarters of the cases in which we observed the transverse colon, we used a 1 meter 80 colonoscope with two-way tip angulation.

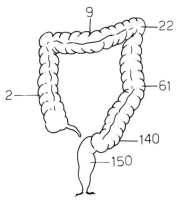

FIG. 6

The gap between the number of observations of the sigmoid flexure and descending colon, 140 and 61 respectively, should not be taken as evidence of a high failure rate in negotiating the sigmoid-colon junction but simply that, in the great majority of cases, the diagnostic problem was at sigmoid level and there was no point in pursuing the investigation higher up.

In only 9 cases, that is 5.8%, did the investigation fail in its purpose: once through intestinal perforation, twice because of abnormal distension of the ileum owing to rapid and continuous passage of air through an ileocolic anastomosis performed previously, once through patient intolerance, and, in the last 5 cases, either the sigmoid stenosis was too severe to permit diagnosis, or there was intestinal kinking, natural or secondary to surgery.

Another point to emerge from our experience is that one should not judge the position of the instrument in the intestine from the length inserted. We have found that to get a full view of the sigmoid we had to insert anything from 25 to 80 cm. This is because of the distensibility of the intestine, and the length and mobility of the meso-sigmoid.

Of our 136 patients, 42 were found after diagnostic investigation and therapeutic check-ups to have malignant tumors. Table 1 summarizes the reliability of radiography, endoscopy and biopsy in this series. Radiography yielded the correct diagnosis in 29 cases, an uncertain or doubtful diagnosis in 5 and missed the tumor in 4 cases. Endoscopy left doubts in 4 cases and missed the tumor in 3. As to biopsy, the 5 false negatives were not the result of misreading of the histologic preparations but mislocation of the biopsy.

TABLE 1   *Figures for X—ray, endoscopic and biopsy examinations in the diagnosis of 42 cases of cancer of the colon*

	X—ray	Endoscopy	Biopsy
Cancer	29	35	31
Doubtful diagnosis	5	4	0
False negatives	4	3	5
Not carried out	4	0	6
Total	42	42	42

TABLE 2   *Diagnostic solutions for doubtful or false negative cases*

		Endoscopic solutions	Histological solutions
Doubtful X—ray cases	5	1	
False negative X—ray cases	4	4	
Doubtful endoscopic cases	4		1
False negative endoscopic cases	3		1
Total	16	5	2

In Table 2 we set out to check the final diagnosis in the doubtful cases or false negatives at X-ray or endoscopy. In 5 of the 9 radiologically-doubtful or false negative cases, endoscopy supplied a solution. In 2 of the endoscopically-doubtful or false negative cases, biopsy supplied the answer. Hence 9 of the 42 tumor cases reached the operating table without a correct diagnosis (21.4%).

More important was the contribution of endoscopy in the detection of polyps. Endoscopy produced the correct diagnosis in 21 of the 24 benign tumors. However, the most striking fact is that in at least 10 cases it showed up polypous formations so small that they had been missed, or might have been missed, on radiologic examination.

In summary, colonoscopy is now an indispensable diagnostic tool, because, by checking or correcting radiologic diagnosis it reduces the incidence of radiologic doubts and errors. It is nonetheless not a simple procedure but one that calls for patience and experience and close cooperation with the radiologist, both in the pre-endoscopic phase and in the actual course of the investigation. Lastly, it permits target biopsies of very high reliability which are essential to the histologic diagnosis of initial conditions that can escape radiologic detection and leave doubts in the mind of the endoscopist.

The case against routine proctosigmoidoscopy

Murray S. Jaffe

Department of Surgery, University of Cincinnati College of Medicine and the Veterans Administration Hospital, Cincinnati, Ohio, U.S.A.

The American Cancer Society has urged routine annual proctosigmoidoscopy for all persons over 40 years of age in an attempt to lower the mortality rate for cancer of the colon and rectum. Cancer developing in these sites will account for an estimated 79,000 new cases in the United States this year. There is an estimated mortality of 47,400 persons this year in the United States from cancer of the colon and rectum (Amer. Cancer Soc., 1973). Since cancer of the colon and rectum is one of the most prevalent and deadly types of cancer, it is easy to understand the desperate need for improvement in results of therapy and for earlier diagnosis.

As a diagnostic procedure, what can reasonably be expected from sigmoidoscopy? Assuming the sigmoidoscope can be inserted its full length of 25 cm, it can reach only 70% of all colonic cancers, whereas, digital examination of the rectum can reach only 13% (O'Donnell et al., 1962). These figures are probably optimal figures and are considerably better than the results I would expect from the practical application of sigmoidoscopy. Those of you who have experience with this technique know that in many instances the colon is not adequately prepared; the patient is apprehensive and tense; there are convolutions in the colon through which the sigmoidoscope cannot be advanced. All these potential difficulties would easily reduce the number of actual colonic cancers found on sigmoidoscopy to well under 50% of all colonic cancer. (Assuming the examination was done on the entire population at risk.)

On the basis of these presumptions, if everyone in the United States over 40 years of age were to have a sigmoidoscopic examination this year, perhaps 40,000 cancers would be discovered. Of these, 8,000 would have been palpable on digital examination, leaving a total of 32,000 cases discovered by sigmoidoscopy alone. In a small series of cases of asymptomatic cancer discovered by routine examination, the 5 year cure rate was 88% (Hertz et al., 1960), whereas, the usual accepted cure rate for cancer of the rectosigmoid is 50% — this difference of 38% of 32,000 cases makes for a potential saving of 12,000 lives. This saving, however, must be balanced against many other factors: unwillingness of the patient to submit to proctosigmoidoscopy, cost, doctor time, complications of sigmoidoscopy, and an unmeasurable sense of false security of patients whose colonic cancer is beyond the reach of the sigmoidoscope. Assuming a patient population at risk of 80,000,000 persons, the incidence of the finding of colonic cancer by sigmoidoscopy is 32,000/80,000,000 or 1 in 2,500 examinations. This figure is borne out by figures collected by Moertel (1966).

At a cost of $25.00 per sigmoidoscopic examination, these figures can be restated as $62,500 per discovered case or a cost of 2 billion dollars a year for performing this procedure for the entire population at risk.

At half an hour per examination, it would require 1250 physician hours to discover a single case of carcinoma, and if the entire population submitted to this examination, it would require 40,000,000 physician hours or roughly 10% of every practicing physician's time.

Complications do occur from sigmoidoscopic examinations. Surgeons do not like to talk about their failures, so little is written about colon perforation during sigmoidoscopy. I asked the 15 surgeons who practice at a Cincinnati Hospital what experience they had had with colon perforation after sigmoidoscopy. Twelve surgeons had at least one experience in treating this complication. Naturally, the more experienced proctologists and large diagnostic clinics have a low incidence of perforations. Gilbertson (1968) reported only 3 perforations in 75,000 examinations. However, others have reported nearly 1 perforation of the colon per 1000 sigmoidoscopic examinations (Kiser et al., 1968). Colon perforations are serious if not recognized. If not promptly recognized and treated, they carry a high risk of prolonged disability and death. If a huge population were subjected to sigmoidoscopy, one would expect a perforation rate closer to the one per thousand figure. Mortality as a result of a routine diagnostic test is a real tragedy. Yet, if one assumes one perforation of the colon per 2,500 examinations, there would be an incidence of 32,000 perforations a year in a population of 80,000,000. Many of these 32,000 patients would die or have serious disability, thereby substantially reducing the significance of those saved by earlier detection.

There cannot be any figures given for the increased colon and rectum cancer mortality due to the false assurance of a negative sigmoidoscopy report. Nevertheless, this factor must be considered by advocates of the routine proctosigmoidoscopy. Many of those 40,000 cancer patients a year, whose colonic cancer was beyond the reach of the sigmoidoscopy, would undoubtedly delay further investigation of their symptoms of colonic cancer out of reluctance to undergo repeated sigmoidoscopy or out of the mistaken assumption they could not have colonic cancer. One would expect the prognosis of these patients to be adversely affected by unnecessary delay (Bolt, 1971).

These figures are convincing enough in themselves to demonstrate that proctosigmoidoscopy as currently practiced is not a practical approach for diagnosis of colonic cancer in asymptomatic patients. Even though many patients would be saved by earlier detection, many others would die from complications of sigmoidoscopy and from false assurance that they did not have colonic cancer. This does not mean that sigmoidoscopy does not have an important place in the diagnosis of colonic cancer. But, in my opinion, sigmoidoscopy should be limited to use in groups of patients prescreened by other simpler and less costly tests, in persons who present an unusually high risk of developing colon cancer, and in patients with any symptoms whatever suggestive of cancer of the colon and rectum.

References

Bolt, R. J. (1971): Cancer (Philad.), 28/1, 121.
American Cancer Society (1973): Cancer Facts and Figures.
Gilbertsen, V. A. (1968): In: Proceedings, Sixth National Cancer Conference, Denver, pp. 439-442. J. B. Lippencott & Co., Philadelphia-Toronto.
Hertz, R. E. L. et al. (1960): Postgrad. Med., 27, 290.
Kiser, J. L. et al. (1968): Missouri Med., 65, 969.
Moertel, C. G. et al. (1966): Proc. Mayo Clin., 41, 368.
O'Donnell, W. E. et al. (1962): Early Detection and Diagnosis of Cancer. C. V. Mosby Company, St. Louis.

Out-patient detection and prevention of cancer of rectum and sigmoid colon

C. A. Muller

Trinity Hospital, Lausanne, Switzerland

We all know that, despite considerable development and sophistication of methods of diagnosis, there has been no significant improvement in the past 40 years in the stage at which cancers of the large intestine are being referred for treatment.

Two reasons for this situation may be suggested: First, proctosigmoidoscopy is still not regarded as a simple extension of a routine physical examination. Most general practitioners and a vast majority of surgeons still rely on their finger to investigate the anal canal and lower rectum, despite the evidence that malignant tumors of the rectum which can be diagnosed by digital examination represent a very small minority (Fig. 1). Consequently, there can be no adequate detection, as far as cancer of the rectum is concerned, without *routine proctosigmoidoscopy*. The second reason, it seems, is the absence of preventive measures in this particular field of medicine.

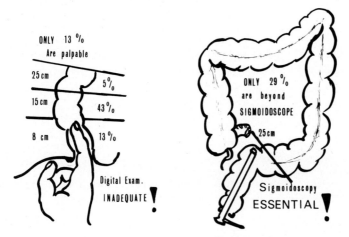

FIG. 1   *Digital examination versus sigmoidoscopy: 7 out of 8 asymptomatic cancers will be missed if sigmoidoscopy is not performed.*

With regard to cancer of the rectum and sigmoid colon, *prevention means routine periodical proctosigmoidoscopy*, and this is precisely the point which is disputed by most people concerned, on the assumption that it is practically impossible to build up a method of proctological check-up which would rely on the patient's memory only.

Therefore, 10 years ago, we put up a program of periodical sigmoidoscopic check-up which we described at our first symposium in Spa, 1968. Briefly, here are some details on which this sort of program depends for its success:

TABLE 1   *Type of checking-card used for periodical proctological check-up*

Name _____   Date of birth _____   Base No. _____

First name _____   Sex _____

Address _____

Tel. No. _____

Date of first examination _____   To be called up : \

Diagnosis _____   Summoned : ✓

Treatment _____   Checked up : ✗

Lost sight of or deceased : ✗ ✗

Year	Jan.	Feb.	March	April	May	June	July	Aug.	Sept.	Oct.	Nov.	Dec.
1968												
1969												
1970												
1971												

In the first place, every patient aged 40 or more will be systematically sigmoidos-coped in the course of his first physical examination. At the end of this, the patient is thoroughly informed about the reasons for this maybe unexpected examination. His attention is drawn to the fact that *2 out of 3 cancers* of the digestive tract are localized precisely in the area that was just examined. Finally we give him all information about our program of preventive rectal check-up, and we invite him to participate in it.

If the patient accepts to be put on our checking list, a checking card is established in his name, with all particulars needed for easy retrieval (Table 1): The lower part of this card is gridded to provide a monthly calendar horizontally and an annual calendar vertic-ally. The date of the next examination is ticked with a particular mark, as shown in the right upper corner of the card, for example: June 1970.

This checking-card is then placed into a card index cabinet comprised of monthly divisions. Every month, the card index is reviewed by the medical secretary. All the cards of the patients to be checked in one particular month are taken out, and an appointment is sent to each of them, together with a self-sealing reply letter on which 3 possible answers are printed, namely:

1. I shall keep the appointment as arranged.
2. The day and time are not convenient. Please arrange another appointment, prefer-ably on the ....., at ..... o'clock.
3. I no longer wish to participate in your program of preventive medicine. Please erase my name from your list.

Signed: .....

Depending upon the patient's answer, the appointment is confirmed or displaced in the diary. Whenever the third answer has been ticked, meaning that the patient does not wish to be examined further, we send him a questionnaire consisting of 9 stereotyped reasons, worded in an everyday simple language, intended to elicit why he has decided to withdraw from our program of prevention, and which he can answer simply by checking the reason of his choice. In addition, a space is provided for any other possible motivation to be mentioned.

As soon as this questionnaire has been returned, or at the latest 3 weeks after it has been mailed, the patient's checking card is removed from the cabinet and stored in his medical chart.

Detection

From January 1 1963, to December 31 1972, 1,842 patients underwent initial proctolo-gical examination and had their checking-card established. Amongst them, 10 had not reached the 40-year limit but were nevertheless listed because an adenomatous polyp had been found and histologically proven at initial sigmoidoscopy. 1,594 cases were entered in the group of diagnostic sigmoidoscopies, because they had been scoped on account of some proctological disorder (Table 2).

In this group, 229 polyps were discovered, of which 110, some 6.9%, were excised and confirmed histologically. 119 (7.5%) were identified but left in place because their dia-

TABLE 2   *Results of 1,594 diagnostic sigmoidoscopies (1963–1972)*

	Total	%
Polyps removed (confirmed histologically)	110	6.9
Polyps identified (not confirmed histologically)	119	7.5
Cancers discovered by scope	33	2.1
Cancers discovered by barium enema (following sigmoidoscopy)	9	0.6

meter was less than 2 mm. 33 cancers were identified by direct vision, an incidence of 2.1%, whereas 9 (0.6%) were diagnosed by means of a barium enema which we had requested on account of a positive occult blood test in suspicious rectal secretions.

In the group of 248 prophylactic examinations, that is in those people where sigmoidoscopy had been performed in the absence of any proctological complaint, 8 adenomatous polyps were excised and examined histologically. One was simply identified, and there was no evidence of cancer (Table 3).

TABLE 3 *Results of 248 prophylactic sigmoidoscopies (1963–1972)*

	Total	%
Polyps removed (confirmed histologically)	8	3.3
Polyps identified (not confirmed histologically)	1	0.4
Cancers identified by scope	0	–
Cancers discovered by barium enema (following sigmoidoscopy)	0	–

Prevention

From January 1 1964 to December 31st 1972, 1,400 patients were sigmoidoscoped in accordance with our program of prevention (Table 4). 64 adenomatous polyps were removed (4.5%); 227 were identified but left in place (16.2%) because their diameter was less than 2 mm. Five cancers were *detected*, an incidence of 0.35%. Two were diagnosed by direct vision and 3 by means of a barium enema which had been ordered on account of suspicious rectal secretions and positive occult blood test.

TABLE 4 *Results of 1,400 preventive sigmoidoscopies, according to program of periodical check-up (1964–1972)*

	Total	%
Polyps removed (diameter: 2 mm or more)	64	4.5
Polyps identified/not removed (diameter less than 2 mm)	227	16.2
Cancers discovered by scope	2	0.1
Cancers discovered by barium enema (following sigmoidoscopy)	3	0.2

Patients lost to follow-up

During the 10 years of our experience, 404 patients withdrew from our program of detection, an incidence of 21.9% (Table 5).

345 refused to attend our appointments. Amongst them 67 died during the period of observation, leaving 278 available for questioning. A questionnaire was sent to all of them and 180 were returned (64.7%), giving altogether 203 answers (Table 6).

We have been surprised by the frequency of the answers appearing under headings 1 and 3. We believe that this unusual quota could be due to inadequate public information about the possibilities offered by preventive medicine in the field of oncology. A particu-

TABLE 5   *Distribution of 404 patients lost to follow-up from a total of 1,842 initial sigmoidos-copies (1964–1972)*

	Total	%
Moved out of town	51	2.8
Followed up by other Institution	8	0.4
Died	67	3.6
Cancer of colon or rectum : 7		
Cancer other than colo-rectal : 31		
Cardio-pulmonary disease : 16		
Other diseases : 13		
Refused further preventive sigmoidoscopy	278	15.1
Total	404	21.9%

TABLE 6   *Reasons for dropping preventive sigmoidoscopies: 180 answers giving 203 reasons*

	Total	%
Are in good health and fail to see purpose of preventive medicine	66	32.5
Deny efficiency of prevention as far as cancer is concerned	13	6.4
Visit general practitioner once a year and think this is good enough	33	16.3
Fear that sigmoidoscopy could reveal presence of a cancer	8	3.9
Find sigmoidoscopy too expensive	30	14.8
On principle against preventive medicine	19	9.4
Too old to care for prevention	16	7.9
Other reasons	18	8.8
Total	203	100.0

larly striking finding must be mentioned here: in the group of 18 'other reasons', 8 patients declared that their family doctor had advised *against* preventive sigmoidoscopy. Careful analysis of these data unfortunately reveals that more than 50% of the patients who abandoned preventive proctological check-up did so for reasons which denote a fundamental ignorance of the improvements realized in modern tumor prophylaxis.

In conclusion, we state that as regards cancer of the rectum and lower sigmoid colon, there can be no detection without routine proctosigmoidoscopy in all patients aged 40 or more. Furthermore, there can be no prevention without regular endoscopic check-up of the rectum. Programming such a periodical check-up is relatively easy, even in private practice. Finally, it is evident that the population at large could still greatly benefit from better information as far as prophylaxis of cancer of the rectum and sigmoid colon is concerned.

Summary

It has been postulated, as far as cancer of the rectum and sigmoid is concerned, that there can be no detection without routine proctosigmoidoscopy in all patients aged 40 or more, as a complement to any physical examination. Furthermore, it has been stated that there can be no prevention without periodical proctological check-up. To this end a method has been set forth which allows us to keep close contact with our patients and makes it easy to retrieve them for check-up, provided they are willing to cooperate. The results obtained with this program are described in detail. It appears particularly striking that in the group of patients who have been checked up regularly during the past 10 years, the incidence of cancer of the rectum and sigmoid discovered was only $3.5^o/_{oo}$, whereas most other statistics record incidences of up to $8^o/_{oo}$. Finally, it appears that the public at large could still benefit from better information regarding prevention of cancer of the rectum and sigmoid colon.

References

Gilbertsen, V. A. and Wagensteen, O. H. (1965): Surgery, 57, 363.
Gilbertsen, V. A. and Wagensteen, O. H. (1967) Surg. Gynec. Obstet., 116, 413.
Hertz, R. E. L., Deddish, M. R. and Day, E. (1961): Postgrad. Med., 27, 290.
Muller, C.-A, (1968): In: Proceedings, 1st International Symposium on Detection of Cancer, Spa, 1968,
    pp. 829-832. Editors: H. Ramioul and A. Liegeois. Sciences et Lettres, Liege.
Muller, C.-A. (1969a): Proc. roy. Soc. Med., 63, 142.
Muller, C.-A. (1969b): Lyon chir., 65, 708.
Stearns Jr, M. W. (1968): Dis. Colon Rect., 11, 1.

Laparoscopy associated with diagnostic localization by radioisotopes in the clinical study of liver tumours

G. Lenzi[1], A. Abbati[2], A. Rossi[3], F.M. Gritti[1], E. Turba[2], A. Grillo[1] and A.L. Bonazzi[1]

[1]Division of Infectious Diseases, [2]Nuclear Medicine Service, and [3]Medical Physics Service, 'Ospedale Maggiore', Bologna, Italy

Anatomical features of the liver have been investigated by many radiological techniques: transhepatic cholangiohepatography, transpapillar cholangiography under laparoscopic control, and splenoportography.

The whole image of the liver, as well as details of its structure, can be detected with other methods. Laparoscopy employs an optical system. Nuclear medicine localizes radioactive colloidal particles fixed by reticuloendothelial cells, such as [198]Au colloidal; or gives information about the distribution of radionuclides selectively absorbed by hepatocytes and excreted in biliary ducts, such as ^{131}I-Bengal-Rose; or it shows retention of positive tumour indicators such as [67]Gallium citrate, in neoplastic cells.

Progress in radioisotope localization studies has been recently achieved through handling the data by an electronic videodisplay processing unit (VDP2) after Ben Porath indication (El Scint, Haifa) and introduced in our hospital by A. Abbati and A. Rossi. This device gives immediate isoactivity colour maps, with an adequate smoothing facility to eliminate statistical fluctuations. It also gives profiles of activity on pre-selected lines, as well as counts over areas of interest. The purpose of this communication is to show the usefulness of these methods for the diagnosis of liver tumours.

Laparoscopy, liver scan, and consequently oriented liver biopsy have a greater diagnostic value than conventional methods (biochemical, roentgenological or clinical) and are often valuable in deciding on the suitability, or otherwise, of surgical intervention.

The main objectives for laparoscopy and liver scan are the following:

(a) To search for the nature of liver enlargement.

(b) To discover localized pathological alterations of the liver, as, for example, cysts and tumours.

(c) To diagnose the different clinical forms of jaundice, using different radio elements. The advantages and characteristics of laparoscopy are well known. It permits oriented needle liver biopsy, which is sometimes necessary to precise diagnosis.

Nevertheless, laparoscopy has some important limitations. Not every patient can undergo the procedure, and neither can we carry out repeated examinations on the same patient. When diffuse peritoneal adherencies and perivisceritis are present, the examination is impossible: neither can deep or posterior hepatic lesions be observed.

Laparoscopy is useful in finding cystic or neoplastic processes on the liver surface, but it is often difficult to distinguish between single or multiple cysts. Parasitic and non-parasitic cysts can be identified or suspected, as well as the true polycystic disease of the liver, but it is often impossible to distinguish cysts of a different nature. However, laparoscopy is important in the recognition of the cystic character of lesions whose nature is doubtful on clinical and scintigraphic examination.

Benign tumours must be differentiated from congenital anomalies, knot-shaped malignant hyperplasias, and other malignancies. Needle biopsy is necessary for the current diagnosis of avascular tumours: angiomas are generally easily recognized by laparoscopy.

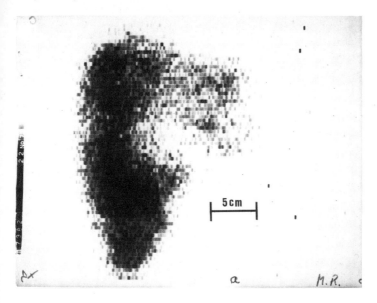

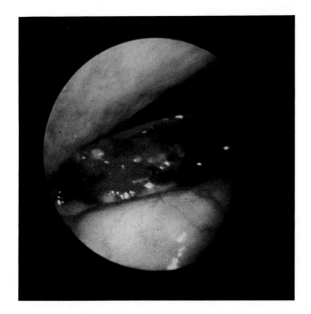

FIG. 1 *Polycystic haemangioma of the liver.*

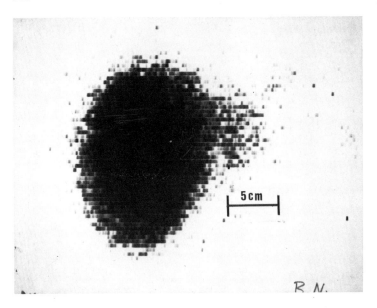

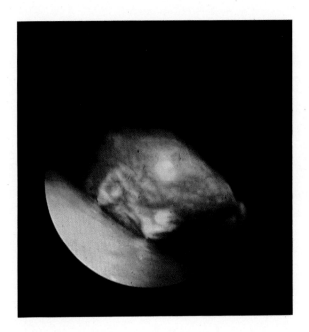

FIG. 2   *Metastases of the left lobe of the liver with malignant lymphangitis.*

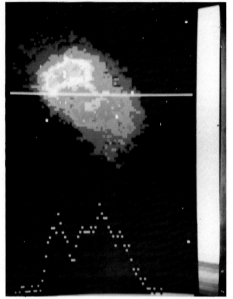

a

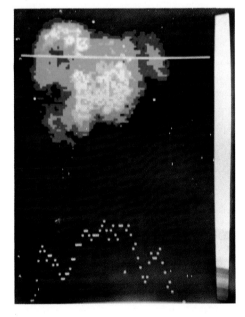

b

FIG. 3   *Metastases of the liver: (a) anterior view, (b) right-lateral view.*

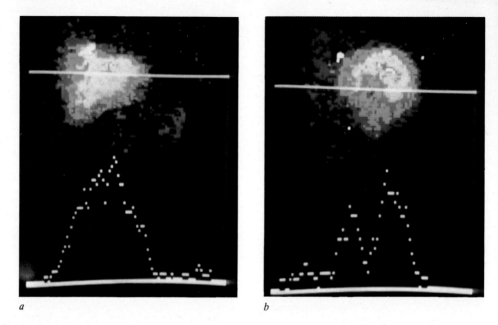

a   b

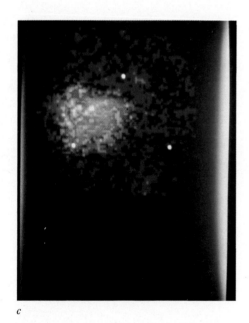

c

FIG. 4   *Liver metastases secondary to rectal adenocarcinoma: (a) anterior view, (b) right-lateral view, (c) [198]Au appears red-coloured; ^{75}Se-methionine shows a blue colour in tissues unable to fix radiocolloidal gold.*

Malignant neoplasms can be nodular or infiltrating. Their macroscopical features are often not specific: needle biopsy is recommended on bulging areas covered by hepatic tissue. When the tumour protrudes through the liver surface, it is generally easily identified (Figs. 1 and 2): cancrocyrrhosis can in many cases be diagnosed by simple laparoscopy.

Biopsy is useful for a correct morphological identification of the tumour. Sarcomas are often infiltrating, adenocarcinomas have generally a nodular distribution. Primitive and metastatic liver malignancies are frequently difficult to differentiate. In practice the simple identification of the tumour is considered a sufficient objective of laparoscopy: the histological picture can help to resolve the problem.

Tumour diagnosis was obtained by laparoscopy in 89% of the cases: malignant tumours have been identified in 93% of the cases. Laparoscopy associated with biopsy gave the correct diagnosis in 98% of the cases. Liver scintigraphy by radiocolloids gave important help in the clinical exploration of the liver. Alterations of its shape and inhomogeneities of the scan have been frequently observed and this technique is necessary when studying the deep and posterior liver areas, which we cannot see by laparoscopy (Fig. 3).

Anterior, right lateral, and in some cases, posterior scans, must be obtained. Isoactivity colour maps and profiles by VDP2 electronic computer have increased the sensitivity of the method and reduced the number of false negative cases previously observed when only conventional analogic monochromatic photoscintigraphy was employed.

Associated pancreas scintigraphy by ^{75}Selenomethionine (Fig. 4), moreover, has proven to be useful in demonstrating inhomogeneities of this organ, which can raise the suspicion of neoplastic localizations in the liver scan. The wax-drop-like liver metastases of carcinomas of the pancreas are often so thin that it is impossible to identify them by the simple liver scan.

Positive neoplasm indication with ^{67}Gallium citrate must also be remembered. It may be present in areas where colloidal particles are not fixed, and pathological alteration is doubtful. An intense Gallium localization, for example, can help to exclude the cystic nature of the investigated lesion.

The physicomathematical premises of the methods, and the clinical experience of our cases, seem to indicate that electronic analysis by VDP2 and associated pancreas scintigraphy have allowed a remarkable increase of sensitivity compared to the conventional liver scan, valued up to only ±20% of false positive and false negative results for lesions larger than 3 cm.

Morphological control by laparoscopy and needle biopsy, which is responsible for definitive and direct diagnostic conclusions, can be prepared and guided by nuclear medical techniques. The techniques give better precision and accuracy, particularly in cases of deep and posterior liver lesions, where sometimes, without a scan, only indirect signs, as increased tension of Glisson's capsule, or local blood perfusion modifications, would have allowed us to suspect a neoplastic localization.

^{99m}Technetium and ^{113m}Indium short-lived sulphur colloids have drastically reduced the radiation burden for the patient. It is now possible, therefore, to study the evolution of hepatic lesions by means of repeated scintigraphic examination: the effects of various treatments can now be thoroughly followed.

In conclusion, both methods discussed here are helpful in the diagnosis of liver tumours, although each has characteristic limitations. They concern mainly the technical condition and interpretation for laparoscopy, and principally, interpretational difficulties for scanning techniques.

Comparison between these two types of examination has shown that a modern and complete hepatological study of the patient (not only for suspected tumours), must include a radioisotope scan, which constitutes a pilot method and an anatomical guide. Laparoscopy, if necessary, will then give confirmation and offer a synergic aid to ultimate diagnosis.

Summary

Laparoscopy and hepatoscintigraphy have been examined in connexion with the diagnosis of liver tumours. Direct liver observation by simple laparoscopy has lead to diagnosis in 89% of the cases. When associated with laparoscopically-oriented needle biopsy, which is necessary in the presence of parenchymal liver protrusions of doubtful nature, diagnosis has been obtained in 98% of cases. Radiocolloid liver scans, associated with pancreatic scintigraphy and positive radioactive tumour indicators, must be considered a technique of first choice in every case of liver enlargement. Advantages offered by the analysis of isoactivity areas in the scans by means of electronic on-line computer devices have been presented.

Laparoscopy gives direct evidence of the explored cold superficial liver areas which are optically accessible: scintigraphy explores also deep and posterior liver regions, which are difficult, or impossible, to investigate by other means.

The combination of both methods provides a diagnostic synergism which is valuable in hepatology.

Early detection of carcinoma of the esophagus

The Co-ordinating Group for the Research of Esophageal Carcinoma, China

The Chinese Academy of Medical Sciences, Peking, China

Carcinoma of the esophagus is one of the most frequent malignancies encountered in North China and it seriously threatens the life and health of the labor population. Statistics revealed that in most patients seen in the city hospitals the disease was already in an advanced stage. Of the patients undergoing surgical intervention, more than half had lymph node metastases and the results were unsatisfactory.

In their endeavor to serve the people, our medical workers have tried to find out an efficient and practical means of detecting early carcinoma of the esophagus in order to study its pathological pattern and improve the therapeutic results.

Since 1959 the medical workers of Honan province and the Chinese Academy of Medical Sciences have jointly started the survey in Linhsien, Honan. They have established local anti-cancer organization and extended to other areas forming an anti-cancer network. They went to the patients, offering medical care right to their homes, and at the same time did much work on anti-cancer propaganda and mass survey of esophageal carcinoma, striving for early diagnosis and early treatment.

After many years' practice it was found that cytological examination has proved to be the method of choice in the early detection of carcinoma of the esophagus. It is simple, accurate, and easily accepted by the patients and fit for mass survey and daily O.P.D. work. At present it is widely utilized both in rural and urban areas.

The purpose of this paper is to report our method and results in the early detection of this disease by cytological examination and to discuss briefly its significance in correlation with clinical, roentgenological and pathological studies.

Method

The apparatus for collecting cytological specimens is a double-lumen rubber tube, measuring about 60 cm in length with an abrasive balloon at the distal end. At the proximal end the double lumen separates into two tubes, one for air injection and the other for suction. The alternative one is a single-tube type.

The person to be examined is instructed to come in the morning with an empty stomach and is asked to swallow the tube until the balloon has passed the cardia. Then, 20 ml of air is injected into the balloon and the tube with the distended balloon is withdrawn gradually. After the balloon has come into the esophagus, the air is partially withdrawn and the traction of the tube continues until it is entirely out. Smears of the exfoliated cells collected on the surface of the balloon are made, stained by Papanicolaou's method and examined microscopically.

Gradings of cytological findings

According to the morphological characteristics, particularly the changes of the nuclei, the epithelial cells of the esophagus are divided into four grades.

1. Normal: The majority of the cells are of the intermediate layer. About 10% are of the superficial layer. Parabasal cells are very rare.
2. Mild dyskaryosis: Cells with dyskaryosis are seen in the smears. Hyperchromatism occurs in both of the intermediate and superficial layer cells. The nuclei are enlarged but not more than thrice the normal cells.
3. Marked dyskaryosis: The size of the nuclei of the intermediate cells is thrice or more than that of the normal. Hyperchromatism is more marked. Dyskaryotic parabasal cells are numerous.
4. Cancer: There are many dyskaryotic cells and squamous carcinoma cells. The latter are usually single, polygonal and comparatively uniform in shape with malignant characteristics in their nuclei. In carcinoma in situ of small size, the carcinoma cells are few in number, while in that of extensive area, especially when accompanied with early infiltration, a large number of carcinoma cells are seen. In advanced carcinoma the malignant cells are often clustered together, with varying degrees of differentiation and shapes.

Mass survey

Mass survey consisted of two groups. In the first group, 7,686 cases with suspected esophageal carcinoma were examined in the years 1963–1969. Carcinoma of the esophagus or gastric cardia was found in 510 cases, and of these, early carcinoma was found in 86 with an incidence of 16.3%.

In the second group, mass survey was conducted in 1970–72 in 11,564 persons over 30 years of age. Carcinoma of the esophagus or gastric cardia was found in 136 cases and out of these, early carcinoma was found in 96 cases, an incidence of 70.6%.

The above figures were compared with 8,528 cases of patients who came to the O.P.D. of the county hospital for upper gastrointestinal diseases (Table 1). Among them, 3,122 cases were found to have carcinoma of the esophagus or gastric cardia, and of these, 212 cases, or 6.8% were in the early stage. It can be seen from the Table that in an area with high incidence of esophageal carcinoma, mass survey provides an effective means for detecting early cases, and is of greater significance among those aged 30 or above.

TABLE 1   *Comparison of the incidence of early carcinoma in mass survey and hospital patients*

	Mass survey of persons with symptoms (1963–1969)	Mass survey of persons aged 30 or above (1970–1972)	Hospital patients (1961–1971)
Total No. examined	7,686	11,564	8,528
No. of proved carcinoma	510	136	3,122
No. of early carcinoma	86(16.3%)	96(70.6%)	212(6.8%)

Roentgenological examinations were carried out in cases either with positive cytological findings, with marked hyperplasia or with symptoms of carcinoma but negative cytological findings. The results were evaluated by a joint group of cytologists, roentgenologists and surgeons and examinations repeated whenever discrepancy existed. Endoscopic cytological examinations were done if necessary. The rate of correct diagnosis had increased gradually from 87.8% in 1961 to 91.93% in 1969. Periodic follow-up cytological examinations of those cases with marked hyperplasia had yielded valuable data for the study of precancerous lesions, as a number of them had subsequently undergone malignant change. During the past 2 years, cytological examinations have been used to locate the lesions of early esophageal carcinoma. For example, when the cytology specimen from a level at 35 cm is negative, while that of lower level positive, the lesion is in the lower third of the esophagus. This had partly replaced endoscopic examinations in cases with positive cytological but negative roentgenologic findings. This method was well checked with pathological examinations of the surgical specimens.

Roentgenological manifestation

Reports on the roentgenological findings of early carcinoma of the esophagus are scanty. Special attention must be paid to the mucosal folds which in early carcinoma may have the following 3 forms:

1. Thickening, interruption and tortuosity of the mucosal folds with irregular and rough margins. These changes are mainly due to the creeping growth of the tumor in the mucosa.

2. Small ulcerations, single or multiple, frequently appear on the thickened mucosa. The diameter ranges from 0.2 to 0.4 cm.

3. Localized filling defect resulting from intraluminal tumor growth, the smallest being 0.5 cm in diameter.

As early cancer is frequently associated with inflammatory changes, there is, in addition to the above findings, spasm of the localized segment of the esophagus, appearing as stiffness of the wall or stagnation of the barium stream.

Pathological examination

In order to verify and improve the cytological examination and to have better understanding of the early carcinoma, meticulous pathological studies were made on 58 surgical specimens. The results are as follows:

1. Gross appearance: As early lesions appear usually as superficial erosions, they are found only on careful examinations. The mucosa of the diseased areas appear more deeply tinged than normal. After fixation it becomes slightly greyish white in color and is then more evident.

2. Microscopic findings: All of the 58 specimens were squamous cell carcinoma, and in one there were, in addition, glandular cells forming a mixed type. Thirty-one cases were carcinoma in situ and the rest were early infiltrative carcinoma limited only to the submucosa. No lymph node metastasis was found. Independent multifocal lesions as many as 8 were found in 92% of the resected specimens. The size of a single carcinoma in situ may reach as large as 4 cm or more. These findings are very useful references for the surgeons in determining the extent of resection of esophagus in early cases.

Discussion

1. According to our observations, the early invasive carcinoma, present either as an independent lesion or as a coexisting lesion adjacent to an advanced carcinoma, is more or less connected to a carcinoma in situ. It is very rare for the basal layer cell carcinoma to invade the deeper tissue forming an infiltrative carcinoma. It is likely therefore that carcinoma in situ is a definite stage through which the epithelium of the esophagus must pass in the course of malignant change and this favors the exfoliative cytological examination in the early diagnosis of carcinoma of the esophagus.

2. A small carcinoma in situ (about 1 cm in size on roentgenologic examination) usually requires 4 to 5 years or even longer to become frankly invasive. Therefore, close

follow-up observations for the suspected cases are justifiable.

3. Recently the method of cytological examinations at different levels of the esophagus in locating early lesions as verified by examination of surgical specimens has been proved to be quite accurate. Endoscopic examination is now less frequently employed.

4. The cure rate had been very much increased for the early cases. Among the 52 cases that underwent surgical resections more than a year ago there were 2 operative deaths. One died a year after operation with recurrence, one 4 years later of carcinoma of cervix and five 4 years later from diseases unrelated to esophageal carcinoma. Of the 43 cases still living, 21 have already reached 5 years. It is worthwhile to point out that during operation for all these cases no tumor mass or obvious abnormality could be palpated on exploration of the esophagus and the extent of resection was determined by cytological, roentgenological or endoscopic examinations.

Conclusion

The criteria, method and results of cytological examination in correlation with roentgenological and other examinations in the early detection of carcinoma of the esophagus are presented and briefly discussed. The cytological examination has a definite place in the early diagnosis and study of the precancerous lesions of carcinoma of the esophagus. This method is simple, convenient, easy to master and especially fit for mass survey in rural districts with high incidence. The cure rate will be very much improved by early discovery and early treatment.

2. Cytological diagnosis of lung cancer

Study of sputum smears in cigarette smokers considered as a high risk population

A. Simatos and A. Cattan

Institut Jean Godinot, Reims, France

Objects

The authors report a study of abnormal bronchial cells observed in sputum from 789 cigarette smokers and 108 non-smokers. They sought the influence, on bronchial cells, of certain characteristics of cigarette smokers (Leuchtenberger et al., 1960). They attempted to classify them in order of importance, with respect to the growth-rate of various abnormal cells. These cells were classified in terms of metaplasia with light, moderate and severe cellular abnormalities (Auerbach et al., 1957; Nasiell, 1966; Saccomanno, 1965; Spain et al., 1970) (Figs. 1, 2 and 3).

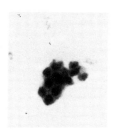

FIG. 1   *Metaplasia with light cellular abnormalities.*

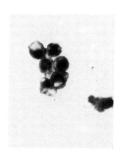

FIG. 2   *Metaplasia with moderate cellular abnormalities.*

Method

The study was carried out on persons who were invited, usually by their factory doctor, to take part in an experiment. They were active people in apparent good health and not suspected of cancer, working under usual conditions in the Paris region. The technique

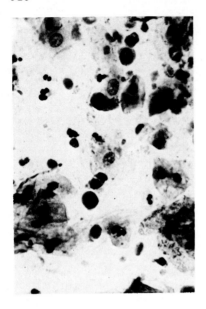

FIG. 3   *Metaplasia with severe cellular abnormalities.*

used was that of sputum smears. For each subject, we examined the early morning sputum on 3 consecutive days. The data were processed automatically on a computer.

Analysis of the cytologic results

The overall results are summarised in Table 1. This table shows that 15% of smokers had given specimens of saliva which were useless. This percentage differed from males to females. It was also modified by the use of tobacco: 29% of non-smokers gave useless specimens of saliva, but only 10%, when the total consumption of cigarettes exceeded 120,000.

Analysis of the result should take into consideration these relatively high levels of useless specimens, to the extent that they caused significant error. The cytologic results were analysed in relation to 6 variables concerning the use of cigarettes, and in relation to 2 variables concerning the smoker's constitutional background.

TABLE 1   *Sputum smears of 789 cigarette smokers*

Useless smears	15%	
Useful smears	85%	
Normal	47%	
Abnormal	53%	– light cellular abnormalities 35%
		– moderate cellular abnormalities 13%
		– severe cellular abnormalities 5%
		– carcinomatous cells 0.4%

1. *Daily consumption of cigarettes*

We compared 4 groups of men with no bronchopulmonary disease. The results are shown in Fig. 4. It appears that these levels of abnormal cases increase with the daily consumption of cigarettes, but the increase is not linear. It occurs in steps: a first step for the low consumptions and a second step for consumptions higher than 20 cigarettes daily.

Furthermore, the effect of this factor may be seen on the type of the cell abnormality. For low daily consumptions, only the frequency of simple metaplasia increased, passing from 19% in non-smokers to 38% in occasional smokers. For higher daily consumptions, the rate of metaplasia was unchanged, but we found a sudden increase in the frequency of severe metaplasia.

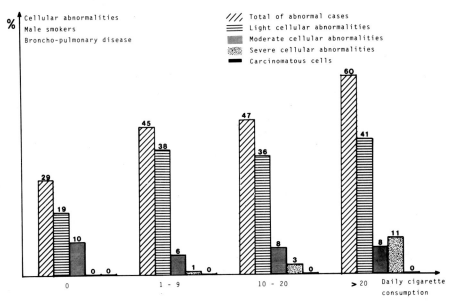

FIG. 4   *Cellular abnormalities related to daily cigarette consumption.*

2. *Earliness of the tobacco habit* (Fig. 5)

As previously, the results were calculated on groups of smokers of the same sex with no bronchopulmonary disease. The population was divided into 2 age groups: below 20, and 20 and above. It was observed that the difference in the rate of severe metaplasia between the two groups was significant. 7% in early smokers as against 2% in the others, whereas the proportions of simple and moderate metaplasia were roughly the same.

3. *Filter*

The results showed that there was a correlation between the use of cigarettes without a filter, and bronchial cell abnormalities (coefficient of partial correlation 0.07, significant to 1%). This correlation did not appear when the subjects used cigarettes with filters.

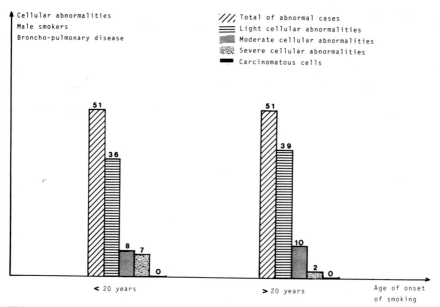

FIG. 5   *Cellular abnormalities related to age of onset of smoking.*

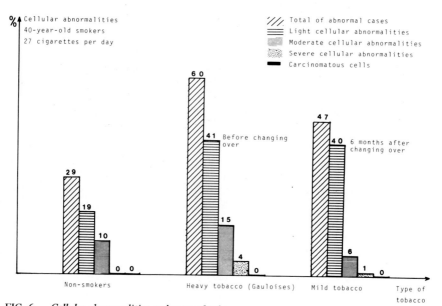

FIG. 6   *Cellular abnormalities and type of tobacco.*

4. *Inhalation of the smoke*

This factor had the same influence as the previous factor. When all other things were equal, it appeared that the bronchial cell abnormalities depended on the use of cigarettes only when the smoke was inhaled.

5. *Type of tobacco*

This factor is probably more important than the 2 previous ones, but the results of our calculations are still debatable and uncertain.

The study of the influence of this factor led us to seek changes in the sputum of smokers who changed their tobacco: we examined the sputum of 100 brown tobacco smokers, of average age 40 years and smoking on average 27 cigarettes daily. After 6 months use of a less toxic type of tobacco, we observed a significant reduction in the levels of moderate and severe metaplasia (Fig. 6).

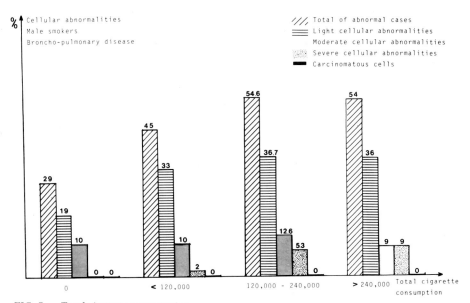

FIG. 7   *Total cigarette consumption.*

6. *Total consumption of cigarettes* (Fig. 7)

The levels of simple metaplasia reached a maximum as soon as the subject became a smoker, and did not vary when this consumption increased. Moderate metaplasia showed a constant level which did not vary in relation to the use of tobacco.

On the other hand, the rate of severe metaplasia progressed with total consumption of cigarettes. We noted that the dependence became significant from 200,000 cigarettes onwards.

7. *Age* (Fig. 8)

The results of smears in relation to age and in relation to total tobacco consumption were not superimposable, although these two factors seem to be intimately linked (Auerbach, 1962). Age seems to induce moderate metaplasia which is absent before the age of 25 years. We observed it in 8 to 10% of older subjects, whether they smoked or not. As for severe metaplasia, we noted that the incidence doubled at about 55 years in smokers.

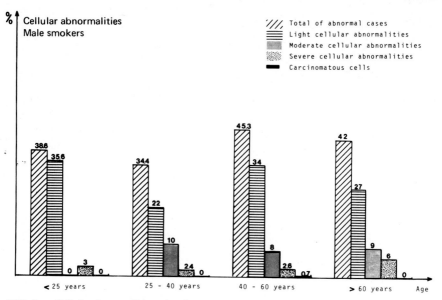

FIG. 8   *Cellular abnormalities related to age.*

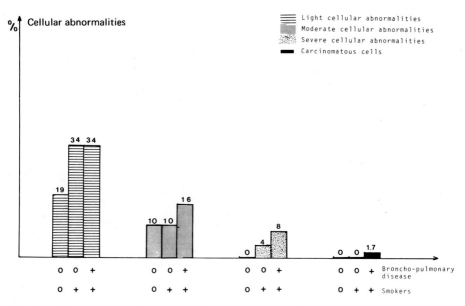

FIG. 9   *Cellular abnormalities related to bronchopulmonary disease.*

8. *Chronic bronchopulmonary diseases*

The influence of these diseases is difficult to determine, because it depends, not only on cigarette smoking, but on climate, pollution, age, cardiovascular disease, etc. (Chretien and Hirsch, 1972; Nasiell, 1968).

We compared the sputum in 100 healthy non-smokers to that of 464 healthy smokers and 174 smokers with chronic bronchitis (Fig. 9). It appeared that the incidence of simple metaplasia is not modified in chronic bronchitis. On the other hand, there were more cases of moderate metaplasia and the cases of severe metaplasia doubled from 4 to 8%. As for carcinomatous cells, we encountered these in 3 smokers with bronchitis, i.e. 1.7% of the cases in this group.

Conclusions

Among the variables studied, there was decreasing order of influence on the number and severity of bronchial cell abnormalities.

The daily consumption of cigarettes was the most important associated factor. Then came, in the following order, the earliness of the tobacco habit, the type of tobacco, chronic bronchitis, age, total consumption of cigarettes when this exceeded 200,000, a filter and inhalation of smoke. Thus, one may draw up the following characteristics of the high-risk smoker: 20 cigarettes daily + onset of smoking before the age of 20 years + chronic bronchitis + present age of 55 years or more.

We are now seeking association with other factors, such as sex, alcoholism, the level of immune reactions, pollution, etc. These results should permit us to discover among smokers, sub-populations with increasingly high risk in order to carry out effective prophylaxis for bronchopulmonary cancer.

Summary

Altered desquamated bronchial cells in the sputum were classified, depending on the degree of severity, into 3 groups: simple, moderate and severe metaplasia. Healthy non-smokers had 19% of simple metaplasia and 10% of moderate metaplasia. A comparable group of smokers had 33% of simple metaplasia, 10% of moderate metaplasia and 4% of severe metaplasia. These differences may be attributed to the effect of the cigarette. The effect of cigarettes was analysed in relation to 8 factors related to the tobacco habit and which were closely connected:

Daily consumption — age of onset of smoking — filter — inhalation of the smoke — type of tobacco — total consumption of cigarettes — age of the smokers and chronic bronchitis.

References

Auerbach, O., Gere, J. B., Forman, J. B., Petrick, T. G., Smolin, H. J., Muehsam, G. E., Kassouny, D. Y. and Stout, A. P. (1957): New Engl. J. Med., 256, 97.
Auerbach, P., (1962): New. Engl. J. Med., 267, 111.
Chretien, J. and Hirsch, A. (1972): Rev. Prat. (Paris), 22, 375.
Leuchtenberger, C., Leuchtenberger, R., Zebrun, W. and Shaffer, P. (1960): Cancer, 13, 721.
Nasiell, M. (1966): Acta Cytol., 10, 421.
Nasiell, M. (1968): Acta Path. Microbiol. Scand., 74, 205.
Saccomanno, G. (1965): Acta Cytol., 9, 413.
Spain, D., Braden, V., Tarter, R. and Matero, A. (1970): J. Amer. med. Ass., 211, 8.

Cytologic investigation of bronchial secretions in bronchopulmonary carcinoma: Detection, early diagnosis, selection

G. Diaconita

Department of Pathology, Tuberculosis Institute, Bucharest, Rumania

Introduction

Of foremost interest in the ever-present problem of cancer and a constant preoccupation in oncology is early diagnosis. This should be established as soon as possible after the onset of the disease, or after it has become suspect. Within the last 10-15 years the number of investigations on the cytodiagnosis of bronchopulmonary carinoma, on the techniques of collecting the material, on morphologic processing procedures, results, interpretation and significance, has greatly increased and are in general well known (Morawetz and Schwetz, 1964; Saccomanno et al., 1963; Nicolescu, 1960; Hattari et al., 1965; Fischmann and Green, 1966; Lanza, 1968; Cardozo et al., 1967; Ebner et al., 1967; Brun, 1969; Mouriquand et al., 1969; Diaconita, 1972*a*). However, with regard to the most precise methods of diagnosing cancer in the early phases, the morphologic procedures are still outstanding (Diaconita, 1972*b*).

Methods

The cytologic technique is most frequently used for the diagnosis of bronchopulmonary carcinomas. It is the least harmful and the most readily accepted by the patient. The cytologic method is easy to perform and it yields a high proportion of positive results. There are two main techniques:

1. *The smear technique* may be considered as a method of orientation and screening of the cases, permitting a diagnosis of malignant neoplasia without establishing the histologic type, except in very rare cases. This method has the advantage of being applicable to the systematic detection of cancer in large communities, without necessitating any special equipment apart from the smears prepared by a technician which can be read by the cytologist in his laboratory. The smear method is in fact the cytologic method.

2. *The embedding technique* may be considered rather as a cytohistologic method of diagnosis which permits not only the early diagnosis of malignant neoplasia, but also a diagnosis of the histologic type in many cases, with a high incidence of positive results.

For very large communities we recommend the smear technique. The Papanicolaou procedure cannot be applied. Giemsa staining gives good results in an early screening survey. The detection of bronchopulmonary carcinomas should be conducted parallel to the mass detection of tuberculosis by microradiophotography. In the cases screened by microradiography and regarded as suspect, cytologic examination of sputum should immediately be carried out by the smear technique which is rapid, practical and economic. In the cytologically-suspect cases, further investigations by the embedding technique will confirm or invalidate the diagnosis. When possible, biopsy has to be performed. In the cases with suspect cytology we recommend sputum collection in a flask with fixative,

5-6 days running, after previously instructing the patient so that the best conditions should be complied with. This is followed by embedding and examination of the sections, in series when necessary.

Results

To demonstrate the significance and efficiency of cytodiagnosis we report the results of our investigations of 2,006 cases of bronchopulmonary carcinomas diagnosed in our laboratory during the last 12 years (Jan. 1, 1961-Dec. 31, 1972). Our material differs from that published in numerous works abroad in that 665 cases were diagnosed by the cytologic method only (33% of the total 2,006 cases); 397 cases were diagnosed cytologically and checked histologically (20%); in 597 cases (30%) the cytologic examination was negative and the diagnosis was made on the basis of an anatomic or biopsy specimen, and in 347 cases (17%) the diagnosis was only histologic, without a previous cytologic examination.

TABLE 1   *The effect of different procedures upon diagnostic accuracy*

Diagnostic methods	No. of cases	%
Cytology alone +	665	33.15
Cytology +; histology +	397	19.79
Cytology −; histology +	597	29.76
Histology alone +	347	17.30
Total	2,006	100.00

TABLE 2   *Histologic type of tumors diagnosed by the cytologic method alone*

Histologic type	No. of cases	%
Epidermoid carcinoma	246	36.99
Macrocellular carcinoma	94	14.14
Microcellular carcinoma	81	12.18
Adenocarcinoma	81	12.18
Undefined carcinoma	163	24.51
Total	665	100.00

These data are summarised in Table 1. Some 1,062 cases (53%) of the total 2,006 cases of bronchopulmonary carcinoma were diagnosed cytologically. For 397 of these 1,062 cases, (37%) histologic confirmation was obtained. The incidence of various histologic types in cases diagnosed only by the cytologic method is summarized in Table 2. The histologic type was determined by the embedding technique. Table 3 gives cytohistologic correlation concerning the histologic type. Cytohistologic agreement concerning the histologic type existed in 270 of the 397 cases (68%). Table 4 shows the incidence of the cases in terms of the number of possible means of investigation.

We had a false-positive cytologic diagnosis of malignant neoplasm in 3 cases in which

examination of the sputum revealed carcinomatous cells, and histologic examination of
the anatomic specimen showed different types of sarcoma. In 8 of our cases the cytologic
method revealed a microscopic cancer on a large bronchus which did not exceed the
bronchic wall.

TABLE 3   Correlation of cytologic and histologic interpretations of tumor type

Histologic type	Agreement		Discrepancy		Total	
	No. of cases	%	No. of cases	%	No. of cases	%
Epidermoid carcinoma	194	48.87	55	13.85	249	62.72
Macrocellular carcinoma	35	8.82	19	4.79	54	13.60
Microcellular carcinoma	17	4.28	7	1.76	24	6.04
Adenocarcinoma	21	5.29	46	11.59	67	16.88
Undefined carcinoma	3	0.75			3	0.76
Total	270	68.01	127	31.99	397	100.00

TABLE 4   Correlation of cytologic findings with the number and type of other diagnostic procedures

Number of procedures	Type of procedures	No. of cases	%
3	Cytology +; biopsy +; anatomic specimen	58	14.99
2	Cytology +; bronchic biopsy	257	66.41
2	Cytology +; anatomic specimen	72	18.60
Total		387	100.00

Discussion

The results of our investigations emphasize the value and significance of bronchic exfoliative cytology for the study of bronchopulmonary carcinomas. This is reflected by the
possibility of:
   1. Significantly increasing the number of cancer cases diagnosed morphologically,
since cytology can be applied in absolutely all cases of bronchopulmonary carcinoma
and has no contraindications.
   2. Increasing the number of early detections, of extreme importance for patients that
may benefit by surgical exeresis if performed in due time. Maltoni and Carretti (1970)
mention dozens of occult bronchic carcinomas published in the literature and diagnosed
cytologically. We likewise had cases in which initially-limited neoplastic lesions were
detected by cytology in the phase of absent clinical and radiologic expression.
   3. Repeating cytologic examination of the sputum an indefinite number of times.
   The discrepancy with other statistics is due to the global approach in the study of our
material. Cases are not specially selected for follow-up histologic checking of the diagnosis
of malignant neoplasia or to check the agreement between the cytologic and histologic
results.

The low incidence of a cytohistologic agreement in our case is due to: the impossibility of performing biopsy in the cases diagnosed only cytologically: the patient's refusal to accept: overdue surgical treatment and death at home of those who asked to be discharged. On the other hand, the high incidence of cases diagnosed only histologically and with a falsely-negative cytology, likewise contributed in large measure to the poor agreement between the cytologic and histologic results. The cytologic examinations considered as falsely-negative were chiefly due to: the deficient processing of the specimens; the fact that the examination was not repeated at short intervals; and also, in part, to the peripheral localization of some of the tumors which do not usually exfoliate.

A difficult problem that may arise in systematic detection surveys in large communities is the great number of cases (603) with inconclusive cytologic results. Some cases of dyskaryosis may perhaps have been interpreted as atypical malignant cellular structures. Experience has shown that the use of the notion of 'atypical cellular structures' in the cases in which nothing precise has been found, is often abused in order to mask the fear and excessive prudence of the cytologist. We consider that this term 'atypical' has too broad a meaning and is too convenient.

In the material of Maltoni and Carreti (1970), mention is made of a large number of suspect and doubtful cases. The relatively small number of subsequent histologic confirmations in this group of cases (18%) lends support of this point of view. Lanza et al., (1970) propose that such cases should be temporarily grouped together as 'dysplasia type'. These authors group in the class of suspect elements, the cells that exhibit morphologic features revealing the existence of histologic lesions with a preneoplastic or paraneoplastic biologic significance (metaplasia and especially dysplasia). It is very likely that in most of the cases labeled as 'atypical' or suspect, either regeneration processes are involved that occur continuously in the bronchial mucosa, or they correspond to metaplasias induced by the varied actions that take place at this level.

As some authors attribute to the epidermoid metaplasia of the bronchial epithelium the character of a precancerous lesion, we consider, together with Maltoni et al. (1966), that the cases in which epidermoid metaplasia was found on examination of the sputum should attend for periodic control.

The cydodiagnostic method has two limitations: (1) technical difficulties and deficient collection of the products to be examined, and (2) the eventual absence of an experienced and rapid cytologist which, in our opinion, is the most serious drawback of the method. The cytologist should initially have a basic training in pathology and only afterwards study cytology. The results must be interpreted without any preconceived ideas.

Conclusion

Cytodiagnosis is the simplest method for detecting bronchopulmonary carcinomas in the stage of operability; it is the most readily applied method in communities exposed to noxious factors with a carcinogen effect, or cocarcinogenic action being performed in ambulatory conditions and by the simplest technique.

The results are certain only in the cases of exfoliating tumors or those which protrude into the bronchial lumen. A monthly radiologic and cytological control is advisable in all cases at microradiographic screening with a suspect, or negative, cytologic examination. The cytologic method should become a mass method of investigation for the early detection of bronchopulmonary carcinomas.

References

Brun, Y. (1969): Poumon, 25, 81.
Cardozo, P. L., DeGraff, S., DeBoer, M. S., Daesburg, N. and Kapsenberg, P. D. (1967): Acta cytol. (Philad.), 11, 101.

Diaconita, G. (1972*a*): Rev. roum. Embryol. Cytol. Sér. Cytol., 9, 75.
Diaconita, G. (1972*b*): Ftiziologia, 21, 349.
Ebner, H., Lederer, B. and Sandritter, W. (1967): Dtsch. med. Wschr., 92, 1901.
Fischman, S. and Greene, G. (1966): Acta cytol. (Philad.), 10, 289.
Hattari, S., Matsuda, W., Sugiyama, T., Terazawa, T. and Wada, A. (1965): Acta cytol. (Philad.), 9, 431.
Lanza, G. (1968): Riv. Pat. clin. sper., 9, 963.
Lanza, G., Cavazzini, L. and Nenci (1970): Riv. Pat. clin. sper., 15, 15.
Maltoni, C. and Carretti, D. (1970): Minerva ginec., 22, 1093.
Maltoni, C., Mattioli, G. and Carretti, D. (1966): Arch. Ostet. Ginec., (Suppl.), Vol. 2, 71, 621.
Morawetz, F. and Schwetz, E. (1964): Krebsarzt, 14, 554.
Mouriquand, J., Brun, J., Rison, H. and Kofman, J. (1969): Poumon, 25, 83.
Nicolescu, P. (1960): Cytological Diagnosis of Pulmonary and Pleural Tumours (In Rumanian). Editura Medicală, Bucharest.
Saccomanno, G., Saunders, R. P., Ellis, H., Arscher, V., Wood, B. and Bekler, P. (1963): Acta cytol. (Philad.), 7, 305.

The potentialities of cytological examination of sputum in diagnosis and typing pulmonary carcinomas

Mariantonia Graziadei, Cesare Maltoni and Donata Carretti

Istituto di Oncologia 'F. Addarii' and Centro Tumori, Bologna, Italy

It is known that sputum cytology is an effective tool for diagnosing pulmonary carcinomas (Foot, 1955; Grunze, 1960; Koss and Durfee, 1961; Russel et al., 1963; Koss et al., 1964).

Sputum cytology is also useful in diagnosing early lung cancers, which are clinically symptomless and radiologically occult. Several of these cases have been previously reported (Papanicolaou and Koprowska, 1951; Umiker and Storey, 1952; Wierman et al., 1954; Woolner et al., 1960; Lerner et al., 1961; Cahan and Montemayor, 1962; Kahlau, 1962; Melamed et al., 1963; Holman and Okinaka, 1964; Pearson and Thompson, 1966; Fullmer and Parrish, 1969; Maltoni and Carretti, 1970). Furthermore, sputum cytology makes it possible to define the histotype of pulmonary tumours (Foot, 1952, 1955; Grunze, 1960; Koss and Durfee, 1961; Russel et al., 1963; Koss et al., 1964).

In our Institute we are applying sputum cytology on a large scale, either for detecting and studying the types and the sequences of cytological precursors of carcinomas and for diagnosing early neoplasias of respiratory tract in heavy smokers or occupational groups exposed to risks, or for ascertaining tumours in clinically or radiologically-suspicious patients. To date, we have performed nearly 100,000 sputum cytologic examinations. Our experience brings further support to the effectiveness of the cytological method in diagnosing and characterizing pulmonary carcinomas.

The present report deals with 6,678 examinations performed on 5,022 pulmonary patients. The final diagnosis of 2,364 was known. Sputum, spontaneously expirated following a cough, was collected, and without any fixation or mucolytic treatment was smeared on 8 slides, and then stained following the Papanicolaou technique.

The general results are shown in Table 1. From these data, we see a high precision of the method for positive results. The significant percentage of false negatives should however be pointed out. This can be explained in part by the insufficiency of sampling and by the fact that in our series of cases, most patients had only one examination.

As mentioned above, cytology may define the histotype of pulmonary carcinomas. The cytological characters of the 3 fundamental types of lung cancer, i.e. adenocarcinomas, squamous-cell carcinomas, and anaplastic carcinomas, are sharply and easily identified by experienced cytologists. Also in our practice a good correlation in characterizing the histotype of carcinomas, has been found between cytology and histology, as can be seen in Table 2.

These data are of value, because the histotype of lung epithelial malignancies is one of the most important parameters for planning therapy and for formulating prognostic judgements.

References

Cahan, W.G. and Montemayor, P.B. (1962): J. Thorac. Surg., 44, 309.

TABLE 1   *General results*

Cytology			Final diagnosis										
Classes	No. of cases	Total	Lung carcinomas		Lung sarcomas		Metastases		Lung benign tumours		Negatives	
			No.	%	No.	%	No.	%	No.	%	No.	%
I, II	3,325	1,522	310	20.37	8	0.53	25	1.64	11	0.72	1,168	76.74
III, IV	275	135	85	62.97	–	–	–	–	1	0.74	49	36.29
V	772	514	511	99.41	–	–	–	–	–	–	3	0.59
		Adenocarcinomas 185										
		Squamous cell carcinomas 185										
		Anaplastic carcinomas 82										
		Mixed or transitional carcinomas 49										
		Undetermined carcinomas 13										
Technically unsatisfactory	650	193	80	41.46	4	2.07	3	1.55	1	0.52	105	54.40
Total	5,022	2,364	986		12		28		13		1,325	

TABLE 2   *Cytological typing of pulmonary carcinomas*

Cytologic diagnosis of histotype		Results of the histological examination	
Results	No. of cases	Results	No. of cases
Adenocarcinomas	49	Adenocarcinomas	26
		Mixed or transitional carcinomas (adenocarcinomas-squamous cell carcinomas)	15
		Squamous cell carcinomas	4
		Anaplastic carcinomas	4
Squamous cell carcinomas	63	Squamous cell carcinomas	57
		Mixed or transitional carcinomas (squamous cell carcinomas–adenocarcinomas)	6
		Adenocarcinomas	–
		Anaplastic carcinomas	–
Anaplastic carcinomas	24	Anaplastic carcinomas	22
		Mixed or transitional carcinomas	1
		Adenocarcinomas	–
		Squamous cell carcinomas	1
Mixed or transitional carcinomas	22	Mixed or transitional carcinomas	13
		Adenocarcinomas	–
		Squamous cell carcinomas	7
		Anaplastic carcinomas	2

Foot, N.C. (1952): Amer. J. Path., 28, 963.
Foot, N.C. (1955): Amer. J. clin. Path., 25, 223.
Fullmer, C.D. and Parrish, C.M. (1969): Acta cytol. (Philad.), 13, 645.
Grunze, H. (1960): Acta cytol. (Philad.), 4, 175.
Holman, C.W. and Okinaka, A. (1964): J. thorac. Surg., 47, 466.
Kahlau, G. (1962): Ther. Ber., 34, 187.
Koss, L.G. and Durfee, G.R. (1961): Diagnostic Cytology and its Histopathologic Bases. Pitman Medical Publ. Co. Ltd., London-Bath.
Koss, L.G., Melamed, M.R. and Goodner, J.T. (1964): Acta cytol. (Philad.), 8, 104.
Lerner, M.A., Rosbash, H., Frank, H.A. and Fleischner, F.G. (1961): New Engl. J. Med., 264, 480.
Maltoni, C. and Carretti, D. (1970): Bull. Sci. med., 4, 346.
Melamed, M.R., Koss, L.G. and Cliffton, E.E. (1963): Cancer (Philad.), 16, 1537.
Papanicolaou, G.N. and Koprowska, I. (1951): Cancer (Philad.), 4, 141.
Pearson, F.G. and Thompson, D.W. (1966): Canad. med. Ass. J., 94, 825.
Russel, W.O., Neidhardt, H.W., Mountain, C.F., Griffith, K.M. and Chang, J.P. (1963): Acta cytol. (Philad.), 7, 1.
Umiker, W. and Storey, C. (1952): Cancer (Philad.), 5, 369.
Wierman, W.H., McDonald, J.R. and Clagett, O.T. (1954): Surgery, 35, 335.
Woolner, L.B., Andersen, H.A. and Bernatz, P. (1960): Dis. Chest, 37, 278.

Bronchial brushing using the flexible fiberoptic bronchoscope

Felix De Narvaez, Arthur D. Boyd and Helen R. Baker

Central Cytology Laboratories, New York City Department of Health, New York, N.Y., U.S.A.

In recent years special emphasis has been placed on preventive medicine and chiefly on one of its increasingly important objectives, the early detection of lung cancer. The Papanicolaou method of cytological examination is one of the most sensitive, widely used and simplest of the techniques currently available for early detection of malignancies of the lower respiratory tract.

The examination of the bronchial tree followed by a brush biopsy of suspicious areas appears to be a desirable method to use in lieu of rigid conventional bronchoscopy when this method appears not advisable.

The use of the flexible fiberoptic bronchoscope appears to be an ideal technique for the diagnosis of neoplastic disease of the lung. It has previously been reported by Fennessy et al. (1970) and Hattori et al. (1971) as well as others.

This technique permits the optical perusal of the bronchial tree. In addition it allows the bronchoscopist to obtain multiple brush smears. By the use of forceps which can be passed through the channel of the bronchoscope multiple small biopsies can also be obtained from any suspicious area.

In order to assess the feasibility and accuracy of this technique, a pilot study was undertaken in conjunction with the Department of Thoracic Surgery of the New York University-Bellevue Medical Center. This report consists of our experience with 140 consecutive cases where the fibroscopic study was done for pulmonary abnormalities. The cases were selected from patients whose age or cardiopulmonary status did not make them good candidates for conventional bronchoscopy.

Material and methods

Patients are required to fast at least 5-6 hr before the examination. They are pre-medicated with codeine 60 mg, Nembutal 100 mg and atropine 0.4 mg about 40 min before the procedure. The pharynx, nose and endolarynx are sprayed with a topical anesthetic (2% Xylocaine). The instrument used is the flexible fiberoptic bronchoscope with an image intensifier model No. BF-5-B-2 manufactured by The Olympus Company of Tokyo, Japan. Both a 4 mm and a 5 mm diameter fibroscope are used. When a biopsy of the lesion is contemplated, we use a biopsy forceps model FB-1-C through the 5 mm scope.

The material thus obtained is smeared by brushing onto a clean glass slide which is immediately sprayed with a fixative solution (Clay Adams, Spray-Cyte).

The biopies are fixed in 10% formalin and sent to the Department of Pathology for processing.

The brushes are rinsed in a small amount of saline to which has been added equal parts of 50% alcohol. The suspended material is sent to the Department of Cytology for further processing. The slides are stained by routine Papanicolaou staining, and the material suspended in saline and alcohol is centrifuged, and the sediment is smeared onto glass slides and processed and stained in a similar manner.

Results

In this study of 140 cases, 83 (59.28%) were negative on cytologic examination. These cases did not have biopsies. Four cases (2.86%) had negative cytology and positive biopsy. Nine cases (6.43%) were positive both cytological and biopsy. Nineteen cases (13.57%) had positive cytology and either negative or unsatisfactory biopsies. Twenty-five (17.86%) cases were unsatisfactory for diagnosis.

Summary

The bronchial washing specimen prepared after the brushing did not increase the diagnostic accuracy of the brushing technique in our experience.

The large number of negatives represents the selection of our patients from TB and pulmonary clinics in which bronchial cancer was not among the most likely clinical diagnosis.

The use of the fiberoptic bronchoscope and the technique of obtaining cells for cytological evaluation, can be utilized for the analysis of many pulmonary lesions. It is useful in the investigation of pulmonary processes such as atelectasis, TB, etc. It can provide material for bacteriologic studies. In our experience the procedure is usually well tolerated by the patients.

References

Fennessy, J.J., Fry, W.A., Manalo-Estrella, P. and Frios, D.V.S. (1970): Acta cytol. (Philad.), 14, 25.
Fry, W.A. and Manalo-Estrella, P. (1970): Surg. Gynec. Obstet., 130, 67.
Hattori, S., Matsuda, M., Nishihora, H. and Horoi, T. (1971): Acta cytol. (Philad.), 15, 460.
Moskowitz, M. and Freihofer, A. (1970): Chest, 57, 426.

Bronchial brushing: A survey on 177 cases

F. Pinet, H. Pison, M. Coulomb, S. Augusseau, J. C. Froment and J. Mouriquand

Hôpital Cardiovasculaire, Lyon, Laboratoire d'Histologie, Faculté de Médecine, Grenoble et Clinique Radiologique, Centre Hospitalier Régional, Grenoble, France

When the clinician is faced with pulmonary lesions for which all the usual diagnostic techniques fail to provide a diagnosis, he is led to try several complementary investigations. Bronchial brushing, which allows the collection of cytological material directly from a selected area, is a valuable method. We report here an analysis of 177 cases.

Technique

The segmental location of the lesion to be brushed is determined as accurately as possible by means of frontal and lateral radiographs. Tomographs may be necessary. Two types of instruments have been utilised:

1. The probe of Pieri, modified by Pinet et al. (1968) is a catheter supplied with a metallic guidewire. Its variable curve may be directed as chosen. A small catheter of Odmann with preformed curve may be introduced in this probe and may catheterize the bronchus as close to the lesion as possible. Once in place in the appropriate segmental bronchus, different types of brushes, linear or flexible, are introduced through this catheter (Pinet et al., 1973).

2. The instruments have been designed by Wilson and Eskridge (1970). They consist of a tracheal catheter and two polyethylene bronchial catheters, one of which can be introduced through the other. A flexible guidewire attached to the brush replaces the probe and is pointed in any direction, by means of a telescopic handhold (Coulomb, 1972).

Brushing is performed under local or general anaesthesia. The largest catheter is introduced under fluoroscopic control up to the appropriate bronchus, lobar or if possible segmental, corresponding to the area to be explored. A second catheter and sometimes a third one, by means of which the brush will reach the region, is pushed into the peripheral bronchial tree up to the lesion. This is the difficult part of the process. Televised frontal and lateral controls give information as to its location with respect to the lesion. After brushing, the brush is withdrawn within the second or third catheter to protect the collected cytological material from contamination by normal cells.

Microscopic slides are prepared immediately by spreading the brush on clean slides which are fixed at once in the fixative solution (ethyl alcohol − ether). It is extremely important to avoid the dessication of cells, which makes interpretation impossible. After brushing, a limited and selective, or global unilateral bronchogram, is performed. This bronchogram is essential as it may provide useful additional information.

Results

Our 177 cases were chosen because of peripheral lesions inaccessible to bronchoscopy and biopsy; and because of repeated negative cytology. Unfortunately, the latter are missing in some cases. Diagnosis relies on surgery and pathological control, or clinical evolution such as metastasis in the case of inoperable cancers, and death. As to benign lesions, the duration of follow-up was at least 10 months.

TABLE 1   *Contribution of bronchial brushing and bronchography to the diagnosis of pulmonary lesions for which all the other methods of investigation had failed*

BENIGN   CANCERS

	20 22.8% negative
	25 28.4% broncho-graphy
89	
	43 48.8% cytology

An analysis of our results is given in Table 1. This report is not a selection of the cases for which the lesion was reached by the brush and the cytologic material collected adequate. All cases submitted to brushing have been taken into account, even if the lesion was extrabronchial, or too peripheral to be reached by the brush, or if the material collected was inadequate for cytology.

Out of 88 cancers for which all other usual diagnostic techniques were negative, 43 gave a positive cytologic brushing. In additon, 25 cases were disclosed by the bronchogram. The false negatives are due to several reasons.

(a) Technical defects (Figs. 1 and 2)

The lesion may be difficult to reach by the brush and a previous bronchogram for guidance may be necessary. Or, by fluoroscopic control, in frontal projection, the brush seems located in contact with the tumor, but is in fact in a different segmental bronchus. The tumor may be too peripheral, out of reach of the brush, or extrabronchial. These technical failures are involved in 26 cases.

(b) Inadequate cytologic material

All the nuclear details on which the diagnosis rests, depend on good fixation performed immediately after brushing, thus avoiding dessication. This is an important source of misinterpretation.

In 10 patients, either the cells were scanty or poorly-fixed. In 5 cases, although the smears were covered with well-stained cells, there was no cytologic evidence of malignancy. One may wonder whether the brush had only reached the margin of the tumor, or whether, in cases of necrosis, no malignant cells may be found (Tsuboi et al., 1967).

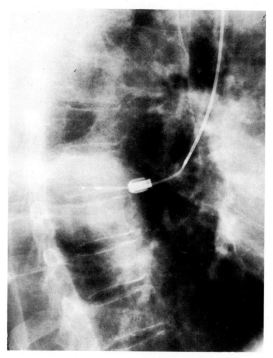

FIG. 1   *Lateral control radiograph showing the brush in place in the right segment of Fowler.*

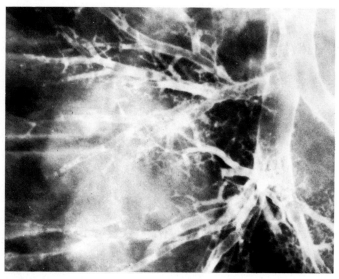

FIG. 2   *DUP... 33 years old. Lesion discovered by routine roentgenogram. The bronchoscopy is negative. The bronchogram shows a typical aspect of stop. Post-operative histological control has shown an epidermoid carcinoma of the right lower lobe.*

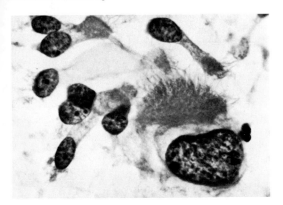

FIG. 3   *Among normal bronchial cells, a large ciliated cell with a hypertrophied nucleus. Gx1250. Reduced for reproduction 39%.*

(c) Problems of cytologic diagnosis

The appearance of cells directly scraped from the bronchus differs, somehow, from that of exfoliated cells. Some types of cell found in bronchial brushings are never found in sputa, such as scraped nuclei, large multinucleated cylindrical cells, groups of hyperplastic basal cells, etc. (Pison et al., 1973). (See Figs. 3 to 5).

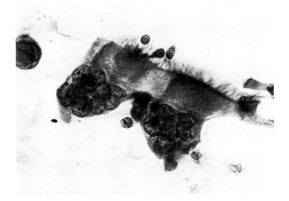

FIG. 4   *Multinucleated bronchial cells. Gx 1250. Reduced for reproduction 39%.*

In four cases, among our first specimens, no malignant cells were reported. After re-examination of the smears, a correct evaluation of severe dyskaryosis as malignant was made. There is no false-positive case in this group of patients.

If the cases of technical failure are discarded, if one takes into account only brushings of intrabronchic lesions, within the reach of the brush, 81.2% of malignant lesions are disclosed by this method (Pison et al., 1973). These results are in agreement with those published in the literature (Fenessy, 1966, 1968; Hattori et al., 1965, 1971; Wilson and Eskridge 1970).

Bronchial brushing is one among other methods of investigating peripheral pulmonary

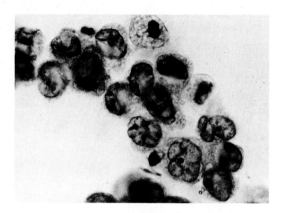

FIG. 5 *Malignant undifferentiated cells. Gx1250. Reduced for reproduction 39%.*

lesions. The more experienced the radiologist who guides the brush in the right segmental bronchus, and the more experienced the cytologist who reads the smears, with the help sometimes of a previous bronchogram with the use of a fibroscope, the number of cases escaping this method will undoubtedly decrease.

References

Coulomb, M. (1972): Ann. Radiol., 15/II–12,863.
Fenessy, J. J. (1966): Amer. J. Roentgenol., 98/2, 474.
Fenessy, J. J. (1968): Dis. Chest, 53/4,377.
Hattori, S., Matsuda, M., Nishihara, H. and Horai, T. (1971): Acta cytol. (Philad.), 15/5, 460.
Hattori, S., Matsuda, M., Sugiyama, T., Wada, A. and Terazawa, T. (1965): Dis. Chest, 48/2,123.
Pinet, F., Amiel, M., Pison, H., Rubet, A., Froment, J. C. and Scheou, A. (1973): Le brossage bronchique associé à la bronchographie. (In preparation).
Pinet, F., Amiel, M., Woehrle, R., Poizat, J. P. and Bonnevie, R. (1968): J. Radiol. Electrol., 49,87.
Pison, H., Augusseau., F., Pinet, F. and Coulomb, M. (1973): Cah. méd. lyon., (In press).
Tsuboi, E., Ikeda, S., Tajima, M., Shimosato, Y. and Ishikawa, S. (1967): Cancer (Philad.), 20,687.
Wilson, J. K. and Eskridge, M. (1970): Amer. J. Roentgenol., 109, 471.

3. *Results of screening campaigns for detection of uterine tumours*

Usefulness of a standardized nomenclature

G. Riotton

World Health Organization International Reference Center for Nomenclature in Cytology, Centre de Cytologie et de Dépistage du Cancer, Geneva, Switzerland

The efforts of the World Health Organization in this regard have now come to fruition and have been published as a book entitled: 'Cytology of the Female Genital Tract' which is accompanied by a set of matched Kodachromes (W.H.O., 1973). This book is No. 8 in the W.H.O. series 'International Histological Classification of Tumours'.

This was only achieved by a great deal of hard work and much discussion among the members of the W.H.O. International Reference Center for Nomenclature in Cytology, who were chosen for their professional competence. They represent different points of view in cytopathology on a world-wide basis.

Some of you will probably question why so much effort is being made to establish an internationally agreed nomenclature. The reason is simple: without adequate communication, progress is hampered, no valuable comparison will be feasible between workers in the same field, for example, between Cancer Registries. Epidemiologic studies cannot be compared, or even made, if the people involved call the same lesion by different names or, as sometimes happens, different lesions by the same name.

This is most important for the clinician who, because of his responsibility to the patient, must always be assured that he understands what the cytologist means.

Needless to say, a prerequisite is an adequate technical procedure, especially of the way in which cytological – and pathological – specimens are worked up. There are still too many so-called 'evaluation of screening programmes' which are totally meaningless and could be very misleading. Most of the time, this is due to inaccuracies of the input of the basic data from the cytopathological laboratory, be it due to inadequate training of personnel, or to a lack of strict criteria for the many aspects of quality control. In this regard, I may cite the absolute necessity of rejecting any inadequate specimens. These errors lead the statistician astray and produce meaningless evaluation and, I quote from the W.H.O. book: 'Although it is widely accepted that effective uterine cancer control can be achieved by means of mass screening, cytodiagnosis can do more harm than good if not properly performed: existing cancers may be missed, so that the patient is given a false sense of security, and the appearance of cells from non-cancerous lesions may be misinterpreted.'

We know that, today, neither cytology nor histology are able to predict accurately the future of many of these lesions. We know too that there may be different types of lesion looking more-or-less alike under the microscope, but having a very different evolution. It is for these reasons that the terms agreed on in cytology must describe a lesion, and should not have a prognostic implication, until we know more about their natural history. I quote again from the W.H.O. book: 'The commonly used system of numerical classification to indicate the cytopathologist's opinion as to the degree of probability that a particular lesion is cancer has led to confusion, because the numerical designation varies from one laboratory to another. Now that cytopathologists are better able to recognize the nature of histological lesions on the basis of cell studies, it is both desirable and feasible that cytology reports should be formulated so as to correspond to the anticipated histological diagnosis.'

Now I want to emphasize, and you should remember, that a nomenclature is never established forever; it is a tentative, more-or-less good, list of definitions on which one may classify for some time, thus permitting data to be compared. However, it can be reevaluated from time to time, as scientific knowledge changes.

Reference

W.H.O. (1973): Cytology of the Female Genital Tract. International Histological Classification of Tumours Series, No. 8, World Health Organization, Geneva.

Cancer of uterine cervix - preventable disease: A study of Indian women

Usha K. Luthra

Indian Council of Medical Research, New Delhi, India

Introduction

Cancer of the uterine cervix is the most frequent neoplasm among women in India, accounting for 20 to 50% of all neoplasms (Chitkara et al., 1966; Khanolkar, 1950; Mali et al., 1968; Paymaster, 1964; Shanta, 1965; Wahi et al., 1969). This information is based upon the relative distribution of cancers. More critical data on incidence in defined populations also verify the high occurrence of cancer of the uterine cervix in India (Jussawalla et al., 1968, 1970).

The concept that cancer of the uterine cervix does not arise from a normal epithelium but is preceded by a spectrum of epithelial abnormalities, which are recognizable, has widened the scope of prevention of this cancer and early detection of such precancerous pathology by exfoliative cytology on a larger proportion of population. Timely detection, follow-up and adequate treatment of these epithelial abnormalities, make prevention of this tumour an acceptable possibility.

The incidence and distribution of this tumour varies in different parts of the country. This variation may be due to differences in habits, customs and socio-economic conditions of the inhabitants of different parts of India (Wahi et al., 1969).

Material, methods and results

Experimental studies

In order to project uterine cancer as a preventable disease, it is essential to understand its natural history, and to realise the extent of reversibility of the precancerous pathological lesions.

To achieve this objective of studying the sequence of epithelial changes during the development of cancer of the uterine cervix, an experimental model was planned, using 150 specially bred, swiss albino, virgin female mice, 2 to 3 months of age. 80 of these were painted intravaginally biweekly with 1% solution of 3:4 benzpyrene in acetone. The remaining 70 mice served as acetone painted controls (Luthra, 1970). Each of the carcinogen-painted mice revealed 'dysplastic' changes in the exfoliated cells. On the basis of cytologic and histologic changes, 4 distinct lesions were encountered during progressive experimental cervical carcinogenesis: (1) acute inflammation of cervical and vaginal epithelium, (2) epithelial dysplastic changes, which depending on the severity and extent of the lesion were classified into mild, moderate and severe dysplastic lesions, (3) epidermoid carcinoma in situ, (4) invasive epidermoid carcinoma.

I will briefly illustrate the important observations of this experimental model.

With continued painting, cervical epithelial dysplastic lesions were encountered. The essential change is in the nucleus which is always enlarged and/or hyperchromatic. The cells show varying degrees of differentiation. By and large more differentiated cell types correspond to the milder forms of dysplasia.

Mild dysplasia   Cells frequently encountered are the superficial or intermediate types and only rarely, a few parabasal cells. Chromatin pattern is always uniform. Numerous small chromocentres may be recognized.

Moderate dysplasia   In addition to superficial and intermediate cells, a fair number of parabasal cells are also seen. Chromatin pattern is coarse. An occasional enlarged chromocentre may be seen.

Severe dysplasia   Cells encountered are mainly of the parabasal and small intermediate type. Chromatin pattern is dense and uniform, with many darkly stained, somewhat enlarged chromocentres. No nucleoli are discerned.

Cells derived from epidermoid carcinoma in situ   These cells are characterized by the presence of poorly differentiated and undifferentiated squamous epithelial cells derived from deeper layers and revealing marked nuclear abnormalities. Nuclear and cytoplasmic ratio is increased. Hyperchromatic and coarsely granular chromatin network is seen. Histologically the entire thickness of the epithelium shows evidence of neoplasia with an intact basement membrane.

Cells derived from invasive epidermoid carcinoma   The cellular sample corresponds to the histologic picture. The most frequently encountered tumours were the keratinizing carcinomas showing a preponderance of abnormal cells with a high degree of pleomorphism characterized by caudate and elongate forms. The chromatin pattern is coarse, irregular and there are several dense chromocentres. Nuclear degeneration characterized by an opaque nuclear mass is an important feature.

These experiments did help in revealing the natural history of a progressive epithelial lesion, but the crucial question, as to at what level the mucosal changes are irreversible – still remained unanswered. With this in mind, another series of experimental design to determine the reversibility of cervical dysplastic lesions in the mouse uterine cervix was designed.

Depending on the number of carcinogen paintings, the evaluation of cervical epithelial dysplastic changes in carcinogen-painted mice could be grouped as follows:

Dyplasia	⟶	Regression to normalcy (7.5%).
Dysplasia	⟶	Persisting (52.2%).
Dysplasia	⟶	Progression to higher grade (8.7%).
Dysplasia	⟶	Carcinoma in situ (10.5%).
Dysplasia	⟶	Invasive carcinoma (21.1%).

TABLE 1   *Evaluation and biological behaviour of experimentally induced cervical dysplasia*

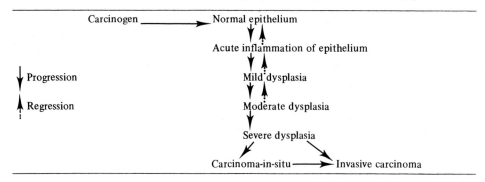

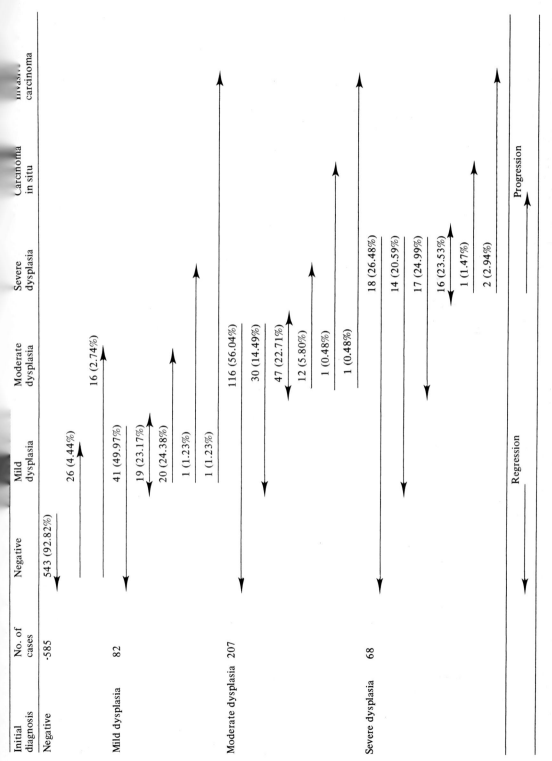

These experiments seem to indicate that several factors are involved in the pathogenesis of experimental cervical carcinogenesis. There appears to be a key point at which progression of cellular atypia does not occur without further stimulation with a carcinogen. There also appears to be a stage beyond which there is a progression to invasive carcinoma even without further stimulation. The variety of physiochemical cellular studies by Christopherson (1969) on cellular and nuclear area, anhydrous nuclear mass, nuclear water content, nuclear DNA and cellular RNA, accurately reflect the stage of atypia beyond which the lesion is irreversible. Dysplastic changes confined primarily to the cytoplasm of the cells are most frequently reversible than the nuclear one. Regression to normalcy occurred up to the stage of moderate dysplasia only in our series of experiments. Finding of markedly dysplastic cells was looked upon with suspicion as they invariably precede cancers in experimental animals. Evolution and biological behaviour of cervical dysplasia can be seen in Table 1.

You would agree with me that application of these results to human females is to be done with caution as the human cervix cannot have a set pattern of reponse to a carcinogen as in the experimental model.

Human studies

We conducted a screening programme for 3 years (1960–63) at the Cancer Research Centre, S.N. Medical College, Agra (Mali et al., 1967). During this period a total of 38,707 women were examined clinically and cytologically. Of these, 676(17.5/1000) showed evidence of invasive epidermoid carcinoma and 17(0.4/1000) showed evidence of carcinoma in situ. All these cases were confirmed on histological examination. 941(24.31/1000) showed evidence of dysplastic lesions.

A second screening programme was conducted for another 4 years i.e. from late 1966 to 1970 in the same population. A total of 26,110 women were screened cytologically. Of these, 162(6.2/1000) showed evidence of invasive epidermoid carcinoma and (0.1/1000) showed evidence of carcinoma in situ. All these cases had histological examination done. 1,641(62.8/1000) cases showed evidence of dysplastic lesions. These results are significant when compared with the results of the first screening programme. In the second study the number of cancer cases had gone up significantly as compared to the first study.

We have carefully followed 357 women with cervical dysplastic lesions along with a control group at the cancer unit, Agra, for a period of 9 years as shown in Table 2.

This follow-up study reveals that a majority of the cases i.e. 66.10% regressed, 22.97% showed persistence of initial lesion, 9.21% progressed to higher grades of dysplasia and 1.6% progressed to malignancy during the period of 4–9 years.

Etiological factors associated with the occurrence of uterine cervical cancer in this investigation are consistent with the findings of other workers (Khanolkar, 1950; Jussawalla et al., 1970).

Prevalence rate of uterine cervical cancer in Hindu females was approximately twice of that in Muslim females (Table 3). This shows that the risk of developing cervical cancer among Muslim females is less than that of Hindu females in spite of early marriage and

TABLE 3   *Frequency distribution and prevalence rate by religion*

Religion	Total No. of women	Cervical cancer cases	Prevalence rate/1000
Hindu	23,850	158	6.62
Muslim	2,186	7	3.20
Christian	74	–	–
Total	26,110	165	6.32

TABLE 4   *Frequency distribution and prevalence rate of cervical cancer cases by age among the total number of women examined and interviewed*

Age (years)	Total No. of women	Cervical cancer cases	Prevalence rate/1000
20–29	12,902	3	0.23
30–39	8,097	42	5.18
40–49	3,482	57	16.37
50–59	1,065	28	26.26
60 and above	564	35	61.83

TABLE 5   *Prevalence rate according to age at marriage*

Age at marriage (years)	Total No. of subjects	Cervical carcinoma	Rate/1000
14 and below	12,090	92	7.61
15–19	12,586	70	5.50
20 and above	1,434	3	2.09
Total	26,110	165	6.32

TABLE 6   *Prevalence rate according to number of pregnancies*

No. of pregnancies	Total No. of subjects	Cervical carcinoma	Rate/1000
(Nullipara)	4,091	3	0.73
1–2	6,814	16	2.35
3–4	5,816	30	5.16
5–6	4,335	31	7.15
7–8	2,638	33	12.50
9 and above	2,416	52	21.52
Total	26,110	165	6.32

higher pregnancies. This major difference of prevalence rates between these 2 religious groups may be due to the custom of circumcision among Muslim males.

This study had also brought out a definite relationship with age. Age specific prevalence rates increase with the advancement of age (Table 4).

Uterine cervix cancer patients had married earlier and had produced more children compared to healthy control women (Table 5).

Early marriage and multipe pregnancies are significant factors for high prevalence of uterine cervical cancer in our study (Table 6).

Discussion

The exact significance of dysplastic changes and their role in the pathogenesis of cervical carcinoma is still not clear. It is tempting to speculate that epithelial dysplastic lesions are intermediary lesions somewhere between the inflammatory lesion and carcinoma of the cervix specially in the pre-invasive stage. We prefer to reserve the term carcinoma in situ for changes in the epithelium that we feel are not likely to revert to normalcy. A majority of our follow-up cases of dysplasia have either regressed or remained stationary over a period of follow-up to 9 years. We thus conceive of dysplasia as a potentially dangerous, but non-carcinomatous lesion, which has not achieved the autonomy of growth that carcinoma in situ has. Dysplastic reactions are quite possible due to a variety of both carcinogenic and non-carcinogenic agents, with evidence favouring the latter in the majority of instances. An important problem the solution of which has eluded till now is the cytological of histomorphological distinction between the two types.

It is postulated that in humans, carcinoma in situ is a lesion produced by a carcinogen. It has attained autonomy of growth and may progress to invasive carcinoma if the lesion is not destroyed provided the life span of the host is sufficiently long. Dysplasia on the other hand, may result from a carcinogenic stimulation, or may arise as a result of a non-carcinogenic stimulation. This could account for the fact that while progression of dysplasia to carcinoma does occur in some cases, it more often does not. A varied biological behaviour of cases of cervical dysplasia emphasizes the need for a careful and prolonged follow-up in these cases.

Summary

Cancer of the uterine cervix is the most frequent neoplasm among women in India. The recognition of biological behaviour of cervical epithelium to a carcinogen with its progressive pathological changes ending in dysplasia, carcinoma in situ and invasive carcinoma, and the recognition of the possible reversible potentiality of the dysplastic lesions, has made cancer of the cervix a preventable disease. However, it implies early detection of the precancerous pathology and its subjection to adequate therapy. Exfoliative cytology has been found to be an extremely useful tool for such detection procedure. Cancer of the cervix is a public health problem today and the mass screening of women should form a part of the regular health check-up.

Epidemiological studies highlight the role of factors like religion, early marriage and multiple pregnancies associated with high prevalence of uterine cervical carcinoma.

References

Chitkara, N. L., Chugh, T. D. and Arya, R. K. (1966): Indian J. Cancer, 3, 94.
Christopherson, W. M. (1969): Obstet. gynec. Surv., 24, 842.
Jussawalla, D. J., Deshpande, V. A., Haenszel, W. and Natekar, M. V. (1970): Brit. J. Cancer, 25, 56.
Jussawalla, D. J., Haenszel, W., Deshpande, V. A. and Natekar, M. V. (1968): Brit. J. Cancer, 22, 623.
Khanolkar, V. R. (1950): Acta int. Un. Cancer, 6, 881.
Luthra, U. K. (1970): Indian J. med.Res., 58, 1.
Mali, S., Wahi, P. N. and Luthra, U. K. (1968): Indian J. Cancer, 5, 269.
Mali, S., Wahi, P. N., Luthra. U. K. and Kapur, V. L. (1967): Cancer, 20, 623.
Paymaster, J. C. (1964): Cancer, 17, 1026.
Shanta, V. (1965): Indian J. Cancer, 2, 142.
Shanta, V. and Krishnamurthi, S. (1969): Brit. J. Cancer, 23, 693.
Wahi, P. N., Mali, S. and Luthra, U. K. (1969): Cancer, 23, 1221.

Cytological mass screening of cancer of the uterine cervix in the province of Florence

Luciano Gambassini

Centro di Medicina Sociale, Provincia di Firenze, Florence, Italy

The cytological mass screening of the uterine cervix is part of a multiphasic screening programme for some social diseases (neoplastic, cardiovascular, dismetabolic and occupational ones) organized by the Province of Florence since 1964. The smears are free of charge executed by midwives in 80 municipal out-patient clinics located all over the Province, by gynecologists and at our Center.

Here the smears are examined, the results sent out and suspected women recalled for colposcopy and eventual biopsy. The family doctor is entrusted with the positive cases and he receives also general directions as to the measures to be taken; moreover the Center sees that these directions are carried out and performs the follow-up of the women.

The smears executed from April 1964 to the 28th of February 1973 were 247,000 but the number of patients the statistical data worked through so far, is 123,491 and it goes from April 15th, 1964 to August the 31st, 1970 (Table 1).

The highest number of smears were taken in the out-patients' clinics by the midwives (32.9%) and at the Center (37.2%) (Table 2). A great majority of the women examined are married (84.70%) (Table 3). The increment of the smears progresses with years, particularly in bigger Communes; however, the women who repeated the exam in the considered period of time were only the 24% and in most cases only once. The highest response has been from those between 31 and 50 years of age and the lowest from those between 51 and 70 years of age (Table 4).

TABLE 1   *Total material studied*

No. of cytological smears examined (April 16,1964–February 28,1973)	247,000
No. of cases statistically studied (April 16,1964–August 31,1970)	123,491

TABLE 2   *Number of cases examined by different out-patient clinics*

Clinic	No.	%
Social medicine centre	45,930	37.2
Midwives	40,580	32.9
Gynaecologists	17,806	14.4
Others	19,175	15.5
Total	123,491	

TABLE 3   *Distribution of women by civil status*

Status	No.	%
Married	76,073	84.70
Unmarried	5,519	5.70
Widows	3,630	4.04
Non-specified	4,993	5.56
Total	89,815	100.00

TABLE 4   *Age distribution of women examined for uterine cancer prevention*

Age group	No.	%
20	1,636	1.8
21−30	16,462	18.3
31−40	25,986	28.9
41−50	25,628	28.6
51−60	11,884	13.2
61−70	4,579	5.2
71−80	1,179	1.3
80	115	0.1
Unknown	2,276	2.6
Total	89,745	100.0

However, since two invasive and two in situ cancers were found in the age-group 21-30, and 66 invasive and 6 in situ in the age-group 30-60, it is important to emphasize the need for a regular and extensive health education activity among the very young and the older age-groups of women.

The morbidity quotient study from 1,000 cases examined according to age-groups, and correlated with the histological diagnosis, shows how invasive cancer increases constantly from 30 (0.08°/oo) to over the 70 year age-group (16.48°/oo) (Table 5).

TABLE 5   *Quotients of morbidity out of 1,000 cases according to age-groups*

Age-group	Invasive cancer	In situ cancer	Dysplasia	Benign pathology	Total
30	0.08	0.47	−	0.35	0.90
31−40	0.91	0.46	0.51	0.88	3.76
41−50	2.51	2.51	0.52	1.42	6.96
51−60	7.04	1.96	0.35	2.36	11.71
61−70	11.31	1.02	0.34	3.42	10.10
70	16.48	1.97	0.66	3.96	23.07
Total	2.79	1.66	0.38	1.31	6.14

On the other hand the lowest morbidity quotient for cancer in situ is under 30 years of age, increasing up to 2.50°/oo , in the 41 to 50 year age-group and decreasing again in the following years.

Dysplasia does not show rough differences in the various age-groups while benign pathology increases progressively with time, passing from 0.35°/oo among the under 30's to 3.96°/oo among the over 70's.

If we consider the distribution in absolute numbers of the histological diagnosis according to the age of the women examined, we once again have confirmation that the highest incidence of invasive cancer is between 41 and 60 years of age, whereas cancer in situ has its highest incidence between 31 and 50 years of age (Table 6).

TABLE 6   *Distribution of histological diagnosis according to age-groups*

Age-group	Invasive cancer	In situ cancer	Dysplasia	Benign pathology	Total
< 30	2	11	–	8	21
31–40	34	54	19	33	140
41–50	98	98	20	55	271
51–60	119	33	6	40	198
61–70	66	6	2	20	94
70 >	25	3	1	6	35
Total	344	205	48	162	759

However, these figures are likely to be influenced by the different rate of response to the screening among the various age-groups and by the natural elimination curve for general mortality in elderly women.

The most meaningful data – with a view to correlate the progressive decrease of invasive cancer of the cervix with the cytological screening – are evident from Table 7, which shows that in our Province the incidence of the invasive cancer passed from 7.95 out of 1,000 cases examined in 1965 to 0.87°/oo in 1970.

TABLE 7   *Yearly quotients of morbidity out of 1,000 cases (1964–1970)*

Year	Invasive cancer	In situ cancer	Dysplasia	Benign pathology	Total
1964	16.20	5.04	0.65	4.81	26.70
1965	7.95	4.08	0.68	2.38	15.09
1966	4.34	3.47	0.39	2.76	10.96
1967	1.54	1.19	0.41	0.62	3.76
1968	2.07	1.04	0.37	1.11	4.59
1969	1.30	1.28	0.22	0.80	3.60
1970	0.87	0.58	0.42	0.87	2.74
Total	2.79	1.66	0.38	1.31	6.14

TABLE 8   *Ascertained cases of cancer and survival rates*

Positive or suspected cases	No.	%
(15/4/1964–31/3/1973)	1,241	10.1

Survival rates for 868 cases after 5 years		
Invasive cancers	269	60
In situ cancers	599	all living

This figure would be even more gratifying if we established as starting point the 16.20°/oo of 1964, but we do not take it into account, because it is assumed that during the first functioning year of the Center there was an attendance of mainly symptomatic women, and often in an advanced stage of neoplastic disease. Cancer in situ too passed from 4.08°/oo in 1965 to 0.58°/oo in 1970. The decrease of cancer in situ is perhaps due to the fall of the benign pathology (cervicitis, trichomoniasis, etc.) which declined from 4.81°/oo to 0.87°/oo in 1970, perhaps because female hygiene standards are getting better.

In the same period, dysplasia has fallen from 0.65°/oo to 0.42°/oo. The relatively short observation time and the rather low number of women who repeated the exam in these years hinder us from seeing whether dysplasia and subsequently cancer in situ reappears frequently.

Morbidity quotient, with histological diagnosis out of 1,000 women examined, shows the 2.79°/oo invasive cancers, the 1.66°/oo cancer in situ and 0.38°/oo dysplasias, as data very close to that in the literature.

Out of the cases examined so far with 255,000 smears, 13,000 women were recalled for colposcopic exam and eventual biopsy; 1,500 operated or suspected women are being followed-up permanently.

Though the period of our cytological service is relatively short to draw definitive conclusions, it seems rather important to establish that 269 women who presented with a cancer in situ are all living, whereas out of the 599 women affected with invasive cancer 40% had already died after 5 years.

In the 123,491 cases statistically examined, the cytological exams have ascertained 10.1°/oo positive or suspected cases for cancer, a figure in accordance with the most important screening programmes in the world (Table 8).

Cytological screening, besides realising an almost total disappearance of invasive cancer, led us to treat most cancer in situ with the conisation, thus preserving the normal function of the uterine cervix. We think it is interesting to point out that the conisation represents an important help to diagnostic definition.

In fact, histological exam of the cone, carried out in 171 cases, has confirmed the presence of cancer in situ in 64.3%, whereas in 8.7% aimed biopsy had already removed all the cellular atypic nest and in the other cases proved to be a matter of dysplasia.

Results of cytological screening for early diagnosis of precancerous changes and tumours of the uterus, in Bologna and Province (1966-1972)

Cesare Maltoni, Anna Palazzini and Maria Teresa Faccioli

Istituto di Oncologia 'F. Addarii' and Centro Tumori, Bologna, Italy

Screening for the early diagnosis of precancerous lesions and tumours of the uterus is performed in Bologna and Province by the Istituto di Oncologia and by Centro Tumori,

TABLE 1   *Distribution of the examined women by cytological classes*

Cytological class	No. of women	$^o/_{oo}$
I and II	220,029	983.86
II–III and III	2,768	12.38
IV	526	2.35
V	316	1.41
Total	223,639*	1,000.00

* 57,304 women underwent one or more examinations

TABLE 2   *Results to date*

Results	No.		$^o/_{oo}$*
Carcinomas	648		2.89
Preneoplastic lesions	420		1.88
Leukoplakias of various degrees		286	1.28
Dysplasias		80	0.36
Leukoplakias and dysplasias associated		54	0.24
Cytologically positive, or suspicious, or doubtful, or abnormal cases not confirmed by biopsy	153		0.68
Cytological classes: V		2	0.01
IV		27	0.12
II–III and III		124	0.55
Cytologically positive, or suspicious, or doubtful, or abnormal cases not yet biopsied	2,613		11.68
Cytological classes: V		36	0.16
IV		139	0.62
II–III and III		2,438	10.90

* With reference to total number of examined cases: 223,639

TABLE 3   *Characteristics of the detected carcinomas*

Localization	No.	%	Extension	No.	%	Histological type	No.	%
Corpus	9	1.39	In situ	5	0.77	Adenocarcinomas	5	0.77
			Invasive	4	0.62	Adenocarcinomas	4	0.62
Cervix	631	97.38	In situ	417	64.35	Squamous cell carcinomas	411	63.43
						Adenocarcinomas	6	0.92
			Microinvasive	61	9.42	Squamous cell carcinomas	60	9.26
						Adenocarcinomas	1	0.16
			Invasive	153	23.61	Squamous cell carcinomas	141	21.76
						Adenocarcinomas	12	1.85
Vagina	3	0.46	In situ	1	0.15	Squamous cell carcinomas	1	0.15
			Invasive	2	0.31	Squamous cell carcinomas	2	0.31
Vulva	5	0.77	In situ	3	0:46	Squamous cell carcinomas	3	0.46
			Invasive	2	0.31	Squamous cell carcinomas	2	0.31

TABLE 4   *Distribution of the detected in situ carcinomas by their cytological type*

Type	Carcinomas definitely in situ No.	Carcinomas in situ in which an early invasive tendency cannot be definitely excluded No.	Total No.
Alpha	132 (59.19%)	44 (37.93%)	176 (51.92%)
Beta	77 (34.53%)	59 (50.86%)	136 (40.12%)
Gamma	14 (6.28%)	13 (11.21%)	27 (7.96%)
Total	223 (100.00%)	116 (100.00%)	339 (100.00%)

with the collaboration of the Local Public Health Service (Hospitals and Open Clinics).

From January 1966 to November 1972, 233,639 women out of the 250,000 in the age-group (over 28) at risk underwent colpocytological examinations. 57,304 had two or more examinations.

The general distribution of the examined women, by cytological classes, is shown in Table 1. The results to date are presented in Table 2. The 38 cytologically positive cases (class V) and the 166 suspected cases (class IV), not yet confirmed, are now under ascertainment. The 2,562 women with abnormal or mildly atypical cytological pictures (classes II-III, III) are kept under frequent examinations. The localization, the extension and the histological type of the 648 carcinomas is reported in Table 3.

TABLE 5   *Distribution of carcinomas and preneoplastic lesions by age*

| Age (years) | Patients with carcinomas | | | | Patients with prenoplastic lesions |
	Total No.	In situ No.	Microinvasive No.	Invasive No.	No.
20 – 29	12 (1.85%)	11 (2.60%)	1 (1.61%)	–	29 (6.90%)
30 – 39	160 (24.69%)	120 (28.37%)	17 (27.42%)	23 (14.11%)	112 (26.67%)
40 – 49	235 (36.27%)	154 (36.41%)	31 (50.00%)	50 (30.68%)	171 (40.71%)
50 – 59	155 (23.92%)	98 (23.17%)	10 (16.13%)	47 (28.83%)	79 (18.81%)
60 – 69	72 (11.11%)	35 (8.27%)	2 (3.23%)	35 (21.47%)	23 (5.48%)
70 – 79	13 (2.01%)	5 (1.18%)	1 (1.61%)	7 (4.30%)	5 (1.19%)
80 – 89	1 (0.15%)	–	–	1 (0.61%)	1 (0.24%)
Total	648 (100.00%)	423 (100.00%)	62 (100.00%)	163 (100.00%)	420 (100.00%)

339 in situ carcinomas have been classified as alpha, beta or gamma, following the cytohistological criteria of Von Haam (Von Haam and Old, 1964; Old et al., 1965) (Table 4) based upon squamous differentiation (of decreasing degree from alpha to gamma). In our series of cases, the number of alpha in situ carcinomas is the highest.

Table 5 shows the distribution by age of tumours and preneoplastic lesions. Both preneoplastic lesions and carcinomas, although not frequent, are however not rare under the age of 30; the largest number has been found between 40 and 50 years.

The colpocytological control in the Bologna Province met with the favour of women and is now a permanent Public Health Service.

References

Old, J.W., Wielenga, G. and Von Haam, E. (1965): Cancer (Philad.), 18, 1598.
Von Haam, E. and Old, J.W. (1964): In: Dysplasia, carcinoma in situ and micro-invasive carcinoma of the cervix uteri, pp. 41-84. Editor: L.A. Gray. Charles C. Thomas, Springfield, Ill.

New ways of reducing morbidity and mortality from cancer of the uterine cervix

L.I. Charkviani, R.A. Chitiashvili, D.D. Gogeliani and T.I. Kvesitadze

Institute of Oncology, Ministry of Health, Tbilisi, Georgia, U.S.S.R.

We have not as yet achieved any appreciable reduction in morbidity and mortality from cancers of the uterine cervix, although the preventive measures taken have been quite extensive and the advances in clinical oncology are obvious.

One of the possible reasons for the growth of morbidity and mortality from malignant tumours in economically developed countries is the significant increase of the average lifespan of people and, consequently, the increase in the number of aged people. However, this cannot be the explanation in the case of cervical cancer because the incidence of malignant tumours in this organ falls sharply at advanced age (Charkviani, 1964; Glebova, 1971; Merkov, 1956; Serebrov, 1968).

The failure of the morbidity and mortality from cervical cancer to decline might be caused by the inadequacy of existing preventive organizational measures. Reconsideration of these measures may be necessary.

If the reduction of morbidity from cervical cancer depends on the discovery and effective treatment of pre-cancerous disease, then the reduction of mortality will primarily depend on the early diagnosis of cervical cancer.

The early diagnosis of invasive cancer is considered to be its discovery at the first stage of the disease. The range of the size of the first stage tumour is quite wide, and some reasons for the difference in the results of first stage cancer treatment in different hospitals might lie in the size of the tumour.

In order to define the concept of early diagnosis 172 patients at the first stage of the disease were studied for the long-term results of complex treatment with respect to the size of the tumour. Depending on the size determined after a thorough examination of the ablated uterine preparation, patients were divided into three groups.

In the first group (17 patients with clinical microcarcinomas) the maximum diameter of the tumour was 0.5 cm. In the second group (92 patients with the first phase of the

TABLE 1   *Long-term results of complex treatment of cancer of the uterine cervix at the first stage, in relation to the size of the tumour*

Size of the tumour	Patients under study					
	3 years			5 years		
	Total	Completely cured		Total	Completely cured	
		No.	%		No.	%
Microcarcinoma $\leqslant$ 0.5 cm	17	17	100	8	8	100
First phase 0.5 – 1.2 cm	92	81	88	50	41	82
Second phase $\geqslant$ 1.2 cm	63	49	77.8	17	12	70.6
Total	172	147	85.5	75	61	81.3

first stage), the size 0.5—1.2 cm; while in the third group (the second phase of the first stage), patients had tumours above 1.2 cm in diameter.

Three years after complex treatment of the 172 patients (Table 1), 147 (85.5%) had completely recovered, 17 (9.9%) had died, while 8 (4.6%) were lost to follow-up. All 17 patients with microcarcinomas were alive after 3 years. At the first phase of the first stage, 81 (88%) patients were completely healthy, and at the second phase, only 49 (77.8%); mortality at the first and second phases was 8.7% and 14.3%, respectively. Of the 75 patients at the first stage of the disease, 81% (61 patients) survived 5 years and were completely healthy, while 10.7% (8 patients) had died; the fate of 8% (6 women) is unknown.

Five years following the complex treatment all the patients with microcarcinoma had survived. At the first phase of the first stage 82% (41 patients) were completely healthy, while at the second stage, only 12 patients (70.6%) were healthy. Therefore, when at the first stage the tumour is small, complex treatment provides a complete recovery, although at the succeeding first and second phases, the effect reduces by 15% and 26.5%, respectively. As a tumour grows, the regional lymphatic nodes become gradually populated by mestastases. Large tumours are mostly observed with endophytic growth and adenocarcinomas. Nowadays we consider the early diagnosis of cervical cancer to be the discovery of the disease when the diameter of the tumour is less than 0.5 cm.

An essential way of avoiding late diagnosis of cervical cancer is the examination of the cervical canal. 256 patients with different stages of cervical cancer were examined and studied to find the reason for late diagnosis. Three were found: an asymptomatic course of the disease (18.1%); carelessness of the patients (42%); specialists working at the maternity welfare centres and gynaecological services lacked experience (39.9%). Therefore, we have established special centres guiding all the activities of prevention and early diagnosis of cervical cancer.

The effect of this new measure has been studied in one district of Tbilisi.

The experimental preventive centres were provided with all the facilities necessary to early diagnosis (colposcopy, cytology, autoradiography, Charkviani-Kharatishvili's cervical speculum). Diathermic surgery is also used extensively in treatment.

Each preventive centre is also provided with a specially trained gynaecologist from the maternity welfare centres. General preventive examinations are carried out at factories and enterprises, while housewives are invited to the centres by mail. All women above 30 are supposed to visit the centres twice a year, free of charge.

The preventive centres arrange a special examination of women with ruptures of the cervix uteri; also, examinations are arranged for patients with precancerous changes of the cervix.

Analysis of the work of the experimental centres of tumour prevention has shown the great effectiveness of this innovation: the number of cases of invasive cancer of the

TABLE 2   *Rate of morbidity of cancer of the uterine cervix in one of the districts of Tbilisi before and after the establishment of preventive centres*

Period	Pre-invasive cancer of the uterine cancer	Cancer of the uterine cervix	Stages			
			I	II	III	IV
Before establishment, 1967—1968	—	47	13 27.6%	24 51.0%	8 17.1%	2 4.3%
After establishment, 1970—1971	10	30	18 60.0%	9 30.0%	3 10.0%	—

cervix has dropped by one third (Table 2), while the diagnosis of the first stage has doubled. Neglected forms no longer occur in this district and finally, in 10 cases the disease was revealed in its pre-invasive form, i.e., at stage zero.

Conclusions

(1) We have concluded that the early diagnosis of cervical cancer is its discovery when the diameter of the tumour is less than 0.5 cm.

(2) The reasons for the late diagnosis of cervical cancer are the following: an asymptomatic course of the disease (18.1%); patients' carelessness in respect of their health (42%); and the lack of experience in oncology of the specialists at the maternity welfare centres and gynaecological services (39.9%).

(3) Organization of special preventive centres headed by specially-trained gynaecologists might sharply reduce morbidity and improve the early diagnosis of cancer of the uterine cervix.

References

Charkviani, L. I. (1964): Nekotozye Voprosy Raka Zhenskikh Polovykh Organov (Female Genital Cancer). Sabchota Sakartvelo, Tbilisi.
Glebova, M. I. (1971): Rak Matki v SSSR (Cancer of the Uterus in the USSR). Thesis, Moscow.
Merkov, A. M. (1956): Vop. Onkol., 6, 752.
Serebrov, A. I. (1968): Rak Matki (Cancer of the Uterus). Meditsina, Moscow.

Evolution, experience and achievements of a uterine cancer detection program in Puerto Rico

I. Martinez

Cancer Control Program, Department of Health, Santurce, Puerto Rico

Introduction

Puerto Rico is an Island of the West Indies located in the Caribbean Sea. Its 3,315 square miles are inhabited by 2,722,000 people, of whom almost half are women (1,388,000). This gives a population density of 821 inhabitants per square mile. Fifty three per cent of the women are 20 years and older (731,000).

The problem

Since 1957, cancer has become the second leading cause of death in Puerto Rico among both men and women.

Cancer of the uterine cervix has been the most frequent malignancy among women, being responsible for 1 out of every 4 malignant tumors in this sex. Among the 5 most frequent sites in women, cancer of the cervix predominates over skin, breast, colon and

TABLE 1   *The five most frequent cancer sites in females (Puerto Rico, 1970)*

Site	No. of cases	%	Rates	
			Crude*	Age-adjusted**
Uterine cervix	628	24.7	45.2	37.9
Skin	469	18.4	33.8	22.4
Breast	272	10.7	19.6	14.9
Colon and rectum	162	6.4	11.7	7.8
Stomach	127	5.0	9.1	5.8
All sites	2,545	100.0	183.3	133.6

*   Crude rates per 100,000
**   Adjusted to 1950 Puerto Rico census population

rectum, and stomach, and this cancer site has always ranked first (Table 1). The incidence of cancer of the uterine cervix has increased steadily with time from 29.6 per 100,000 women in 1950, to 45.2 in 1970 (Table 2). However, mortality from cancer of the uterus has decreased very significantly in the last 21 years: from 20.6 deaths per 100,000 in 1950, to 12.5 in 1970 (Table 3).

TABLE 2   *Incidence of cancer of the uterine cervix (Puerto Rico, 1950–1970)*

Year	No. of cases	Rates	
		Crude*	Adjusted**
1950	321	29.6	29.6
1955	315	28.1	26.7
1960	379	33.9	28.4
1965	515	38.7	35.3
1967	572	41.9	38.2
1968	504	36.6	32.0
1969	519	37.1	32.5
1970	628	45.2	37.9

*   Crude rates per 100,000 females
**   Rates adjusted by age to 1950 census of Puerto Rico

TABLE 3   *Mortality from cancer of the uterus (Puerto Rico, 1950–1970)*

Year	Deaths	Rates	
		Crude*	Age-adjusted**
1950	228	20.6	20.6
1955	199	17.9	16.3
1960	182	16.4	13.3
1965	152	11.4	9.3
1967	163	11.9	9.4
1968	175	12.7	10.0
1969	155	11.1	8.5
1970	173	12.5	8.8

*   Crude rates per 100,000 females
**   Adjusted to Puerto Rico census population 1950

The program

In 1952, the Detection Program started with a demonstration and training clinic at the School of Medicine of the University of Puerto Rico. The number of women screened during the first 5 years was limited to a few thousand per year, and the yield of cancer cases was very high (10 per 1,000). Personnel were sent outside the country for training.

In 1957, the Department of Health fully supported this activity as a part of the Cancer Control Program and started a School of Cytotechnology in collaboration with the Department of Pathology of the same School of Medicine. An average of 7,000 women were screened every year.

In 1960 this activity was expanded to each of the 5 regions of the Island. The number of women examined has increased every year, as more personnel and other resources have become available. During 1962, 11,752 women were examined in contrast to 142,795 during 1971 an increase of a factor of 12. In addition, an estimated 30,000 women had Pap smears through private practice last year, to give a round total of 176,000 women examined by Pap smears during 1971. This figure shows that we are now screening 24% of the female population aged 20 years and above in one year.

TABLE 4   *Control of patient with uterine cervix cytologies*

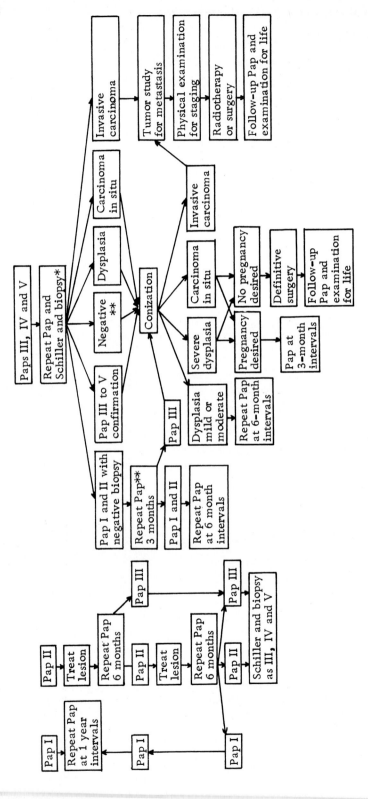

* Biopsies from yellow areas. In case all areas are stained brown, perform biopsies from the 4 quadrants.

** If the patient is a high surgical risk with initial Pap III and negative biopsy, and secondary Pap II or I, repeat Pap from curettage and aspiration from endocervix instead of conization.

The sources prompting women to get examined have been multiple. They range from an Island-wide Pilot Clinic where patients arrive through their own initiative, to inclusion of groups of women receiving other services such as prenatal, post-partum, family-planning, diabetes, and special detection clinics.

The personnel who take the smears consist mainly of graduate obstetric nurses where physicians are either not available or are overburdened with other duties. Clerks fill out the forms, and send appointment notices. The follow-up of patients with abnormal cytologies is done by Medical Social Workers, assisted by the above-mentioned nurses, in order to complete the diagnosis and send patients for treatment.

The flow of patients follows a standard accepted methodology (Table 4) modified according to our experience, resources and difficulties of controlling classes II and III.

TABLE 5   *Detection of cancer of the uterine cervix (Puerto Rico, July 1962–December 1971)*

	Initial cytology	Second cytology	Third cytology	Fourth cytology	Fifth cytology	Total cytology
Women examined	447,890	85,648	71,429	50,429	68,024	723,420
Average age	33	34	34	36	39	35
Total	1,583	71	45	26	53	1,778
Cancer cases discovered						
Invasive cases	687	16	6	5	11	725
In situ cases	896	55	39	21	42	1,053
Cancer cases per 1,000	3.5	0.8	0.6	0.5	0.8	2.5
Ratio, In situ/Invasive	1.3:1	3.4:1	6.5:1	4.2:1	3.8:1	1.5:1

Findings

Before women from family-planning clinics were included in the detection program, the yield of cancer cases was of the order of 10 per 1,000 women examined (Table 5). In general from 1962 to 1971 we have had an average yield of 3.5 cancer cases per 1,000 in almost half a million women initially screened; 0.8 per 1,000 in 85,000 who had a Pap test a second time; 0.6 per 1,000 in 71,000 who had the third Pap test; 0.5 per 1,000 in 50,000 of fourth Pap test, and 0.8 per 1,000 in 68,000 with the fifth, or more, annual

TABLE 6   *Yield of cancer cases by initial cytology, by age-group (Puerto Rico, July 1962– December 1971)*

Age-group (yr)	No. examined	Cases per 1,000		Total	Ratio In situ/ Invasive
		In situ	Invasive		
All ages	447,890	2.1	1.4	3.2	1.5:1
15-29	227,973	0.6	0.1	0.7	6:1
30-44	140,289	3.2	1.2	4.4	2.7:1
45 and above	79,558	6.7	11.8	18.5	0.6:1

Pap test. Altogether the average yield has been of 2.5 per 1,000. The median age of women examined was 33 for the initial examination, but 34 to 39 for subsequent examinations.

The yield increases with the age of the examinees: 0.7 cancer cases per 1,000 women screened in the age-group 15-29 years, to 18.5 per 1,000 for the group aged 45 years or more (Table 6).

At the first Pap test, the ratio of carcinoma in situ to invasive carcinoma has been 6:1 among the youngest women; 2.7:1 in the 30 to 44 years group, and 0.6:1 among the oldest group (45 years and above). For all ages combined, the ratio is 1.5:1.

The yield of cancer differs between geographical areas (Table 7). The highest occurs in the Northern Region (7.8/1,000), the lowest is for the Northeastern Region, University Hospital (1.6/1,000). Age and socio-economic patterns are responsible for these differences.

Quality control of laboratory work and adequate follow-up of patients with abnormal cytologies have been our main concern in the program.

TABLE 7   *Yield of cancer cases by initial cytology, by area (Puerto Rico, July 1962–December 1971)*

Area	No. examined	Cases per 1,000		
		In situ	Invasive	Total
All areas	447,411	2.0	1.5	3.5
Northeast (S. Juan)	235,231	1.9	1.0	2.9
South (Ponce)	62,585	2.7	1.7	4.4
East (Fajardo)	60,862	0.9	1.3	2.2
North (Arecibo)	51,787	4.1	3.7	7.8
West (Mayaguez)	30,249	1.2	0.6	1.8
Central (Caguas)	6,697	1.2	0.5	1.7

TABLE 8   *Cancer cases of the uterine cervix by stage (Puerto Rico, 1950–1970*)*

Year	In situ		Invasive		Ratio In situ/ Invasive
	No.	%	No.	%	
1950	16	5.2	305	94.8	0.05:1
1955	41	13.2	303	86.8	0.14:1
1960	84	22.7	195	77.3	0.43:1
1965	219	42.4	297	57.6	0.74:1
1967	270	47.2	302	52.8	0.89:1
1968	204	40.5	300	59.5	0.68:1
1969	242	46.6	277	53.4	0.87:1
1970	314	50.0	314	50.0	1:1

*   Information obtained from the Puerto Rico Cancer Registry

Conclusion

We may put the question: How much has been the contribution of this screening program towards the reduction of mortality from cancer of the uterus in Puerto Rico? While several other factors — such as improved socio-economic conditions, better medical care for obstetrical and gynecological conditions, family planning programs, etc. — have contributed significantly in reducing the mortality rate, we believe that early diagnosis has played the leading role in this matter. In 1950 carcinoma in situ was only 5% of the total cases of cancer of the uterine cervix as against 50% in 1970 (Table 8). Moreover, the stages of invasiveness of the cases have also changed: up to 1956 cases at Stage III predominated, while today Stages I and II are the most commonly found.

From the above findings we may conclude that a modest detection program for cancer of the uterus like ours, can help in decreasing significantly the mortality from cancer of this organ.

Summary

Although the incidence of cancer of the uterine cervix in Puerto Rico rose from 29.6 cases per 100,000 women in 1950 to 45.2 in 1970, reported mortality from cancer of the uterus decreased from 20.6 in 1950 to 12.5 in 1970. Carcinoma in situ was diagnosed in 5% of all cases of cancer of the cervix in 1950, in comparison with 50% in 1970. In invasive cases, Stage III predominated up to 1956 as against Stages I and II in 1970. The Pap test screening program is the most important factor responsible for this change.

Experience with cancer detection in Jamaica (1966-1972)*

D.C. Watler and K. Robinson

The Jamaican Government Clinico-Pathological Services, Kingston, Jamaica

Introduction and statistical background

A Cancer Registry was started in Jamaica in 1958 to ascertain the frequency of cancer in the island, to compare findings with populations having different ethnic and environmental backgrounds, and to highlight those most frequently occurring cancers.

The incidence study was confined to the urban area of Kingston and St. Andrew where medical facilities are better developed than in the rural areas. A census in 1960 and in 1970 showed the population of this area to be 419,416 in 1960 (189,768 males and 229,648 females), and approximately 527,600 in 1970 (244,700 males and 282,900 females).

Table 1 shows the leading cancers in Jamaica in males for the period 1958—1963, and compares this with figures for the period 1964- September 1972. This information has been taken from the records of the Jamaica Cancer Registry (Brooks and Watler, 1972). More detailed discussion on regional differences in the earlier period is given by Bras et al. (1965).

Gastric cancer remains the commonest malignancy in males with little change in the incidence. However, cancer of the lung which was the fourth commonest tumour in the earlier period is the second commonest tumour in the latter period. Moreover the trend has continued, as for the last 2 years of registration lung cancer exceeds stomach by 65 cases to 61.

Table 2 shows the leading cancers in the female where the relative frequency of the various cancers have remained unchanged. There has, however, been a small percentage fall in cervical cancer, as well as a fall from 41.8/100,000 population in 1960 to 35.3/100,000 in 1970. The incidence of mammary carcinoma has remained the same.

Mortality statistics indicate that deaths from cancer have risen from 5.3% of all deaths in 1955 to 10.1% in 1969 becoming after cardiovascular disease, the second single most common cause of death in Jamaica.

Material and methods

No cancer detection work was attempted until 1966, but it was clear that emphasis particularly should be placed on trying to detect, and prevent the 3 common cancers in Jamaica i.e. cervix, breast and lung by using methods proven elsewhere.

A cytological screening programme for cervical cancer began in 1966, when the Jamaican Government with assistance from the American Agency for International Development (A.I.D.) set up a National Family Planning Board and as a part of this programme it

* Financial assistance has been provided for this work through grants from Cancer Research Campaign, the Jamaica Cancer Society and the United States Agency for International Development (A.I.D.).

TABLE 1　　*Commonest cancers in Jamaica in males*

6 year period			8¾ year period		
Years (1958–1963) – Total 1100 cases			Years (1964–September 1972) – Total 2082 cases		
Site	No. of cases	% of all tumours	Site	No. of cases	% of all tumours
Stomach	160	14.5%	Stomach	269	12.9%
Skin	103	9.4%	Lung	233	11.2%
Oesophagus	87	7.9%	Prostate	203	9.8%
Lung	83	7.5%	Colon and rectum	154	7.4%
Colon and rectum	76	7.0%	Skin	147	7.1%
Prostate	72	6.5%	Oesophagus	96	4.6%
Penis	62	5.6%	Penis	79	3.8%
Annual rate per 100,000 population (1960) 95.3			Annual rate per 100,000 population (1970) 108.3		

TABLE 2　　*Commonest cancers in Jamaica in females*

6 year period			8¾ year period		
Years (1958–1963) – Total 1798 cases			Years (1964–September 1972) – Total 3202 cases		
Site	No. of cases	% of all tumours	Site	No. of cases	% of all tumours
Cervix	522	29.0%	Cervix	828	25.9%
Breast	315	17.5%	Breast	588	18.4%
Colon and rectum	131	7.3%	Colon and rectum	218	6.8%
Skin	109	6.1%	Stomach	178	5.6%
Stomach	91	5.1%	Skin	175	5.5%
Ovaries	78	4.3%	Ovaries	147	4.6%
Body of uterus	40	2.2%	Body of uterus	142	4.4%
Annual rate per 100,000 population (1960) 146.7			Annual rate per 100,000 population (1970) 146.3		

TABLE 3   *Cases from family planning clinics. Age groups in abnormal smears found for years 1966–1971. Total smears examined 73,238*

Age groups	10–14	15–19	20–24	25–29	30–34	35–39	40–44	45–49	50+	Age not stated	Totals
Mild to moderate dysplasia		50	246	286	209	125	52	19	29	75	1091
Very severe dysplasia } Borderline carcinoma-in-situ }		10	29	69	35	24	11	4	16	23	221
Malignant		2	9	38	41	22	15	12	12	19	170

Of the 221 cases of very severe dysplasia borderline for carcinoma, 67 were biopsied and 43 were positive for carcinoma-in-situ (64%); 16 were very severe dysplasia (24%); 4 unsatisfactory biopsies, and 4 showed severe cervicitis with atypicality. Of the 170 positive smears, 120 were biopsied, and 100 confirmed malignant (mainly carcinoma-in-situ with about half showing endocervical glandular involvement — i.e. 83%). 12 showed very severe dysplasia, (10%); 6 were unsatisfactory biopsies, and 2 were not confirmed histologically.

was decided that cervical cytology be offered to all women atttending the Family Planning Clinics (F.P.C.). Technical assistance was provided by A.I.D. through a training programme for cytotechnologists. Apart from examining patients from the Family Planning Clinics (F.P.C.) smears were encouraged from other sources.

In May 1972, the Jamaica Cancer Society began a Detection Clinic confining the examinations to breast and cervix cancer. At this clinic any woman can attend for a breast and Pap. smear examination carried out by a qualified nurse with all suspicious cases being referred weekly to volunteer doctors for further assessment. At all clinics Pap. smears were taken from the external os using the Ayre spatula.

With regard to lung cancer extensive efforts are being made to secure the help of Government in not only supporting the anti-smoking campaign of the Jamaica Cancer Society, but by enacting definite legislation as is done elsewhere. So far, no method of early detection has been tried.

Results

For the period 1966–1971 a total of 123,406 Pap. smears were examined of which 73,238 were new cases from F.P.C. Some slight statistical readjustment in the new cases for 1971 may be necessary on final rechecking.

Table 3 shows the breakdown of the abnormal smears by age group. From this table it can be seen that there were 391 very suspicious or positive smears giving an approximate incidence of 5–6 per 1,000 population. This overall figure is low compared to a smaller study done within this group where the percentage was 1.0% from 3,585 cases screened, and in cases from sources other than the Family Planning Clinics the incidence was about 1.2% or even higher. The low incidence in cases from the Family planning Clinics may be due to poorer sampling techniques in the rural areas and the fact that many cases attending the clinics are from better educated and higher socio-economic groups and are therefore to some extent selected. We feel that the overall incidence of carcinoma-in-situ in Jamaica in females over 20 is 8–10 per 1,000 of the population. Of the 391 positive or very suspicious smears from the National Family Board only 187 returned for biopsy follow-up (i.e. 48%). On the approximate 400 new cases detected outside the F.P.C. the follow-up is about the same.

With regard to cervical and breast cancer screening from the Cancer Society Detection Clinic, results of the project so far are shown in Table 4. This is the first attempt being made to detect early breast cancer in Jamaica and examination is limited to clinical palpation only along with an intensive educational programme.

TABLE 4   *Jamaica cancer society screening clinic. May, 1972 – December, 1972.*

Cervix uteri

Total number of cases examined	Positive cases	% age positive	Histology	Follow-up data
588	6	1% approximately	All confirmed	5 Treated

Breasts

Total number of cases examined	Lumps discovered	Malignancy found	Follow-up
588	35	3	2 Treated 1 Never returned

Discussion

Cancer detection in Jamaica is still in its infancy, with a discouraging feature being the poor follow-up in the early cervical cancer cases. This is partly due to lack of education in a population where there is still about 50% illiteracy combined with a scarcity of trained staff. A massive literacy campaign has been started by the Jamaica Government, and if this is successful the population will be more easily receptive to a cancer educational programme.

Lung cancer is not yet as serious a problem in Jamaica as in North America and Europe, but its rapid increase is ominous.

There is need to emphasize the importance of detection of breast cancer, as this cancer is common in Jamaica, and experience elsewhere is beginning to show the value of breast detection clinics, especially using other modalities than simple palpation (Shapiro et al., 1971).

Summary

Cervix, breast, and lung cancers are the commonest cancers in Jamaica. Cytological screening for cervical cancer was begun in 1966, and more recently a simple breast cancer detection programme has been attempted. The incidence of carcinoma-in-situ of the cervix is approximately 1%. Follow-up of early cervical cancer cases has so far been poor.

Acknowledgments

We are grateful for the very great assistance of Dr. Sophia Bamford, who, through the facilities offered by the A.I.D. helped in initiating the cytology programme, and for her technical assistance and advice over many years.

References

Brooks, S.E.H. and Watler, D.C. (1972): Annual Report of the Jamaican Cancer Registry. University of West Indies, Kingston, Jamaica.
Bras, G., Watler, D.C. and Ashmeade-Dyer (1965): Brit. J. Cancer, 19, 681.
Shapiro, S., Strax, P. and Venet, L. (1971): J. Amer. med. Ass., 215, 1777.

A mass survey of gynecologic cancer in Korea

J. K. Lee, S. W. Kim, K. Y. Rah, J. K. Choi, T. H. Lee, Y. S. Choi and
B. K. Moon

Radiological Research Institute, Seoul, Korea

According to a report issued in 1968 by the Korean Society of Pathology, cancer of the uterine cervix is the most frequently encountered malignancy in Korea. Among 21,921 cancers confirmed by biopsy, 23.5% (5,157 cases) were of this type, which represents 44.9% of all cancers among Korean women. In contrast, cancer of the corpus uteri accounts for only 1.08% (237 cases), or 2.06% of all female cancers. The report also pointed out that the incidence of cervical cancer tends to increase every year. Our institute initiated and has conducted a mass survey of gynecologic malignancy in Korea since July 1969, financed by the Government.

During the first year, 5 regional detection centers were established in the 5 national university hospitals, which carried out only the stationary survey. In the next year, 6 mobile clinics were introduced, and the detection centers were expanded to 6 teams, adding the Korean Cancer Society, which cooperated well with the regional health centers. Each team consisted of 2 gynecologists, 1 cytologist, 4 technicians, 4 nurses, 2 administrators, and 1 driver. The examination was done free of charge, mostly for women of low socio-economic standing. The vaginal and cervical smears were examined cytologically and classified by the Papanicolaou method. Each woman was notified of the results, and the positive cases were requested to be reexamined, sometimes with biopsy. During a period from July 1969 to December 1972, a total number of 160,121 women were surveyed. The total expenses for this project were $295,310, including 430,000 worth of printed materials for public education: therefore, it averaged $1.84 per person.

The number of cases of Classes I and II were 156,482(97.7%); Class III, 2,631 (1.64%); and Classes IV and V, 1,008 (0.63%) (Table 1). Some 62,065 women were examined at the stationary centers over a period of 42 months and 98,056 by the mobile clinics over a period of 30 months, but the survey numbers over the same 30-month period were 44,549 and 98,056 respectively. The cervical cancer cases found were 807 (1.30%) by the former and 201 (0.21%) by the latter. Just over half of the women were in their thirties (50.9%), and the highest incidence was noted in the age group 40 to 44 (Table 2 and Fig. 1). A remarkably higher incidence was present in the Kwangju area, almost twice the average. A positive correlation between incidence and increase of age was noted (Fig. 2). An epidemiological study in the area, where 283 cancer cases out of 43,345 women were found, showed that the sex- and age-adjusted incidence rate was 35.1 per 100,000 women; the age of marriage was mostly before 21 (Fig. 3); the socioeconomic standing was low (99.5%); and the educational background was poor (90% under the primary school). The incidence became higher with increasing parity (Fig. 4), which, however, had no correlation with the number of abortions, either spontaneous or induced. No single case of cancer of the corpus uteri was found in the present study.

It has been stated that cancer of the uterine cervix is more frequently encountered among women with low socio-economic standing, early sexual experience and high parity. In a city-wide study in the United States, the incidence of cervical cancer was reported to be 26.4 for white, 49.4 for black, and 2.9 for Jewish women per 100,000. A preliminary mobile survey of gynecologic cancer in one area of Japan, which is quite similar to ours, showed that there were 90 cervical cancer cases out

TABLE 1 Mass survey of gynecologic malignancy in Korea (1.7.1969–31.12.1972)

Area	Survey	No. of women	%	Class					
				I and II	%	III	%	IV and V	%
Seoul	S	11,830		11,528		209		93	
	M	19,101		18,930		142		29	
	T	30,931	19.9	30,458	98.5	351	1.13	122	0.39
Daegu	S	20,505		20,048		196		261	
	M	22,840		22,785		33		22	
	T	43,345	27.1	42,833	98.8	229	0.53	283	0.65
Kwangju	S	18,340		17,360		626		354	
	M	13,570		13,277		277		16	
	T	31,910	19.9	30,637	96.0	903	2.82	370	1.16
Busan	S	5,889		5,519		301		69	
	M	24,732		24,318		354		60	
	T	30,621	19.1	29,837	97.4	655	2.14	129	0.42
Daejon	S	5,501		5,312		159		30	
	M	7,645		7,326		297		22	
	T	13,146	8.2	12,638	96.1	456	3.47	52	0.40
Kangwon	M	10,168	6.4	10,079	99.1	37	0.36	52	0.51
	S	62,065	38.8	59,767	96.3	1,491	2.4	807	1.30
	M	98,056	61.2	96,715	98.6	1,140	1.2	201	0.21
Grand Total		160,121	100.0	156,482	97.7	2,631	1.6	1,008	0.63

TABLE 2   *Incidence of gynecologic cancer by age groups*

Age group	No. of women	Class					No. Ca	%
		I	II	III	IV	V		
20 – 24	5,330	4,232	1,081	15	2	0	2	0.04
25 – 29	21,481	16,770	4,594	110	4	3	7	0.03
30 – 34	39,414	28,815	10,098	442	41	18	59	0.15
35 – 39	42,073	28,608	12,658	643	110	54	164	0.39
40 – 44	28,192	17,915	9,420	606	159	92	251	0.89
45 – 49	13,540	8,110	4,813	422	118	77	195	1.44
50 – 54	5,758	3,197	2,229	191	93	48	141	2.45
55 – 59	2,666	1,272	1,185	122	46	41	87	3.26
over 60	1,667	737	748	80	52	50	102	6.12
Total	160,121	109,656	46,826	2,631	625	383	1,008	0.63

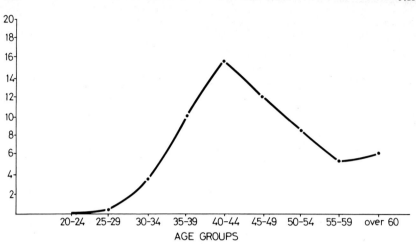

FIG. 1   *Corrected age incidence.*

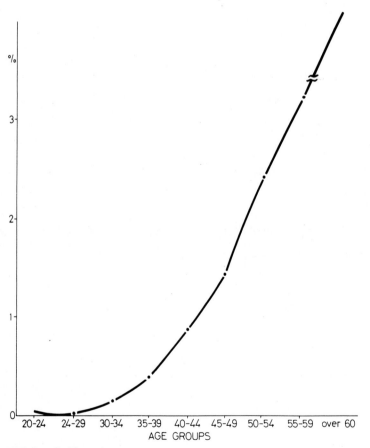

FIG. 2   *Incidence in age groups.*

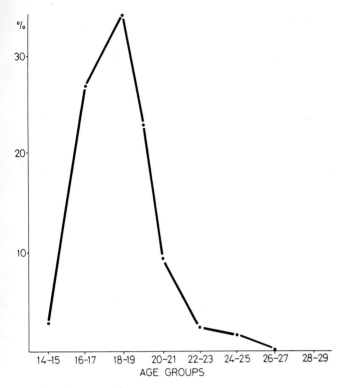

FIG. 3   *Age at marriage.*

of 20,327 women (0.44%). The result obtained in our study seems to be higher than this, but it may be attributed to the fact that a very high incidence was noted in the stationary survey. It is lower when the result of the mobile survey alone is compared.

A survey of this type would not show the real incidence, as the women who visit the detection centers or mobile clinics would tend to have some symptoms which may be related to gynecologic malignancy. As the average age of marriage of Korean women is reported to be 22, the cancer cases had married at an earlier age.

As the first trial for the mass survey of gynecologic cancer in Korea, 160,121 women were surveyed by the Papanicolaou method at a fairly cheap cost. The survey was carried out by the stationary and mobile teams placed in the university hospitals and cancer society which cover most parts of the country. Of all the women examined, 1,008 cases (0.63%) were found to have cancer of the uterine cervix. In respect of the number of women examined, the mobile survey seems to be twice as effective as the stationary survey; however, about 2.7 times more positive cases were detected by the latter. A fairly even distribution was noted throughout the country except for one area, the reason for which is difficult to explain. The sex- and age-adjusted incidence rate was 35.1 per 100,000 women. It was confirmed in the present survey that the higher incidences were noted among the women who married earlier, had more parity, were uneducated, and had lower socio-economic standing. A positive correlation between incidence and increasing age was present. No single case of cancer of the corpus uteri was found in the present study. It is felt that the survey work of this type is very useful as it will also serve to educate the public about cancer.

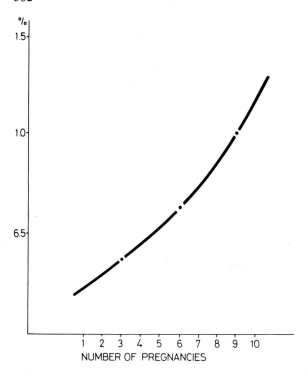

FIG. 4   *Incidence and parity.*

References

Colo, S. (1964): Obstet. and Gynec., 23, 274.
Kurokawa, T. (1968): Report of the Miyagi Prefecture Cancer Society, Japan.
Lee, C. K. (1968): Research Report E 68–62, Ministry of Science and Technology, Republic of Korea.
Moon, H. S. (1971): Report of the Korean Institute for Family Planning: Fertility-Abortion Survey, 1971.

Statistical analysis of observer errors in cervical screening

A. Lambourn and H. Lederer

Department of Community Medicine, The University of Sheffield, Sheffield, and Pathology Department, Doncaster Hospital Management Committee, Doncaster Royal Infirmary, Doncaster, United Kingdom

The present study has evolved from a review of cervical screening in an English District Hospital during a 5-year period. This had consisted of an analysis of cervical smears from about 40,000 women and of histological diagnoses of about 3,000 specimens obtained by hysterectomy or conisation (Table 1). Methods and results of the investigation have been published.

TABLE 1   *Analysis of cervical cytology: 5-year period 1966 – 70 (Doncaster Royal Infirmary)*

Area population	: 250,000
Females over 25 years	: 84,000
Total number of cervical smears : 44,201	
Total number of gynaecological operation specimens : 3,141	
Rate of Grade IV smears : 5.5/1,000	
(Sheffield Region : 3.2/1,000)	
Rate of Grade III smears : 4.8/1,000	

We were dissatisfied with the high false-positive and false-negative error rate and decided to check our results. We selected 100 smears from patients in whom a histological diagnosis had subsequently been made. The selection was made in such a way that Grade I–IV smears were approximately equally represented. These smears were re-examined blindly in our laboratory and then sent to two cytology laboratories of high reputation. Histological specimens pertaining to these smears were similarly reviewed in our Department and sent to one of the cyto-histology laboratories. (As some of the 100 smears referred to the same patient, only 80 operation specimens were available for histological analysis.)

TABLE 2   *Cytological grading by 3 cytologists*

Grade	D	A	.B
IV	23	37	23
III	18	16	17
II	28	39	29
I	30	7	25
Unsatisfactory	1	1	6
Total	100	100	100

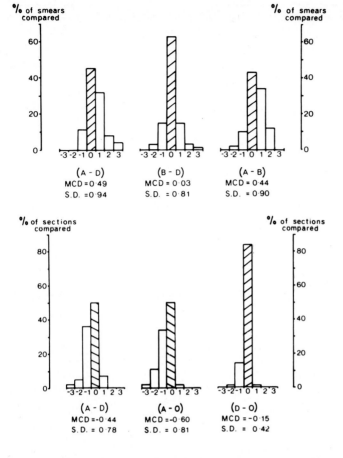

FIG. 1   *Pair-wise comparisons of cytological (upper portion) and histological (lower portion) diagnosis.*

In Table 2 we tabulate the *cytological gradings* of the three centres. There appears to be close concordance between D and B while A is more severe in its gradings.

However, on determination of the Mean Class Differences of three observers it is clear that the apparent close agreement between D and B is the result of scatter and not due to any specific trend (Fig.1). A is consistently more severe in classifying cytological changes and there is closer concordance between A and B than between B and D. Using the same analytical approach to *histological* changes, we graded them into 4 classes: invasive carcinoma (including microinvasive carcinoma); carcinoma in situ; severe dysplasia; and mild dysplasia and normal in one class. Note that A is consistently less severe in his histological gradings than D, although more severe in his cytological gradings. In the histogram D−O, D represents the review grading in our laboratory in 1971 based on morphological criteria of the working party of the RCOG (Govan, 1969), and O the original histological gradings during the period 1966—70. It shows a trend to less severe grading of the review specimens.

Observer differences of this range are generally acceptable for a large number of laboratory tests. We decided, however, to assess their *implications on population screening.* To do this, we combined the cytodiagnoses of all 3 laboratories and grouped them

TABLE 3   *Variations in histological diagnoses*

Histologist	Grading	Total cases		Total smears		Combined cytodiagnoses					
						(III or IV)			(I or II)		
						No.	%		No.	%	
	Invasive carcinoma	10		30		25	83		5	17	
			23		69			77		16	23
O	In-situ carcinoma	13		39		28	72	53	11	28	
	Severe dysplasia	16		48		19	40		29	60	
	Mild dysplasia or normal	3		9		4	44		5	56	
	Invasive carcinoma	8		24		19	79		5	21	
			18		54			85		8	15
D	In-situ carcinoma	10		30		27	90	46	3	10	
	Severe dysplasia	21		63		29	46		34	54	
	Mild dysplasia or normal	3		9		1	11		8	89	
	Invasive carcinoma	6		18		15	83		3	17	
			12		36			78		8	22
A	In-situ carcinoma	6		18		13	72	28	5	28	
	Severe dysplasia	16		48		36	75		12	25	
	Mild dysplasia or normal	14		42		12	29		30	71	

according to their *clinical significance* into grades III and IV and grades I and II (Table 3). These groups were then checked against the *histodiagnosis* of the 3 observers O, D, A. Observer O confirmed invasive carcinoma in 83% of Grade (III—IV) smears, observer D in 79 and observer A in 83%. If we combine all malignancies, then the results are 77—85 and 78%. The results for false-negative smears are 23, 15 and 22 in this series.

Variations in *cytological* diagnoses by the 3 cytologists were found in a similar way by comparing the cytodiagnosis of the individual cytologist against the diagnosis of individual histologists. Observer variations of a similar order were found.

The efficiency of any laboratory test in detecting abnormalities may be expressed by its sensitivity. This is the proportion of the particular abnormality investigated, which is detected by the particular test. Alternatively, the 'false-negative error rate' is simply the proportion of the particular abnormality not detected.

Table 4 shows the results of our *analysis of observer variation*. On the right side, the cytodiagnoses of 3 individual cytologists have been compared against the histodiagnosis of observer D. The sensitivity of the cervical smear test in detecting cervical malignancy in

TABLE 4   *Variations in sensitivity caused by differences in cyto-histological grading*

Conditions detected	Histology			Mean sensitivity	Maximum variation	Cytology Grades III - IV			Mean sensitivity	Maximum variation
	O	D	A			D	A	B		
Invasive and in-situ carcinoma	77	85	78	80	8	72	84	88	81	16
In-situ carcinoma	72	90	72	88	18	87	87	93	89	6
Severe dysplasia and in-situ carcinoma	54	60	74	63	20	52	69	57	59	17

cytology laboratory D was 72, in A, 84 and in B, 88, giving a mean of 81 and a maximum variation of 16; sensitivity for detecting both dysplasia and in situ carcinoma was 52, 69, and 57 respectively, a mean sensitivity of only 59 maximum observer variation of 17.

On the left side of the Table the cytodiagnoses of all 3 cytologists have been combined and compared against the histodiagnoses of 3 individual histologists. The result shows maximal variations of 8 for all malignancies, 18 for carcinoma in situ and 20 for a combination of carcinoma in situ with severe dysplasia.

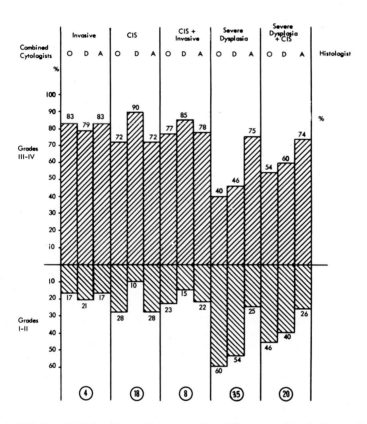

FIG. 2   *Variations in sensitivity caused by differences in histological grading.*

In the last histogram we have summarised these variations in sensitivity based on differences in cyto-histological diagnoses (Fig. 2). The ringed figures at the bottom of each column give the *maximum observer variation* found in different cervical abnormalities. This, as expected, is particularly large for conditions referred to by some authors as 'borderline cases', namely severe dysplasia and combination of severe dysplasia with carcinoma in situ.

The results of this analysis indicate that observer variation is at least partly responsible for the *discrepancies of opinions* on the significance of epithelial abnormalities of the cervix, on the concept of progression from dysplasia to carcinoma in situ and invasive carcinoma, on the therapeutic value of conisation, and lastly, on the efficacy of mass screening in reducing morbidity and mortality from cervical carcinoma.

Our analysis may be criticized on two accounts (*a*) the smallness of the sample and (*b*) the selection of a sample which does not represent the prevalence of cervical abnormalities in the population. We hope that our findings presented here will stimulate a larger and wider investigation of this problem along the lines we have indicated.

Reference

Govan, A.D.T. (1969): J. clin. Path., 22, 383.

Re-screenings for cervical cancer

M. Grönroos and R. Punnonen

*Department of Obstetrics and Gynecology and Radiumkoti of Turku, Turku
University, Turku, Finland*

The Finnish Cancer Society has developed over the last 10 years a permanent organisation
for the early detection of cervical cancer. Re-screening became increasingly common
towards the end of this active decade.

The longest and most comprehensive screening in an individual town in Finland is the
one in Turku which has a total population of 156,000. The screening studies were
commenced in 1963 and by the end of 1971 a total of 40,538 women had been screened
once. If the number of women examined twice or thrice is added to this, 65,286 cytologic smears have been examined so far. Re-screening began in 1967.

Table 1 shows the number of patients examined and the final histologic finding in the
different cytologic classes in the first screening in Turku. In the first re-screening, the total
finding rate is 3.9 per thousand (Table 2). This number includes dysplasias and other

TABLE 1 *The first screening in Turku (1963-1971). Correlation of the cell findings with the final
diagnosis*

Cell findings	Total number of cases		Patients studied by a gynecologist							
			Dysplasia No./1000		Ca in situ No./1000		Ca invasive No./1000		Total No./1000	
	No.	%								
I	39,420	97.2								
II	741	1.8	38	51.2	21	28.3	8	10.8	67	90.4
III	217	0.6	76	350.2	36	165.8	12	55.2	124	571.4
IV	77	0.2	21	272.7	26	337.7	26	337.6	73	948.0
V	83	0.2	12	144.5	33	397.5	38	457.8	83	1000.0
Total	40,538	100.0	147	3.6	116	2.9	84	2.1	347	8.6

TABLE 2 *The second screening in Turku (1967-1971). Correlation of the cell findings with the
final diagnosis, smears taken 3 years after the first cytological sample*

Cell findings	Total number of cases		Patients studied by a gynecologist							
			Dysplasia No./1000		Ca in situ No./1000		Ca invasive No./1000		Total No./1000	
	No.	%								
I	16,387	96.0								
II	587	3.4	11	18.7	2	3.4	1	1.7	14	23.8
III	80	0.5	27	337.5	6	75.0	3	37.5	36	450.0
IV	13	0.1	6	461.5	6	461.5	1	76.9	13	1000.0
V	3	0.02			1	333.3	2	666.6	3	1000.0
Total	17,070	100.0	44	2.6	15	0.9	7	0.4	66	3.9

invasive carcinomas, in addition to carcinoma of the cervix. If erroneous cytologic inter-pretations in the first screening and processes outside the cervix (a vaginal, an endometrial and an ovarian carcinoma) are eliminated (Table 3), the number of new invasive processes developing in the cervix is reduced to two preclinical cervical carcinomas. Hence, the total incidence of lesions which probably originated during the interval between the screenings is 2.8 per thousand.

The number of women screened thrice in the Turku mass screening was 7,678 by the end of 1971 (Table 4). It appears from the results that no invasive cervical carcinomas originated during the interval between the screenings. If only the cervical processes are considered, the incidence of lesions originating during the interval was only 1.4 per thousand. Re-examination of the earlier cytologic specimens from the cases in which lesions had originated showed that there were no cytologic interpretational errors in any of the earlier screenings. The proportion of Papanicolaou classes III-V decreased from 1% at the first screening, to 0.6% at the second screening and to 0.3% at the third screening.

All the cases detected in the mass screenings in Turku were treated at the University Central Hospital, Turku. The same applies to the cases diagnosed during the same period

TABLE 3 *Analysed results at the second screening; A = possible new cases of premalignant and malignant lesions, B = false negative findings at the first screening*

Cell finding in the second screening	Final diagnosis					
	Dysplasia		Ca in situ		Ca invasive	
	A	B	A	B	A	B
II	10	1	2		1[1]	
III	22	5	4	2	3[1,2,3]	
IV	4	2	6		1[2]	
V			1		1[3]	1[4]
Total	36	8	13	2	6	1

1[1] Ca colli ut. gr. Ia

1[2] Ca colli ut. gr. Ia

1[3] Ca corporis ut. gr. I

1[4] Ca corporis ut. gr. II

3[1] Ca vaginae prim.

3[2] Ca colli ut. gr. IV

3[3] Ca ovarii seminal. gr. III

(typus endom.)

TABLE 4 *The third screening in Turku (1967-1971). Correlation of the cell finding with the final diagnosis, smears taken 3 years after the second cytological sample*

Cell finding	Total number of cases		Patients studied by a gynecologist				
	No.	%	Dysplasia	Ca in situ	Ca invasive	Total No./1000	
I	7,468	97.3					
II	182	2.4	3			3	
III	26	0.3	6	1		7	
IV	1	0.01			1*	1	
V	1	0.01	1			1	
Total	7,678	100.0	10	1.3	1	0.13	1	0.13	12	1.6

1* Ca corporis ut. gr. II

TABLE 5   *Variation of the clinical stage and occurrence of cervical cancer in Turku patients at the Department of Obstetrics and Gynaecology, University of Turku, during a mass screening January 1, 1963 – December 31, 1970, in Turku*

Year	Clinical stage								Total	Share of Turku patients (%)
	0		I		II		III-IV			
	No.	%	No.	%	No.	%	No.	%		
1961-1962	2	4	15	29	16	31	19	37	52	36.4
1963-1964	55	44	51	41	7	6	11	9	124	67.8
1965-1966	51	45	42	37	11	10	9	8	113	52.6
1967-1968	16	50	11	34	1	3	4	13	32	19.3
1969-1970	20	56	7	19	3	8	6	17	36	26.7
Total	144		126		38		49		357	

TABLE 6   *Incidence and mortality of cervical cancer, cases/100,000 (1961-1970)*

Years	Turku		Finland	
	Incidence	Mortality	Incidence	Mortality
1961-1962	36.1	7.9	19.8	
1963-1964	47.5	17.9	18.9	7.4
1965-1966	41.2	18.6	17.8	6.5
1967-1968	10.2	5.7	16.4	6.4
1969-1970	9.7	6.7	15.8	6.5

by the gynecologists of the town, but not included in the mass study. The material of the hospital may thus be considered to reflect the true cervical carcinoma morbidity rate in the town of Turku. Table 5 indicates that the total frequency of pre-invasive and invasive cervical carcinoma during the years immediately before the mass screening (1961-1962) was considerably lower than during the first 4 years of the mass study. It can also be seen that the proportion of Turku residents among the patients increased sharply. The pronounced change in the distribution of grade is also typical: the share of pre-invasive carcinoma and carcinoma of stage I increased appreciably; 90% of the pre-clinical invasive carcinoma cases came under treatment through screening, but only 18% of the patients with clinical carcinoma did so. The decrease in the total frequency of lesions during the past 4 years is partly due to the high proportion of re-screened patients examined during this period.

We analysed more closely the surprisingly large number of cases with clinical carcinoma of the cervix that came under treatment without participating in the mass screening. Eight per cent had not received the invitation to attend, owing for example to a change of address. Only 4% stated that they had neglected to attend although they had received an invitation. During the first years of the mass study, many cervical carcinoma patients developed symptoms before the invitation to attend for screening reached them; the number amounted to 43%. The 16% who belonged to age-groups not included in the screening study also argues for the inadequate scale of the mass examination. Eleven per cent had been screened earlier with negative results. All these factors which are associated to a smaller or greater extent with the negative aspects of screenings can be largely eliminated by making different arrangements and organizational changes.

Summary

All considered, it may be said that the screening study has decreased the incidence of cervical carcinoma in the town of Turku and improved its distribution by grade (Table 6). Nothing can be said so far about mortality from cervical cancer in Turku, although the trend appears to be a declining one. It seems that a 3-year interval between individual examinations is an unnecessarily short period outside the risk age-groups.

References

Christopherson, W. (1966): Acta cytol. (Philad.), 10, 6.
Dickinson, L., Mussey, M. and Kurland, L. (1972): Mayo Clin. Proc., 47, 545.
Dickinson, L., Mussey, M., Soule, E. and Kurland, L. (1972): Mayo Clin. Proc., 47, 534.
Pedersen, E., Høeg, K. and Kolstad, P. (1971): Acta obstet. gynec. scand., Suppl. 11.

Fate of women with detected cancer of the genital organ during mass examinations (1966-1968 to 1971-1972)

Stefan Soszka, Wanda Alicja Kazanowska, Danuta Filipowska and Jerzy Goszczyński

Department of Prophylaxis of Female Genital Organ Cancer, National Institute of Mother and Child Care; Institute of Obstetrics and Gynecology, Medical Academy Białystok; and Białystok Oncological Centre, Białystok, Poland

Mass examination of women residing in the Białystok Province was initiated in 1966-1968. Bearing in mind the principle postulates of prophylaxis in neoplastic illness, which are the detection of early cancer developmental stages and the simultaneous increase in curability, it was decided to follow-up the results of mass examinations related to those women in whom cancer of the genital tract was detected.

The examinations were carried out in 319,836 women, representing 96.4% of all the female population over 20 years of age, residing in the Białystok Province. Out of the total examined women, cancer of the genital tract was detected in 531. The highest proportion, i.e. 70.8% represented patients with diagnosed cancer of the uterine cervix. Table 1 summarizes the cancer sites of the genital tract found in the examined women.

TABLE 1   *Absolute and relative values of the prophylactic oncologic examinations of women in Białystok district in 1966–1972*

Years	No. of neoplasms of female genital organ	Cancer of the uterine cervix		Cancer corpus uteri		Ovarian cancer		Cancer vulvae		Cancer vaginae	
		No.	%	No.	%	No.	%	No.	%	No.	%
1966 1968	531	376	70.8	74	13.9	53	9.9	19	3.6	9	1.8
1969 1970	314	236	75.2	39	12.4	30	9.6	8	2.5	1	0.3
1971 1972	322	200	62.1	69	21.4	35	10.9	10	3.1	8	2.5

The highest number of patients with cancer of the uterine cervix was found in 1967, i.e. in the second year of the examinations. This refers to all clinical stages. The highest percentage of detected cancers was between 1969-1970. Between 1966-1968 the frequency of detected cancers of the uterine cervix was 0.11% and in 1971-1972, it was 0.06%.

As the period over which mass examinations are carried out gets longer the groups of clinical advancement of the neoplastic process shift towards $0°$ and $I°$ stages (Figs. 1 *a, b, c*). In the group of invasive cancer, an increase in cancers requiring radical surgical treat-

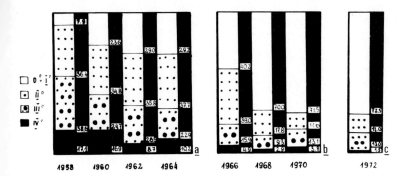

FIG. 1a,b,c *Graphic illustration of the actual occurrence of cancer of the uterine cervix before and during mass examinations. (a) Before prophylactic mass examinations; (b) results of mass examinations of women in Białystok district, 1966-1970; (c) actual occurrence of cancer of the uterine cervix in Białystok district, 1972.*

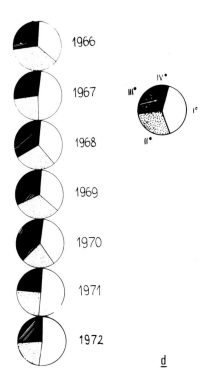

FIG. 1d *Graphic illustration of an increase in cancers referred for radical surgical treatment.*

ment is also seen (Fig. 1*d*). The greatest age group in the presented material comprises women below 50 years of life (Table 2). Only 69 were less than 30 years of age.

From the group of 812 patients with cancer of the uterine cervix (according to the scheme of therapeutic procedure accepted in Poland) 576 patients ($0°$ and $I°$) were chosen for surgical treatment. However, only 564 patients were cured by this treatment. The remainder (12) were not operated upon, because of the lack of consent of patients (5), or a general systemic disease. The ailments were: circulatory failure, hyperthyroidism

TABLE 2   *Age groups in women with detected carcinoma of the cervix*

Years	20–30	31–40	41–50	51–60	> 60
1966	8	21	17	8	2
1967	16	26	20	14	2
1968	7	29	47	36	1
1969	11	28	36	26	15
1970	12	29	39	24	16
1971	5	22	34	23	12
1972	8	24	33	25	14

and (unbalanced) diabetes. These patients underwent conservative treatment with radium and X-rays. The operative procedure in most of the patients was radical hysterectomy according to Wertheim. This type of operation was performed in 312 patients. Less extensive hysterectomy according to Freund was carried out in 117 patients. The least radical operative procedure, high amputation of the uterine cervix, was performed in 135 patients.

Women treated by the Wertheim method (312) had supplementary therapy in the Oncologic Centre in Białystok, 14-21 days after the operation. As a rule, radium in vaginal applicators was administered, according to the modified Parisian method, and X-rays were used from 4 cervical gynecological fields. From the total of 312 patients — 90.7% are well without any signs of recurrence and 9.3% died (Fig. 2). In histopathologic diagnoses of the deceased, the picture of carcinoma solidum was mostly found, and in lymphatic nodes metastatic foci were detected.

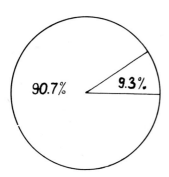

FIG. 2   *Graphic illustration of the therapeutic results (total operated 100%; dead 9.3%; living 90.7%).*

236 women with diagnosed cancer of the uterine cervix in stage II, III, and IV were treated conservatively in the department of gynecological oncology. As a rule, radium in vaginal applicators was used as well as a lineal catheter into the uterine cavity. Roentgeno-therapy in conventional conditions was applied from 4 utero-gynecological fields. In stage IV, 23 patients were treated. The treatment consisted of palliative irradiation with X-rays. Of 236 patients treated in this way, 52.7% of women survived 3 years, all of them being under constant control of the Oncologic Centre. From this group, 47.3% died in a period of 3 months to 3 years.

The second largest group were women with cancer of the uterine body. During pro-

TABLE 3   *Age groups of women with detected carcinoma of corpus uteri*

Years	< 30	31–40	41–50	51–60	> 60
1966	0	0	4	12	2
1967	0	1	8	10	3
1968	0	1	10	17	2
1969	0	1	5	15	4
1970	0	0	4	10	4
1971	1	4	8	12	10
1972	0	3	8	14	9

phylactic examinations in 1966-1968 to 1971-1972 carcinoma corpus uteri was detected in 182 women. The age of the patients in whom cancer of the uterine body has been found is shown in Table 3. From this Table we see that cancer of the uterine body has been found most frequently in women aged 50-60 years. In 12 of them the coexistence of diabetes, obesity and hypertension was encountered, representative of a so-called hormonal profile of woman suffering from cancer of the uterine body.

The treatment of these patients consisted of hysterectomy with adnexae, according to Freund, and subsequent irradiation with X-rays and radium in the same way as with the group described before. 32 patients died in the first year following treatment. The cause of death was associated with neoplastic disease, mainly with distal metastases to lungs. The observation period enables us to state that 90.2% of women with carcinoma corpus uteri detected during mass examinations live and feel well after 3 years (Table 4).

TABLE 4   *Illustration of the therapeutic results*

Years	No. of women	Dead women	Living women No.	Living women %
1966	18	5	13	72.2
1967	24	6	18	75.0
1968	30	9	21	70.0
1969	21	5	16	76.1
1970	18	3	15	83.3
1971	34	3	31	88.5
1972	34	1	33	97.1

The third group is composed of 118 patients in whom ovarian carcinoma has been detected. The incidence of detected ovarian carcinoma by the end of 1968 was 0.017%. In the majority of this group (32 women) I° and II° stages of the clinical cancer advancement was found. The same index in 1971-1972 was 0.012%. The largest age group in the presented material is between 41-60 years of age (Table 5).

Radical hysterectomy according to Freund was performed in 59 patients. Supravaginal amputation of the uterus, together with adnexae, was made in 38 women. Explorative laparatomy only was done in 21 patients. Operative treatment was supplemented by

TABLE 5   *Age groups in women with detected ovarian carcinoma*

Years	No. of women	Age of women					> 60
		< 20	21–30	31–40	41–50	51–60	
1966	12	1	2	2	4	2	1
1967	24	1	1	4	5	9	4
1968	17	1	1	4	3	4	4
1969	16	1	0	0	4	6	5
1970	14	0	0	1	10	3	0
1971	15	0	0	1	6	4	4
1972	20	1	1	4	8	4	2

irradiation from ovarian fields in doses of 3000 rads on the upper field and 3500 rads on the lower field. 21 patients (stages III and IV) were treated only conservatively. Thirteen were irradiated with X-rays in the manner analogous to that formerly described. The presence of fluid in the peritoneal cavity of 45 women required administration of cytostatics (Endoxan, Trenimon, Dactinomycin). The drugs were given intraperitoneally (following fluid aspiration) and intravenously, 200 mg/24 hr.

Four patients were irradiated with X-rays 6 weeks after the end of chemical treatment. In the whole group of 118 patients with diagnosed ovarian cancer, the 3-year survival was 33.8%. In 19.4% recurrence was found at about 6 months following treatment. They are under systematic control at the oncologic clinic and periodic chemotherapeutic treatment. The remaining 41.8% have died because of local recurrences and distant metastases (Fig. 3).

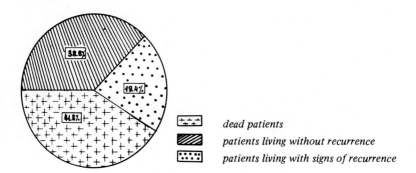

dead patients

patients living without recurrence

patients living with signs of recurrence

FIG. 3   *Graphic illustration of the therapeutic results.*

The design and consistent application of mass examinations of women in the Białystok Province have achieved their objective. This may be seen from:

(a) almost all the female inhabitants in Białystok Province, 20 years old and more have been examined;

(b) increased detection of malignant tumours of the genital tract, this being greatest in the second year of continued examinations;

(c) increased detection of the early developmental stages of neoplasms.

Although these findings apply with special force to cancers of the uterine cervix, they are also relevant to cancers of the corpus uteri. Similar findings for the detection of these cancers have been published by authors carrying prophylactic mass examinations in Italy, Finland, Yugoslavia and other countries. It may also be presumed that an increased detection of other cancers of the genital tract has been achieved, although it is difficult to be certain that early detection has been attained.

The introduction of complex treatment seems to be most important for women in whom cancer of the genital tract has been detected. Undoubtedly, the material presented cannot be regarded as a discussion of all results of treatment although it has an essential importance from the epidemiologic point of view and that of rehabilitation of patients.

Our observations justify the statement that the most favourable outcome has been for women operated upon for cancers of the uterine cervix, or of the uterine body, as in these two groups 90% survived the period of follow-up without any recurrence of symptoms.

With reference to ovarian cancer, in agreement with the majority of the authors dealing with this problem, difficulties must be emphasised. We lack well-devised methods and a satisfactory model for early detection. These deficiencies reduce the efficacy of therapy.

To sum up, it should be presumed that systematically carried-out prophylactic mass examinations, early complex treatment, and careful follow-up of the fate of referred women will enable us to minimize the number of cancers, especially at an advanced stage.

Summary

The purpose of this paper is to follow-up the results of mass examinations of those women in whom genital neoplastic disease was detected.

Our observations justify the statement that the most favourable outcome has been for women operated upon for cancers of the uterine cervix, or of the uterine body. In these two groups, about 90% survived the period of follow-up without any recurrences. With reference to ovarian cancer, only 38.8% of women survived the 3 year period of follow-up without recurrences. In 19.4% recurrence was found at about 6 months following treatment. The remaining 41.8% have died because of local recurrences and distant metastases.

References

Audy, S., Bacic, M., Bagovic, P. and Bolanca, M. (1970): Minerva ginec., 22, 22.
Cameron, Ch. S. (1969): In: Proceedings, World Conference on Cancer of the Uterus, New Orleans, La., 1969.
Giacobbie, E. (1971): Minerva ginec., Vol. 23, No. 2.
Kolsted, P. (1971): Acta obstet. ginec. scand., Suppl. 11.
Nuzollilo, L. (1970): Minerva ginec., 22.
Soszka, S. (1970): Pol. med. J., Vol. 9, No. 4.
Timonen, S. (1971): Minerva ginec., 23.

Observations on the evolution of cervical lesions in women

P. Bagović, M. Bačić, Jasna Ivić, M. Bolanča, I. Vodopija and Silvana Audy

Gynecological Clinic Hospital, Zagreb, Yugoslavia

Introduction

Gynecological examinations are aimed not only at the detection of suspicious lesions and of cancer, but also at the prevention of such conditions. The purpose of such work is the treatment of all pathological changes of the cervix uteri after excluding cytologically and colposcopically all alterations that might be suspected of malignancy. The treatment of inflammations, erythroplakias, tramautic and other benign lesions can be conservative or surgical.

Most important are continuous clinical, cytological and colposcopical follow-ups of all patients with changes of the uterine cervix. This report presents the results of a 5-year follow-up of such patients in a campaign for the early detection of gynecological cancer in Medveščak, Zagreb, Yugoslavia (Audy et al., 1971).

Materials and methods

From 1966-1968, a total of 10,334 women, age 18 years and above, were examined for the first time. Normal clinical, cytological and colposcopical conditions were found in 5,607 women while some clinical, cytological and colposcopical changes were found in 4,727 cases. During the following period of 5 years, the majority of these women were regularly controlled (Table 1).

TABLE 1   *Clinical, cytological, and colposcopical findings on the cervix uteri in 10,334 women during the first examination*

No. of examined women	Normal findings	Changes of the uterine cervix
10,334	5,607	4,727

Results

The group of women with clinical, cytological and colposcopical changes of the cervix, could be divided up as shown in Table 2. Out of these 4,727 women, 4,616 had benign, and 111 had suspicious colposcopical changes of the cervix uteri. Patients in Papanicolaou Groups IV and V are not included in this report: we present our follow-up examinations on the following 3 groups.

TABLE 2   *Clinical, cytological and colposcopical changes found in the controlled group*

Cytological findings	No. of women	Colposcopical findings	
		Benign	Suspicious
Papanicolaou Groups I and II	4,504	4,469	35
Abnormal cells	93	89	4
Papanicolaou Group III	51	37	14
Papanicolaou Groups IV and V	79	21	58
Total	4,727	4,616	111

The first group

This comprises 4,504 women in whom there were clinical and colposcopical changes as well as a cytological finding in Papanicolaou Groups I or II. Colposcopical benign changes were found in 4,469 women, while in 35 cases findings were atypical. Of these 4,504 women 2,922 were treated while the remaining 1,582 were not treated because they refused electro-coagulation, or an operation. Conization of the cervix uteri was performed in 35 women with suspicious colposcopical findings, while the other 2,887 were electrocauterized (Table 3).

TABLE 3   *Treatment procedures in 4,504 women where benign changes in the cervix uteri were diagnosed*

Total no.	Treated	Conization	Electro-cauterization	Not treated
4,504	2,922	35	2,887	1,582

The histopathological diagnosis of the operated cone in 35 women were as presented in Table 4. Of the 2,887 women in whom the cervix was electrocoagulated, 2,715 were regularly controlled during the next 5 years. The clinical colposcopical and cytological findings at the follow-up examinations were normal. There were 172 women who did not come for their follow-up control.

The situation in the group of 1,582 women in whom the clinical and colposcopical examinations revealed benign changes of the exocervix, was quite different. Cytological findings revealed Papanicolaou Groups I or II. After the follow-up of controls during the

TABLE 4   *Histopathological diagnosis of the operated cone in 35 women*

Diagnosis	No. of cases
Erosio glandularis inflammata	19
Leukoplakia	15
Dysplasia	1
Total	35

TABLE 5   Progress of clinical and cytological changes of cervix uteri in a group of 7 women

Patient	Years of observation										Operation	Patho-histological diagnosis
	1 Pap	Colp	2 Pap	Colp	3 Pap	Colp	4 Pap	Colp	5 Pap	Colp		
S.R.	II	E–TZ	II/III	E–TZ	–	–	–	–	–	–	Conisation	Ca in situ
K.E.	I	E–TZ	I	E–TZ	II	E–TZ	III/IV	E–TZ	–	–	Conisation	Ca in situ
P.C.	II	E–TZ	II	E–TZ	II	E–TZ	III	E–TZ	IV/V		Extirpation uteri	Ca in situ
O.F.	II	E–TZ	II	E–TZ	II/III	E–TZ	IV	E–TZ	–	–	Extirpation uteri	Ca in situ
B.J.	I	E–TZ	I	E–TZ	I	E–TZ	II	E–TZ	III	E–TZ	Under observation	
A.S.	I	E–TZ	I	E–TZ	II	E–TZ	III	E–TZ	III	E–TZ	Under observation	
I.J.	I	E–TZ	I	E–TZ	II	E–TZ	II	E–TZ	III	E–TZ	Under observation	

5-year period, the progression of cytological findings from Papanicolaou Group II to Papanicolaou Groups III, IV and V was observed in 7 patients. Four of these women were operated on and the histopathological finding was carcinoma in situ in two of the cases; the third had microinvasive carcinoma of the cervix; and the last had adenocarcinoma of the cervix (Ib). The remaining 3 are under constant control in our dispensary. The full cytological and colposcopical changes are presented in Table 5.

The second group

In this group of 93 women in whom abnormal cells were found during the first examination, 89 had inflammation, or *Trichomonas vaginalis*. Among the 89 women, the colposcopical picture was benign and 4 atypical colposcopical changes of the exocervix were found.

In 39 women, after the treatment of inflammation, and two consecutive findings of cells of Papanicolaou Groups I and II, electro-coagulation of benign changes of the cervix uteri was performed. Among that group, we controlled 34 women for the next 5 years and the results were always normal. Five women did not attend for the controls after their first check-up. The whole picture of the work with this group is presented in Table 6.

There were 12 women in whom surgical intervention was necessary. In 9 cases, conization was performed. In 2 cases extirpation of the uterus was done and in one woman, the radical Wertheim operation was performed. Histopathological diagnosis was as follows: carcinoma in situ in 6 women, invasive carcinoma of the cervix in one woman, 2 women had leukoplakia, and in 3 cases inflammation was found.

In this group, 42 women were not actively treated because after the inflammation was cured, the changes of the exocervix receded, and the cytological findings reversed to Papanicolaou Groups I or II. The clinical findings were normal and we are still controlling this group of women. From this entire group, 6 women dropped out because they did not return for control examinations.

The third group

This group has 51 women, in whom the first cytological examination revealed Papanicolaou cell group III. Inflammation was found in 49 women. After treatment, the cytological findings showed a return to Papanicolaou cell groups I or II in 17 of the women. After cytological findings showed improvement, and following 3 controls separated by 3-6 months, electro-coagulation was performed in 11 of the 17 women with benign changes of the exocervix. The follow-up through the next 5 years indicated that there was no deterioration of these results. Also, we did not find any cytological progression in a group of 19 women who did not undergo electro-coagulation. The full picture is presented in Table 7.

The remaining 21 patients, who showed progression towards Papanicolaou groups IV and V, had to be surgically treated during the follow-up period of 3-5 years. In 17 women conization was performed, while in 4, total extirpation was undertaken. This radical surgical step was taken because of other gynecological conditions and not because of the cytological findings. The follow-up controls after these interventions in the above-mentioned group showed that there was no change towards malignant progression in the clinical and cytological findings. Three women were lost from the series because they did not come for their control examination.

Discussion

The optimal protection of women from carcinoma of the uterine cervix can be obtained only if benign changes of the cervix are treated at first detection (Bagović et al., 1970). Experience in many countries indicates that the healthy uterine cervix is less likely to be affected (Fluhman, 1961; Cristopherson, 1966; Zinser, 1968). Even the 7 cases which had

TABLE 6   *The treatment and histopathological findings in 93 women with abnormal cells*

Treatment	Without inflammation	With inflammation	After complete treatment Pap		Cauterization	Conization	Extirpation uteri totalis	Operation sec. Wertheim	Under control
			Cells I & II	Abnormal cells					
Erosio glandularis inflammata	4	89	81	12	39	9	2	1	42
Leukoplakia						2	1		
Dysplasia						2			
Ca in situ cervix uteri						5	1		
Carinoma invasive cervix uteri (Ib)								1	

TABLE 7   *Findings for 51 women with Papanicolaou cell Group III*

Treatment	Without inflammation	With inflammation	After treatment for inflammation Pap		Cauterization	Conization	Extirpation uteri totalis	Further control
			I–II	III				
Erosio glandularis inflammata	2	49	30	21	11	17	4	19
Leukoplakia						1	2	
Dysplasia						6	1	
Ca in situ cervix uteri						2		

a confirmed progression towards malignancy accord with this statement. Over a period of 1-5 years, we had the opportunity to observe cytological changes from the benign type to malignant cells. However, the treated group of women did not show any suspicious changes towards malignancy.

For physicians who work in the field of prevention and detection of gynecological cancer, cytological findings are most important for proper diagnosis and therapeutic procedures (Bengt, 1969; Benz and Glatthar, 1972). For that reason, it is of particular importance to have all women under continous control, especially those in whom benign changes of the uterine cervix were not completely clinically cured (Bagović, 1972). From our report, it appears that there are 3 possibilities of cytological changes.

First, the Papanicolaou cell group III shows a regression towards cell groups I and II after proper treatment. Secondly, cells of group III may remain unchanged for a longer period, and thirdly, they may show a progression towards cell groups IV and V.

It is thus particularly necessary to have continuous control of those women with clinical and colposcopical changes of the exocervix which have not been completely cured. In that group, progression towards malignancy should be observed more frequently than in those women where the uterine cervix was completely healed.

Conclusion

This report stresses the importance of continuous control and follow-up of the examined female population in the campaign for the detection of gynecological cancer. It is not enough to detect women with suspected changes and those with obvious carcinomas of the uterine cervix; it is just as important to provide adequate treatment for inflammatory lesions. Systematic observations over an extended period may detect changes progressing towards malignancy. It is interesting to note that out of our group of 1582 women, who were not subjected to treatment of the changes in their uterine cervix, and in whom no electrocoagulation was performed, progression towards malignancy was observed in 7 women.

References

Audy, S., Bačić, M., Bagović, P., Bolanča, M., Urbanke, A. and Vodopija, I. (1970): Minerva med., I, 117.
Bagović, P., Ivić, J., Rajhvajn, B. and Zimolo, A. (1970): Minerva med., I, 71.
Bagović, P., (1972): Libri oncologici, 1/1-2, 5.
Bengt, B., (1969): Acta obstet. Gynec. scand., Suppl. 48/6, 1.
Benz, J. J. and Glatthaar, E., (1972): Geburtsh. u. Frauenheilk., 32/3, 176.
Cristopherson, W. M. (1966): Acta cytol., (Philad.), 10, 15.
Fluhman, C. F. (1961): In: The Cervix Uteri and its Diseases, Vol. I., Chapter II, pp. 155-162. W.B. Saunders Co., Philadelphia, Pa.
Zinser, H. K. (1968): 'Folgerungen aus den Ergebnissen eines Zytologischen Krebssuch-Programmes,' Zbl. Gynäk., 90/26, 904.

4. Screening for breast cancer

The value of clinical examination in breast diseases

Christer Johnsén, Nils Bjurstam, Kersti Hedberg, Arvid Hultborn and Nils Johansson

Department of Surgery II, Department of Radiology II, Department of Cytology and Department of Pathology I, Sahlgren's Hospital, University of Gothenburg, Gothenburg, Sweden

There are nearly 3,300 new cases of mammary carcinoma in Sweden every year. 25% of all female cancer is breast carcinoma (National Board of Health and Welfare, 1970). The results of treatment have not become much better during the last decades. We believe that an earlier and more accurate diagnosis of breast carcinoma is one way of improving these results. The chief aim of this study is to compare and evaluate different diagnostic methods. We have studied clinical examination, soft tissue X-ray examination of the breast (so called mammography), fine needle aspiration biopsy and thermography. This paper reports the results of clinical investigation: the results of the other methods are presented in separate papers.

The study was performed by a special diagnostic group consisting of 3 surgeons, a radiologist, a cytologist and a pathologist, formed to ensure optimal investigating conditions. All examinations were performed by members of the group. Our ambition was to study a consecutive series of patients seeking medical care for breast symptoms in the Gothenburg region. The material was collected in 15 months and the majority of patients with breast complaints seeking medical care during this time was referred to our diagnostic group. All patients were examined by thermography, clinical examination and mammography on the same day. No investigator knew the results of the other methods. Patients with clinically or mammographically demonstrated lesions were referred for fine needle aspiration biopsy. Even in cases of non-palpable tumors, we have tried to do aspiration biopsy by directing the needle after instructions from the radiologist. Results of the clinical examination, thermography, fine needle biopsy and mammography have been pooled and evaluated. If surgical biopsy, or some sort of mastectomy, was necessary the majority of these operations were performed by members of the group. All surgical specimens were analysed by X-ray before examination by the pathologist.

Material

The material consists of a consecutive series of 1,310 women with breast complaints, and 241 women without breast symptoms as a control group. All patients are examined by thermography, clinical examination and mammography. In cases of circumscribed lesions, fine needle aspiration biopsy was carried out. In 397 cases surgical biopsy or some sort of mastectomy was performed. 181 had malignant breast tumors and 784 had palpable benign lesions.

Figure 1 shows the age-distribution, the number of patients operated upon and the number of patients with cancer.

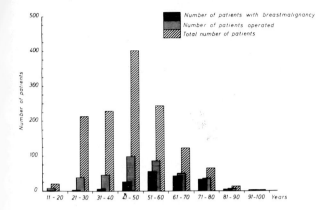

FIG. 1   *Age distribution of 1,310 women seeking medical care for breast symptoms.*

Methods

The clinical examination was standardized as far as possible. As a rule, 2 investigators were present. We started with a record of the patient's history according to a special scheme. The patient was then examined, first sitting and then supine, by inspection and palpation. The axillary, supra- and infraclavicular glandular regions were examined. The clinical examination was made according to Haagensen. Immediately after this examination we classified the results on a 4-graded scale from malignant, probably benign to benign. This was done without knowledge of the results of the other diagnostic methods. We established that all cases clinically judged as malignant, probably malignant, or probably benign must have a surgical biopsy performed in order to exclude or prove malignancy. This initial decision for surgical biopsy was thus based solely on the results of clinical examination, but was later modified when we learned the results of the other diagnostic methods. Thus, recommendation for surgical biopsy based on clinical examination alone did not always lead to an operation if the results of mammography and fine needle aspiration biopsy revealed that the lesion was genuinely benign.

Results

As seen in Table 1, 181 patients have malignant breast tumors. In 4 cases there is synchronous bilateral carcinoma, which means that the material consists of 185 breasts with malignant tumors. Included in these figures are 2 cases of malignant lymphoma and one of metastases in the breast from a spinocellular carcinoma with the primary tumor in the

TABLE 1   *185 malignant breast tumors (Figures in per cent)*

	Malignant	Probably malignant	Probably benign	Benign or inconclusive	Total	No. of patients not examined
Clinical examination	37.8	34.0	18.4	9.8	100	–
Mammography	83.0	9.3	5.4	2.3	100	2
Aspiration biopsy	74.1	12.1	8.3	5.5	100	3

mouth. In Table 1, the results of clinical examination, mammography and aspiration biopsy are compared. In 18 cases, clinical examination had failed to reveal a malignant tumor. This means that if we had relied on clinical examination alone, not more than 90% of the cancer cases would have been correctly diagnosed.

Table 2 presents the results of clinical examination of 185 malignant breast tumors, of which 169 were palpable and 16 were not palpable, or occult. Of the 169 palpable tumors, 5 were clinically misinterpreted as benign lesions and biopsy was not recommended. Of the patients with the 16 non-palpable tumors, 3 had Paget's disease of the nipple and 4 had clinically involved axillary nodes. In 9 cases there were thus no signs of malignancy whatsoever. In these 9 cases, mammography alone diagnosed the carcinoma and in the 3 cases of Paget's disease and the 4 cases of clinically involved nodes without palpable tumor in the breast, mammography localized the lesion.

In Table 3 we present the results of clinical examination, mammography and fine needle aspiration biopsy of 784 palpable lesions subsequently proven benign. In 226 cases, or 29%, it was not possible to exclude malignancy by clinical examination alone and surgical biopsy was recommended. However, many of these cases were not operated because mammography and aspiration biopsy revealed the genuinely benign nature of the lesions.

Discussion

Our results stress the well known fact that clinical examination alone is not capable of providing an exact diagnosis in either malignant, or benign, lesions. It is not possible to find directly comparable figures in the literature. Table 4 presents the accuracy of pre-operative clinical diagnosis according to several authors. The diagnostic accuracy ranges between 75 and 85% of the cancer cases.

Our results, and these results from the literature, show clearly that if we want to improve our diagnostic accuracy we cannot rely on clinical examination alone, but have to introduce other diagnostic methods such as mammography and fine needle aspiration biopsy. Our results with thermography, mammography and fine needle aspiration biopsy

TABLE 2   *Results of clinical diagnosis in 185 malignant breast tumors*

Palpable tumor		Occult tumor			
Biopsy recommended	Biopsy not recommended	Biopsy recommended involved axillary nodes	Paget's disease	Biopsy not recommended no signs of malignancy	Total number
164	5	4	3	9	185

TABLE 3   *784 benign palpable lesions (Figures in per cent)*

	Malignant	Probably malignant	Probably benign	Benign	Incon-clusive	Total	No. of patients not examined
Clinical examination	0.5	2.9	25.4	71.2		100	
Mammography	0.1	0.1	5.6	94.2		100	2
Aspiration biopsy	0	1.0	10.0	76.2	12.8	100	52

TABLE 4   *Results of preoperative clinical diagnosis in breast carcinoma*

Author	Year	Accuracy % correct diagnosis
Arcari and Wilson	1961	85
Wright	1962	79
Farrow	1963	85
Leis	1965	75
Forrest et al.	1970	85
Haagensen	1971	81

are presented in separate papers. They indicate that thermography does not contribute to the diagnosis in patients with breast symptoms, but that a combination of clinical examination, mammography and fine needle aspiration biopsy can result in:

1. Earlier diagnosis.
2. Improved planning of treatment:
   (*a*) Better chances of judging surgical curability.
   (*b*) In cancer: Direct radical mastectomy without prior surgical biopsy and frozen section.
3. The elimination of unnecessary surgical biopsies of clearly benign conditions.

Without mammography it is not possible to detect so-called occult or preclinical cancer tumors in the breast. Among patients with breast symptoms we can expect to find an occult carcinoma in more than one out of 100 patients. With the aid of mammography and fine needle biopsy the planning of treatment can be improved. In cancer, it is possible to perform radical mastectomy directly without prior surgical biopsy, which is an advantage. By combining these 3 methods we have avoided surgical biopsies of clearly benign lesions. In the literature (Montgomery et al., 1961) 5-10 times as many surgical biopsies are performed on benign lesions as on maliganant ones, as compared to our ratio of 2:1. This clearly indicates that our diagnostic procedures have reduced the number of unnecessary operations bringing benefits to the individual and reduction of the costs for society. We have now observed and checked all our 1,310 patients for a period of 3-4 years. During this period, 2 of the patients have developed malignant breast tumors. In neither of these 2 cases did the tumor develop in a circumscribed lesion earlier interpreted as benign at the first combined examination.

Even if we introduce mammography and fine needle aspiration biopsy, clinical examination remains the fundamental basis for the diagnosis of breast carcinoma. It is the doctor performing the clinical examination who has to evaluate the results of mammography and aspiration biopsy and combine this with information from the patient's history and the clinical examination. From this information, the individual case can be evaluated and each patient can be given the best possible treatment.

Summary

1,310 patients with breast symptoms were examined by thermography, clinical examination and mammography. In all clinically or mammographically detected lesions fine needle aspiration biopsy was performed. Clinical examination alone failed to diagnose 9.8% of the cancer cases. The majority of these cases were non-palpable or occult carcinomas diagnosed by mammography. A combination of clinical examination, mammography and fine needle aspiration biopsy can improve the diagnostic accuracy in many ways and this might lead to a better prognosis for patients with breast carcinoma.

References

Arcari, F. A. and Wilson, G. S. (1961): GP, 23, 82.
Farrow, J. (1963): Surg. Reporter, 1, 3.
Forrest, A. P. M., Gleave, E. N., Roberts, M. M., Henck, J. M. and Gravell, I. H. (1970): Proc. roy. Soc. Med., 63, 11.
Haagensen, C. D. (1970): Diseases of the Breast. Second Edition. W. B. Saunders Company, Philadelphia, Pa.
Leis Jr, H. P. (1965): Hosp. Med., 1, 27.
Montgomery, T. L., Bowers, P. A. and Kittleberger, W. C. (1961): J. Obstet. Gynec., 17, 112.
National Board of Health and Welfare (1970): Cancer Incidence in Sweden 1970. The Cancer Registry, Stockholm 1970.
Wright, H. K. (1962): Arch. Surg., 85, 1021.

Thermography in the diagnosis of breast diseases: A preliminary report

Christer Johnsén, Nils Bjurstam, Kersti Hedberg, Arvid Hultborn and Nils Johansson

Department of Surgery II, Department of Radiology II, Department of Cytology and Department of Pathology I, Sahlgren's Hospital, University of Gothenburg, Gothenburg, Sweden

Thermography is an electro-optical means of translating variations of surface temperature into a visual image. The skin emits infrared radiation as a function of its temperature and emissivity according to Stephan-Boltzmann's Law. Minor changes in the emissivity of the skin have been reported, but in most instances it is considered to be very close to unity. Thus, although available thermographs do not reveal minor changes in the emissivity, highly reliable temperature measurements can be obtained with this technique. The temperature of the skin is a result of the dynamic equilibrium between the heat gained through blood circulation and conduction from the inner parts of the tissues, versus the heat loss from the skin surface by radiation and evaporation. Thermal changes from pathological processes may therefore be caused by one or more factors such as decreased or increased blood circulation, changes in thermoconduction in the tissues and locally increased metabolic activity.

There have been great expectations for thermography as a method for detecting the thermal radiation from an increased metabolism in malignant tumors and especially breast cancer. Many authors do indeed report good results with thermography in breast cancer diagnosis.

In 1968 we began to study different diagnostic methods in connection with breast diseases. The chief aim of the study was to compare and evaluate thermography, clinical examination, mammography and fine needle aspiration biopsy. To do this properly, we set up a breast service group including 3 surgeons, a radiologist, a cytologist and a pathologist. Almost every patient in the Gothenburg region consulting a doctor for breast complaints during a period of 15 months was referred to our group and examined with thermography, clinical examination and mammography on the same day. If the clinical examination, or mammography, discovered circumscribed lesions the patient was referred for aspiration biopsy. Results of thermography, clinical examination, mammography and aspiration biopsy were then reviewed together and if surgical biopsy and/or some sort of mastectomy was recommended the majority of the operations were performed by our group. Surgical specimens were sliced and examined by X-ray before the microscopic investigation.

Material and methods

The clinical material consisted of a consecutive series of 1,310 women with breast complaints. As a control group, we had 241 healthy women without breast symptoms (see Fig. 1, p. 405).

Thermography was performed with an AGA-thermovision equipment. We constructed a special room for thermography with facilities for constant temperature and humidity. All possible draughts were excluded and the patient was examined sitting in a chair with her arms above her head after 15 min equilibration time. Frontal and oblique ther-

mograms were taken. The interpretation of the thermogram was made directly from the
screen and written on a special protocol for further computer analysis. Photographs were
taken of all thermograms. The thermographic investigator had no knowledge of the
patient's history or symptoms and signs when making the interpretation. Directly after
the thermographic examination, the patient was sent for a standardized clinical examination. After that, mammography was performed with a so-called Senograph. Aspiration
biopsies were performed in all patients with lesions detected by clinical examination or
mammography. Results of clinical examination, mammography and fine needle aspiration
biopsy are presented in separate papers.

Results

Of 1,310 patients with breast complaints, 181 had malignant breast tumors. In 4 cases,
bilateral synchronous malignant disease was found. We also found 784 palpable benign
lesions. The thermographic results for precancerous lesions and circumscribed non-
palpable benign lesions detected by mammography are not presented here.

In the preliminary interpretation, thermograms were classified as normal or negative,
or abnormal or positive. 31.7% of the cancer cases had normal thermograms and among
all the patients in the material without breast malignancy, 46% had abnormal or positive
thermograms. Among these 46%, patients with benign breast lesions and patients without
signs of breast abnormality are included (Fig. 1).

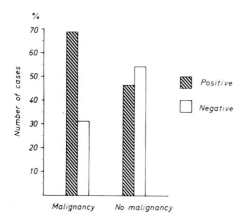

FIG. 1   *Results of thermography.*

The results of thermography are influenced by many factors such as the type of
thermographic equipment, the room of the examination and the equilibration time. The
age of the patient, co-existing benign lesions, previous mastectomy, pregnancy and lactation, use of contraceptive pills or other types of hormonal treatment, may all influence
the results. The biological properties of the tumor, its vascularisation, the diameter,
depth, and localisation of the tumor can influence the results of thermography.

In the present study we have tried to analyse some of the factors mentioned above.
When we started in 1968 we had no previous personal experience with thermography. We
chose as a criterion for an abnormal or positive thermogram a measurable temperature
increase of one degree Celsius or more in one part of the breast as compared with the
same part of the other breast. This criterion has been used by several authors (Gershon-
Cohen et al., 1965). With our criteria for normal and abnormal thermograms we included
in the abnormal group not only patients with so-called 'hot spots' but even patients with
asymmetrical thermal patterns, because these patterns will in most instances give a measurable temperature difference of one centigrade or more between comparable parts of both

the breasts. We intend to divide our thermograms into different groups according to Draper and Jones, 1969, and Bourjat and Gautherie, 1970 in order to study how these and other interpretational criteria might influence the results of thermography.

Table 1 illustrates how the choice of different temperature levels to separate normal from abnormal thermograms influences results. In this table we compare the cancer cases with the group of patients with different benign lesions and a group of patients with normal breasts. It is evident that if we increase the temperature difference from 1 up to 1.5 or 2 degrees Celsius, we increase the number of false-negative results although the number of false-positive results is decreased.

TABLE 1   *Thermographic results with different temperature levels (All figures in percent)*

	Control		Benign		Malignant	
	Negative	Positive	Negative	Positive	Negative	Positive
> 1°	62	38	55	45	32	68
> 1.5°	68	32	68	32	47	53
> 2°	78	22	82	18	58	42

In Table 2, results of thermography in the left breast versus the right breast are presented. From this table it is clear that the number of positive thermograms in the left breast are much higher than in the other breast irrespective of whether the breast is normal or contains a malignant tumor. This means that the number of false-negative cancer cases in the left breast is 20% compared to 49% in the right breast. We do not know the reason for this and we have not been able to find comparable figures in the literature.

TABLE 2   *Thermographic results in left breast versus right breast*

	Cancer		Control	
	Negative	Positive	Negative	Positive
Left	20%	80%	67%	33%
Right	49%	51%	94%	6%

TABLE 3   *Breast cancer: Relation between thermographic results and age of the patient*

Age (yr)	Thermography	
	Negative	Positive
< 50	39%	61%
50–60	35%	65%
> 60	29%	71%

In Table 3, results of thermography in relation to the age of the patient are presented. There is a tendency for a more accurate thermographic diagnosis with increasing age of the patient. An explanation for this might be the fact that benign lesions such as fibro-adenoma and chronic cystic disease, which are known sometimes to give a measurable temperature increase, are less common in the higher age groups.

From Table 4 and Figure 2 it is evident that there is some relation between tumor diameter and the measured temperature increase. From these results we think it is correct to conclude that the smaller the tumor, the more inaccurate is thermography as a diagnostic method.

TABLE 4   *Realtion between TNM classification of tumor and thermographic results*

	Thermography	
TNM	Negative (%)	Positive (%)
T_0	57	43
T_1	40	60
T_2	43	57
T_3	25	75
T_4	21	79

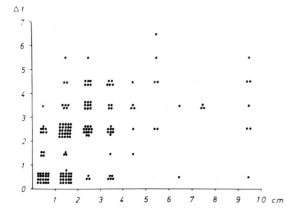

FIG. 2

Relation between the temperature difference and the size of the carcinoma. Tumor diameter measured in the surgical specimen.

A high metabolic activity in the tumor increases the vascularisation in the tissue surrounding the tumor and such cases should appear as an abnormal thermal pattern on the thermographic picture. We have tried to estimate the grade of vascularisation around the tumor on the mammogram compared with the results of thermography. From Table 5 it is evident that highly vascularised tumors are more easily detected by thermography.

Discussion

The results presented here indicate multifactorial influences on the thermogram. We intend to analyse in more detail how different interpretational criteria, the histologic grading of a tumor, depths of the tumor in the breast, co-existing benign disease, etc.,

TABLE 5   *Breast cancer: Relation between the grade of vascularisation around the tumor (estimated from the mammogram) and the thermographic results*

Vascularisation	Negative (%)	Positive (%)
Not increased	55	45
Moderately increased	36	64
Much increased	20	80

influence the results of thermography. According to our experience so far, thermography does not help to diagnose breast cancer beyond the information received from a combination of clinical examination, mammography and fine needle aspiration biopsy. Thermography is far too inaccurate, especially for small tumors, to be used as a screening procedure.

Summary

1,310 women with breast complaints and 241 women without breast symptoms were examined by thermography, clinical examination and mammography. More than 30% of the cancer cases had normal thermograms. A positive correlation between tumor size and results of thermography was found, i.e. the smaller the tumor the more inaccurate is thermography as a diagnostic method. The conclusion is drawn that thermography, in its present state, does not contribute to diagnosis in breast diseases.

References

Bourjat, P. and Gautherie, M. (1970): Electromedica, 1, 17.
Draper, J. W. and Jones, C. H. (1969): Brit. J. Radiol., 42/498, 401.
Gershon-Cohen, I., Haberman-Brueschke, J. A. P. and Brueschke, E. E. (1965): Radiol. Clin. N. Amer., 3, 403.
Gershon-Cohen, I., Hermel, M. B. and Murdock, M. G. (1970): Cancer (Philad.), 26, 1153.
Hitchcock, C. R., Hickok, D. F., Soucheray, I., Moulton, T. and Baker, C. R. (1963): J. Amer. med. Ass., 204/6, 99.
Isard, H. J., Ostrum, B. J. and Shilo, R. (1969): Surg. Gynec. Obstet., 128, 1289.
Nathan, B. E., Burn, I. I. and MacErlean, D. P. (1972): Brit. med. J., 2, 316.

Practical aspects of early diagnosis of breast cancer with the aid of thermography and mammography

Olaf Melander

Karolinska Hospital, Stockholm, Sweden

When trying to compare the results of different examinations of the breasts with the aid of thermography, one often finds it difficult to explain the differences in results. The first reason is that the group of patients examined is not clearly defined and second, there is often no clear definition of the reason for classifying a finding as positive or negative. About the groups of patients examined, I should suggest three main groups:

1. Patients with a clinically obvious cancer.
2. Patients with breast symptoms, but not clearly cancer.
3. 'Asymptomatic' patients.

Examinations on patients from the first group are often made, not only in order to learn the temperature distribution of a breast cancer, but also to follow the results of a given treatment. The second group are the patients asking their doctor for a breast examination because of unclear symptoms. Here the thermographic picture can be a good help in reading the mammogram, and in the clinical examination. The third is the type of patient examined in the health screening in Gävle. By 'asymptomatic' is meant that the patient had not noticed any changes in the breasts before the screening, even if she later proves to have a clear palpable tumor.

Our experience of the temperature distribution in breast cancer is built mainly on the first group. Measuring the temperature differences between symmetric areas, one finds a clear difference between cancer and benign diseases. We therefore chose to regard those between zero and one degree centigrade as negative, those between one and two as suspect, and those more than two degrees difference as positive. In the first group, out of 518 patients operated upon, 92% were positive and 6% false-positive in an earlier examination at Radiumhemmet.

From earlier examinations of patients of the second group (those with unclear symptoms), we learnt that there is also often an atypical picture in cases with fibroadenomas, in mastitis and in duct papillomas. Papillomas, when not calcified, can generally not be seen on the mammogram. On the thermogram there are in those cases often atypical warm vessels to the areola regions. When there is bleeding from the nipple, the duct opening can often be localized and contrast medium can be injected with a tiny silver cannula. Thus masses of big papillomas can be seen filling out the dilated ducts. Careful examination of the mammogram over exactly the same area does not reveal any sign of the papillomas. In the same way, adenomas can be hidden in a dense parenchyma or considered to be cysts. In health screening, papillomas will remain undetected, when not bleeding. From an earlier study on patients with symptoms, we found that for thermography 80% of 72 cases operated upon and with proven cancer were true positive, but the number of false-positive and suspect cases among 178 cases without proven cancer was as high as 45%. Among these cases cancer later appeared and the follow-up of this study is still going on. However, it is already clear that such a suspect group on thermography is a high-risk group that must be followed for years with repeated controls. This examination was a comparative study between different methods for the diagnosis of breast cancer and a drawback in such a study is, that one method cannot be used to help the other to diagnosis.

When combining the different methods, trying to explain the atypical thermogram with the aid of not only the mammogram, but also case history, clinical examination and perhaps needle biopsy, very early cases can be detected. To exemplify this, three cases with a similar thermogram, with a small warm area in the upper lateral part of the right breast could be demonstrated, all without a palpable lump.

The first case has a difference between symmetric areas of three degrees, read in the color thermogram from white to violet. In the mammogram, a slightly more dense area is seen in one projection containing some small calcification. Compressing the actual warm area with a small tube, the tumor is no longer hidden by the normal parenchyma. The second case is a patient with bleeding from the nipple and a hot spot in the same area as the earlier case. Also here the tumor is difficult to see before the area is locally compressed. In galactography the ducts in this area are obliterated. The third case has also a hot spot in the same area, but in the mammogram a crown of small subcutaneous vessels is seen, indicating the hot spot as an artefact.

Another problem is how to do a needle biopsy on these not-palpable tumors. We have therefore made a special stereo-attachment to the Senograph, which is fixed to the apparatus and independent of the movements of the tube. The breast is separately compressed by a plate and needle biopsy can be performed through holes in this plate. By moving the tube three degree in each direction, a stereopicture is obtained. The use can be exemplified with a case with a cyst, seen by galactography, where there is an irregularity in the posterior wall. First a leading needle is stuck as close to the actual area as possible and thereupon stereopictures are taken. With the aid of the leading needle, a second needle can then be stuck into the actual area and a sample obtained.

Mammography in the diagnosis of breast cancer

Nils Bjurstam, Kersti Hedberg, Arvid Hultborn, Nils Johansson and Christer Johnsén

Department of Radiology II and Department of Cytology and Department of Pathology I and Department of Surgery II, Sahlgren's Hospital, University of Gothenburg, Gothenburg, Sweden

Soft tissue X-ray examination of the breast has been one of the diagnostic methods in a study initiated to evaluate the roles of clinical examination, thermography, mammography and fine needle aspiration biopsy in diagnosing breast diseases. In this paper the results of the X-ray examination are presented. The results of the other methods are given in separate papers.

Material

The material consists of a consecutive series of 1,310 women with breast complaints. Seven patients were not examined by mammography. All but these 7 patients were examined with thermography, clinical examination and mammography and in cases of circumscribed lesions, with fine needle aspiration biopsy. 397 cases were operated on. 181 patients had malignant breast tumors, 4 of whom had synchronous bilateral carcinoma.

Only the patients with a clearly benign or clearly malignant status are reported in this paper. The so-called pre-cancerous lesions in the material will not be discussed here.

The age-distribution, the number of patients operated upon and the number of patients with cancer in different age-groups, is shown in Figure 1, p. 405.

Method

In mammography, as in no other area of roentgenologic study, diagnostic accuracy depends on obtaining excellent films with optimal detail and contrast.

Before starting the study in 1968, we made a thorough investigation of different mammography techniques and soon found that Gros' technique was superior to others. The first, and at that time the only available, specifically designed apparatus built on the principles of this technique was the Senograph made by CGR in France which was used in this study. One of the advantages of Gros' technique is that the spectrum of X-rays emitted by the molybdenum target is optimally suited for soft tissue roentgen examination of the breast. Another advantage of great importance is that the Senograph permits maximum compression of the breast under standardized conditions with minimal discomfort to the patient. The tube can be rotated through 360 degrees so that the entire examination can be made with the patient seated. As a routine, three views were taken of each breast — one craniocaudal, one mediolateral and one medial oblique. If necessary, additional views and spot films were taken. In addition, each axilla was examined with one projection. The procedure is rapid and readily reproducible and the standardized projections permit accurate localization of any lesion in the breast. Nonscreen, automatically developed 'industrial' type film was used for the examinations (Kodak Crystallex).

TABLE 1   *185 malignant breast tumors (Figures in percent)*

	Malignant	Probably malignant	Probably benign	Benign or inconclusive	Total	No. of patients not examined
Clinical examination	37.8	34.0	18.4	9.8	100	
Mammography	83.0	9.3	5.4	2.3	100	2
Aspiration biopsy	74.1	12.1	8.3	5.5	100	3

TABLE 2   *784 benign palpable lesions (Figures in percent)*

	Malignant	Probably malignant	Probably benign	Benign	Inconclusive	Total	No. of patients not examined
Clinical examination	0.5	2.9	25.4	71.2		100	
Mammography	0.1	0.1	5.6	94.2		100	2
Aspiration biopsy	0	1.0	10.0	76.2	12.8	100	52

Results

In Table 1, the results of clinical examination, mammography and aspiration biopsy of 185 breasts with malignant tumors are compared.

Each investigator had to classify the diagnosed lesion in one of four different groups — malignant, probably-malignant, probably-benign and benign. In the first three groups, biopsy was recommended so that the cancer diagnosis would not be missed. Thus the fourth group represents the false negatives. The Table shows that four cases, or 2.3% of cancers, appearing benign radiographically were proved to be cancer on biopsy. On the other hand, clinical examination failed to reveal a malignant tumor in 18 cases. That means that almost 10% of the breast malignancies were not suspected clinically.

Table 1 also shows that mammography enables diagnosis of the cancer with a higher accuracy than the other methods. Thus in 83% of the malignant cases the radiologist interpreted the lesion as cancer without doubt. The corresponding figure for clinical examination was 38%.

Table 2 shows the results of clinical examination, mammography and aspiration biopsy in 784 palpable lesions subsequently proved to be benign. In this Table, the fourth group with lesions classified as benign represents the true positives, while in lesions classified in the other groups, biopsy was recommended. These latter groups therefore represent the false-positives.

Thus, with mammography, malignancy could be excluded in 94% — only in 6% of these benign lesions did the radiologist recommend biopsy.

Discussion

Our results stress the important role of soft tissue X-ray examination in the early detection of breast cancer. In more than one out of a 100 patients with breast complaints, the X-ray examination revealed malignant tumors that were not suspected clinically. It is also evident that with mammography it is possible to distinguish better between benign and malignant disease. Another contribution of the X-ray examination is the additional information on the nature and the extent of the disease — for example, accurate information is given about the growth pattern, localization and extension of a lesion. In impalpable lesions this information is a necessity for fine needle aspiration biopsy as well as for the surgical biopsy. Also, in palpable lesions, mammography has proved to be of value by giving accurate information about the localization of the lesion to facilitate the biopsy procedure.

Thus clinical examination, mammography and fine needle aspiration biopsy must be regarded as complementary diagnostic methods and by combining them, as has been done in this study, it is possible to improve diagnostic accuracy. This is evident from the results of a 3-year follow-up which shows that only two additional cancers have developed during this period. These two cancers developed 2 and 3 years respectively after the initial study. This indicates that our diagnostic system has a very high degree of accuracy.

Summary

A series of 1,310 unselected consecutive patients with breast complaints have been studied by clinical examination, mammography, thermography and in cases with circumscribed lesions, by fine needle aspiration biopsy. When comparing the results of the radiological examination to that of other methods and histopathological findings, it is evident that mammography makes it possible to diagnose malignant tumors that were not suspected clinically. Almost 10% of the malignant tumors in this series were so-called clinically occult carcinomas.

The results also show that with mammography it is possible to distinguish between benign and malignant disease with a higher accuracy as compared to the other methods. The

X-ray examination is also of value for the localization of the tumor to facilitate fine needle aspiration biopsy and surgical biopsy.

References

Egan, R. L. (1960): Radiology, 75, 894.
Gershon-Cohen, J. (1970): Atlas of Mammography. Springer-Verlag, Berlin-Heidelberg-New York.
Gros, C. M. (1967): J. Radiol. Electrol., 48, 638.
Haagensen, C. D. (1970): Diseases of the Breast. Second Edition. W. B. Saunders Company, Philadelphia, Pa.
Leborgne, R. A. (1953): The Breast in Roentgen Diagnosis. Impresora Uruguaya S.A. Montevideo.

Mammography screening for breast cancer in the province of Florence

G. C. Maltoni and M. Cappellini

Centro per le Malattie Sociali e la Medicina Preventiva, Provincia di Firenze, Florence, Italy

19,178 women were examined, divided into age-groups as shown in Table 1. The total number of tests performed, however, were 21,786 as some women underwent mammography more than once. Since June 1971 mammographic screening has been used for first investigation; from this date on, this procedure has been given up as the number of the suspected cases at the screening was too high (around 30%), and as, mammographic screening as initial execution, in our opinion, presents the risk of many false-negatives especially when we are faced with cancer in the initial phase—that which reveals itself with microcalcifications.

TABLE 1   *19,178 examined women divided into age-groups*

Age groups	1–10	11–20	21–30	31–40	41–50	51–60	61–70	71–80	Non-specified age
No. of examined women	2	23	224	2,716	8,504	4,678	2,675	367	89

In our group we separated patients who had no symptoms, even subjective, from those who had a subjective and/or objective symptomatology. Women with no symptoms numbered 12,286 (64.06%) and others 6,892 (35.93%).

The highest number of asymptomatic women were found among those examined by the mobile unit. From among the total examined (19,178 women) we found 280 cancers (1.46%). Among these, 251 (89%) were found among the positive and the radiologically suspected and the rest among those subjected to the radiological test, being of benign pathology or non-readable (Table 2).

Table 2 shows the coefficient of breast cancer stage in the different age groups. From the distribution of these coefficients it is possible to see a direct relation between the age of the patient and mammary cancer, which develops progressively with age. We also wanted to verify the relation between radiological and histological diagnosis of breast cancer. Table 3 shows that there is a good accordance between these two types of diagnosis with a very low percentage of false-positives (8.52%).

TABLE 2   *The coefficient of breast cancer stage according to age-groups*

Age groups	31–40	41–50	51–60	61–70
Specific coefficients for 100 women examined	7.00	10.60	16.89	20.93

TABLE 3   *Relation between radiological and histological diagnosis of breast cancer*

Radiological diagnosis	No. of tests	Histologically verified cases		Not followed	False positives	
		No.	%		No.	%
Positives	223	199	89.24	5	19	8.52
Suspected	221	52	23.53			
Benign pathology	4,612	12	0.26			
Non-readable	2,600	17	0.65			
Negatives	11,522	–	–			
Total	19,178	280	1.46			

TABLE 4   *Relation between radiological diagnosis of the cancer and the presence of a clinical objectivity*

Radiological diagnosis	Histologically verified cases	Objectivity		
		Positive	Negative	Unknown
Positives (223)	199	175	9	15
Suspected (221)	52	48	4	
Benign pathology (4,612)	12	12		
Non-readable (2,600)	17	17		
Total	280	252	13	15

Note the high number of non-readable cases (2,600 of 19,178 women tested). We consider as non-readable, those cases in which a thick corpus mammae or diffused mastosis does not permit a premature diagnosis of the cancer; this is the limitation of mammography.

We have also tested the relation existing between radiological diagnosis of the cancer and the presence of a clinical objectivity (Table 4); this having been possible, because all the women affected by cancer were submitted to an extensive examination by the surgeon.

The number of asymptomatic women affected by cancer of the breast is very high: 13 out of 12,286 asymptomatic cases (0.1%).

The above-mentioned results confirm, in our opinion, the validity of mammography for the premature diagnosis of cancer of the breast.

Importance of mammography in cancer detection: Contribution of cytology. A radio, anatomo, cyto and clinical confrontation

A. Vandenbroucke-Vanderwielen, M.A. Sergent-Millet and H. Maisin

Cancer Institute, University of Louvain, Louvain, Belgium

One of our cancer detection centers has possessed a senograph since the beginning of 1972. After a very detailed interrogation about complaints and mammary symptoms shown by the patient and the control of obstetrical and gynecological antecedents, a careful inspection and palpation of the breasts and its ganglionic zones is effected. A radiological examination of the breasts is proposed to those patients who present a clinical anomaly of the breasts and also to those who complain of symptoms. On the other hand, some radiological examinations have been carried out on patients who had no symptoms or clinical signs, in order to reassure the worried patient.

At the end of 1972, 436 examinations had been effected on 415 patients: 21 of them had 2 examinations and 18% of all the women who have undergone an examination for cancer detection submitted to mammography. The protocols of the radiological examinations have been codified. In fact, it takes the clinical examination into consideration (Mazy et al., 1972). The left side of Table 1 shows the codification and on the right, we see the results of the 436 radiographical examinations. We shall pay attention to categories IV, V and X and analyse the indications of the clinical examinations and the results of further investigations of those cases.

TABLE 1   *Codification and results of 436 radiological examinations*

Examination	Codification and results		
	Class	No.	(%)
Normal	I ⎫		
Banal	II ⎭	355	(81.50)
Doubtful (necessitating a clinical or radiological control in the next months)	III	58	(13.30)
Suspicious (necessitating a biopsy excision)	IV	11	(2.52)
Positive	V	3	(0.69)
Uncertain	X	9	(2.06)

The clinical interpretation of the criteria are shown in Table 2. Our attitude towards a clinically 'suspicious' case differs completely from the one we adopt towards a clinically 'doubtful' case. Indeed, when a case is clinically 'suspicious', we propose an exeresis

TABLE 2   *Clinical interpretation of the criteria*

Examination	Interpretation
Nothing special	banal
Presence of one or more hard, movable, uniform and well-determined nodules, without other signs or in a dysplastic breast	doubtful
Presence of a hard, irregular, adherent, not well-determined nodule. Signs such as a more visible venous circulation and retraction confirm the suspicion. (Two of these signs are enough to classify the case as suspect.)	suspicious
Association of a hard, irregular, adherent nodule with cutaneous phenomena such as orange skin and retraction	positive

TABLE 3   *Radiologically positive cases (class V)*

Patient file no.	Clinical examination	Anatomo-pathological
72.2972	S	Glandular epithelioma
72.3885	D	Comedocarcinoma
72.5593	+	Infiltrating duct epithelioma

TABLE 4   *Radiologically suspicious cases (class IV)*

Patient file No.	Clinical examination	Anatomo-pathological examination	Other forms of follow-up
67.2898	D	−	Rx control : intradermal benign anomaly
68.0424	(−)	−	Rx control : status quo - probable F.A.
69.6107	(−)	Fibrous dysplasia + adenosclerous lesion	−
68.5291	S	−	−
72.3131	D	Fibromatous nodule	−
69.5648	S	Epithelioma	−
72.4788	D	Glandulo-cystic mastopathy	−
70.3617	(−)	Epithelioma in situ	−
72.4791	D	Fibrous dysplastic lesion	−
72.5807	(−)	Scirrhous cancer	−

TABLE 5   *The 9 cases for which radiological uncertainty was total*

Patient file No.	Clinical examination	Anatomo-pathological examination	Other forms of follow-up
71.4199	D	–	Rx control : (–)
69.0675	D	–	Rx control : lesion of type fibro-myxolipoma
72.0169	D	–	Rx control : (–)
72.1209	(–)	–	Rx control : status quo
68.4459	S	Fibrocystic masto-pathy - focus of epithelial intraductal proliferation	
68.1903	(–)	–	Clinical examination : status quo
72.4318	D	–	Rx control : (–)
72.5592	D	–	Rx control : status quo
72.5458	S	–	Clinical and cytological control : status quo

biopsy of the tumor, whatever the results of the other examinations may be (mammography and cytology). This point is essential for the consistency of our statement.

Tables 3, 4 and 5 analyse the information obtained from the radiological examination. In Table 3, which refers to the radiologically positive (class V) cases, we see that 3/3 cases are revealed to be cancerous at the histo-pathological examination. The clinical examination shows the following:

   – positive (+)   = 1 X
   – suspicious (S) = 1 X
   – doubtful (D)   = 1 X

(The number in the left column of the table indicates the patient's file number.)

In Table 4, which refers to the radiologically suspicious cases (class IV), we see that 3/10 cases were revealed to be cancers at the histopathological examination, whereas in 5 cases benign tumors were found. In 2 of these cases no biopsy has been effected, but the radiological examination made by the same radiologist points to a benign lesion. In this series, the clinical examination revealed 2 suspicious cases (S) and in the others it was either doubtful (D) in 4 or negative in 4.

(N.B.: the table gives 10 radiologically suspicious cases; in the first table (1) there were 11 such cases. This is due to the fact that one patient had 2 radiologically suspicious examinations.)

In Table 5, we see that among the 9 cases for which the radiological uncertainty was total, only one had to undergo an exeresis biopsy and this had declared itself as a benign tumor (BT). The other cases have radiological or clinical control (or both), and they showed no evolution with time: 2 of these cases were clinically suspicious (S); 5 clinically doubtful (D); and, 2 clinically banal (B).

Out of a total of 436 examinations, 6 cases (1.4%) of cancer have been discovered (Table 6). Mammography has confirmed malignancy in 3 cases, and there was a suspicion for 3 others. We must emphasize that in 3 of these cases (50%) the clinical examination did not suggest malignancy, and the intervention has been effected on the basis of mammography. Thus radiography has revealed that 0.7% of cancers are not suspicious at the clinical examination.

TABLE 6   *Radio-clinical correlation of the 6 cancer cases discovered out of a total of 436 examinations*

Patient file No.	Mammography	Clinical examination
69.5648	S	S
70.3617	S	–
72.5807	S	–
72.2972	+	S
72.3885	+	D
72.5593	+	+

A feeling of distrust is noticeable for the radiologically suspicious cases: 5(50%) of them have been revealed to be BT by the anatomo-pathological examination, and in 2 cases the radiological control examination has revealed a benign lesion. On the other hand, one case was described as radiologically benign, but the anatomo-pathological examination revealed a cancer.

Clinical and radiological mammary examinations have in certain cases been followed by cytological examination. The cytological examinations carried out in the same cancer detection center are not numerous enough to consider them in isolation, so we added them to the results obtained in our main center at Louvain. We consider here patients selected by systematic examination, because they presented certain clinical anomalies.

Table 7 indicates that in the years 1970, 1971 and 1972, 10,486 women have been examined in our centers of cancer detection, and 726 (about 7%) of these have required special mammary investigation. In all these cases, mammography has been carried out after questioning and a clinical examination: in certain cases a cytological examination has also been made. In consequence, 167 exeresis-biopsies have been made. In 57 cases (32%) the tumor was malignant, and this represents 0.54% of the total number of examined women. We did obtain complete clinical, radiological and cytological information in 30 cases of exeresis-biopsy, in which 18 were malignant tumors.

TABLE 7   *Results from examinations of 10,486 women during 1970–72*

Examined women	10,486
Mammary investigation	726 (7%)
Biopsy excision	167
Malignant tumor	57
Complete clinical, radiological and cytological information	30

Table 8 shows the cytological details of 18 cases of cancer.

However, we must indicate that in 2 other cases of doubtful cytology (III) the histopathological examination was negative. In one, a fibrocystic mastosis of Reclus was found; in the other case, a benign mammary dysplasia with multiple sources of sclerosing adenosis was diagnosed, associated with galactophoritis. We did not obtain any cytological false-positive result.

TABLE 8   *The cytological details of 18 cases of cancer*

Condition	No. of cases
Acellular	4
Benign (Papa Cl. I–II)	6
Doubtful (Papa Cl. III)	3
Suspicious or malignant (Papa Cl. IV – V)	5

TABLE 9   *Comparison between clinical, radiological and cytological results for cases that were more-or-less suspicious*

Patient file No.	Clinical	Radiological	Cytological	
70.1931	S	(–)	IV	a–b
66.1139	D	S	V	n–d
71.0426	D	D	VI	a–b
71.0999	D	D	III	n–d
71.5466	+	+	IV	a–b
69.3799	D	(·)	III	a–b
69.5648	S	S	V	a–b
72.0353	S	D	III	n–d

N.B.   : a–b = aspiration-biopsy
        n–d = nipple discharge

Table 9 compares clinical, radiological and cytological results, for those cases that were more or less cytologically suspicious (8 cases of class III, IV, V). In 5 of these cases, the clinical and/or radiological examination did suspect the malignancy, but it is very interesting to note that in 3 cases, it was neither the clinical examination, nor the mammography that pointed strongly to malignancy, but the result of the cytological analysis.

Discussion

Our preliminary experience in mammography on patients at our cancer detection centers has been based on women on whom mammography was carried out because they presented a clinical anomaly. We have compared mammography with our clinical and pathological findings. The results are interesting and they allow us to assess the value of mammography but the number of false-negative and uncertain findings reduce its value (Maisin et al., 1971, Vandenbroucke -Vanderwielen and Maisin, 1972).

By practising mammography on clinically-dubious cases or on patients presenting with symptoms or in need of reassurance we are able to enhance the value of mammography performed in a detection center. Under these conditions, we have detected cancers in breasts which are clinically entirely negative and most often in old patients with involuted breasts. The value of mammography seems to us to be greater in clinically-negative breasts than in certain positive ones and poses the issue of systematic mammography as a matter of principle at the first screening consultation, as already claimed by Le Treut (1972).

What is the value of cytological examination?

In our opinion, this examination must be regularly practised but a negative result must be interpreted in the light of clinical and radiological results and not considered in isolation. On the contrary, a positive or dubious result must always be considered an important finding notwithstanding negative, clinical or radiological data.

This point of view is also held by Zajdela et al. (1972), whose experience bears on more than 2,000 examinations of malignant, benign and inflammatory cases, compared cytologically and histologically. These authors point out the number of false-negative cytological examinations (about 4%) but also the ones which are positive or suspect (3.4%) notwithstanding a clinically-negative examination.

Donegan and Perez-Meza (1972) have shown that cytological examination is very important, for example, in the diagnosis of early cancer in the second breast of patients with lobular carcinoma, which is very often bilateral. In such cases, they were able to discover 35% of cancers — 8% of them invasive and 25% in situ — on the basis of systematic and repeated cytological examination in a series of 20 clinically-normal patients.

Conclusion

Mammography is indicated every time there is the slightest doubt and even when the clinical examination is normal. On the other hand, cytological examination is an essential complementary diagnostic aid, but a negative examination may not be decisive. Diagnosis must be completed by an exeresis-biopsy when there is the slightest doubt of malignancy, either through clinical or radiological examination.

Summary

One of our cancer detection centers has possessed a senograph since the beginning of 1972. 18% of all women who have undergone an examination for cancer detection have been submitted to mammography. We have performed 436 radiological breast examinations, with the following results:

81.5% were radiologically normal or benign;
13.3% asked for a clinical or radiological examination after 2 to 6 months;
2.52% were radiologically suspect and required a biopsy;
0.69% were radiologically malignant;
2.06% gave an uncertain result.

Overall, 6 cancers were discovered — which corresponds to 1.4% of the radiological examinations: in 3 of these cases, clinical examination did not suspect malignancy. Thus breast radiography revealed 0.7% of cancers, which were clinically non-suspicious.

Clinical and radiological mammary examinations have also been, in certain cases, completed by cytological examination.

The cytological examinations carried out in the same cancer detection center were not numerous enough to consider them in isolation, so we added the results to those obtained in our main center at Louvain.

During the last 3 years, out of a total of just over 10,000 women screened, 167 mammary biopsies have been effected; in 57 cases (32%) or 0.54% of the examined women, we found a malignant tumor.

We have obtained clinical, radiological and cytological information in 18 cases of malignant tumors.

Cytology has given the following information:
grade IV-V: 5 cases
grade III: 3 cases

grade I-II: 6 cases
acellular: 4 cases (classification according to Papanicolaou).
In 3 malignant tumors, the biopsy was made only on a positive cytological finding.

To conclude, we believe that radiological examination of the breast is essential for cancer detection, as well as the gynaecological smear which we usually carry out.

On the other hand, we believe that systematic cytology can, with advantage, complete clinical and mammographical examination.

If we look for the reliability of these different examinations, clinical examination remains the most reliable.

References

Donegan, W. L. and Perez-Mesa, C. M. (1972): In: Proceedings, Symposium sur les Thérapeutiques non mutilantes des Cancéreuses du Sein, Strasbourg. In press.
Le Treut, A. (1972): In: Proceedings, Symposium sur les Thérapeutiques non mutilantes des Cancéreuses du Sein, Strasbourg. In press.
Maisin, H. (1967): Louvain Méd., 86, 273.
Maisin, H. Vandenbroucke-Vanderwielen, A., Salamon, E., Van de Merckt, J., Pham, H. Q. and Mazy, G. (1968): In: Proceedings, Premier Symposium International sur le Dépistage du Cancer, Spa, p. 650. Editor: A. Liégeois. Sciences et Lettres, Liege.
Maisin, H., Vandenbroucke-Vanderwielen, A., Van de Merckt, J. and Salamon-Dargent J. (1970): Arch. belges Méd. soc., 6, 411.
Maisin, H., Vandenbroucke-Vanderwielen, A., Mazy, G. and Van de Merckt, J., (1971): Minerva ginéc., 23, 377.
Mazy, G., Jeanmart, L. and Fassin, Y. (1972): In: Proceedings, Symposium sur les Thérapeutiques non mutilantes des Cancéreuses du Sein, Strasbourg. In press.
Vandenbroucke-Vanderwielen, A., and Maisin, H. (1972): In: Proceedings, Symposium sur les Thérapeutiques non mutilantes des Cancéreuses du Sein, Strasbourg. In press.
Zajdela, A., Pilleron, J. P., Ennuyer, A. and Maublanc, M. A. (1972): In: Proceedings, Symposium sur les Thérapeutiques non mutilantes des Cancéreuses du Sein, Strasbourg. In press.

Needle aspiration cytology in the diagnosis of breast cancer

K. Hedberg, N. Bjurstam, A. Hultborn, N. Johansson and C. Johnsén

Sahlgrens Hospital, University of Gothenburg, Gothenburg, Sweden

During a period of slightly more than a year a systematic comparison between different methods in diagnosing breast cancer has been undertaken in Gothenburg, Sweden. The survey comprises 1,310 patients with breast complaints referred to us by doctors in the Gothenburg region. On the first day of the examination they underwent thermography, clinical examination and mammography. The surgeon in charge decided whether an ordinary clinical follow-up was sufficient or if an aspiration biopsy should be performed. Thus, 69% of the patients were selected for aspiration biopsy. The material was obtained by the method described by Franzén and Zajicek and stained by May-Grünwald-Giemsa. Any liquid aspirate was processed according to the Millipore filter method. To identify the lesions properly, a localization system was devised where the nipple-tumour distance was measured both horizontally and vertically, as well as the approximate skin-tumour distance. The same patient could have more than one palpable, or impalpable, lesion. Aspiration biopsy was performed in 1076 lesions.

Table 1 shows the cytological report on the different lesions. There is no clearcut difference in the distribution of the cytological diagnoses among the 985 palpable lesions and the 91 radiologically detected impalpable lesions. There is one slight difference between the groups of suspected carcinoma and of cytologically proven carcinoma. We believe that this difference might depend partly on the fact that it is more difficult to obtain diagnostic material from impalpable lesions, but partly on the fact that the cytologist when performing a biopsy on a palpable lesion might be influenced by the palpation and by the tissue resistance at puncture. In cytologically borderline lesions this might lead to more conclusive diagnosis of carcinoma than in impalpable lesions.

Table 2 shows a comparison between the cytological and the histopathological diagnoses in the cases with clinically detected, palpable lesions. There are no false positives. This figure does not include 20 cases of advanced cancer with conclusive evidence of malignancy at clinical examination, mammography and cytology. These patients were given radiotherapy only: we have no histological report. If we include these 20 cases, we get about 8% false negatives. Among the false negatives is one case of intraepidermal carcinoma with no cancer of breast tissue. Another is a case of Paget's disease with no palpable lesion, no lesion detected by mammography and no ductal carcinoma behind the nipple. A small scirrous carcinoma was situated very deeply. Most of the other false

TABLE 1   *Cytologic findings in the different lesions*

Cytologic findings	Palpable lesions		Impalpable lesions	
Benign or unsatisfactory	757	(77%)	68	(75%)
Cellular atypia	78	(8%)	11	(12%)
Suspected cancer	9	(1%)	5	(5%)
Cancer	141	(14%)	7	(8%)
Total number	985		91	

TABLE 2   Cytologic findings in 349 cases with a histologically diagnosed and clinically palpable mammary gland lesion

Cytologic findings	Histologic findings			Total number
	Benign	Atypia	Cancer	
Benign or unsatisfactory	174	11	13	198
Cellular atypia	20	6	2	28
Suspected cancer	—	3	6 ⎫(90%)	9
Cancer	—	—	114 ⎭	114
Total number	194	20	135	349

TABLE 3   Impalpable lesions

Cytologic findings	Histologic findings			Total number
	Benign	Atypia	Cancer	
Benign or unsatisfactory	10	1	5	16
Cellular atypia	5	2	4	11
Suspected cancer	—	1	4	5
Cancer	—	—	7	7
Total number	15	4	20	39

negatives were, as in all the impalpable lesions, small carcinomas situated 2—5 cm underneath the skin, with an average diameter of 7 mm, the smallest being 4 mm.

Even with palpable lesions, close cooperation between the radiologist and cytologist is of great help. Small scirrous carcinomas can evoke a reactive response in the surrounding breast tissue, resulting in a large palpable lump. In these cases we not infrequently obtained no cancer cells when the needle was directed by the clinician's instructions, but definite proof of cancer was forthcoming when the needle was directed by instructions from the radiologist.

Table 3 shows the cytological versus the histopathological diagnoses in the 39 cases of the impalpable lesions where we have a histological report. The remainder were followed clinically. There are no false-positives. Among the impalpable cancers, 5 of 20 are false-negatives; in 11 cases the cancer diagnosis was certain or suspected; in 4 additional cases there was atypia, prompting surgical biopsy.

TABLE 4   Cytologic findings in palpable and impalpable cancer

Cytologic findings	Palpable cancers	Impalpable cancers
Benign or unsatisfactory	13	5
Cellular atypia	2	4
Suspected cancer	6 ⎫(90%)	4 ⎫(55%)
Cancer	114 ⎭	7 ⎭
Total number	135	20

Table 4 shows a comparison between the cytological findings in palpable versus impalpable cancers. The percentage of false negatives is greater among impalpable cancers which was to be expected. For practical purposes, all cases with a positive mammogram and the slightest suspicion of malignancy should have a surgical biopsy regardless of the cytological report. Also specimen radiography should be done to ensure that the actual lesion is excised. But it is of interest that it is sometimes possible to give a positive cytological diagnosis even in these very difficult cases.

To conclude, where palpable lesions are concerned close cooperation between the radiologist and cytologist is of great value in directing the needle to the centre of the lesion. For the impalpable lesions, such cooperation is essential and even small, impalpable cancers can be diagnosed, making a direct mastectomy possible. Our preliminary results show that it is worthwhile to try to get a cytological diagnosis even in impalpable lesions, but a negative cytological report must not prevent the surgeon from making at least a local excision in these cases. Judging from our results, mammography is the safest method for diagnosing breast carcinoma, while thermography was not an effective screening procedure. Aspiration biopsy did not come far behind mammography in diagnostic accuracy. As the false negatives in mammography and in cytology are not identical, a combination of these methods, in addition to clinical examination, enables palpable or impalpable breast cancer to be diagnosed with a high degree of accuracy.

The results of screening in Ravenna and Province for early diagnosis of preneoplastic lesions and tumours of the uterus and the breast

Gianfranco Buzzi, Alessandra Amadori, Maria Casotti, Anna Maria Uguzzoni and Cesare Maltoni

Centro Tumori, Ravenna, Italy

The screening for early diagnosis of preneoplastic lesions of the uterus and breast is performed in Ravenna and Province by the Centro Tumori. Uterus screening is carried out by the Centre, in collaboration with Open Clinics of the Local Public Health Service.

The uterus mass-screening program began in the second half of 1965. A first report on the results up to 1969 has already been published (Sega et al., 1969). Up to December, 1972, 39,644 women were cytologically examined (75,266 examinations). The general results are presented in Table 1. The localization, the extension and the histological type of the 179 detected carcinomas are shown in Table 2.

A comment should be made on these figures: when compared to the number of cervical carcinomas, the endometrial cancers are far below the expected number (the ratio of cervical to endometrial epithelial malignancies being usually 8:1). To avoid missing the diagnosis of endometrial carcinomas, it has now been planned to adopt, in the age-groups of women at risk, the jet-washer technique for cytological endometrial sampling.

Screening for breast preneoplastic lesions and tumour detection started in May 1971, with the same technical program adopted as in the Istituto di Oncologia of Bologna, which has been described during the conference. That is, screening is based upon a clinical examination and on cytological examination of nipple discharges, followed, in selected cases, by mammography, galactography, cytological examination of needle aspiration material and biopsies (nodulectomy or galactophorectomy). The results of breast screening are shown in Table 3.

TABLE 1   *General results of screening for the detection of uterine preneoplastic lesions and tumours*

Type	No.	%*	
Carcinomas	179	4.52	
Dysplasias	243	6.13	
Leukoplakias of II and III degree	53	1.34	
Cytologically atypical cases	67		
Class IV		63	
Class V		4	

* Referred to 39,644 examined women

TABLE 2   *Distribution of the detected uterine carcinomas by extension and histology*

Localization	No.	%	Extension	No.	%	Histological type	No.	%
Corpus	13	100.00	In situ ca	6	46.15	Adenocarcinomas	6	46.15
			Invasive ca	7	53.85	Adenocarcinomas	7	53.85
Cervix	166	100.00	In situ ca	105	63.25	Squamous cell ca	103	62.05
						Adenocarcinomas	2	1.20
			Microinvasive ca	27	16.27	Squamous cell ca	27	16.27
			Invasive ca	34	20.48	Squamous cell ca	31	18.67
						Adenocarcinomas	3	1.81

TABLE 3   *Results of screening for detection of breast preneoplastic lesions and tumours*

Type	No.	
Carcinomas	44	
Intraductal papillomas	3	
Fibroadenomas	17	
Fibrocystic mastopathy	1,861	
Cytologically atypical cases*	59	
III		44
IV		11
V		4

* Cytology on nipple discharges and needle aspirations. These cases are under ascertainment and frequent controls

    The high percentage of benign mastopathies and malignancies is due to the fact that the group of women examined are self-selected; in no way do they represent the general population which, in that area, accounts for more than 100,000 women within the age-group at risk.
    Among the cancers, we had one case of Paget's disease of the nipple with serous discharge, in which galactography showed ductal abnormalities that were proved at biopsy to be due to cancer. The three intraductal papillomas (all seen by galactography), presented areas of dysplasia at the histological examination.
    Nearly all the cases of breast carcinoma in our series were found in women who came to our Center because of self-detected lumps or other mastopathies. It was, therefore, not unexpected that most of our cases were at stage III or IV (UICC classification). The few carcinomas at stage I were in fact detected in apparently normal breasts.

Reference

Sega, E., Uguzzoni, A. M. and Settepani, R. (1969): Romagna Med., 21/4, 421.

Breast screening of executive women at the B.U.P.A. medical centre*

Jane Bomford Davey, Bernard Hugh Pentney and Annabel Mary Richter

The Medical Centre, London

Introduction

The Women's Screening Unit at the B.U.P.A. Medical Centre, in London, is a department in a general diagnostic screening centre. It is financed by private health insurance as part of its Policy towards preventive medicine. Patients pay for this service and may either have the breast and cervical cytology examination alone, or participate in the full comprehensive scheme.

Access to these facilities is open and although most people attending are symptom free, several patients have one or more symptoms in the breast and some are specially referred; to this extent, therefore, our patients are selected. Availability is important because the number of patients dying from breast cancer is approximately 4 times that of carcinoma of the cervix. The most recent figures show that breast cancer is increasing.

Results

The Women's Screening Unit was opened in 1970. Since then 7,118 patients have been seen, and 51 cancers of the breast detected. This is 7. 2/1,000. Originally, apart from clinical examination of the breast, we only had an Aga Thermovision Unit.

In an 18-month period, after obtaining a Senograph mammography unit, 4,412 patients were seen in the unit, and 36 cancers of the breast were detected – 8. 2/1,000.

These patients were mostly from the upper social groups and ranged in age from 15 to 85, although the majority were in the age group of 35–64.

Methodology

Our Breast Screening consists of a full history and 3 investigations: clinical examination; infrared thermography; and X-ray senography (on selected patients).

The clinical examination is undertaken by nursing sisters who have been trained by us and at the Royal Marsden Hospital Breast Unit. Findings can always be confirmed by the medical staff before referral to a surgeon. Self Examination is discussed with the patient and leaflets are available.

Thermovision pictures are taken of all patients, using the Aga Thermovision Unit S/N 624. The patients are unclothed to the umbilicus and cooled at 19° C for at least 10 min, during which time the history is taken. The scan is recorded by polaroid film by the same nursing sister who examines the patient. This investigation is undertaken prior to the clinical

* This presentation is reproduced by kind permission of The Editor, The Practitioner, wherein it first appeared (*The Practitioner*, 1969, *210*, 541).

examination. Three views are recorded, one with the patient facing the camera, and two lateral views. Black represents areas of thermal activity and white shows cold areas.

The results of our thermography on 4,412 patients were: Normal — 3,085; Equivocal — 947; Suspicious — 380.

There is a high percentage of suspicious and equivocal scans, but it is too early, as yet, to say whether some of these so-called false positives may not form part of the high risk group of the future. To keep spurious patterns to a minimum it is essential to ensure that patient cooling is carefully monitored. The machine is extremely reliable, and is quick, and simple to use. We recognise that each individual has a baseline pattern which will fluctuate according to her hormonal state.

Thermography is especially valuable in the screening of patients with clinically nodular breasts. Nodularity is a common finding, especially in the premenstrual state and if there is no abnormal thermal activity at this stage it is likely to be due to pre-menstrual fluid retention and the patient need only be reviewed, clinically, in mid-cycle. But, further investigations are indicated if there is any area of excess thermal activity, or if, on subsequent screening there is any change from her previous baseline pattern. The cost of thermography is comparitively small, i.e. £0.51 per patient.

Senography is undertaken for the following reasons:

1. All patients over the age of 40
2. Family history of maternal breast cancer
3. Previous malignancy in the patient
4. Breast symptoms
5. Large breast
6. Clinical abnormality
7. Abnormal thermovision.

Approximately 2/3 of the patients coming for screening have an X—ray of the breast.

The machine is very reliable and compact. The radiation dose per exposure is approximately 2. 5 rads.

The results of the X-ray senography are as follows:

Total patients X-rayed	3,380
Benign calcification	149
Malignant calcification	20
Other malignant	32

It is, as yet, difficult to differentiate with certainty benign from malignant type microcalcification, but further studies into this are being undertaken. The immediate value of senography is to make a diagnosis in a lesion which is not clinically palpable. The cost of X-ray senography is approximately £ 3.25 per patient.

Discussion

In the 36 cases of breast cancer that were found in 4,412 patients, i.e. 8. 2/1,000, we find that:

29 cases were suspicious on clinical examination
19 cases were suspicious on thermography
27 cases were suspicious on senography

Although 14 patients were positive on all 3 investigations, when we compare and evaluate each investigation individually, we find that the positive rate for each modality falls within such a close range that it becomes not statistically significant. The diagnosis of cancer becomes more accurate if 2 or more of the investigations are positive. Therefore, to give the highest rate of breast cancer detection, all 3 investigations should be employed.

Conclusion

To obtain the optimum yield from screening, each investigation has its individual value and follow up is essential with comparative records.

The cost makes screening the whole population impractical; for this reason we have tried to identify a high risk group in whom the positive pick-up rate would be at its greatest:

High Risk Group:
1. Family history of maternal breast carcinoma
2. Previous malignancy in patient
3. Late first pregnancy or nulliparous
4. Late menopause
5. Previous benign breast biopsy
6. All women reaching the age of 50

Also we would ask that breast screening is undertaken, routinely, whenever cervical cytology is done.

We feel that every effort should be made to try and check the increase in the incidence of breast cancer, both by exploring all new fields of early detection, and by encouraging surgeons to deal with cancers that are small and often still impalpable. To do this localization techniques must be improved. It is in this way that we shall improve the prognosis and hopefully keep mutilating procedures to a minimum.

Summary

Over 7,000 patients attended the Women's Screening Unit and 42 patients were proved to have breast cancer.

Clinical examination of the breasts by specially trained State Registered Nurses and thermography was used on all patients. Selected women underwent X-ray mammography. It is shown that each component of screening is valuable and individually complimentary, but no method should be utilized alone if the optimum results are to be obtained.

Selection of X-ray mammography is undertaken on grounds of irradiation risk and cost. The reasons for the choice of patients selected are discussed as well as details of cost.

Follow-up of all cases shows the need for baseline observations and gives useful information about quality of records and standardization of technique. Access to this clinic is entirely open but with increasing popularity the possibility of restricting those screened to those in a high risk group is discussed and a high risk group identified.

Early breast cancer detection in a Swedish city

A preliminary report on health screening of half the population of a medium sized Swedish city

Sören Jakobsson[1] , Olof Melander[2] , Bengt Lundgren[3] and Torsten Norin[3]

[1] *Department of Health Screening and Preventive Medicine, County Council, Gävle;*
[2] *Department of Roentgen Diagnostics, Karolinska sjukhuset, Stockholm; and* [3] *Department of Radiotherapy, Gävle sjukhus, Gävle, Sweden*

1. The screening

(S. Jakobsson)

During the last two decades, there has been an increasing interest in mass screening and an increasing demand by the public for low cost periodic health examinations. However, until now only limited evidence regarding the benefit of health screening has been demonstrated. Testing this means many years of research concerning not only the efficiency of health screening but also that of medical care. Entering such a study it is essential to know the degree of accuracy of the screening instrument.

In the city of Gävle, Sweden, a research project concerning this subject began in October 1969. The most important objectives of the investigation were:

— to analyse the ability of different screening methods to indicate people with current need of medical care;

TABLE 1   *The screening program*

Questionnaires
Urine tests
Automated laboratory tests
EKG
Blood pressure
Chest X-ray (ODELCA 100)
Lungs, cardiac size
Breast cancer screening

— to make possible advanced statistical analyses of collected data and to evaluate methods for mass screening with special regard to breast cancer detection by thermography in combination with self administered medical history, automated chemical laboratory tests and computerized EKG evaluation.

Gävle has about 62,000 inhabitants. The study population comprises 24,171 men and women born in 1944 or earlier and living in the largest of the two parishes in the city. The breast cancer study covered all women aged 35 and over, totalling 10,591. The first screening took place in 1969-1970 and until now the population has been screened twice with a 2-year interval and will be further observed.

This report concerns the 1969-1970 part of the breast cancer study. The breast cancer study formed an integral part of a general screening program (Table 1). All routines were adapted to electronic data processing. Table 2 demonstrates the number and the rate of participation in the health survey. Almost every 10-year group comprises nearly 2,000 females. The highest participation rate, about 88%, appears in the 40 to 59 year group.

TABLE 2   *Gävle health survey: Number of examined women, rate of participation (%) and age distribution*

Age groups	Number	%
35–39	948	88
40–49	2,361	88
50–59	2,260	87
60–69	1,780	79
70 and over	1,024	51
Total	8,373	79

In the breast cancer study 8,242 subjects participated, that is 78% of those invited. The breast cancer screening was performed using a questionnaire and grey tone thermography with isotherms. A mark sense sheet was designed to carry all relevant information. Specially trained technicians performed the examination and a radiologist, Dr Melander, Stockholm, interpreted the thermograms. Optimum screening capacity was 100 subjects a day using 2 thermography units and 3 technicians. Ideal interpretation capacity was much lower, about 50 a day. The breast cancer data were processed together with other screening data by Uppsala University Data Center.

The data processing was based on off-line routines and included weekly input of acquired information, filing of data and computerized selection of subjects who were to be checked up. The letters to subjects, screening reports and so on were printed automatically. Those with abnormal screening results and a control group were invited to a secondary examination by breast X-ray and clinical examination.

It must be stressed that results of each type of examination were separately and independently reported. When lesions were confirmed either by cytological or surgical biopsy, subjects were referred for surgery and radiotherapy. The design of the study makes it possible to analyse the sensitivity and the specificity of the screening method as well as to estimate the sensitivity of clinical examination compared to that of breast X-ray.

It is natural to consider clinical examination as the standard reference method in this connection. But if, as happened in our study, a method with higher sensitivity and specificity is revealed by growing experience, this latter method — breast X-ray — must be used as a new reference. However, it is important to underline that clinical examination in this study was performed by very experienced oncologists.

2. Criteria and methods for selecting subjects for secondary examination

(O. Melander)

When trying to compare different studies of thermographic breast examinations, one often finds it difficult to explain the extraordinary variation in results. One reason for this is that the population examined is seldom clearly defined, and secondly, there is almost never a clear statement as to the criteria used for classifying a find as positive or negative.

For future studies, we would like to suggest three main categories of populations:
1. Patients with clinically evident cancer.
2. Patients with vague breast complaints, but no clinical signs of cancer.
3. Non-selected population screenings of asymptomatic subjects.

Examinations of patients of the first type are often done in order to learn the heat picture in breast cancer, and also to follow-up results of treatment. In the second category the thermographic picture can be a good help in reading mammograms and for the clinical examiner. The third category is the object of the present study.

The theoretical and practical background of the thermographic screening procedure was as follows: Our experience of the breast cancer heat picture was based mainly on 518 patients of the first category above. When measuring temperature differences between symmetric areas, there was a marked difference between cancer and benign disease. We chose to call those with a difference of zero to one degree centigrade 'negative', one to two degrees 'suspect' and those with more than two degrees difference 'positive'.

In the Gävle screening we tried to use this experience by letting technical assistants measure temperature differences between warmest as well as coldest areas in the two breasts. This was done after alcohol spray and fan cooling for 10 min. Eleven isotherm-indicated pictures were obtained in frontal and oblique views. We found, however, that a degree of experience, much higher than the assistants had, was necessary: false measurement values were not unusual.

From earlier studies of 72 symptomatic cancer patients we knew that 80% were true positive on thermography. On examination of 178 cases without proven cancer the false positive percentage was as high as 45, but among these 'false' positive cases a few cancers appeared later. Thus we felt it was important to keep such subjects under close observation.

In this screening there were 3 sources of information available for the selection procedure:
The questionnaire.
Information from assistants.
The thermograms.

The questionnaire was printed on a mark sense sheet. Three questions had absolute selecting power when answered in the positive:
Previous breast cancer.
Palpable lump.
Dark discharge from the nipple.

Other questions with a more relative value were tumor in another site, breast pains, colourless discharge, earlier treatment for benign breast disease and cancer heredity.

Questionnaire, thermograms and assistant's annotations were mailed to me.

Before arriving at the decision whether to select or not, there were thus many factors of varying importance to consider. First, the thermogram:

1. Breast configuration.
2. Vascular patterns. Symmetry and assymmetry.
3. Temperature differences (described earlier).

1. The relative sizes of breasts are readily estimated and size differences are often combined with temperature differences. Most subjects with size difference have been selected. General configuration is important as skin retraction with the thermographic 'edge' sign, can be thus easier to discover than on direct inspection.

2. Vascular patterns are classed as to type of 'normal' appearance in a thermogram. Four types were recognized: with few vessels; vascular type; mottled type; 'hormonal' type.

These were further sub-typed as 'moderate', 'typical' or 'marked'.

The symmetrical vascular type was weighed against age and general medical history. In case of bad agreement, subjects were selected. In an assymetric picture suspect areas are easier to localize. Sometimes a single atypical vessel is at hand, at other times several vessels point at one specific area. An increased number of vessels in one of two breasts of equal size or an area with irregular vessels were also reasons for selection.

3. Temperature increase without visible vessels, is explained in several ways:

Hot spot – less than two centimeters.

Limited zone – two to five centimeters.

Extended warm areas – more than five centimeters.

A retrospective study has been done by Dr B. Lundgren concerning important selection parameters in thermography on our 34 cancer cases, from 200 selected and 200 not selected subjects. It was found that temperature differences are of much less importance than was earlier believed. 'Pathological picture' and hot spot appear only slightly more frequently among cancer cases than among the others.

It was also found that the skin – tumor distance as well as tumor size as measured by the pathologist were of great importance. The conclusion was that the bigger the tumor and the more superficial it was, the more suspect the heat picture. Even if measured temperature values were important help in interpretation of thermograms, it was found to be of no use for selection. This has been a disappointment, since there were high hopes that in thermography we had a simple tool suitable for later adaption to automated breast cancer screenings.

It is perhaps not quite fair to make a direct comparison of the examination methods used in this project. Thermography was part of the screening of an unselected population, while clinical examination and breast X-ray dealt with the selected group and controls. Also surgery was only performed on cases indicated by clinical or X-ray examination, never on screening results alone. Subjects with high strength suspicions on thermography are still followed with regular examinations. So far no cases of cancer have been revealed among them, after about three years' observation.

In conclusion, among asymptomatic subjects thermography does not diagnose cancer, nor does it differentiate benign from malignant disease. Still, in this project a marked concentration of cancer cases among selected subjects was obtained, and abnormal thermograms can be considered as indications for more exhaustive diagnostic examinations. The disadvantages are the high percentage of just under 30's selected for secondary examination, and that this selection must be performed by highly trained physicians. The heat picture in very early stages of cancer growth is not distinct enough for safe diagnosis and localisation. A combined reading of thermogram and mammogram increases the possibility of early diagnosis.

3. Secondary examination of selected cases and control group

(B. Lundgren)

As stated in a former section, 8,242 women participated in this screening. From these, 2,401 subjects were selected to a secondary examination, either giving positive answers to one or more of three relevant questions in the questionnaire, or by the thermographic procedure described earlier. In a number of cases both criteria were present:

Positive history		4%
Positive thermogram	(at least)	25%
Total percentage selected		29%

Of the 2,401 subjects selected, 103 refused for various reasons. Thus the refusal or 'drop-out' percentage was 4.3 making the number actually participating in the secondary examination 2,298.

The secondary examination was organized in two, or rather three, separate stages:

1. Breast X-ray, using the Senograph, industrial X-ray film (Kodak 'Industrex C'), Pakorol processing machine and with an assistant obtaining three views of each breast, namely: cranio-caudal, oblique, 30 degrees from the medial horizontal and lateral.

2. Clinical examination was the second stage (see following section).

3. Pooling of information was the last stage, in which the oncologist decided on further management of the subjects.

We feel it is important to stress that all reports were made separately and independently. Thus the radiologist did not palpate and had no information on screening reports. The oncologist doing clinical examination had no access to screening or X-ray reports until after he had delivered his own.

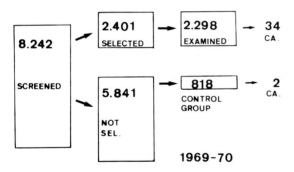

FIG. 1   *Results of breast cancer screening, Gälve, 1969-70.*

Figure 1 summarizes what happened to the population during screening. In the secondary examination 34 cases of cancer were detected among selected subjects. Two cases of cancer were found in the control group of 818 women. The reasons for selection, as stated earlier, were either positive history or thermography, or a combination of both. Another factor found in a number of cases was that the technical assistants performing thermography, though not required to, sometimes passed on their observations to the interpreter. In Table 1 the 34 cancer cases have been grouped as to selection reasons. In 24 cases, apart from the thermography picture no other information was available at the time of interpretation. Table 2 shows how the 2,298 selected subjects were classed according to suspicions of malignancy. In a way, however, most women selected, except the few with

TABLE 1   *34 cancer cases grouped according to reasons for selection (Gävle, 1969–70)*

A. History only:	
Palpated a lump	1
Previous breast cancer	2
B. History or assistant's observation	
combined with abnormal thermogram	7
C. Thermography alone:	
Abnormal in wrong breast	8
Abnormal in right breast:	
Report code 2 (low strength)	8
Report code 3-5 (high strength)	8
Total	34

TABLE 2   *2,298 selected subjects classified according to suspicion of malignancy and resulting verification (Gävle, 1969)*

	Screening		Secondary examination			
	Thermography		Breast X-ray		Clinical examination	
Report code	Total No. of women	No. of cancers detected	Total No. of women	No. of cancers detected	Total No. of women	No. of cancers detected
1. Normal 2. Benign	1,530	19	2,102	4	2,117	14
3. Malignancy not excluded	636	9	146	1	158	8
4. Strong suspicions	114	4	26	6	14	3
5. Cancer	18	2	24	22	9	9
Total		34		33		34

positive history alone, can be regarded as suspicious because of their abnormal thermograms.

19 cases of cancer were regarded as either normal or had some slight abnormality in the thermogram, but only two of the 34 were declared as 'certain' cancers. Among the 'normal/benign' subjects there were no less than 8 where vague signs of abnormal heat pattern were found in one breast, whereas a cancer was found in the other, thermographically normal, breast. On clinical examination 9 cases were regarded as 'certain' cancers, 3 had strong suspicion of malignancy and 9 were coded 'malignancy cannot be excluded'.

14 cases of cancer were clinically normal or benign. These were detected by X-ray. Most of them were very small, the smallest measuring 4 mm in diameter in the specimen. As can be seen in Table 2, 22 cases were considered to be certain malignancies roentgenologically, 6 were strongly suspect, and one was in the group 'malignancy cannot be

TABLE 3   *Cancer frequency and prevalence by age-groups according to WHO, 1969*

	Selected			Controls		
	Total No.	Cancer		Total No.	Cancer	
		No.	$^o/_{oo}$		No.	$^o/_{oo}$
Young (35–44)	566	4	7.1	321	–	–
Middle-aged (45–64)	1,231	18	14.6	374	2	5.3
Elderly (65 and over)	381	12	31.5	121	–	–
Total	2,178	34	15.6	816	2	2.5

excluded'. Four cases were not detected on X-ray. In error, one of the 34 cases was not X-rayed.

Table 3 depicts cancer frequency and prevalence by age-groups according to WHO. Prevalence among the older women was very high, 4-times as high as in the 'young' group. Prevalence in the selected group was 15.6 per thousand, and among the controls 2.5 per thousand. The relative cancer prevalence in the population, were its age distribution identical with that of a standard population, would be 16.1 per thousand in the selected group and 2.8 per thousand in the control group. The conclusion of a statistical analysis is that this difference is probably caused by the selective capacity of the screening procedure.

Cancer frequency in the total screened population, counting only cases found immediately on screening, was 4.37 per thousand. Within one year after the last day of screening, a further 11 cases of cancer were found in the target population, with equal distribution in selected and not selected groups.

A most encouraging feature of this screening has been the ability of breast X-ray to detect very small, and supposedly early, cancers. Had only clinical examination been used in the secondary stage, results of this screening would have been insignificant. Since the majority of palpable breast cancers are quite advanced, technical means like X-ray must be used in screening if early detection is the objective.

4. Role of clinical examination: Conclusions

(T. Norin)

As previously mentioned, those women selected by questionnaire and thermography as well as the control group were reexamined by mammography and they were also invited to clinical examination. This examination consisted of ocular inspection, palpation in sitting and lying positions without any knowledge of the results from thermography and mammography.

After recording the result of this clinical examination in the 5 code-group-patients mentioned earlier, who had a suspicious finding in either thermography, mammography or palpation, were further investigated through fine needle aspiration biopsy a.m. Franzén for cytology. This method and the possibility of positive results also in preclinical cancers were reported in an earlier paper.

About 2,300 women were clinically examined at which 181 showed signs of suspected or had clinically evident cancer (Fig. 1). In 20 of these women cancer was verified but 14

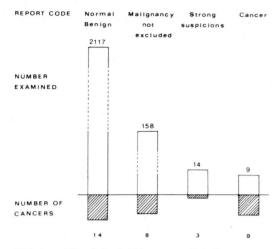

FIG. 1   *181 of the 2,300 women clinically examined, showing signs of suspected, or clinically evident, cancer.*

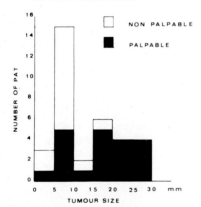

FIG. 2   *An analysis of 14 cancers showing that all except two were roentgenologically smaller than 10 mm in diameter.*

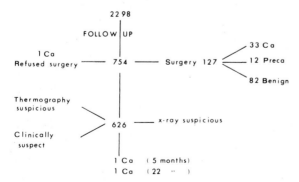

FIG. 3   *Reasons for follow-up in 754 of the 2,300 women examined.*

further cancers were found among those who were regarded as normal on palpation. An analysis of these 14 cancers shows that all except two were roentgenologically smaller than 10 mm in diameter (Fig. 2).

In four patients the palpation revealed cancer in spite of the fact that mammography showed no indication of cancer. The fine needle aspiration biopsy showed cancer in 19 of the 34 cases and was positive in 6 of the non-palpable tumors where fine needle aspiration was performed on the basis of the X-ray findings.

Of the 2,300 women examined, abnormal findings by thermography, mammography and palpation were the reason for follow-up in 754 patients (Fig. 3). Of these patients 127 have undergone surgery, either local biopsy for histological examination or, in clinically and cytologically proved cancer cases, primary simple mastectomy. 33 of these 127 operated patients had cancer, 12 precancer and in 82 patients the histological examination has shown a benign lesion. One patient diagnosed by cytology refused operation. This patient was treated with irradiation. Skeletal metastases, more than 3 years later, have further confirmed the diagnosis.

In addition to these 128 women we have regularly followed 626 who have shown an abnormality which indicates a possibility of cancer in the future, e.g. thermography with high suspicion of cancer. In none of these thermographically suspect cases has cancer appeared during the 3 years following primary examination. In the X-ray group one cancer has been found five months after the primary examination and still another after 22 months. From the group with palpable findings a great number of cases have been excluded as benign e.g. benign cysts, necrosis of the fat tissue and lipomas.

According to the TNM-system 14 patients belong to the TONOMO group and 13 to T1-T2-T3 with no signs of lymphnode -or distant-metastases. Another 7 patients of T2 and T3 group had lymphnode metastases and one of them skeletal metastases (Table 1). The age distribution of the preclinical — non-palpable — cancers has a mean of 64 years compared to 56 years in the clinical — palpable — cancer group, and 52 years in the X-ray negative group (Table 2). The treatment of patients with cancer has been simple mastectomy followed by irradiation of the axilla, parasternal and medial supraclavicular area.

TABLE 1   *Clinical staging according to the TNM—system (1969)*

T0 N0 M0		14
T1 N0 M0	7	
T2 N0 M0	4	13
T3 N0 M0	2	
T2 N1 M0	3	
T3 N1 M0	3	7
T2 N1 M1	1	

TABLE 2   *Age distribution among different cancer groups*

Group	Cancers	Mean age
Preclinical and presymptomatic (X-ray detection only)	14	64
Presymptomatic (but clinical detection)	15	56
Symptomatic (and clinical detection)	5	52
Total	34	58

TABLE 3   *Results of follow-up after 30 months*

Group	No. of patients	Symptom free	Recurrence	Dead
Positive X-ray, non-palpable	14	13	1	0
Positive X-ray, palpable	15	8	5	2
Negative X-ray, palpable	4	1	2	1

TABLE 4   *An indicator of the importance of early diagnosis*

	Average No. of days of illness
Non-palpable cancer	67
Palpable cancer	115

The main purpose of screening for breast cancer is to attain better survival by an early diagnosis. The ultimate answer however, cannot be obtained until after a very long period of time. As an indication of a trend, follow-up of the cancer patients after 30 months has given the following results:

In the non-palpable tumour group all 14 patients are still alive; one of these, however, has had a recurrence (Table 3). In the 15 patients with palpable tumours 2 have died of cancer and another 5 have had recurrences, 8 are still living symptom free. An indicator of the importance of an early diagnosis is the average number of 'days of illness' recorded by the public health insurance (Table 4). The non-palpable group had an average of 67 days of illness compared to 115 in the palpable group.

The breast screening of these, about 8,000 women has been repeated during 1971 – 1972 and will be repeated during a long period within two or three years interval and we hope that repeated examinations will give us more definitive information about the possibility of reducing the mortality of breast cancer in a screened population.

In this study of 8,242 women a rather high proportion of cancer of the breast has been found. Thermography has been the main selection method. The high selection rate, 29%, created a great demand for an expensive follow-up organization. The high selection rate has also put an extra psychological pressure on those women selected.

The interpretation capacity has been rather low and the specificity of the method has been doubtful, e.g. in 8 cancer cases the thermography was positive in the wrong breast.

Because of the abovementioned factors we have come to the conclusion that thermography is not a suitable method for breast screening on a big population; at least not in its present stage of development. This opinion has been confirmed during the second screening of the same population.

Scheduling of examinations for early detection of breast cancer

R. L. A. Kirch and M. Klein

Clinical Unit of Memorial Sloan-Kettering Cancer Center, Memorial Hospital for Cancer and Allied Diseases, New York, N.Y., U.S.A.

Annual examination programs for early breast cancer detection have been demonstrated to find smaller cancers with fewer axillary nodal metastases (Venet et al., 1971; Gilbertson and Kjelsberg, 1971) than those generally seen by the surgeon. These screening programs have been associated with significantly improved survival rates. Schedules proposing more frequent examinations to detect breast cancer earlier have been proposed (Gershon-Cohen et al., 1967). The experimental evaluation of such schedules by extensive field trials is impractical. Hence, we have developed a mathematical model (Kirch and Klein, 1972, 1974) to provide a method for theoretically evaluating examination schedules. This model can also be used to construct 'optimal' schedules which are slightly more efficient.

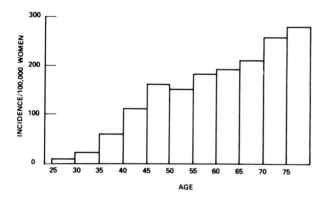

FIG. 1   *Annual breast cancer incidence rates as a function of age (for white females in Connecticut 1963).*

The increasing incidence rate of breast cancer with age (Fig. 1) has suggested that there should be a tendency towards concentrating examinations in the older age range when breast cancer becomes a significant problem.

We have characterized schedules in terms of the length of time between the first point at which a malignancy could theoretically be detected (if an examination had happened to be performed at that time) and the point at which it is actually detected during an examination or by the patient (Fig. 2). This is called the detection delay. Clearly one would like to make this as short as possible.

As most women will not get breast cancer, the expected number of examinations per

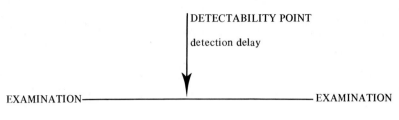

FIG. 2   *Illustration of terms.*

woman should be limited. If mammography is employed, cumulative radiation exposure might impose such a limit. The economic, social and organizational difficulties associated with mass screening would also tend to be limiting factors.

When such a limit on number of examinations has been imposed, the mathematical model enables one to choose a schedule with a minimum expected detection delay. These optimal schedules are non-periodic with a gradual shortening of the inter-examination intervals with increasing age (Fig. 3). They produce an advantage of about 3 to 5% shorter detection delay for the same number of examinations as schedules with regular periodicity (Table 1).

It has been suggested that better patient education to minimize the delay between possible discovery of cancer and its medical diagnosis is of major importance. The average patient delay has been estimated as 20 months (Hutchinson and Shapiro, 1968). It must be noted that there are several components in this factor of patient detection presenta-

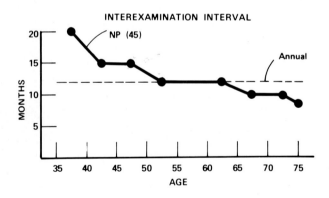

FIG. 3   *Non-periodic schedule NP (45) compared with annual schedule P (12).*

TABLE 1   *Expected detection delay for non-periodic schedule NP (45) and annual schedule P (12)*

	NP (45)	P (12)
Expected number of examinations	38.6	38.4
Expected detection delay (months)	6.0	6.3

(examinations starting at age 35)

tion delay. First, asymptomatic breast cancer may at present be detectable only by mammography or thermography. Next, a woman's effectiveness in detecting breast cancer may be related to the physical characteristics of her breast (Thiessen, 1971) as well as to proper training and motivation. Finally, given the detection of a breast mass, additional delay before presentation for an examination may be due to patient procrastination. Our calculations have shown that the effect of this factor is relatively small for examination schedules beginning by age 40 (Table 2). However, its effect is significant when regular examinations are not begun until age 45 or 50. This effect is of course largest in magnitude for those women who are never screened.

TABLE 2   *Effect of patient detection delay on expected detection delay*

Annual examinations start at:	Patient delay of	
	12 months	24 months
Age 35	6.1	6.4
Age 50	7.6	10.8
No examination	12.0	24.0

The age of starting examinations has also been investigated. We have found that the expected detection delay increases as the age at which the examinations start is increased (Fig. 4). This effect, however, is quite small when examinations begin by age 35 to 40. Thus our calculations support the general practice of deferring regular examinations until this age range.

The mathematical formulation is not affected by whether the examinations are single or multi-modal except inasmuch as this would change the error probability factor. Under reasonable assumptions, the lengthening of the expected detection delay associated with a 10% error will be in the range of 20%.

Calculations also indicate that a semi-annual program may detect cancer on the average 3 months earlier than annual examination programs. This is of the magnitude of

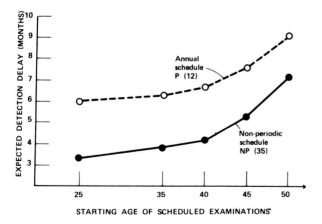

FIG. 4   *Expected detection delay as a function of the starting age of scheduled examinations (with patient presentation delay equal to 18 months).*

the estimated doubling time for breast cancers and may be significant. This suggests that large scale experiments with semi-annual examination schedules should be conducted.

In summary, our calculations support the idea of beginning regular breast examinations by the age of 35 to 40. Further, the advantages of non-periodic examination schedules are relatively small. It should be noted, however, that the slight advantage of optimal non-periodic schedules could lead to substantial savings in a mass screening program.

Finally, it is suggested that experimental evaluation of semi-annual examinations may be warranted on theoretical grounds.

References

Gershon-Cohen, J., Ingleby, H., Berger, S. M., Forman, M. and Curcio, B. M. (1967): Radiology, 88, 663.

Gilbertson, V. A. and Kjelsberg, M. (1971): Cancer (Philad.), 28, 1552.

Hutchinson, G. B. and Shapiro, S. (1968): J. nat. Cancer Inst., 41, 655.

Kirch, R. L. A. and Klein, M. (1972): Surveillance Schedules for Medical Examinations. Operations Research Group, Columbia University, School of Engineering and Applied Science, Technical Report No. 53 (to appear in Management Science).

Kirch, R. L. A. and Klein, M. (1974): Examination schedules for breast cancer. Cancer (May, 1974).

Thiessen, E. U. (1971): Cancer (Philad.), 28, 1537.

Venet, L., Strax, P., Venet, W. and Shapiro, S. (1971): Cancer (Philad.), 28, 1546.

The results of screening in Bologna and Province, 1967-72, for early diagnosis of preneoplastic changes and tumours of the breast

Cesare Maltoni, Giuseppe Corradi, Feliceantonio Grosso and Laura Pieri

Istituto di Oncologia 'F. Addarii' and Centro Tumori, Bologna, Italy

The screening for early diagnosis of preneoplastic changes and tumours of the breast is performed in Bologna and Province by the Istituto di Oncologia and by the Centro Tumori, with the collaboration of the Local Public Health Services (Hospitals and Open Clinics). The screening is based upon a clinical examination and on the cytological examination of nipple discharges, followed, in selected cases, by mammography, galactography, cytological examination of needle aspiration material and biopsies (nodulectomy or galactophorectomy).

Galactography is always carried out when abnormal, doubtful, suspicious or positive cells are observed in the nipple discharges. Cytological examination of needle aspirates is always made on clinically or radiologically detected nodules of whatever type: in our experience this method has shown a high precision, mainly when the results are positive. Nodulectomy is performed for all benign, doubtful or suspicious nodules, but not when lumps are clinically or radiologically positive. Galactophorectomy is undertaken as a conservative diagnostic-therapeutic measure when suspicious cells are present in nipple discharge with, or without, irregularity of galactophores elicited by galactography. We routinely employ nodulectomy, enlarged nodulectomy and galactophorectomy with good results. The surgical specimens following nodulectomy and galactophorectomy are then examined histologically in serial sections.

From January 1967 to November 1972, 82,536 women out of the 250,000 at risk age (over 28) were examined at least once. The number of examinations performed and the results obtained are shown in Tables 1 and 2. The high percentage of in situ carcinomas and the large rate of invasive carcinomas without metastases should be pointed out. However, it will not be possible to assess the full significance of our mass screening until

TABLE 1   *Exams*

Women clinically examined	82,536
Cytological examinations of nipple discharges	5,100
Cytological examinations of needle aspirations	2,050
Mammographies	5,042
Galactographies	213
Nodulectomies	273
Galactophorectomies	14

TABLE 2   *Results to date (November, 1972)*

Type	No. (%)		%*
Carcinomas	290		3.51
Histologically examined by us:	138	(100)	
in situ	44	(32)	
microinvasive	4	(3)	
invasive (total)	90	(65)	
without metastases		57	
Precancerous lesions	65		0.79
Cytologically atypical cases**:			
Class III	54		
Class IV	105		

 * Referred to 82,536 examined women

** Cytology on nipple discharges and on needle aspirations. These cases are under ascertainment or frequent controls

at least 10 years of periodic controls have been made on detected cases, and until mortality figures in our Province, before and after screening, can be compared.

Mass screening in Bologna and Province for the early detection of oncological lesions of the breast is now becoming widespread and it represents a permanent Public Health Service.

Eight years of experience in prevention and detection of breast cancer

I. Mlinarić, M. Bašić and Š. Knežević

Surgical Clinic, Institute of Radiology and Radiotherapy and Institute of Pathology, M. Stojanović Hospital, Zagreb, Yugoslavia

Modern team work on the early detection and prevention of breast cancer started in our hospital 23 years ago. At that time, for the purpose of early detection and adequate treatment of breast tumour, an extemporaneous biopsy (Knežević and Knežević, 1963), was carried out for the first time in Zagreb, and close collaboration was established between the surgeon and pathologist.

However, after the application of mammography to the diagnosis of breast cancer (Bašić, 1963), a team was formed 16 years ago in which there was close collaboration between the surgeon, the radiologist and the histopathologist. Such organised collaboration has shown itself to be particularly effective in making a faster and more exact diagnosis, and in selecting and performing adequate therapy, organising preventive action and raising public health consciousness.

The complexity of the problems which arose in the course of the work of the unit demanded further extension of team work to the consultative specialist service (Mlinarić et al., 1972). During the last 2 years this attained its definitive form as is shown schematically in Figure 1.

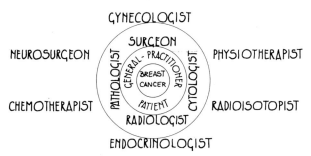

FIG. 1   *Team for detection, therapy and prevention of breast cancer.*

In our present organisation, we start from the relation between the patient and the general practitioner as shown on the drawing by the central circle. We underline this on account of the fact that for an early detection of pathologic changes in the breast, and in view of the difficulties in organising systematic examinations of all threatened age-groups of women, we continue to attach priority to self-examination by women, who in over 90% of cases are the first to notice changes on the breast (Haagensen, 1958). They then consult their general practitioner. Should the finding turn out to be positive, the patient is sent for further diagnostic examination to the specialists of the second circle. This is the level at which definite diagnosis is made and an adequate method of treatment is decided upon. Only close collaboration at this level can, in our experience, contribute to a speedy and efficacious diagnostic and therapeutic intervention. Nevertheless, and this is also our experience, it has been shown in a certain percentage of cases that it was also necessary to consult the specialists of the third circle who, in their respective fields, participate and are dovetailed in the execution of a specific treatment. Throughout this time, and after completion of therapeutic procedure, the course of the patient's sickness is followed by her general practitioner. According to need, he sends the patient to undergo control examinations and executes ambulatory medicinal therapy in accordance with the instructions of the specialist.

The physicians of the second circle of our scheme have performed during the last 8 years a relatively large number of primary examinations of breast diseases as seen in Table 1.

TABLE 1   *Confrontation of the examinations carried out on lesions of the breast during a period of 8 years (1965 – 1972)*

Surgical examinations	5049
Mammographies	8548
Histological examinations	6000
Cytological examinations	60*

* Only for a period of one year (1972)

The difference between the number of surgical examinations amounting to 5049, and the number of mammographies amounting to 8,548, arises because mammographies at our hospital are also made for other medical institutions which have not the necessary apparatus for that purpose. We wish to point out that, so far, more than 20,000 mammographies have been made at our hospital, and that thanks to the experience and efforts of our radiologists, mammography was introduced as far back as 1957 as a routine procedure in Yugoslavia.

A strikingly large number of intraoperative biopsies of breast tumours amounting to over 6,000 as compared with surgical examinations, is the consequence of the collaboration of our Institute for Pathology with other surgical departments outside our Hospital. We would like to emphasize that for more than a year, our Institute for Pathology differentiates between benign and malignant intraductal epitheliosis of the breast, by means of the histochemical reaction to β-glucuronidase, which is positive for malignant epithelium. When urgent diagnosis is needed, an important part is played by the cryostat and the contrast-phase microscope which will be reported upon at the congress of the German Society for Pathology in Karlsruhe.

Based on the clinical examination, mammography and extemporaneous biopsy, we have been successfully diagnosing breast cancer for years, while availing ourselves of the experience of others (Zajdela and Rousseau, 1970). We began using puncture biopsy for ambulatory cases in the course of last year, which explains the small number of cytological examinations, i.e. 60 in all.

We are satisfied that our experience and the positive results achieved in early detection and therapy of breast tumour prompted the foundation of similar teams in other hospitals. We hope that the experience gained in other towns and other countries, which we hope to learn about at this symposium, will contribute to the still better functioning of our team.

Conclusion

Lack of understanding of the etiology of breast cancer compels us to search for suitable organisational schedules in the fight against this disease, which on the average, attacks about 6% of women. The chief aim of such organisations is the establishment of teams which are able efficiently to carry on prevention and early detection of breast cancer. We began such work in our Hospital 23 years ago. The experience gained and some of the results of our work are presented in the form of the attached organisational scheme and the number of examinations made in the course of the last 8 years.

References

Bašić, M. (1963): Anali Bolnice 'Dr. M. Stojanović', Zagreb, Vol. 2, Suppl. 6.

Haagensen, C. D. (1958): Carcinoma of the Breast, p. 7. American Cancer Society, Inc., New York, N.Y.

Knežević, M. and Knežević, Š. (1963): Anali Bolnice 'Dr. M. Stojanović', Zagreb, 2, 5.

Mlinarić, I., Bašić, M., Knežević, S., Knežević, M. and Kvakan, D. (1972): Libri oncologici, 3, 1319.

Zajdela, A. and Rousseau, J. (1970): Bull. Soc. méd. (Paris), 4, 1.

Early detection of breast cancer in Israel

Z. Teva and N. Trainin

Department of Surgery, Kaplan Hospital, and Department of Cell Biology, The Weizmann Institute of Science, Rehovot, Israel

In 1966 the Israel Cancer Association began to develop a network of clinics for the early detection of breast cancer. These clinics are attached to Government, Kupat Holim (Sick Fund) and Hadassah hospitals. Their number at the end of 1972 reached eleven, and they are dispersed over the map of Israel in proximity to the regional medical centers. The clinics are staffed by a team of surgeons experienced in the detection of breast cancer, aided by a nurse who is in charge of registrations and appointments. Suspected cases are hospitalized and undergo biopsy, and where necessary, definitive surgical treatment. The use of auxiliary diagnostic methods such as thermography and mammography was not general, and was applied in special cases only. The main clinical diagnosis was accordingly based on the physical examination.

The women reached the clinics by invitation on the basis of the official Population Registry, and apart from a few exceptions, only women aged 34 and over were invited. The clinics were also open to any woman of any age who wished to be examined, and also served as advisory clinics to family doctors. Over the years they have become more and more popular in the areas in which they operate, and the percentage of women sent to them by family doctors for advice, or who came on their own initiative, has increased yearly. Part of the women examined returned annually for a routine reexamination, while others presented themselves again for checking of suspicious findings. Thus the percentage of women who reappeared increased each year.

Table 1 gives a summary of the activities of the clinics during the years 1966–1972. These figures reflect a very selective group in relation to age and frequency of the pathological findings, and of course no conclusions can be reached from them on the general morbidity incidence in the entire population.

The data for the years 1970–72, which included 56,648 women who underwent examinations, were processed with the aid of a computer. In 12,713 cases, i.e. 22.4%, some physical findings were detected, mostly in the form of palpable lumps, and less frequently, discharges from the nipple or changes in the areola and nipple. Figure 1 shows the frequency of the above findings according to age groups. It can be seen that the incidence in the different age groups fluctuates between 29% at the age of under 34 and 14% at the age of 55–60. There is a clear indication that the incidence is greater in the young age groups, but as stated, these figures do not represent a section of an entire population. However, when the incidence of cancer cases among the detected physical findings is examined, it is obvious that the percentage of malignant cases increases stead-

TABLE 1   *Summary of work performed during 7 years (1966–1972)*

No. of examinations	157,701
No. of women examined	79,586
Repeated examinations	78,115
Biopsies	3,961
Positive cases	895

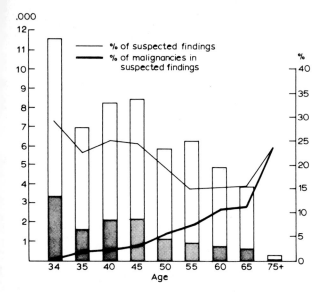

FIG. 1 *Age distribution of suspected findings and malignancies in total population examined (56,684) - 1970–1972.*

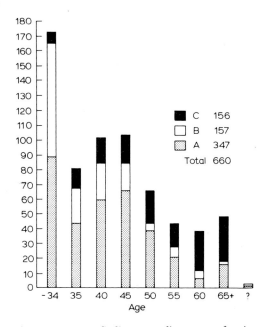

FIG. 2 *Biopsy findings according to age of patients (1972).*

ily with age. While in the age group under 34 years only 0.34% of the physical findings showed a malignant process, this percentage reached 24% at the age of 75 and over.

This conclusion is further corroborated when the biopsy results are analysed. In 1972, 660 biopsies were performed among 20,461 women examined. Figure 2 shows the histological findings according to the classification of W.H.O., and Figure 3 the relative distribution of these findings according to age.

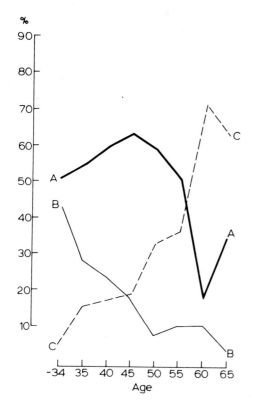

FIG. 3   *Distribution of pathological findings according to age (1972).*

(*a*) In 347 cases the following diagnosis was made:
Benign mammary dysplasias, which contained mainly cysts, adenosis, regular typical epithelial proliferations in ducts or lobules, and duct ectasias and fibrosclerosis.

(*b*) In 157 cases benign or apparently benign tumors were found, i.e. duct papillomas, fibroadenomas and adenomas of breast.

(*c*) In 156 cases, malignancies, i.e. carcinomas of different types, were diagnosed.

The incidence rate in the above 3 groups is different for the different age groups. While the incidence of benign mammary dysplasias is high at young ages, and decreases with age, the incidence of malignancy increases steeply with age. Only 4.6% of the biopsies at the age of 34 and under demonstrated a malignant process, while this percentage reached 63.3% at the age of 65 and over. In other words, with the increase in age of the women examined, each palpable lump acquires a more serious diagnostic significance.

Table 2 divides the findings according to ethnic origin in Israel. Though the population of Israel is composed of immigrants from all 5 continents, we divided them into 4 main groups, i.e. those born in Israel, immigrants from the Western countries, which include Europe and North and South America, from Asia, and from Africa. The number of women examined from each origin is not proportional to the percentage in the general population. It can be assumed that the readiness to visit the clinic was greater on the part of immigrants from the Western countries than of immigrants from Asia and Africa. There is also a difference in the composition of the age groups. Immigrants from Europe include higher age groups, while those born in Israel belong to the younger age groups, most of which have not reached the age at which the incidence of breast cancer is highest. Accordingly, no final conclusions can be reached from these figures. It is nevertheless

TABLE 2   *Distribution of suspected cases and malignancies according to ethnic origin (1970-1972)*

	Israel	Europe and America	Asia	Africa
Total examined	6,858	30,828	5,401	5,956
Total suspects	1,891	6,415	1,230	1,002
Per 10,000	2,700	2,080	2,280	1,680
Total malignancies	29	326	46	35
Per 10,000	42	106	85	59
Malignancies suspected (%)	1.5	5.1	3.7	3.5

interesting to note that suspicious physical findings exist in a large percentage in all the ethnic groups, and they fluctuate between 16.8% in the women examined from Africa, and 27% in those born in Israel. On the other hand, the incidence of breast cancer increases sharply in women from the Western countries. In women of African origin, it is 59 for every 10,000 examined, and it reaches 106 for every 10,000 women from the Western countries. The low incidence in women born in Israel again reflects the young age of this sector of the population. An attempt to divide the incidence in the different ethnic groups according to age produced groups too small to have statistical significance. We may be able to present clearer conclusions in only a number of years' time, when the different age groups will be more homogenous.

Figure 4 presents the division according to pathological stages of 459 cases which were proved to be malignant following histological examination. 41% of the cases were at clinical stage I, another 29.93% were still operable, i.e. at stage II. On the other hand, 12.85% were at stage III, and 5.22% at stage IV. The high number (11%) at an unknown stage is due to the fact that we have not yet succeeded in processing all the data of the histological examinations for the year 1972. These figures are not impressive from the

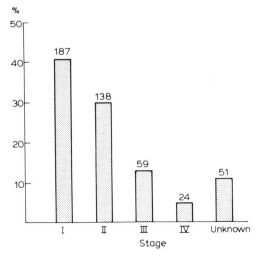

FIG. 4   *Pathological staging of breast cancer (1970–1972).*

viewpoint of the early detection of cancer, and they are due to the fact that the majority of positive cases was found in women sent for consultation by the family doctor (67 out of 1321), or in women who came on their own initiative (48 out of 3611), while only 3 cases (out of 3061) were discovered in women who visited the clinic by invitation.

The conclusion should not be drawn from the above data that the work of the clinics for the early detection of breast cancer, as carried out in Israel, does not contribute to earlier diagnosis. Since the establishment of these clinics, the awareness of the significance of abnormal findings in the breast has increased both among the female population and among general practitioners, and the ease with which every woman can obtain advice and professional assessment certainly prevents the postponement of diagnosis and suitable treatment. We intend during the present year to organize clinics in which thermographies and mammographies will be performed routinely. This will probably contribute to the earlier detection of malignant cases.

5. Identification of high risk groups

Prediction of cancer incidence in Finland for the year 1980

T. Hakulinen, L. Teppo and E.A. Saxén

The Finnish Cancer Registry, Helsinki, Finland

The main use of cancer incidence trends has been in the search for possible aetiological factors and the evaluation of the effect of different public health programmes. Trends may also be applied to the prediction of the future incidence of cancer. Hence it is possible to plan large-scale preventive, diagnostic and therapeutic measures in a given country. This is a report on an attempt to predict the incidence and the number of new cases of different types of cancer that will occur in Finland in 1980.

Prediction of the trends was based upon the incidence data of the Finnish Cancer Registry for the 12-year period, 1957-1968 (Finnish Cancer Registry 1963-1971). The Registry covers the whole country and obtains information on all cancer patients. Regression analysis (linear or exponential, depending on the specific site) was applied to the age-adjusted annual incidence rates. The rates were adjusted for the estimated population in Finland in 1980, forecast by the Central Statistical Office of Finland (1972).

Results

It is expected that no change will occur in the total cancer incidence (Fig. 1), although both increasing and decreasing trends will be apparent within the age-specific incidence rates. The most marked changes are the increases in children and in age groups of 80 years and over.

A decreasing trend is expected with respect to cancer of the stomach (in all age groups), oesophagus, mouth, pharynx and lip (Fig. 2). The increase in the incidence of cancer of the colon, rectum and pancreas (Fig. 2) does not compensate for the diminution in the incidence of cancer of the stomach and oesophagus. Consequently, a diminu-

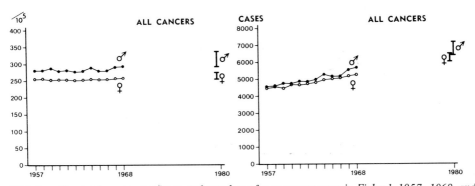

FIG. 1   *The total cancer incidence and number of new cancer cases in Finland, 1957–1968, and the corresponding predictions (90% confidence intervals) for 1980.*

tion should be apparent in the incidence of cancer of the digestive organs.

An increase should occur in the incidence of lung cancer in males (Fig. 3). The increase is most marked in more advanced age groups; it is expected that no change will take place in groups below 50 years of age. According to this prediction, no change will occur in the incidence of lung cancer in females.

In addition to the above-mentioned sites, increases should be observed in the incidence of cancer of the prostate, female breast, urinary organs and the skin (especially melanoma) as well as in Hodgkin's disease, lymphoma and multiple myeloma.

No significant change should occur in the incidence of cancer of the uterine cervix if the

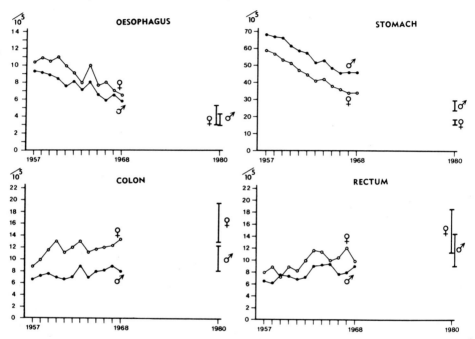

FIG. 2   *The incidence of the commonest cancers of the gastrointestinal tract in Finland, 1957–1968, and the predicted incidence (90% confidence interval) for 1980.*

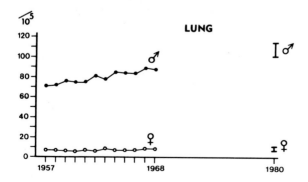

FIG. 3   *The incidence of lung cancer in Finland, 1957–1968, and the predicted incidence (90% confidence interval) for 1980.*

data from the whole period 1957-1968 are employed as a basis for estimation. However, from the 1960's, large-scale population screening has been carried out for the early detection of cancer of the uterine cervix: subsequently, during the years 1965-1968, a uniform decrease has been observed in the incidence of cancer at that site, excluding carcinoma in situ (Fig. 4). On the basis of these figures, the predicted incidence rate will be nearly one-half of that observed in 1968.

In 1957, the number of new cancer patients in Finland was nearly 9,000, the figure in 1968 was about 11,000 and the prediction for 1980 is 13,000 (Fig. 1). This increase is mostly attributable to the increase in the population of older groups.

In 1980, lung cancer should constitute more than one-third of all cancer cases in males

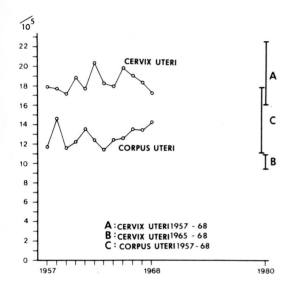

FIG. 4   *The incidence of cancer of the uterine cervix (in situ carcinoma excluded) and that of the corpus uteri in Finland, 1957–1968, and the predicted incidence (90% confidence interval) for 1980. Cancer of the cervix has been predicted in two ways.*

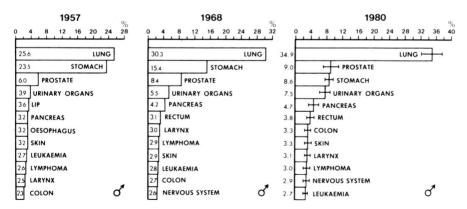

FIG. 5   *The 12 commonest cancer sites in males in Finland in 1957, 1968, and as estimated for 1980 with 90% confidence intervals.*

(Fig. 5). Cancer of the stomach consisted of more than 20% of all cancer in the 1950's, while in 1980 the proportion of this type of cancer should be less than 10%. Cancer of the colon and rectum will, on the contrary, probably become commoner. In females, the commonest type of cancer should be that of the breast (one-fifth of all cancer patients in 1980) (Fig. 6). The proportion of cancer of the stomach has diminished, and is expected to decline markedly in females, too. Other changes will be minor if the possible effect of mass screening is excluded as in Figure 6.

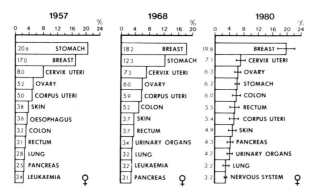

FIG. 6   *The 12 commonest cancer sites in females in Finland in 1957, 1968, and as estimated for 1980 with 90% confidence intervals.*

Discussion

The estimates presented here are based on the assumption that during the 1970's no abrupt change will occur in the incidence rates for cancer of any site. This assumption may, however, be incorrect. Increased smoking among young people and in females may invalidate the estimates of lung cancer incidence; for instance, the femal incidence has already started to rise in Connecticut. It is also difficult to evaluate the effect of mass screening programmes for the early detection of cancer of the uterine cervix upon the incidence of cervical cancer. Similar measures have been practised in British Columbia, where subsequently a diminution in the incidence of invasive cancer has taken place (Fidler et al., 1968). To date, the effect upon incidence has been less striking in Finland. The decrease in the incidence of cancer of the stomach, oesophagus and lip is expected to slow down, as has been observed in Connecticut (Connecticut Tumor Registry, 1971). This has also been taken into account when choosing the method of estimation for these forms of cancer.

Summary

The data of the Finnish Cancer Registry have been used to predict the incidence rates and the number of new cases of cancer of various sites in Finland in 1980. The total incidence is expected to remain approximately unchanged. The annual number of new cancer cases should, however, increase. Increases should also be observed in the incidence of cancer of the lung (in males), colon, rectum, pancreas, prostate, urinary organs, skin, and also in Hodgkin's disease, lymphoma and multiple myeloma.

A decreasing trend is expected with respect to cancer of the stomach, oesophagus, mouth, pharynx and lip. The commonest types of cancer should be lung cancer in males (35% of all) and breast cancer in females (20% of all).

References

Central Statistical Office of Finland (1972): Projection of Population in the Communes to the year 2000, Statistical Publication Series No. 49, Helsinki.

Connecticut Tumor Registry (1971): Cancer in Connecticut 1966-1968. Connecticut State Department of Health, Hartford, Conn.

Fidler, H. K., Boyes, D. A. and Worth, A. J. (1968): J. Obstet. Gynaec. Brit. Cwlth., 75/4, 392.

Finnish Cancer Registry (1963-1971): Cancer Incidence in Finland 1957-1968, Helsinki.

Cancer in young Connecticut adults, aged 15-29 years, 1950-1969*

Barbara Christine, Paul Sullivan and John Flannery

The Connecticut Tumor Registry, Connecticut State Department of Health, Hartford, Conn., U.S.A.

Introduction

The connection between maternal exposure to estrogen and the development of adeno-carcinoma of the vagina in offspring (Herbst et al., 1971) has suggested a need to evaluate the temporal occurrence of cancer in young people which might have a hormonal basis and compare it with that which does not. Changes in the incidence of several such sites were therefore studied over a 20-year period 1950–1969 utilizing the data of the population-based Connecticut Tumor Registry. The latter collects information on all malignant tumors and specified benign tumors diagnosed in Connecticut residents primarily through the reporting of hospital tumor registries. The public health statistics section of the Connecticut State Department of Health also forwards to the registry all death certificates mentioning cancer. Those not matched against reported cases are included in the registry as 'death certificate only' cases and the year of death is considered to be the year of diagnosis. The latter have made up less than 3% of cases registered annually in recent years. All malignant tumors are included as incident cases whether or not they are microscopically confirmed. However, microscopic confirmation was obtained for 90% of cases in 1965–1969.

Method

Young Connecticut men and women 15–29 years of age were taken as a study group. The age specific incidence rates were examined by sex, all ages combined and by 5-year age groups 15–19, 20–24, 25–29. The 20-year study period was broken into quinquennia.

The sites chosen for study were vulva, vagina, cervix and corpus uteri, ovary, breast, prostate, testis, kidney, melanoma, colon, thyroid, and other endocrine glands. In order to investigate genital organs fully the sites designated as 'uterus not otherwise specified', 'other female genital', and 'other male genital' were included. Also reviewed were data for brain, bone, and leukemia. As would be expected the numbers of cases were very small for some tumors.

Discussion

The greatest increase in rates of genital tumors for the age group 15 to 19 years from 1950–1954 to 1965–1969 were noted for cancer of the ovary and testis with peak rates actually occurring in the third period, 1960–1964 (Table 1). Other tumors showing noticeable gains were tumors of brain and bone in both sexes and with the exception of

---

* Supported by National Cancer Institute Contract NO1 CP 43203.

bone tumors in females, peak rates for these sites also occurred in the third period. Minimal rate gains were noted in females for malignant melanoma, thyroid, and leukemia. Cancers of the vagina and 'other female genital organs' and 'other male genital tumors' were not diagnosed in this age group until the period 1965–1969 when one case was reported for each site.

In young adults aged 20–24 sites whose rates showed the greatest increase from first to last period were ovary, thyroid in both sexes, brain and bone in males. Peak rates were noted in the fourth period for all of these except for brain cancer which was at a maximum in 1955–1959 and cancer of the bone for which the rate was highest in 1960–1964. Minimal increases were noted for large intestine, brain and bone in females, prostate and leukemia in males.

The greatest increase in rate from first to last study period in those aged 25–29 was that of tumors of the thyroid gland in females. Tumors which showed slight increases were malignant melanoma and bone tumors in both sexes; testis, thyroid, brain, and leukemia in males; and uterine corpus and breast tumors in females. Highest rates occurred in the fourth period for tumors of the corpus, thyroid, and malignant melanoma in females and leukemia in males. Minimal increases were found for large intestine and prostate in males, uterus N.O.S., and vulva in females.

Although rates for in situ cancer of the cervix rose slightly in 15–19 year olds and markedly in the two older age groups as well as in all ages combined from the first to the last period there were no cases of invasive cervical cancer in the 15–19 group in any period and rates decreased for the other two age groups.

For all ages combined, 15–29, thyroid tumors in females showed a significant increase in rate from 1950–1954 to 1965–1969. Sites which increased to a lesser extent were ovary; brain and leukemia in males; and bone in both sexes. Minimal increases of 0.1 to 0.2 were recorded for vulva, vagina, corpus, uterus N.O.S., and brain in females and prostate and testis in males.

Comparison with California

Linden and Henderson (1972) recently reviewed the California Tumor Registry data for the periods 1950–1962, 1963–1969 to investigate changes in the occurrence of cancer of the breast and genital organs in those aged 10–19 and 20–24 as well as non-genital tract sites — bladder, stomach, colon, and rectum. In persons 10–19 they reported increases in numbers of cases of the vagina, corpus uteri, prostate, testis, and bladder (in males) and in those 20–24 increases in tumors of the vulva and testis.

For slightly different time periods, 1950–1959 and 1960–1969, data for the Connecticut age group 10–19 years showed an increase in number of cases of tumors of the large intestine, ovary, cervix, and vagina in females; rectum, prostate, and testis in males; and bladder in both sexes. Except for ovary, testis, and large intestine (female) all sites had only 3 tumors or less reported in 1960–1969. Age-specific rates also increased except for large intestine and bladder in females. Thus Connecticut failed to show an increase in cancer of the corpus noted in California but showed an increase in tumors of the ovary and cervix in females and rectal tumors in males not found there.

Connecticut young adults aged 20–24 failed to show increased age-specific rates of cancer of the vulva and testis (although the number of tumors of the testis increased) for which this age group showed increased numbers of cases in the California registry. Cancer of the ovary had an increase in rate of 1.2 and cancer of the large intestine in females and bladder in males showed rate increases of less magnitude. Minimal increases in incidence rates of 0.1 to 0.2 from one decade to the next were noted in Connecticut for cancer of the stomach, rectum, vagina, and bladder in females and stomach and prostate in males.

TABLE 1　Number of cancer cases and age-specific incidence rates per 100,000 population for selected sites among persons aged 15-29 years, by sex and period of diagnosis, Connecticut, 1950-1969

ICD* No.	Primary site	Sex	No. of cases				Rate per 100,000			
			1950-1954	1955-1959	1960-1964	1965-1969	1950-1954	1955-1959	1960-1964	1965-1969
					Age 15–19					
175.0	Ovary	F	1	2	10	10	0.3	0.5	2.1	1.7
173,175.1-175.9, 176.7-176.9	Other female gen.	F	–	–	–	1	–	–	–	0.2
176.1	Vagina	F	–	–	–	1	–	–	–	0.2
178	Testis	M	2	4	8	8	0.6	1.0	1.7	1.4
179	Other male gen.	M	–	–	–	1	–	–	–	0.2
193.0	Brain	M	2	5	11	11	0.6	1.3	2.3	1.9
	Brain	F	1	7	5	6	0.3	1.8	1.1	1.0
196	Bone	M	3	6	9	10	0.9	1.5	1.9	1.7
	Bone	F	4	1	6	10	1.2	0.3	1.3	1.7
					Age 20–24					
175.0	Ovary	F	3	9	9	17	0.8	2.5	2.2	3.2
193.0	Brain	M	4	7	7	10	1.2	2.1	1.9	2.0
	Brain	F	4	4	3	8	1.1	1.1	0.7	1.5
194	Thyroid	M	–	1	3	9	–	0.3	0.8	1.8
	Thyroid	F	7	6	13	23	1.9	1.7	3.2	4.3
196	Bone	M	2	4	6	7	0.6	1.2	1.6	1.4
	Bone	F	–	3	2	3	–	0.8	0.5	0.6
					Age 25–29					
170	Breast	F	28	28	31	34	6.6	7.0	7.5	7.1
172	Corpus	F	1	2	3	5	0.2	0.5	0.7	1.0
178	Testis	M	18	13	22	23	4.5	3.4	5.6	5.1
190	Malignant melanoma	M	9	10	13	13	2.3	2.6	3.3	2.9
	Malignant melanoma	F	12	11	9	16	2.8	2.7	2.2	3.3
193.0	Brain	M	5	8	9	9	1.3	2.1	2.3	2.0
	Brain	F	8	6	6	9	1.9	1.5	1.5	1.9
194	Thyroid	M	1	6	3	5	0.3	1.6	0.8	1.1
	Thyroid	F	7	11	15	22	1.6	2.7	3.6	4.6

196	Bone	M	—	3	2	3	—	0.8	0.5	0.7
		F	—	5	1	3	—	1.2	0.2	0.6
204	Leukemia	M	10	5	12	16	2.5	1.3	3.1	3.5
		F	6	5	6	5	1.4	1.2	1.5	1.0

Age 15–29

175.0	Ovary	F	20	23	28	41	1.8	2.0	2.2	2.6
176.0	Vulva	F	—	3	1	3	—	0.3	0.1	0.2
176.1	Vagina	F	—	—	1	1	—	—	0.1	0.1
177	Prostate	M	—	—	1	2	—	—	0.1	0.1
178	Testis	M	34	27	39	51	3.2	2.4	3.2	3.3
193.0	Brain	M	11	20	27	30	1.0	1.8	2.2	1.9
		F	13	17	14	23	1.2	1.5	1.1	1.4
194	Thyroid	M	1	7	8	15	0.1	0.6	0.6	1.0
		F	15	22	37	49	1.3	1.9	2.9	3.1
196	Bone	M	5	13	17	20	0.5	1.2	1.4	1.3
		F	4	9	9	16	0.4	0.8	0.7	1.0
204	Leukemia	M	27	19	36	45	2.5	1.7	2.9	2.9
		F	17	19	17	20	1.5	1.6	1.3	1.3

* International Classification of Diseases, seventh revision, 1955, World Health Organization.

TABLE 2　Number of cancer cases and age-specific incidence rates per 100,000 population for selected sites among persons aged 10-24 years by sex and period of diagnosis, Connecticut, 1950–1969

ICD* No.	Primary site	Sex	Age 10–19				Age 20–24			
			No. of cases		Rate per 100,000		No. of cases		Rate per 100,000	
			1950–1959	1960–1969	1950–1959	1960–1969	1950–1959	1960–1969	1950–1959	1960–1969
151	Stomach	M	1	–	0.1	–	1	2	0.1	0.2
		F	1	1	0.1	0.04	–	1	–	0.1
153	Large intestine	M	2	2	0.1	0.1	2	3	0.3	0.3
		F	3	5	0.2	0.2	3	8	0.4	0.9
154	Rectum	M	–	2	–	0.1	4	1	0.6	0.1
		F					1	2	0.1	0.2
170	Breast	F	3	3	0.2	0.1	12	7	1.6	0.7
171	Cervix (invasive)	F	–	1	–	0.04	10	8	1.4	0.9
172	Corpus uteri	F	–	–	–	–	3	3	0.4	0.3
175.0	Ovary	F	7	26	0.5	1.1	12	26	1.6	2.8
176.0	Vulva	F	1	–	0.1	–	1	1	0.1	0.1
176.1	Vagina	F	–	1	–	0.04	–	1	–	0.1
177	Prostate	M	–	2	–	0.1	–	1	–	0.1
178	Testis	M	6	17	0.4	0.7	24	29	3.5	3.3
181.0	Bladder	M	–	3	–	0.1	6	11	0.9	1.3
		F	1	2	0.1	0.1	4	7	0.5	0.7

* International Classification of Diseases, seventh revision, 1955, World Health Organization.

Conclusion

Selected tumors which showed the greatest increase in incidence rates from 1950–1954 to 1965–1969 in young Connecticut residents aged 15–19 were those of the ovary in females and brain in males. Ovarian and thyroid tumors in females led with the greatest rise in 20–24 year olds while thyroid tumors in males ranked second. In the age group 25–29 the largest increase in rate from first to last period was that of thyroid tumors in females.

With all ages combined, 15–29 years, the greatest increases in incidence rates from first to last period were noted for thyroid in both sexes and ovarian tumors in females. In sites not expected to be influenced by hormonal factors all except leukemia in females showed increased rates with the largest noted for tumors of the brain in males and bone in both sexes.

A comparison of data from California and Connecticut tumor registries for persons aged 10–24 utilizing slightly different time periods revealed that although the numbers of cases were for the most part small, Connecticut showed both increased numbers and increased rates of tumors of the vagina, prostate, testis, and bladder in males in the 10–19 age group correlating with the increased number of cases in those sites noted in the California registry. Increases in other sites did not correspond for the two registries. The leading increases in incidence rates found in Connecticut residents aged 20–24, for ovary and large intestine in females and bladder in males, did not correspond to the California report of increased numbers of cases of vulva and testis.

References

Herbst, A.L., Ulfelder, H. and Poskanzer, D.C. (1971): New Engl. J. Med., 284, 878.
Linden, G. and Henderson, B.E. (1972): New Engl. J. Med., 286, 760.

Cancer rates for uterine cervix and breast, observed at an early detection clinic: Presentation of some characteristics of these two populations of cancers

Y. Fassin

Early Detection Clinic, Institut Jules Bordet, Brussels, Belgium

Material

During a 7-year period (1965-1971), 43,505 women have been examined at our Early Detection Clinic. Of these, 24,240 were seen for the first time and 19,265 came for a second or a third clinical examination. The time lapse between two examinations ranged from 1 to 2 years. All women attending for the first clinical examination come spontaneously; most of them are alerted through a public education programme, relying on the distribution of pamphlets, or the holding of conferences in social communities or work centres. Those attending for re-examination are called up by personal invitation, through the use of a computerized system.

Figure 1 presents the comparison, by 5-year age-groups, between the female population at first examination and that coming for re-examination. This shows that the examined population is mostly comprised of women aged from 30 to 49 years. This group represents more than 60% of all women attending the clinic. It is representative of the informed population, and demonstrates the special receptiveness of these age groups to sanitary education.

Rates of cancer detection (uterine cervix and breast)

The general results of screening are presented in Table 1. This table gives the rates per 1,000 women examined at first examination, compared to those for re-examination. For all cancers (cervix invasive and stage 0 as well as for breast), the rates of discovery decrease in the population seen at re-examination.

Presentation of the population of cancer

(a) Comparison of cancer population detected at first examination with that detected at re-examination

We collected at first examination 143 cases and only 53 at re-examination. Figure 2 shows the age distribution by 5-year groups of all cancer cases; it shows the different stages for cervical and breast cancers. At first examination, cervical cancer stage 0 represents 69% of all cervical cancers; breast cancer stage 1 comprises about 51% of all breast cancers discovered. At re-examination, cervical cancer stage 0 rises to 77% of all cervical

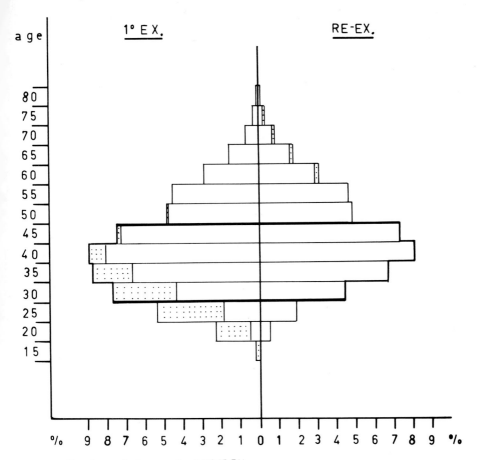

FIG. 1   *Female population examined (1965-71).*

TABLE 1   *Comparison of rates (uterine cervix and breast, per 1,000 women examined)*

	At first examination (0/00)	At re-examination (0/00)
Cervical carcinoma (stage 0)	2.269	1.038
Invasive cervical carcinoma	1.031	0.311
Breast carcinoma	2.599	1.401
Total	5.899	2.750
No. of examinations	24,240	19,265

DIB. 1965–1971

cancers discovered; on the other hand, breast cancer stage 1 rises only to 41% of the breast cases.

It must be emphasized that very few cases have been detected in the population under 30 years of age (4 cases in total) and all of them are cervical cancers. At the other end of the age-range, there is a higher number of breast cancer cases in the population over 65 years of age at first examination. This fact may be the reflection of self-selection among women coming spontaneously; this does not seem to be the case for a population called for re-examination.

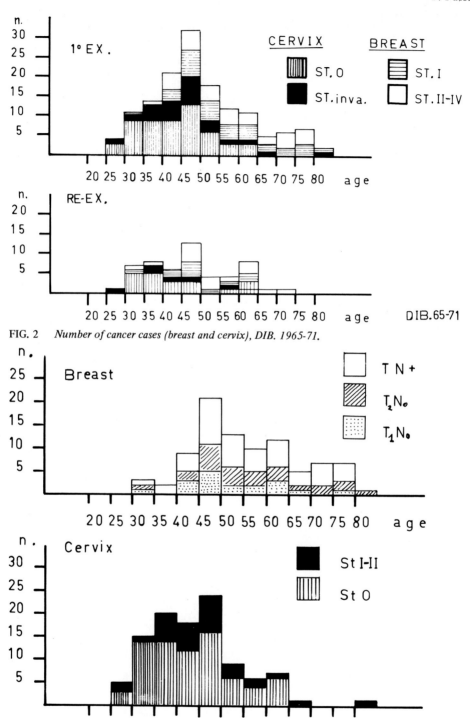

FIG. 2   *Number of cancer cases (breast and cervix), DIB. 1965-71.*

FIG. 3   *Cancer cases populations, DIB. 1965-71.*

(*b*) *Comparison of cancer population by each type of cancer*

Figure 3 compares, by 5-year age-groups, the population of 90 breast cancer cases and the population of 106 cases with cervical cancer. This presentation shows the age differences both for stage and type of cancer, compared with those presented in Figure 2.

TABLE 2   *The differences of mean age for the different stages of carcinoma of cervix and breast*

		No.	%	Mean age
Cervical cancer	Stage 0	75	70.8	42.5
	Stage I A	10	9.4	39.9
	Stage I – II	21	19.8	48.8
	Total	106	100.0	43.7
Breast cancer	Stage I	43	47.8	54.9
	Stage II	26	28.9	55.0
	Stage III – IV	21	23.3	57.6
	Total	90	100.0	55.6

Table 2 demonstrates the differences of mean age for the different stages of carcinoma of cervix and breast. The mean age for cervical cases is 43.7 years and as would be expected, the mean age for breast cancer is higher: 55.5 years.

Presentation of some characteristics of the two cancer populations

(*a*) *Cancer heredity declared by patients*

The results of the inquiries regarding cancer heredity are presented in Table 3. The consideration of cancer heredity has been limited to mother, aunts and sisters. 109 women knew of no cancer cases in their family members. The comparison for cervical cases and breast cases does not show any difference between these 2 populations.

(*b*) *Age at first menstruation declared by patients*

The results of this inquiry depend mostly on memory and it is noted that in 5 cases for women aged over 65 years, we were unable to collect answers. The comparison of the mean age at first menstruation in the 2 cancer populations does not give any appreciable difference (cervical cancer: 12.99 years; breast cancer: 12.88 years).

(*c*) *Habits of breast feeding*

88 women declared they had not breast fed their children (38% of the cervical cases and 52% of the breast cancers): this difference is not found to be significant.

(*d*) *Differences in parity and gestation*

The 2 cancer populations are described in Table 4 with regard to parity (P) and abortion (AB). The duration of pregnancy is evaluated: 9 months for a pregnancy ending in normal

TABLE 3   *Results of inquiries regarding cancer heredity*

	Cervical cancer		Breast cancer	
	No.	%	No.	%
None	52	49.0	57	63.3
Other cancers	39	36.8	21	23.4
Breast cancer	9	8.6	8	8.9
Uterine cancer	6	5.6	4	4.4
Total	106	100.0	90	100.0

TABLE 4   *Average duration of all pregnancies*

Cervical cancer %	n	P	$\frac{P}{n}$	AB	$\frac{AB}{n}$	$\frac{P+AB}{n}$	
14.15	15	0	–	0	–	–	
6.60	7	0	–	9	3.8 m	–	
51.89	55	92	15.0 m	0	–	–	17.9 m
27.36	29	69	21.4 m	51	5.3 m	26.7 m	
100.00	106	161	13.7 m	60	1.7 m	15.4 m	

Breast cancer %	n	P	$\frac{P}{n}$	AB	$\frac{AB}{n}$	$\frac{P+AB}{n}$	
32.22	29	0	–	0	–	–	
5.56	5	0	–	12	7.2 m	–	
42.22	38	70	16.5 m	0	–	–	18.0 m
20.00	18	38	19.0 m	30	5.0 m	24.0 m	
100.00	90	108	10.8 m	42	1.4 m	12.2 m	

n = number of women who had been pregnant;
1 P = 9 months;
1 AB = 3 months.

delivery, and 3 months for an abortion. For the two cancer populations, we have collected the declarations of 269 pregnancies (161 for cervical carcinoma and 108 for breast carcinoma).

The only highly significant difference we have found between the two cancer populations, is in relation to nulli-parity (P=0), combined with no abortion (AB=0). For cervical cancer, 15 women out of 106 (14%), and for breast cancer, 29 women out of 90 (32%) fell in these categories. On the other hand, if we consider the cumulative duration of pregnancies in the two populations for the cases who have been pregnant, no significant difference is seen (cervical carcinoma average cumulative exposure: 17.9 months; breast cancer: 18.0 months).

Summary

The results of 43,505 examinations are presented. The rates of cervical cancer and breast cancer discovered among these women are given in relation to the first examination and re-examination.

The two cancer populations have been compared with regard to different criteria. We find differences in the age distribution of the cases. No difference was found concerning cancer heredity, age of first menstruation, and habits of breast feeding.

Although we have been unable to prove any difference of pattern in the average cumulative duration of pregnancies for women who have been pregnant, we have found a highly significant difference between the two populations for women who have never been pregnant.

Relative rates of breast and cervix cancers in mass screening: Evaluation of high-risk groups

H. Maisin, A. Vandenbroucke-Vanderwielen, M. A. Sergent-Millet and J. Van de Merckt

Cancer Institute, University of Louvain, Louvain, Belgium

Introduction

Our aim was to determine the groups at high risk of cancer in a population of asymptomatic women examined through mass screening by a clinical examination. To achieve this objective, we have investigated:

the relative frequency of cancers
the relative rates of small and large cancers of the breast and of in situ and invasive cancers of the cervix
the relative frequency of cancer diagnosed at first and second examinations
the influence of virginity, nulliparity and pregnancy
the influence of the age at first pregnancy
the influence of a previous mastopathy
the influence of menopause
the influence of a cancerous heredity
the influence of the social environment

Material and method

Our experience bears on 25,004 women examined at least once: it covers 7 years (1966 to 1972). To obtain a representative sample, we have chosen only women examined in urban and rural communities (20,774), and nuns (4,230). We have excluded women examined in business concerns because they are generally younger and have a lower rate of cancer (Maisin et al., 1968, 1970). At the beginning of our survey, we advised a screening examination every two years, but for the last year, in the light of experience, we have recommended a breast examination at least annually.

Each examination includes a complete physical examination and a vaginal smear. The method has already been described (Maisin, 1967). We now practise a full examination every two years and in between, we carry out a breast examination only. We always request mammography if we find an anomaly in either breast. When we discover a mammary anomaly, we repeat the examination twice a year, but we describe it as a control examination and not a new screening examination. 31.4% of the examined 'women' and 22.8% of the nuns have undergone two or more examinations. We have examined women from the age of 25, but for the last year, on the basis of our experience, we suggest that they do not come before the age of 30. (When we use the term 'women' we refer to women examined in urban and rural communities.) To analyse certain of the selected data we were obliged to choose at random a representative sample of 1,000 women living in urban and rural communities. We used this sample to study the influence of the age at first pregnancy, and the relation to social environment. These questions are now systematically included in the questionnaire.

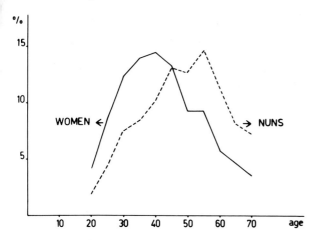

FIG. 1   *Age distributions of the 'women' and the nuns examined.*

TABLE 1   *The number and overall rate of cancers in 'women' examined during mass screening in urban and rural communities, and in nuns.*

	No. of examinations	Cancers confirmed by biopsy							
		Total Ca		Breast Ca		Cervix Ca		Other Ca	
		No.	$^o/_{oo}$	No.	$^o/_{oo}$	No.	$^o/_{oo}$	No.	$^o/_{oo}$
Urban and rural communities	20,774	184 (100%)	8.8	98 (53%)	4.7	43 (23.4%)	2	43 (23.4%)	2
Communities of nuns	4,330	50 (100%)	11.8	29 (58%)	6.8	0	0	21 (42%)	4.9

Results

The age distributions of the 'women' and the nuns are given in Fig. 1. The nuns, on the average, are at least 10 years older. Table 1 gives the number and overall rate of cancers in 'women' examined during mass screening in urban and rural communities and in nuns. Nuns have substantially more cancers: $11.8^o/_{oo}$ versus $8.8^o/_{oo}$; more breast cancers, $6.8^o/_{oo}$ versus $4.7^o/_{oo}$ and more 'other cancers', $4.9^o/_{oo}$ versus $2^o/_{oo}$, but do not present with cancer of the cervix.

The overall relative rates of breast cancer, cervical cancer and of 'other cancers', and the rate of onset of those cancers in relation to the age of the women examined in urban and rural community, are shown in Figure 2. The biggest risk of cancer in asymptomatic women examined in mass screening is clearly breast cancer. It increases throughout life. The overall risk presented by cervix cancer, or 'other cancer', is in each instance, less than half.

Cancers of the cervix appear most frequently before and after the menopause. We shall refer to this later. 'Other cancers' appear throughout life. This graph implies that there is no advantage in examining women before the age of 30. With nuns, the rates of onset in relation to age for breast cancers and of 'other cancers', are raised, but comparable. We shall refer later to cancer of the breast in nuns. (Remember we have detected no cervical cancer in nuns.)

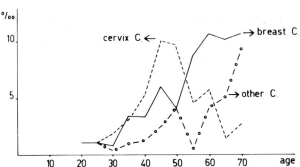

FIG. 2   *Overall relative rates of breast cancer, cervical cancer and of 'other cancers', and the rate of onset of those cancers in relation to the age of the women examined in urban and rural community. (Total rate: breast cancer – 4.7°/₀₀; cervical cancer – 2.1°/₀₀; other cancers –2.1°/₀₀.)*

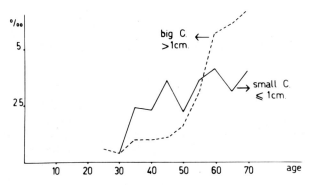

FIG. 3   *Comparison of the rate and age of onset of small cancers as against big cancers. (Total rate: small cancers – 2.3°/₀₀ (50%); big cancers – 1.8°/₀₀ (37%).)*

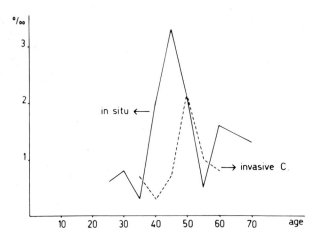

FIG. 4   *Comparison of the rate of in situ and invasive cervical cancer in an asymptomatic population. (Total rate: in situ – 1.2°/₀₀ (69%); invasive 0.6°/₀₀ (31%).)*

Small breast cancers (less than, or equal to, 1 cm) — see Figure 3 — are more numerous, and appear much earlier, than cancers larger than 1 cm. Because most cases (80%) do not present with axillary nodes, this shows the importance of early and regular screening of the breast and provides a good indication of the natural history of breast cancer. In the case of the breast, it is therefore risky not to examine women regularly above the age of 30.

As expected in an asymptomatic population (Fig. 4), cervical cancer is infrequent and 69% are in situ. In our sample, about 10 years separates the age-specific onset of cancer in situ from that of invasive cancer. This is generally accepted but is now confirmed for an asymptomatic population.

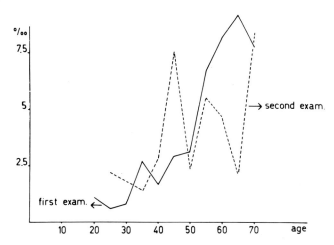

FIG. 5 *The rate of onset of breast cancer in 'women', as at first and following examinations. (Total rate: first examination – 3.3⁰/₀₀; second examination – 3.3⁰/₀₀.)*

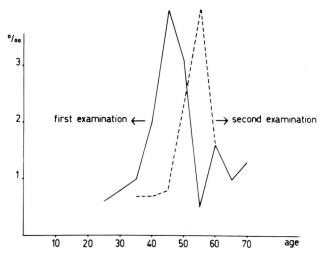

FIG. 6 *Comparison of the overall rate of cervical cancer discovered at second examination, as against breast cancer. (Total rate: first examination: 1.4⁰/₀₀; second examination – 1.0⁰/₀₀ (21%).)*

The rate of onset of breast cancer in 'women', as at the first and following examinations, is very interesting (Fig. 5). Overall, many cancers are discovered at each examination, but the rate under 50 is particularly elevated at the second examination; over 50 the finding is reversed. This confirms the fact that breast cancer rates increase faster with age in young women, and emphasizes the great advantage of annual examination of the breast, and especially the systematic repetition of the examination, even twice a year, if an anomaly is detected. The results are similar for the nuns.

For cervical cancer, the overall rate discovered at the second examination is proportionally less elevated than for the breast, and cancers discovered during the second examination are detected at a more advanced age, on the average 10 years later (Fig. 6). Most are in situ. This seems to show that it should be practicable to reduce the frequency of screening of the cervix, for example to every two or three years.

The overall rate of breast cancer in the nuns and in the 'women' who did not get pregnant, compared with that of 'women' who bear children, shows that women bearing children get less cancer than the other, and that it appears at a later age (Fig. 7). But, bearing more than 4 children does not necessarily protect the mammary gland. In our sample, these women seem to have about the same risk as childless women.

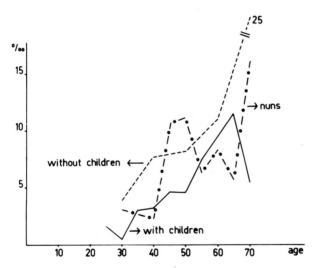

FIG. 7   *The overall rate of breast cancer in the nuns and in the 'women' who did not get pregnant, compared with that of 'women' who bear children. (Total rate: nuns − 6.8°/$_{00}$; women without children − 6.5°/$_{00}$ (32.8%); women with children − 4.1°/$_{00}$ (67.2%). (≤4 children − 3.8°/$_{00}$; >4 children − 5.8°/$_{00}$.)*

Non-virgin women who did not bear children have more cervical cancer (2.3°/oo) than those who marry and bear children (1.9°/oo). The rate increases with age in both groups (Fig. 8). Among women who bear children, those who bear many have the most cervical cancer. The nuns and the 'women' who remain virgins do not, it will be recalled, develop cervical cancer. For breast cancer, 32.8% appeared in 'women' who did not bear any children; they represented 23% of the total. For cervical cancer, this proportion was 23% but as this cancer did not affect virgins, it represents 17% of the total.

When we consider the influence of age of the first pregnancy on the age of onset of breast cancer (Fig. 9), women who have borne a child at or before the age of 20, have less breast cancer (upper part of Fig. 9). In our sample, rates are similar for those bearing their

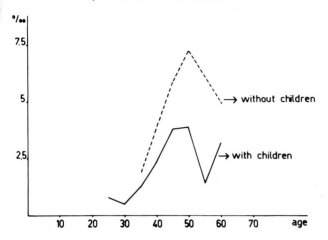

FIG. 8   *Showing that non-virgin women who did not bear children have more cervical cancer than those who marry and bear children. (Total rate: nuns − 0; virgin women − 0; non-virgin women without children − 2.3°/$_{00}$ (23%); women with children − 1.9°/$_{00}$ (77%). (≤4 children − 1.7°/$_{00}$; >4 children − 4.7°/$_{00}$.)*

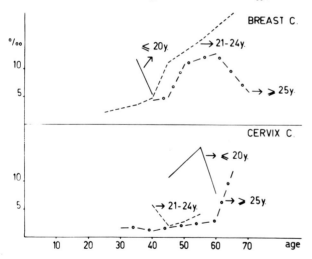

FIG. 9   *The influence of age of the first pregnancy on the age of onset of breast cancer (upper part), and cervical cancer (lower part). (Total rate for breast cancer: ≤ 20 years − 2.2°/$_{00}$; 21−24 years − 4.9°/$_{00}$; ≥ 25 years − 4.0°/$_{00}$; no children − 6.5°/$_{00}$.) (Total rate for cervical cancer: ≤ 20 years − 3.0°/$_{00}$; 21−24 years − 1.9°/$_{00}$; ≥ 25 years − 1.8°/$_{00}$; non-virgins without children − 2.3°/$_{00}$; virgins − 0.)*

child above the age of 20. However, for cervical cancer, the bearing of a child at or before the age of 20 is associated with an increased risk (lower part of Fig. 9).

A mastopathy is associated with a markedly increased risk of cancer. In the population of 10,486 women examined between 1970 and 1972 we found 5.45°/oo cancers of the breast. Among these women, 795 or 7% presented a breast anomaly that called for mammography or a control examination. In these patients the rate of mammary cancer was found to be more than 70°/oo. We have not yet had the opportunity to study systematically all the charts and thus we cannot describe the outcome in those mammary glands in relation to the type of mastopathy.

We did investigate the possible relation of the menopause to onset rate of cancers of the breast and cervix.

Influence of menopause

Breast cancer	Yes:	$7.8^0/_{00}$	No:	$2.9^0/_{00}$
Cervix cancer		$2.4^0/_{00}$		$1.7^0/_{00}$

The overall rate of breast cancer is much higher in menopausal than in non-menopausal women. We can draw a similar conclusion for cancer of the cervix. Thus, the menopause constitutes a higher risk for both cancers.

Heredity was also studied in breast and cervix cancer. The rates found are shown in Table 2. For breast cancer, it was known that breast heredity has an undeniable influence, and this is verified in our mass screening patients; for cervical cancer, cervix heredity seems also to have an important influence. This is less well known, but may be the consequence of the economic level of certain families.

TABLE 2   *Influence of cancer heredity*

	Without heredity ($^0/_{00}$)	With heredity except of breast and cervix Ca ($^0/_{00}$)	With breast cancer heredity ($^0/_{00}$)	With cervix cancer heredity ($^0/_{00}$)
Breast cancers	4.5	4.5	7.8	3
Cervix cancers	1.8	1.6	no data	3.5

Finally, we investigated the possible influence of socio-economic factors. We considered only the influence of education and established two levels:

1 : primary and low secondary school education

2 : high secondary school and university education. The results are shown in Figure 10. The rate of breast cancer is higher and appears earlier in women of high educational attainment (upper part of Fig. 10); the reverse is found for cervical (lower part of Fig. 10).

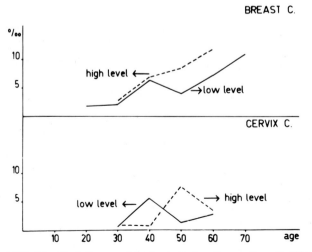

FIG. 10   *The influence of the level of education on the rate of breast cancer (upper part), and cervical cancer (lower part). (Total rate for breast cancer: low level – $4.5^0/_{00}$; high level – $5.1^0/_{00}$.) (Total rate for cervical cancer: low level – $2.2^0/_{00}$; high level – $1.7^0/_{00}$.)*

TABLE 3   *High risk groups of cancer*

	Breast cancer		Cervix cancer	
	High	Low	High	Low
Compared incidence	+			−
Cancer volume	+ ≤ 1 cm 30–40 years + > 1 cm older than 50		+ in situ 35–45 years + invasive older than 45	
1st and 2nd examination	*Second* 40–45 years *First* older than 50		*First* 35–50 years *Second* older than 50	
Virgins – Nuns	+			0
Nulliparity (non virgins)	+		+	
Pregnancy ≤ 4 > 4	more or less +		more or less ++	
Age at 1st pregnancy	older than 20	20 years or less	20 years or less	older than 20
Mastopathy	+++			
Cervix (pre-cancer)			no data	no data
Menopause	+		+	
Cancer heredity	breast heredity	cervical heredity	cervical heredity	no data
Education level	high		low	

Discussion

Consider first the data in Table 3. Contrary to the views of some investigators, breast cancer can be detected in an asymptomatic population (Maisin et al.,1968, 1970). But to find breast cancer, examiners must be strongly motivated. General practitioners who collaborate with our institute, find very few cases of breast cancer — one tenth of those found by our medical team (Maisin et al., 1968, 1970, 1971).

It is interesting that small breast cancers can be detected and that most of these are found in young women. It may be concluded that cancers appearing in young women are more aggressive and that there is little advantage in detecting them. We should be cautious before drawing such conclusions because most small cancers are not associated with affected axillary nodes. A definitive answer will be given by the results of follow-up after adequate treatment. In our view, cancer screening should be carried out at about the age of 30. It must be done regularly — at least every year for young people — because we found more cancer in young people at the second examination. For older women, the interval between two examinations can be longer but we must bear in mind that the later the cancers are detected, the bigger they are, the more likely they will have spread to axillary nodes, and the poorer the prognosis will be. Finally, we must recall that in our sample the risk of discovering a cancer after the menopause is high, which shows the importance of regular examination of post-menopausal women. Onset rates of breast cancer in our sample increase up to, and after 70 years of age, as shown previously (Berkson et al., 1957). If pregnancy protects the breast against cancer — as has already been assumed (Smithers et al., 1952) — very early pregnancy at or before 20 years of age is effective, as shown by MacMahon et al. (1970). Moreover, an increase in the number of pregnancies is accompanied by an increase in cancer, as MacMahon (1958) found.

We can confirm the high rate of cancer of the breast found previously in nuns (Maisin et al., 1967, 1968, 1971; Taylor et al., 1959). Their rate is similar to that found in childless women, as suggested by Smithers et al., 1952. Women suffering mastopathy are a particularly high-risk group, but more studies must be done in our cases to determine which type of mastopathy is most dangerous.

In our sample, a family history of cancer of the breast is associated with high risk (Macklin, 1959; Lilienfeld, 1963), but more work must be done to determine associations with factors such as blood groups (Hems, 1970). In our sample high level education is associated with a high risk of cancer of the breast. In our population, the level of education seems to be a good index of socio-economic level; other parameters studied by Clemmesen and Nielsen (1951) and Stocks (1955), are of little interest in our highly developed population. In our sample of asymptomatic women we have been able to show a good relation between women who develop cancer of the breast and most of the high risk groups previously recognized (Zippin and Petrokis, 1971). This emphasizes the importance of mass screening in the high-risk groups.

The chance of detecting cancer of the cervix in asymptomatic women is low (Maisin et al., 1968, 1970). The reverse is found for women examined by general practitioners who collaborate with our Institute. They find 2 to 3 times more cervical cancer (most cases being invasive) than we do, because women report symptoms (Maisin et al., 1968, 1970, 1971). Most of the cancers of the cervix found in our asymptomatic sample are in situ and are detected at the first examination. The frequency of examination of the cervix can thus be less than that for the breast. The menopause is associated with an increased risk.

In our sample, virgins and nuns who are virgins have not developed cancer of the cervix (Maisin et al., 1967, 1968, 1970, 1971). This confirms the findings of Taylor et al. (1959) for North American nuns. Women in our sample who are not virgins frequently develop cancer of the cervix, especially if they are not married (Stocks, 1958).

Pregnancy increases the rate of cancer of the cervix in proportion of the number of pregnancies. To be pregnant before the age of 20 definitely increases the rate. It appears that sexual activity may be an important factor in cervical cancer (Terris et al., 1967). Heredity may also be involved in cancer of the cervix, but the association may be with low education level. This needs to be investigated.

Conclusion

The risk of cancer of the breast in our asymptomatic population of women is twice as high as for cancer of the cervix.

Systematic screening should start at the age of 30 and should be more frequent for the breast than for the cervix — at least once a year for breast — the number of detected cancers at the second examination proves it — and every two or three years for the cervix. Small cancer of the breast without spread to axillary nodes can be found in young women, even at the second examination, which thus remains a valuable one. Small cancers are more numerous. Most of the cervix cancers found are in situ.

To have children protects the breast; the high rate of cancer in nuns and in childless women, married or not, supports this view. To protect, the age at first pregnancy should be 20 years or less, but in our sample, to have too many children fails to protect.

Nuns and virgins do not develop cancer of the cervix. Women who are not virgins have a high risk of cervical cancer. To have a child before the age of 20, and to have many children, increase the risk.

Mastopathy and menopause are high risk factors where cancer of the breast is concerned. The menopause is also a high risk factor for cancer of the cervix.

With asymptomatic women, breast heredity remains a reliable index for increased risk of breast cancer; a similar finding seems to hold for cervix heredity and cancer of the cervix.

A high level of education is associated with a high risk of cancer of the breast; and low level is associated with a high risk of cancer of the cervix.

Summary

Among 25,000 asymptomatic women, aged over 20, examined in mass screening, we have compared the rate of breast, cervical and other cancers with married and unmarried women; more than 4,000 of them were nuns.

We have investigated the influence of parity and the age of the first pregnancy, on the age of onset of cancer. The volume of the cancer, the compared interest of the first and following examination, the existence of mastopathy, the influence of menopause, heredity and education level were also studied.

Cancer of the breast is by far the most frequent; it can be detected in young women, when the cancer is always very small without axillary nodes, even at the second examination. Breast cancer is more frequent in nuns and women without children. Pregnancy protects, but particularly before and at 20 years of age. Furthermore, we found out a simultaneous increasing between fertility and cancer. Mastopathy, menopause, breast cancer heredity and education level, increase the rate of breast cancer.

Cervix cancer does not occur in virgins and nuns; early pregnancy, before the age of 20, and an increasing number of pregnancies increases the rate of cervix cancer. Most of the cancers detected are in situ. The rate of cervix cancer increases with menopause and cervix cancer heredity and decreases with education level.

Cancer detection in women must not start before the age of 30; yearly examination is essential for breast; an examination every two years is sufficient for the cervix.

References

Berkson, J., Harrington, S. W., Clagett, O. T., Kirklin, J. W., Dockerty, M. B. and McDonald, J. R. (1957): Proc. Mayo Clinic., 32, 645.
Clemmesen, J. and Nielsen, A. (1951): Brit. J. Cancer, 5, 159.
Hems, G. (1970): Brit. J. Cancer, 24, 226.
Lilienfeld, A. M. (1963): Cancer Res., 23, 1503.
Macklin, M. T. (1959): J. nat. Cancer Inst., 23, 1179.
MacMahon, B. (1958): Cancer (Philad.), 11, 250.
MacMahon, B., Cole, P., Lin, T. M., Lowe, C. R., Mirra, A. P., Ravnihar, B., Salbery, E. J., Balaores, V. G. and Yuasa, S. (1970): Bull. Wld. Hlth. Org., 43, 209.
Maisin, H., Van de Merckt, J., Maldague-Pham, H. O., Mazy, G., Col-Debeys, C. and Salamon, E. (1967): Arch. belges Méd. soc., 8, 529.
Maisin, H. (1967): Louvain Méd., 86, 273.
Maisin, H., Vandenbroucke-Vanderwielen, A., Salamon, E., Van de Merckt, J., Maldague-Pham, H. Q. and Mazy, G. (1968): In: Comptes Rendus, 1er Symposium International Sur le Dépistage du Cancer, Spa, 1968. Sciences et Lettres, Liège.
Maisin, H., Vandenbroucke-Vanderwielen, A., Van de Merckt, J. and Salamon-Dargent, J. (1970): Arch. belges Méd. soc., 6. 411.
Maisin, H., Vandenbroucke-Vanderwielen, A., Mazy, G. and Van de Merckt, J. (1971): Minerva ginec., 23, 8, 377.
Smithers, D. W., Rigby-Jones, P., Galton, D. A. G. and Payne, P. M. (1952): Brit. J. Radiol., Suppl. 4, 1.
Stocks, P. (1955): Schweiz. Z. alg. Path., 18, 706.
Stocks, P. (1958): Cancer, III/4, 137. Editors: R. W. Raven Butterworth & Co (Publishers) Ltd., London.
Taylor, R. S., Carrol, B. E. and Lloyd, J. W. (1959): Cancer (Philad.), 12, 1207.
Terris, M., Wilson, F., Smith, H., Sprung, E. and Nelson Jr, J. H. (1967): Amer. J. publ. Hlth., 57, 840.
Zippin, C. and Petrakis, N. L. (1971): Cancer (Philad.), 28, 1381.

Some possibilities for establishing risk groups in the female population by mass screening for gynecological cancer

I. Vodopija, P. Bagović, M. Bačić, Jasna Ivić, M. Bolanča and Silvana Audy

Institute of Public Health, City of Zagreb, Zagreb, Yugoslavia

Although mortality from certain types of cancer, such as of the uterus, is decreasing in many countries (De Haas, 1967), there is still a need for better understanding of this trend. The techniques that might help to speed up this trend should also be improved. This applies particularly to the areas where mass screening campaigns for the detection of gynecological cancer are in progress.

Not only medical, but also socio-economic factors require new approaches. Because of financial limitations in many instances, it has been impossible to implement fully many of the tested and proven procedures. Therefore, as a necessary solution in such circumstances, the search for high risk groups offers good prospects.

Available resources and personnel should be directed to the screening of those sections of the population where, under local conditions, certain types of cancer are expected, or are more likely to be found. In this paper we describe an attempt to define more precisely high risk groups of women in relation to gynecological types of cancer.

TABLE 1   *Number of women examined, by age group, and type of gynecological cancer, per thousand*

Age groups	No. of examined women	Uterine cervix carcinoma				Breast carcinoma	
		In situ		Invasive			
		No.	per 1000	No.	per 1000	No.	per 1000
19	342	0	0.0	0	0.0	0	0.0
20 – 24	1732	1	0.7	0	0.0	0	0.0
25 – 29	1776	8	4.5	0	0.0	1	0.6
30 – 34	1634	23	14.1	2	1.2	1	0.6
35 – 39	2300	19	8.3	3	1.3	5	2.2
40 – 44	2922	22	7.5	13	4.4	10	3.4
45 – 49	2596	22	8.2	13	4.8	7	2.6
50 – 54	1674	2	1.2	10	6.0	6	3.6
55 – 59	1866	5	2.7	7	3.8	9	4.8
60 and over	3058	9	2.9	11	3.6	11	3.6
Total	20,000	111	5.6	59	3.0	50	2.5

Results

A campaign to detect gynecological cancer in the City of Zagreb started in 1966. The study area covers a part of the city where some 20,000 women aged 18 or over are living (Bačić et al., 1967; Audy et al., 1971.). The results of the whole campaign are presented in Table 1. It is quite clear that the highest rate of carcinoma in situ of the uterine cervix is in the age-group 30-34 years and of the invasive type of cervical cancer, in the age group 50-54 years. As to breast cancer, the group with the highest risk is 55-59 years of age. We see a peak in the age-group 40-44 years, followed by continuing upward trend with increase of age above 50.

The rates of births and abortions in relation to cervical and breast cancer are shown in Tables 2 and 3. From Table 2 we see that the highest number of cases of carcinoma in situ is found among the women with two births: the invasive type of cervical cancer is. commonest among those who had three births. The risk of breast cancer is also highest in women with three births.

The data in Table 3 show a distinctive tendency for all three types of cancer to increase with the number of abortions. However, we still lack a proper explanation for the rather high number and rates of these types of cancer in women without a single abortion.

TABLE 2   *Number of births in relation to the number and rates of gynecological cancer in examined women*

No. of births	No. of examined women	Uterine cervix carcinoma				Breast carcinoma	
		In situ		Invasive			
		No.	per 1000	No.	per 1000	No.	per 1000
0	6254	15	2.4	7	1.1	12	1.9
1	6406	40	6.2	22	3.4	17	2.7
2	4944	47	9.5	11	2.2	11	2.2
3	1488	8	5.4	15	10.1	5	5.4
4	544	1	1.8	3	5.5	2	3.7
5 or more	364	–	–	1	2.7	9	0.0
Total	20,000	111	5.6	59	3.0	5.0	2.5

TABLE 3   *Number of abortions in relation to the number and rates of gynecological cancer in examined women*

No. of abortions	No. of women examined	Uterine cervix carcinoma				Breast carcinoma	
		In situ		Invasive			
		No.	per 1000	No.	per 1000	No.	per 1000
0	6962	41	5.9	27	3.9	15	2.2
1	6774	26	3.8	15	2.2	13	1.9
2	3184	19	6.0	7	2.2	11	3.5
3	1558	11	7.1	4	2.6	6	3.9
4	652	5	7.7	3	4.6	3	4.6
5 or more	870	9	10.3	3	3.4	2	2.3
Total	20,000	111	5.6	59	3.0	50	2.5

TABLE 4   *Relationship of cervical cancer and of breast cancer to the eye pigmentation of examined women*

Colour of eyes	No. of women examined		Uterine cervix carcinoma				Breast carcinoma	
			In situ		Invasive			
	No.	%	No.	%	No.	%	No.	%
Dark	11,278	56.39	60	54.0	23	39.0	27	54.0
Blue	8,722	43.61	51	46.0	36	61.0	23	46.0
Total	20,000	100.00	111	100.0	59	100.0	50	100.0

Table 4 shows the relationship of cervical and breast cancer to eye pigmentation. In the groups of women with cervical cancer there is a significantly higher proportion of blue-eyed women among those with invasive type of cervical cancer, while the proportions of women with dark eyes among those with carcinoma in situ and breast cancer are similar to that in the total female population.

Discussion and summary

If the risk of cancer increases with age as seen in Table 1, then this should apply to the whole female population in the observed area. We have no explanation for the significantly higher risk of invasive type cervical cancer in blue-eyed women. Although we are aware that the increased number of births and abortions may be risk factors we still lack a proper understanding of the complex processes underlying these manifestations.

However, these findings might lead to the development of criteria for identifying those persons who, because of their genetic constitution, may stand an increased risk of developing cervical cancer.

References

Audy, S., Bačić, M., Bagović, P., Bolanča, M., Urbanke, A. and Vodopija, I. (1971): Minerva ginec., 23/1, 20.
Bačić M., Bagović, P., Bolanča, M., Karačić, M. and Vodopija, I. (1967): Zdrav. novine, 20/3–4, 105.
De Haas, J. H. (1967): In: Health of Mankind, Chapter 4, pp. 79–102. Editors: C. Wolstenholme and M. O'Connor. J. & A. Churchill Ltd., London.

The epidemiology of invasive carcinoma of the cervix in Georgian SSR (1965-1971)

D.A. Gvamitchava, L.I. Tcharkviani, Z.J. Khitarishvili and T.I. Kvesitadze

The Research Institute on Oncology, Ministry of Public Health, Georgian SSR, Tbilisi, USSR

The study of regional peculiarities of prevalence of malignant tumours has great importance for the discovery of aetiological factors of cancer and for planning practicable prophylactic measures (Tchaclin, 1963; Tcharkviani, 1964; Serebrov, 1968; Droll, 1971).

The epidemiology of cancer of women's genitals in Georgia has been studied since 1955 (Tcharkviani, 1964) and highly interesting results have accumulated. Our present contribution is concerned with the organization of the All-Union Centre of cancer epidemiology of women's genitals, and the working out of procedures for the scientific investigation of the problem (Tcharkviani et al., 1973).

Georgia is not a large country, but taking into account its climatic, geographic and demographic peculiarities, it provides a very interesting 'natural experimental laboratory' for the study of the regional peculiarities of malignant tumours.

The Georgian SSR is located in the middle and western parts of the Caucasus, between the latitudes 43°07' and 43°47' North, and the longitudes 40°01' and 46°44' East, in the South of the European part of the USSR. It borders on Turkey in the South and occupies 69,700 sq.km. Georgia is notable for a wide range of altitudes and many types of climate.

Georgia has 44 cities, 54 settlements and 4,600 villages; it is divided into 67 rural regions. According to the census of 1970, the total population of the GSSR is 4,686,400, with 2,483,800 women.

In studying the epidemiology of carcinoma of the cervix, we did not adhere to the modern administrative divisions, but to the ethnic divisions, which were formed in Georgia in ancient times. These divisions determine peculiarities of manners and customs.

In 1965-1971, the standardised rate of cervical carcinoma in Georgian SSR was 18.49 per 100,000. The female population, according to the census of 1970, was used as a standard (Table 1).

A certain lowering of the rate in Georgia has been recorded with time. For instance, in 1965 the rate was 19.05 per 100,000, and in 1971 the rate was 15.65 per 100,000. The maximum rate was recorded in 1967. The lowering of morbidity can be explained by the wide and effective prophylactic measures which are carried out in the republic.

TABLE 1   *The rate of carcinoma of the cervix in Georgian SSR per 100,000 women (standard index)*

Year	1965	1966	1967	1968	1969	1970	1971	Average for 7 years
Carcinoma cervix	19.05	18.96	20.54	20.21	19.06	15.94	15.67	18.49

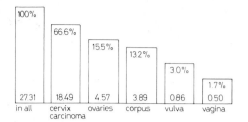

FIG. 1   *Cancer rates for women's genitals in GSSR per 100,000 women according to the standard indexes (1965-1971).*

Carcinoma of the cervix is the commonest cancer of female genitals in Georgia (Fig. 1). The rate of carcinoma of the cervix in Eastern Georgia was somewhat lower (16.77) than in Western Georgia (20.91). More marked differences are discovered in relation to ethnic regions (Fig. 2). For instance, the minimum rate of carcinoma of the cervix, 7.9 per 100,000, was found in Meskhet-Javakheti, and the maximum rate, 37.9 per 100,000, was found in Abkhazia. Southern Ossetia, Mengrelia and Imereti were closer to the average index for the republic.

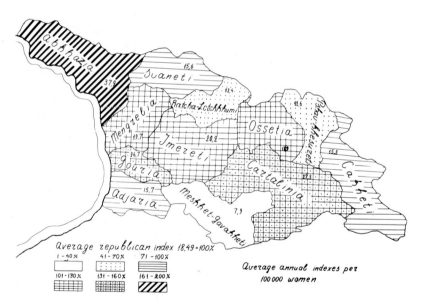

FIG. 2   *The rates of carcinoma of the cervix in GSSR according to ethnic regions (1965-1971).*

Taking the average rate of cervical carcinoma as 100%, the rate in Abkhazia was 204.9%; in Meskheti 42.7%; and in South Ossetia, Mengrelia and Imereti the rate fluctuated from 101.1% to 103.8%.

Carcinoma of the cervix was more frequent in cities (23.23) than in villages (15.76). The rate recorded in Tbilisi (a big industrial city) was 22 per 100,000. The native population did not often suffer from the disease (Georgian women: 15.8 cases, Armenian women: 19.38 cases, and Russian women: 29.46 cases, per 100,000).

The age dependence of carcinoma of the cervix is shown in Figure 3. The maximum rate — 54.6 — is found in the 50-59 year-age-group. Up to 30 years, only 0.93 per

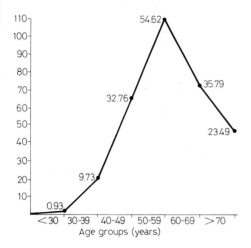

FIG. 3   *The rates of carcinoma of the cervix according to age in GSSR, per 100,000 women (1965-1971).*

100,000 suffered from carcinoma of the cervix. At 70 and above, the rate was 23.49 per 100,000.

In 1965-66, 1.84 per 100,000 women under 30 years suffered from carcinoma of the cervix, but in 1970-71 the rate had declined to 0.37 per 100,000. An analogous fall in the morbidity rate over the same period of time was observed in age groups 30-39 and 40-49 (17.9 to 7.26 and 47.6 to 29.8 respectively). The decrease was not observed in the older age-groups.

Summary

1. In 1965−71, the standardised rate of invasive carcinoma of the cervix averaged 18.49 per 100,000 in Georgian SSR. The rate varied from 7.41 to 37.9, according to nationality and place of residence.

2. A decreased rate was recorded with time in Georgia (1965−19.05; 1971−15.67); the maximum rate −20.54− was recorded in 1967.

3. The maximum age-specific rate − 54.62 − was recorded in the 50−59 year age-group. The change of the rate in the older age-groups with time is noted, and is evidently the consequence of wide prophylactic measures.

References

Droll, R. (1971): Prevention of Cancer Pointers from Epidemiology. Publishing House 'Medicine', Moscow.

Serebrov, A. I. (1968): Cancer of Womb. Zdorovie, Leningrad.

Tchaclin, A. B. (1963): The Regional Peculiarities of Prevalence of Malignant Tumors. State Publishing House of Medical Literature, Leningrad.

Tcharkviani, L. I. (1964): Some Questions on Cancer of Women's Genitals. Publishing House 'Sabtchota Sacartvelo', Tbilisi.

Tcharkviani, L. I., Khitarishvili, Z. J. and Gvamitchava, D. A. (1973): The Principles of Organization and Methods of Epidemiological Study of Cancer of Women's Genitals. Tbilisi.

Further studies in the aetiology of uterine cervical cancer in South India

V. Shanta and A. Ramachandra

The Cancer Institute, Adyar, Madras, India

Material

This report is based on a retrospective analysis of 1730 cervical cancer cases and 2815 controls interviewed and examined during the period 1969–1972. All the cervical cancers were in-patients at the Cancer Institute, Madras. 2161 of the controls were drawn from an apparently healthy adult female population interviewed and examined during the rural and urban screening programmes carried out by the Institute during the same period. A further 654 controls were drawn from women with carcinoma of the upper alimentary tract (U.A.C.), admitted to the Cancer Institute concurrently. All the cervical cancers and controls were consecutive cases admitted or seen during the period mentioned: no special attempt was made to match any of the parameters under study. All the cervical cancers were squamous cell carcinomas.

Methods

The interviews were carried out by two trained medical social workers, one male and one female, according to a prepared questionnaire.

All the cases and controls were examined by a gynaecologist specially appointed to the project. Vaginal and cervical smears were examined in every case. All the cancers were confirmed by biopsy also. All the controls with the least suspicion of an unhealthy cervix or endometrial pathology were biopsied to exclude epithelial dysplasias or carcinomas-in-situ. All the smears and tissues were reported from our cytology and pathology laboratories, and the haematological and biochemical investigations were carried out in our clinical pathology and biochemical laboratories.

The parameters studied were age, religion, ethnic group, regional (rural or urban) distribution, educational status, socio-economic status, menstrual history (menarche, rhythm, and menopause), marital history (age at marriage, widowhood, parity, abortions, medical attendance during labour etc.), pre-existing pathology, family history of cancer, occupation, diet, blood group, genital hygiene, circumcisional status of husband, gynaecological pathology in co-wives, if any, and the use of contraceptives.

The data obtained are shown in the Tables 1–17.

Commentary:

(*a*) The study group and the controls were nearly matched as regards age distribution.

(*b*) The large number of Tamils in the series is because the Institute is situated in the Tamil region and does not signify any special ethnic predisposition.

(*c*) Region (rural or urban), occupation, diet and blood groups did not seem of any aetiological significance.

(*d*) As in most other reported series the lower socio-economic classes and the uneducated were the most affected. But the incidence in the poorer and ignorant classes seemed to follow closely the socio-economic and educational pattern of the general population. Their significance, therefore, as an aetiological factor is a matter for doubt.

We have, however, never come across a carcinoma of the cervix in a university educated woman though 3% of our breast cancer patients belonged to that category.

(*e*) The menstrual history did not reveal any significant difference between the study group and the controls.

TABLE 1   *Age (figures are percentages)*

Decade (years)	Ca. Cx.	Controls	
		Hospital (U.A.C.)	Population (healthy)
10–19	nil	0.1	8.5
20–29	3.4	2.2	53.5
30–39	24.1	13.0	23.6
40–49	30.0	28.2	9.5
50–59	24.2	33.9	2.7
60–69	8.0	19.4	1.9
70–above	1.0	3.3	0.9

TABLE 2   *Age incidence*

	Ca. Cx. (years)	Controls	
		U.A.C. (years)	Population (healthy) (years)
Mean Age	45.5	45.5	45.5
Youngest	20	11	15
Oldest	86	85	86

TABLE 3   *Religion (figures are percentages)*

Religion	Ca. Cx.	Controls		
		U.A.C.	Population (healthy)	Indian census 1971
Hindu	92.4	88.8	86.9	89.02
Moslem	4.5	8.7	7.7	5.11
Christian	2.7	2.3	5.2	5.75
Others	0.23	nil	0.1	0.12

TABLE 4   *Ethnic group (figures are percentages)*

Ethnic derivation	Ca. Cx.	Controls	
		U.A.C.	Population (healthy)
Tamils	64.8	71.1	100
Andhras	26.9	21.1	nil
Keralites	6	6.4	nil
Others	2.0	1.2	nil

TABLE 5   *Region (figures are percentages)*

Region	Ca. Cx.	Controls	
		U.A.C.	Indian census 1971
Rural	66.6	70	71
Urban	33.4	30	29

TABLE 6   *Education (figures are percentages)*

Standard	Ca. Cx.	Controls	
		U.A.C.	Indian census 1971
Illiterate	69.8	82.5	85.0
School	30.1	17.4	16.0
University	nil	nil	0.185

TABLE 7   *Socio-economic status (figures are percentages)*

Class	Ca. Cx.	Controls		
		U.A.C.	Population (healthy)	Indian census 1971
Labour	67.1	79	65.8	data not available
Middle class	29.5	18.3	30.4	
Upper class	3.3	2.9	3.6	

TABLE 8   *Occupation (figures are percentages)*

Occupation	Ca. Cx.	Controls		
		U.A.C.	Population (healthy)	Indian census 1971
Housewife	86.7	70.3	95.4	85.0
Cooly	11.4	27.4	4.4	13.0
White collar workers	1.6	1.9	–	1.9
Professionals (teachers, etc.)	0.3	0.4	0.2	0.08

TABLE 9   *Diet (figures are percentages)*

Diet	Ca. Cx.	Controls	
		U.A.C.	Population (healthy)
Vegetarian	12.3	16	Data not available
Non vegetarian	87.7	84	–do–

TABLE 10   *Menstrual history (figures are percentages)*

Menarche Age in years	Ca. Cx.	Controls	
		U.A.C.	Population (healthy)
9	0.1	nil	nil
10	0.2	0.15	0.2
11	2.1	1.2	2.9
12	18.5	19.4	13.2
13	36.6	34.4	29.2
14	22.1	20.6	27.1
15	11.3	15.6	14.8
16	5.9	5.2	7.5
17	1.4	1.0	3.1
18	1.0	1.5	1.0
19	0.05	nil	0.37
20	0.15	0.3	0.09
24	nil	0.15	nil
25	nil	0.15	nil

TABLE 11 (*a*)   *Marital history (figures are percentages)*

	Ca. Cx.	Controls	
		U.A.C.	Population (healthy)
Not married	nil	0.3	nil
Married	100	99.7	100

TABLE 11 (*b*)   *Age at marriage (figures are percentages)*

Age (years)	Ca. Cx.	Controls	
		U.A.C.	Population (healthy)
< 10	8.2	11.5	2.0
11–15	48.4 ⎱ 88.4	45.8 ⎱ 83.7	37.5 ⎱ 89.9
16–20	40.0 ⎰	37.9 ⎰	52.4 ⎰
> 20	3.2	4.4	8.1

(f) All the cervical cancer patients were married, but so were 99.7% of the upper alimentary tract cancer patients and 100% of the healthy controls from the general population.

88.4% of the cervical cancers, 83.7% of the upper alimentary tract cancers and 89.9% of the healthy controls had their first sexual experience between the ages of 11 and 20 years.

Marital history did not thus reveal any significant difference between the study group and the controls in regard to spinsterhood, age at marriage, or widowhood. There was no case of divorce though a few women were deserted after they developed the cervical cancer. No history of pre-marital or extra-marital sexual relationship was given by the women either in the study group or controls. History in regard to intensity of sexual intercourse could not be reliably elicited.

It is, however, of significance that there was not a single case of cervical cancer in an unmarried woman, though 3.17% of breast cancers were from that category.

Parity did not seem to play any significant role in cervical carcinogenesis. The percentage of nulliparous women was certainly lower in the cervical cancer group than in the controls, but the risk in nulliparous women and in women who had borne 11 children or more appeared to be very nearly the same. Abortions did not seem of any significance either, nor did the age at the first childbirth. Medical assistance during labour was slightly higher in the study group than in the controls.

The only pre-existing pathology of significance seemed to be leucorrhoea, but it could not be definitely ascertained whether this was a consequence or a cause of the malignant process. Syphilis, diabetes, anaemia and tuberculosis were not of any aetiological significance.

TABLE 12   *Parity (figures are percentages)*

Parity	Ca. Cx.	Controls	
		U.A.C.	Population (healthy)
0	2.4	9.6	5.9
1	7.1	11.0	14.9
2	10.2	14.0	15.0
3	14.0	11.9	18.8
4	14.3	11.9	12.8
5	12.7	13.0	9.9
6	11.9	9.0	8.2
7	9.3	6.2	5.2
8	7.9	6.2	3.9
9	4.0	3.0	1.9
10	3.4	3.0	1.2
11 and more	2.0	2.0	2.2

TABLE 13   *Abortion (figures are percentages)*

	Ca. Cx.	Controls	
		U.A.C.	Population (healthy)
Abortions	17.4	12.3	16.9

TABLE 14   *Medical assistance during childbirth (figures are percentages)*

Medical assistance	Ca. Cx.	Controls	
		U.A.C.	Population (healthy)
Assistance available	19.0	11.9	Data not available
No assistance	81.0	88.1	—do—

TABLE 15   *Pre-existing disease or pathology (figures are percentages)*

Disease	Ca. Cx.	Controls	
		U.A.C.	Population (healthy)
Syphilis (positive serology)	1.6	1.4	Data not available
Leucorrhoea	74.8	2.7	–do–
Diabetes mellitus	7.2	13.4	–do–
Anaemia	2.1	14.5	–do–
Pulmonary tuberculosis	3.9	5.6	–do–

TABLE 16   *Family history of cancer (figures are percentages)*

Tumour site	Ca. Cx.	Controls	
		U.A.C.	Population (healthy)
Cervix	1.15	0.15	0.18
U.A.C.	0.05	0.30	nil
Stomach	0.35	0.15	0.09
Breast	0.15	0.15	0.20
Others	0.55	1.50	0.59
All sites	2.4	2.2	1.1

TABLE 17   *Blood groups (figures are percentages)*

Blood group	Ca. Cx.	Controls	
		U.A.C.	Population (healthy)
A	25.2	19.7	Data not available
B	24.0	29.8	–do–
O	44.4	43.5	–do–
AB	6.2	6.0	–do–

The cervical cancer group gave a significantly higher family history of cervical cancer in a near blood relative than the controls, but yet it occurred only in 1.15% of all the cervical cancers.

Our previous study (Shanta and Krishnamurthi, 1969) had shown a strikingly low frequency of cervical cancer in the Moslem women of South India – 0.8%. In the present study, however, 4.5% of the cervical cancers were in Moslem women which is close to their general population trend of 5.11% (Chandrasekhar, 1971). As a matter of fact the incidence is lower in Christian women (2.7%) compared to their fraction in the general population viz. 5.75. The cervical cancer frequency in Hindus is also in consonance with their population distribution. It is, therefore, a matter for doubt whether religious customs like ritual circumcision in the Moslem male babies are of any significance in the aetiology of carcinoma of the uterine cervix. Ritual circumcision is not practised amongst either the Christians or Hindus in South India.

Sexual abstinence during menses and for nearly 3 months after delivery is the usual rule amongst the population of South India, whatever the religious denomination.

None of our study cases or our controls gave a history of practising contraception in any form. None of them practised douching either.

0.45% of our cervical cancers and 0.3% of our controls had co-wives. None of these co-wives of our cervical cancer patients has developed a cervical cancer so far.

Note on preliminary experimental studies

An attempt was made by the virus research unit of Dr. A. Ramachandra Rao at the Infectious Disease Hospital to culture the Herpes virus hominis on CAM from 68 cases of proved carcinoma of the uterine cervix in collaboration with the Cancer Institute. Cervical biopsies and cervical swabs were taken and cultured. 63 cases were negative in the first passage itself. In 5 other cases the membranes were hazy in the first passage, but the cultures were all negative in the second passage. To verify the reliability of the technique similar cultures of swabs taken from clinical genital herpes in 7 women were carried out. All were positive for the herpes virus. Despite these discouraging results the studies are continuing.

Discussion

The information derived from the present study has been largely negative.

The only positive fact seems to be that cervical cancer does not occur in the absence of coitus. There is also a suggestion of an inherent local tissue susceptibility in some individuals.

None of the other factors studied including the age at first coitus, parity, the age at first childbirth, poverty, malnutrition or absence of medical attention seem to play any significant role in aetiology.

As the number of cases studied grew larger the apparent differential incidence in the different major religious communities in South India seemed to disappear. As a matter of fact the incidence was proportionately less in the Christian than in the Moslem community. The Christian like the Hindu male is an uncircumcised individual. Ethnically, socio-economically, culturally and in their habits and customs the South Indian Hindu, Christian and Moslem are very much alike. Only the Hindu will not eat beef, the Moslem will not eat pork and the Christian will eat both. The Moslem male baby is also ritually circumcised, while the other babies are not. The value of circumcision of the male partner in the prevention of carcinoma of the cervix in the female is, therefore, according to our present study, doubtful. The role of poor genital hygiene in aetiology seems also equally in doubt.

The attempt to culture the Herpes virus, class II, from cervical cancers on chicken chorio-allantoic membrane has also proved futile.

None the less, the association of a long standing vaginal discharge with cervical carcinoma would suggest the possible role of a low grade chronic infective process in oncogenesis. It is possible that the stagnant exudates and the products of cellular disintegration generated by such a process in the compound glands of the endocervical mucosa induce a pathological alteration in an inherently susceptible epithelium, passing in turn through the phases of metaplasia, dysplasia, and carcinoma-in-situ to invasive cancer. This impression is strengthened by the observation that the squamous cell carcinomas of the uterine cervix are a distinct histological entity by themselves, often exhibiting imperfect glandular elements containing mucin. We believe that the infective process is non-specific and that no particular virus or bacterium is involved. All other factors are only incidental and contributory to this infective process.

Summary

1730 cervical cancers and 2815 controls concurrently interviewed and examined between the years 1969–1972 are analysed. The parameters studied were age, religion, ethnic derivation, regional (rural or urban) distribution, educational status, socio-economic status, menstrual and marital history, parity, pre-existing pathology, family history of cancer, occupation, diet and blood group.

In addition an attempt was made to culture the Herpes virus hominis on CAM.

The analysis suggested that the most likely aetiological factor was a chronic non-specific low grade infective nidus, consequent on coitus, in the compound racemose glands of the endocervical mucosa acting on a susceptible epithelium.

References

Chandrasekhar, A. (1971): Census of India, 1971, Series I, Papers 1 and 2 of 1972.
Shanta, V. and Krishnamurthi, S. (1969): Brit. J. Cancer, 23, 693.

Ethnic and geographic factors in high buccal pharyngeal cancer rates in Canada*

D. L. Anderson

Division of Clinical Sciences, Faculty of Dentistry, University of Toronto, Toronto, Ontario, Canada

Buccal pharyngeal cancer mortality rates for every year have been much higher in Quebec than in any of the other 9 provinces of Canada. This excess in Quebec is seen only in males, and only for malignancies of the upper digestive and respiratory tract. For males the mean buccal pharyngeal cancer mortality rate from 1950 to 1969 was 7.5 per 100 thousand population per year, in contrast to 3.5 for the other provinces, according to the Dominion Bureau of Statistics (1966, 1964-1970).

Does Quebec differ from the other provinces? Geographically, it is adjacent to the cluster of states which Burbank (1971) showed to have the highest buccal pharyngeal cancer mortality rates for white males in the U.S.A. Another factor is ethnic origin. Quebec is the only province whose population is predominantly French in origin (Dominion Bureau of Statistics, 1962) (Fig. 1). That this could be a pertinent factor is suggested by the male buccal pharyngeal cancer rates of Segi et al. (1969) for Europe. France has the highest rate. Also, in Ontario, the province adjacent to Quebec on the west, Cook et al. (1972b) found a higher than expected number of oral cancers in those with French names.

Materials and methods

To determine if French origin is an important factor in the high rates in Quebec, the records of the Quebec Tumour Registry were examined. Although ethnic origin was not specified, it was possible with the assistance of Cook and Hewitt to separate those with French names from those with non-French names. Cook et al. (1972a) have shown this to be a useful and reliable method for use in Canada.

Results

Statistics Canada (1973) report that 81% of the males of Quebec are French in origin. 81% of the intraoral cancers (ICDA List nos. 141, 143-146) in Quebec males in 1969 and 1970 occurred in those with French names. But of the 19% non-French in the province, two-thirds (13%) live on the island of Montreal. In comparison, only one-quarter of the French live there. From the two large cities of the province, Quebec City and Montreal Island, the French males account for only 27% of the total male population of the province, but they have 45% of the province's intraoral cancers.

Incidence rates per 100 thousand population per year 1969-70 for Quebec males with French names with intraoral cancer, including oropharynx, were 12.7 for Montreal Island and Quebec City, 5.9 for the Montreal suburbs and 4.8 for the remainder of the province (Fig. 2).

---

* Grant in aid from the Ontario Cancer Treatment and Research Foundation.

n/100,000/yr.

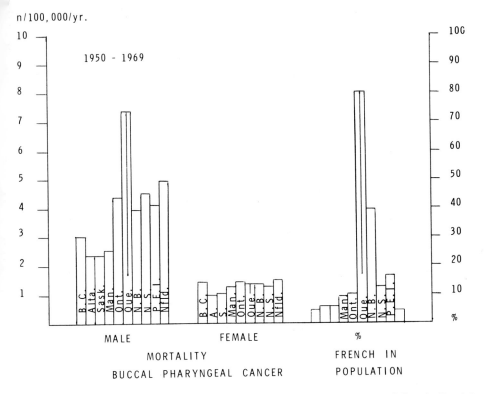

FIG. 1   *Buccal pharyngeal cancer mortality rates by sex for the Provinces of Canada, Dominion Bureau of Statistics (1966 and 1964-70); and the percentages of the population who are of French origin, Dominion Bureau of Statistics (1962).*

In contrast, the rates for those with non-French names were respectively 7.5, 7.7 and 8.0.

The rates for individual oral sites for the males with French names are listed in Table 1.

The rates for Quebec City are very similar to those for Montreal Island. The rates for Montreal suburbs (census divisions of Chambly, Chateauguay, Deux-Montagnes, Ile Jesus, Laprairie, L'Assomption, Terrebonne and Vaudreuil), are similar to those for the less densely populated remainder of the province; and are approximately one-half the rates of the two large cities.

TABLE 1   *Incidence of intraoral cancers in Quebec males with French names*

ICDA site	No./100,000/year 1969–1970			
	Quebec city	Montreal island	Montreal suburbs	Other parts of province
141 Tongue	3.0	4.0	1.8	1.0
143 Gingiva	1.0	0.9	0.6	0.4
144 Floor	2.3	2.0	0.9	0.9
145 Other mouth	1.3	1.9	0.9	0.9
146 Oropharynx	4.3	4.2	1.7	1.6

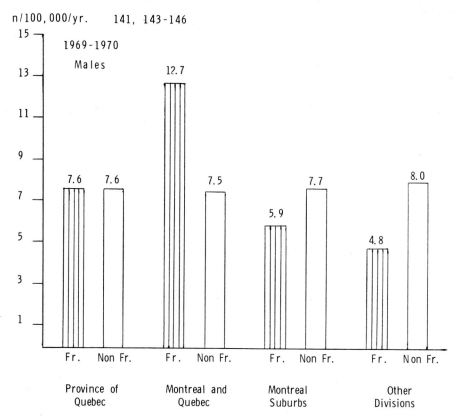

FIG. 2   *Intraoral cancer incidence rates by ethnic origin and residence for Quebec males.*

Discussion

High buccal pharyngeal cancer mortality rates in males in North America are clustered in the north-eastern states of the United States and in the nearby Canadian Province of Quebec. Ethnic groups appear to be involved. Seidman (1971) in New York City and Lombard and Doering (1929) in Boston found the Irish migrants to have particularly high rates. In the present investigation in Quebec, it appears to be the French Canadians who are particularly susceptible.

The increased susceptibility seems dependent on a large urban environment. This relationship of increasing incidence of intraoral cancer with increase in urban size has also been noted in Connecticut by Eisenberg (1967) and in Denmark by Clemmesen and Nielsen (1956) and Clemmesen and Schultz (1960). This is illustrated in Figure 3.

The low male buccal pharyngeal cancer mortality rate for the Province of New Brunswick, which adjoins Quebec to the east and is 39% French in origin (Fig.1), can be accounted for by the finding that the high rates occurred only in the large cities; New Brunswick has no large cities.

The large urban environment, however, did not influence the intraoral cancer rates in the non-French in Quebec; nor did it equally affect the various migrant groups in New York City. Jews especially were noted by Newill (1961) and by Seidman (1971) to have quite low mortality rates from cancer of the upper digestive and respiratory tracts.

Thus it seems that it is not the general environment of the large cities which increases upper digestive and respiratory cancer incidence and mortality. More likely it is a cultural-

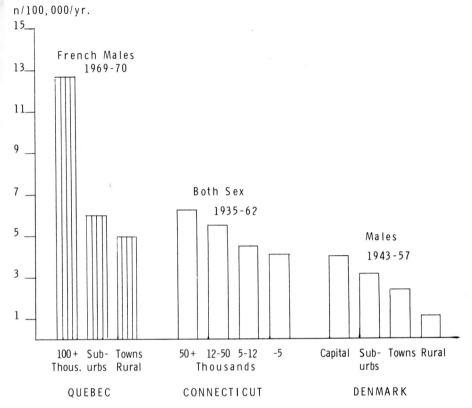

n/100,000/yr.

FIG. 3 *Intraoral cancer incidence by residence for Quebec French; Connecticut according to Eisen-berg (1967); and Denmark according to Clemmesen and Nielsen (1956) and Clemmesen and Schultz (1960).*

ly related exposure which is greater in the large cities. Such an assumption of course does not rule out the possibility that the French and the Irish are also genetically susceptible. The factors in the large urban environment which are significant to the French Canadian on Montreal Island may, or may not be the same as those that are significant to the Irish in New York City. That the situation indeed may be somewhat different is suggested by the observation that esophageal cancer mortality rates are high in males in the same north-eastern states in the U.S.A. (Burbank, 1971, 1972) and in the Irish in New York City (Seidman, 1971); but not in Quebec (Dominion Bureau of Statistics, 1966, 1964-1970). On the other hand, male laryngeal cancer mortality rates are especially high in Quebec as well as in the north-eastern states and in the New York Irish.

Conclusions

Consistently high mortality rates for buccal pharyngeal cancer in males in the Province of Quebec, Canada, appear to be due to high cancer incidence of these sites in the French Canadians of the large cities of the province.

Summary

Buccal pharyngeal cancer mortality rates during the past 20 years in Quebec have been consistently double that of rates in the other provinces of Canada. Quebec is geographically near the states which have the highest rates in the U.S.A. Quebec differs from the other provinces in having a population predominantly French in origin. Because France has the highest rates in Europe, and Ontario in Canada had a higher than expected number of oral cancers in those with French names, the records of the Quebec Tumour Registry were examined to determine rates for those with French and non-French names. The rate per 100 thousand per year for 1969-70 in males with French names for intraoral cancers (ICDA 141, 143-161) was 7.6 for the province, 12.7 for the large cities of Montreal Island and Quebec City, 5.9 for Montreal suburbs and 4.8 for the remainder of the province. In contrast, the rates for the males with non-French names were 7.6, 7.5, 7.7, and 8.0 repectively. Although French males in the large cities of Quebec comprise only 27% of the total male population of the province, they had 45% of the intraoral cancers. Thus the high buccal pharyngeal cancer mortality rates in Quebec appear to be due to high buccal pharyngeal cancer incidence in French males of the two large cities.

Acknowledgements

The author acknowledges the assistance of Drs. G. Martineau and M. Blanchet-Patry of the Quebec Tumour Registry who gave permission to obtain data from the Registry; and Dr. Cook and D. Hewitt, who participated in the selection of the French and non-French names.

References

Burbank, F. (1971): Nat. Cancer Inst. Monogr., No. 33. Superintendent of Documents, Washington.
Burbank, F. (1972): Amer. J. Epidem., 95/5, 393.
Clemmesen, J. and Nielsen, A. (1956): Dan. med. Bull., 3/2, 33.
Clemmesen, J. and Schultz, G. (1960): Dan. med. Bull., 7/6, 168.
Cook, D., Hewitt, D. and Milner, J. (1972a): Amer. J. Epidem., 95/1, 38
Cook, D., MacKay, E. N. and Hewitt, D. (1972b):Canad. J. publ. Hlth, 63/2, 120.
Dominion Bureau of Statistics (1962): 1961 Census of Canada. Population, General Characteristics. Queen's Printer, Ottawa.
Dominion Bureau of Statistics (1966): Cancer Mortality by Site. 1950-1963. Queen's Printer, Ottawa.
Dominion Bureau of Statistics (1964-1970): Vital Statistics, Malignant Neoplasms. Annual. Queen's Printer, Ottawa.
Eisenberg, H. (1967): Cancer in Connecticut. Incidence characteristics 1935-1962. Connecticut State Department of Health, Hartford, Conn.
Lombard, H.L. and Doering, C. R. (1929): J. prevent. Med., 3/5, 343.
Newill, V. A. (1961): J. nat. Cancer Inst., 26/2, 405.
Segi, M., Kurihara, M. and Matsuyama, T. (1969): Cancer Mortality for Selected Sites in 24 Countries, No. 5, 1964-65. Tohoku University School of Medicine, Sendai, Japan.
Seidman, H. (1971): Environ. Res., 4/5, 390.
Statistics Canada (1973): 1971 Census of Canada, Population, Specified Mother Tongues for Census Divisions and Subdivisions. Information Canada, Ottawa.

Some high risk groups in cancer of the oesophagus

J. C. Paymaster*, P. Gangadharan and D. Nagaraj Rao

Tata Memorial Centre, Bombay, India

Health problems in developing countries are vastly different from those of developed countries. Collection of data on health problems in developing countries like India is faced with many difficulties. The majority of the population in India live in villages which are scattered over large areas widely separated from each other. Almost 90% of the villages have a population of less than 2,000 persons, and inadequate facilities of communication and transportation make it difficult to obtain medical assistance. Lack of health awareness of the population, illiteracy, poverty, inadequate modern medical facilities, prevalence of indigenous systems of medicine often hinder the collection of data on any disease, including cancer.

Incidence data on cancer are not yet available in India, except for a few sites in certain selected small areas of the country. The available data on cancer in the country are obtained from some of the large and well equipped general hospitals in the country. Such data, in spite of limitations have provided important and useful information regarding the pattern of cancer. It must be mentioned that generalizations regarding the pattern of cancer in India should be attempted with caution because of the size and geographic features of the country, and also the great variations in the ethnic groups, habits and customs of the people. However, in most parts of the country, oral cavity, oropharynx, hypopharynx and cervix are affected with cancer in large proportions (Paymaster, 1964). Cancer of the oesophagus has also a high frequency rate (Paymaster et al., 1968).

In Greater Bombay, the age adjusted incidence rate (adjusted to world population) of cancer of the oesophagus was 13.0 per 100,000 male population and 11.3 per 100,000 among females; the crude rates being 6.1 and 5.1 per 100,000 for males and females respectively. The corresponding age adjusted rates for Connecticut were 5.7 and 1.4 per 100,000 (U.I.C.C., 1970). In Greater Bombay, 10% of all deaths due to cancer were from cancer of the oesophagus, the crude annual mortality rate being 4.15 per 100,000 population (Paymaster and Gangadharan, 1971). At the Tata Memorial Hospital, cancer of the oesophagus formed 10% of all cancer in males and 7% in females. It ranked 3rd in order of frequency among all cancer cases seen, and annually almost 800 cases of cancer of the oesophagus were recorded at this hospital.

In the past, several studies in India have demonstrated statistical association of the habits of chewing *pan* and smoking with cancer of the oral cavity and pharynx. As the oesophagus is an organ contiguous with the oral cavity and the pharynx, it would be of special interest to study the association of the habits of chewing *pan* and smoking with cancer of the oesophagus.

The habits of chewing *pan* and smoking are prevalent in a large section of our population. *Pan* is made of betel leaf, betel nut, slaked lime, acacia catechu, with or without tobacco and other ingredients. These are made into a bolus and chewed frequently. The juice obtained by masticating the bolus is often swallowed but when tobacco is added, a

---

* Present address: Medical Research Centre, Bombay Hospital, Marine Lines, Bombay 400020, India.

part is spat out. There is a tendency on the part of some to keep the quid in the gingivo buccal groove for hours and sometimes even while asleep. In our country a vast majority of those who indulge in smoking smoke *bidi*, the Indian form of cigarette made by rolling by hand a small quantity of tobacco placed in dried leaves of a tree of the ebony family instead of the usual cigarette paper. A *bidi* is usually 5 cm in length and contains on an average 0.216 g of tobacco, whereas a regular cigarette is 7 cm long and holds an average of 0.973 g of tobacco. This means that when a person smokes 45 *bidies*, he has smoked a quantity of tobacco equivalent to that in 10 cigarettes.

The data on the habits of chewing and smoking presented here were collected routinely from patients attending the Tata Memorial Hospital for the first time during 1963 to 1971. There were 3,255 interviewed cases of cancer of the oesophagus and 5,266 controls were selected from the non-cancer patients attending the hospital during the same period. All the patients were interviewed as far as possible before the medical examination. The cases formed only 58% of all cancer cases of the oesophagus recorded at the hospital during the same period. Patients who were too ill with advanced disease, could not be interviewed. The controls were selected from the non-cancer group of persons above the age of 35 years, attending the hospital. The selected controls had either no evidence of any disease or were those who had minor infectious or inflammatory diseases of the mouth and throat, cervix etc. There was no case of benign tumour or cancer at any site included in the control group.

For planning therapy and assessing the end results it is customary to consider the 3 segments of the oesophagus, viz.

Upper one-third: The post-cricoid region (the pharyngo-oesophageal junction, where the lesion cannot be visualised on indirect laryngoscopy). The cervical and supra-aortic portions.

Middle one-third: The retro-aortic, hilar and infrahilar portions.

Lower one-third: Supradiaphragmatic, infradiaphragmatic portions and the cardio-oesophageal junction.

In this paper the association of the habits of chewing *pan* and smoking with cancer in the different segments of the oesophagus i.e., post-cricoid, upper one-third, middle one-third and lower one-third are evaluated.

The distribution of cases in the 4 segments of the oesophagus in males and females are presented in Table 1.

The cases and controls had similar distribution with regard to several characteristics. The mean age for cases and controls are presented in Table 2.

The composition of cases with regard to the various religious communities of Western India were as follows: Hindus from Maharashtra 40%; Hindus from Gujarat 15%; Moslems 16%; Christians 4%; Parsis 0.4%; other religious communities 20%; and the controls had the following distributions: Hindus from Maharashtra 36%; Hindus from Gujarat 16%; Moslems 14%; Christians 7%; Parsis 2%; other religious communities 25%.

TABLE 1   *The distribution of cancer in the oesophagus among males and females. Tata Memorial Hospital (3255 cases)*

Site of cancer	Males		Females		Total	
	No.	%	No.	%	No.	%
Post-cricoid	121	5.3	65	6.9	186	5.7
Upper-third	348	15.1	102	10.8	450	13.8
Middle-third	996	43.1	396	41.9	1392	42.8
Lower-third	460	19.9	231	24.4	691	21.2
Unclassified*	385	16.7	151	16.0	536	16.5
Total	2310		945		3255	

* Where exact location could not be ascertained or where the lesion involved more than one segment

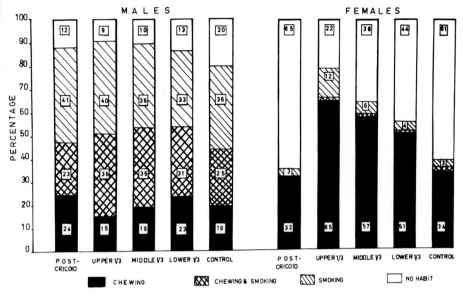

FIG. 1   *Percentage distribution of chewing and smoking habits among cases and controls in males and females.*

The proportion of cases and controls with habits is presented in Figure 1. It may be observed that the proportion with habits is more among cases than among controls in both sexes. The habit pattern in cancer of the post-cricoid region differs in some ways from that of other segments of the oesophagus. The percentage of cases with habits decreases as the lesion is observed lower down the tract in both sexes. The proportion of smokers was more in the upper third of the oesophagus.

Many studies have indicated an association of cancer of the oesophagus with alcohol consumption, especially with the use of heavy spirits (Tuyns, 1970). On account of the enforcement of prohibition in most parts of our country, the data regarding the use of alcohol were obtained with difficulty and in many instances the information was found to be scanty. Hence, no detailed analysis could be attempted. The data on smoking alone, chewing alone and the combined habits of chewing and smoking, all without alcohol habit, was further analysed. Comparing cases and controls, the relative risk was calculated using the Mantel-Haenszel formula for matched samples (Mantel and Haenszel, 1959).

Assuming the risk to be 1 among the no-chewing, no-smoking, no-alcohol group of persons, the relative risks among the 3 habit categories for the different segments of the

TABLE 2   *Mean age and standard deviation in cases and controls*

Site of cancer	Males		Females	
	Mean	Standard deviation	Mean	Standard deviation
Post-cricoid	50.1	12.3	49.1	10.9
Upper one-third	55.1	10.1	54.1	10.3
Middle one-third	53.2	10.1	52.3	10.4
Lower one-third	53.5	10.7	53.1	10.2
Control	51.0	10.1	48.8	9.2

oesophagus were calculated. These are presented for males and females in Tables 3 and 4. There were no females with the combined habit in certain categories, hence the relative risk could not be presented. The overall pattern of risk levels is presented in Figure 2.

The statistically significant relative risk levels observed among those who chewed only could be due to the presence of one or the combination of factors constituting the *pan* viz. the betel leaf, slaked lime, betel nut, and tobacco. Sufficient data were available to analyse the risk among those who chewed *pan* with and without tobacco compared with the no-habit group. The relative risks for the groups who chewed *pan* with tobacco and those without tobacco are presented in Table 5 with their statistical significance. Similar data for those who smoked only were analysed to study the role of *bidi* compared with the no-habit group. The relative risks for those who smoked *bidi* and those who smoked cigarettes were obtained and these are presented in Table 6. Amongst those with the

TABLE 3   *Relative risk among chewers and smokers – Males*

(a)   *Chewing habit only*

	Cancer		Control		
Site	Chewing only	No habit[1]	Chewing only	No habit[1]	Relative risk
Post-cricoid	25	15	477	568	1.9
Upper one-third	50	31	477	568	2.0**
Middle one-third	174	97	477	568	2.1**
Lower one-third	94	61	477	568	1.8**
All cases[2]	420	240	477	568	2.1**

(b)   *Smoking habit only*

	Cancer		Control		
Site	Smoking only	No habit[1]	Smoking only	No habit[1]	Relative risk
Post-cricoid	41	15	770	568	2.0*
Upper one-third	106	31	770	568	2.5**
Middle one-third	272	97	770	568	2.1**
Lower one-third	124	61	770	568	1.5*
All cases[2]	635	240	770	568	1.9**

(c)   *Chewing and smoking habit*

	Cancer		Control		
Site	Chewing and smoking	No habit[1]	Chewing and smoking	No habit[1]	Relative risk
Post-cricoid	22	15	480	568	1.7
Upper one-third	91	31	480	568	3.5**
Middle one-third	258	97	480	568	3.1**
Lower one-third	111	61	480	568	2.2**
All cases[2]	587	240	480	568	2.8**

* = p<.05; ** = p<.01
[1] = no chewing, no smoking, no alcohol
[2] = including unclassified

combined habit of chewing and smoking, similar analyses were undertaken for males and these are presented in Table 7. The trends in the relative risks in the various habit groups are presented in Figure 3.

The habits of chewing *pan* and smoking are believed to be high risk factors in cancer of the oesophagus in India (Sanghvi et al., 1955; Paymaster et al., 1968; Jussawalla and Deshpande, 1971). Among the cases, 10% of the males and 39% of the females did not have these habits. The statistically significant relative risks obtained indicate that the risk is almost 2 to 3 times only in those with habits when compared with those without these habits. The role of these habits in cancer of the post-cricoid seems to be minimal. The general pattern indicates that the risk levels reduce as the lesion is observed lower down the tract and also there is an additive effect of the habits of chewing *pan* and smoking among males. The role of tobacco has not been consistent. Among *pan* chewers, the

TABLE 4   *Relative risk among chewers and smokers – Females*

(a)   Chewing habit only

Site	Cancer		Control		Relative risk
	Chewing only	No habit[1]	Chewing only	No habit[1]	
Post-cricoid	21	42	826	1480	0.9
Upper one-third	66	23	826	1480	5.1**
Middle one-third	224	142	826	1480	2.8**
Lower one-third	118	102	826	1480	2.1**
All cases[2]	501	368	826	1480	2.4**

(b)   Smoking habit only

Site	Cancer		Control		Relative risk
	Smoking only	No habit[1]	Smoking only	No habit[1]	
Post-cricoid	2	42	82	1480	0.9
Upper one-third	11	23	82	1480	8.6**
Middle one-third	20	142	82	1480	2.5**
Lower one-third	9	102	82	1480	1.6
All cases[2]	58	368	82	1480	2.8**

(c)   Chewing and smoking habit

Site	Cancer		Control		Relative risk
	Chewing and smoking	No habit[1]	Chewing and smoking	No habit[1]	
Post-cricoid	–	42	30	1480	–
Upper one-third	–	23	30	1480	–
Middle one-third	7	142	30	1480	2.4
Lower one-third	2	102	30	1480	0.9
All cases[2]	12	368	30	1480	1.6

** = p < .01
[1] = no chewing, no smoking, no alcohol
[2] = including unclassified

TABLE 5 Relative risk among pan chewers with and without tobacco

Site	Cases			Controls			Relative risk	
	Pan with tobacco	Pan without tobacco	No habit[1]	Pan with tobacco	Pan without tobacco	No habit[1]	Pan with tobacco	Pan without tobacco
Males								
Post-cricoid	23	2	15	389	88	568	2.2*	0.9
Upper one-third	42	8	31	389	88	568	2.0**	1.7
Middle one-third	147	27	97	389	88	568	2.2**	1.8*
Lower one-third	80	14	61	389	88	568	1.9**	1.5
All cases[2]	361	59	240	389	88	568	2.2**	1.6*
Females								
Post-cricoid	17	4	42	608	218	1480	1.0	0.6
Upper one-third	52	14	23	608	218	1480	5.5**	4.1**
Middle one-third	181	43	142	608	218	1480	3.1**	2.1**
Lower one-third	92	26	102	608	218	1480	2.2**	1.7*
All cases[2]	402	99	368	608	218	1480	2.7**	1.8**

* = p < .05; ** = p < .01
[1] = no chewing, no smoking, no alcohol
[2] = including unclassified

TABLE 6   *Relative risk among bidi smokers and cigarette smokers*

Site	Cases			Control			Relative risk	
	Bidi	Cigarette	No habit[1]	Bidi	Cigarette	No habit[1]	Bidi	Cigarette
Males								
Post-cricoid	30	7	15	575	139	568	2.0*	1.9
Upper one-third	90	12	31	575	139	568	2.9**	1.6
Middle one-third	232	23	97	575	139	568	2.4**	0.9
Lower one-third	103	15	61	575	139	568	1.7**	1.0
All cases[2]	536	67	240	575	139	568	2.2**	1.1
Females								
All cases[2]	55	1	368	65	6	1480	3.4**	0.7

* = $p < .05$; ** = $p < .01$
1 = no chewing, no smoking, no alcohol
2 = including unclassified

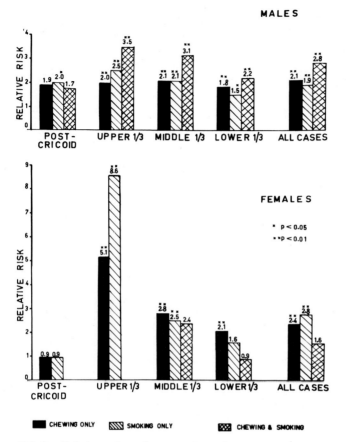

FIG. 2   *Relative risks and statistical significance among pan chewers and smokers in males and females.*

presence of tobacco in *pan* increased the risk, but the *bidi* smokers who were also *pan* chewers without tobacco had higher risk than those who chewed tobacco. *Bidi* smokers had a greater risk than cigarette smokers, which is compensated by the chewing habit and it must be mentioned that cigarette smokers in our country can be classified as only light smokers by western standards.

In our studies we have observed that there are definite variations in the distribution of cancer among the major religious communities of Western India (Paymaster, 1967). The proportion of cancer of the oesophagus is particularly high among Hindus from Gujarat attending the Tata Memorial Hospital (Fig.4). As yet we do not have any incidence data to study the pattern of cancer in these populations but the relative frequencies obtained from some of the large hospitals indicate that cancer of the oesophagus is a major problem in Gujarat (Fig. 5). This may have a bearing on the habits prevalent in these populations. In this connection it is pertinent to observe the differences in the habit patterns among the Hindus from Maharashtra and Gujarat. The proportion of chewers, smokers and those with the combined habit among the no cancer group (controls) are indicated in Table 8 and Figure 6. Those who were from Maharashtra had a higher percentage of chewers among them; whereas those who were from Gujarat indulged in smoking more often.

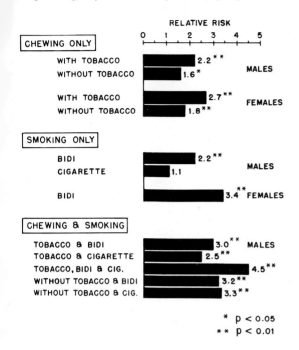

FIG. 3   *Relative risks and statistical significance among different categories of pan chewers and smokers.*

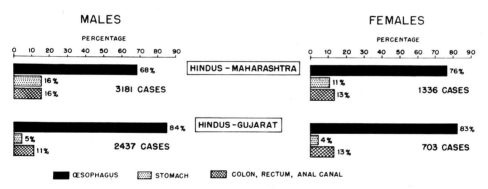

FIG. 4   *Relative frequency distribution of cancer within the gastrointestinal tract among Hindus from Maharashtra and Gujarat attending the Tata Memorial Hospital, Bombay.*

Further, distribution of cancer in the oesophagus also shows some variations between communities (Paymaster and Gangadharan, 1970). Amongst Hindus, Moslems and Christians attending the Tata Memorial Hospital, the disease is more often observed in the upper $\frac{2}{3}$rd of the oesophagus; whereas, amongst the Parsis, a majority of whom are non-smokers and non-chewers, the lower $\frac{1}{3}$rd is more often affected (Fig. 7).

The data presented so far indicate that chewers and smokers are high risk groups for cancer of the oesophagus. The risk levels are not that high to warrant any drastic public health measures. It may be mentioned here that the controls we have used are hospital

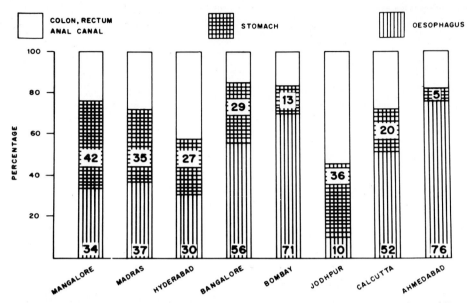

FIG. 5   *Relative frequencies of cancer in the segments of the gastrointestinal tract observed in some of the major hospitals in the country. (From Paymaster et al., 1973. Courtesy of the Editors.)*

TABLE 7   *Relative risk among chewers and smokers (males)*

	Cases		Control		
Habit	With habit	Without habit	With habit	Without habit	Relative risk
Tobacco chewing and *bidi* smoking	306	240	245	568	3.0**
Tobacco chewing and cigarette smoking	49	240	46	568	2.5**
Tobacco chewing and *bidi* and cigarette smoking	23	240	12	568	4.5**
Chewing *pan* without tobacco and *bidi* smoking	159	240	116	568	3.2**
Chewing *pan* without tobacco and cigarette smoking	28	240	20	568	3.3**

** = $p < .01$

TABLE 8   *Distribution of chewers and smokers among Hindus from Maharashtra and Hindus from Gujarat (control group)*

	Hindus from Maharashtra		Hindus from Gujarat	
Habits	No.	%	No.	%
Chewers	306	38.0	61	16.0
Smokers	281	34.0	204	53.0
Chewers and smokers	226	28.0	119	31.0
Total	813		324	

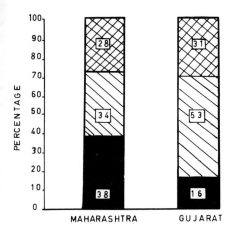

FIG. 6 *Proportion of persons with the habit of pan chewing, smoking, and the combined habit of chewing and smoking, among Hindus from Maharashtra and Gujarat (males). For explanation of symbols see Fig. 1.*

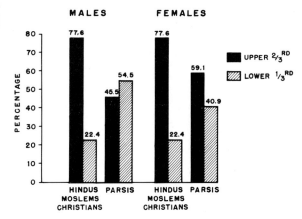

FIG. 7 *Distribution of cancer in the oesophagus among Hindus, Moslems, Christians and Parsis (From Paymaster and Gangadharan, 1970. Courtesy of the Editors.)*

patients.It was thought that if some of the mouth and throat infections were associated with chewing and smoking, the relative risk among the cases would be low, when compared with such controls. But a perusal of the characteristics of the general population controls which have been used in some studies (Jussawalla and Deshpande, 1971) indicate that our controls were comparable to the population controls and did not have a higher percentage with the habits. In this connection it is important to study the distribution of cancer within the oesophagus in the absence of any of the habits. The distribution of cancer in the oesophagus among the no-habit group is presented in Table 9.

It might be observed that compared with all cases (Table 1) the distribution among the no-habit group shows an excess of cases of the lower third in males whereas amongst females the percentage of cases in the post-cricoid region was markedly increased. In the no-habit group of registered cases, the sex ratio for each segment is just the opposite of that observed among all cases (Table 10). The incidence of cancer of the oesophagus is almost equal among males (6.1) and females (5.1) of the Greater Bombay population; whereas the habits of chewing and smoking are predominantly observed among males. Hence, it could be that our female population has a higher incidence of cancer of the

TABLE 9   *Distribution of cancer in the oesophagus in the 'no-habit' group*

	Males		Females	
Site	No.	%	No.	%
Post-cricoid	15	6.0	42	11.0
Upper-third	31	13.0	23	6.0
Middle-third	97	40.0	142	38.0
Lower-third	61	25.0	102	28.0
Unclassified*	36	15.0	59	16.0
Total	240		368	

* Where exact location could not be ascertained or where the lesion involved more than one segment

TABLE 10   *Sex ratios among all registered cases of cancer of the oesophagus and among the no-habit (no chewing, no smoking, no alcohol) group of persons*

	Sex ratios	
	Registered cases	No-habit group
Site	Male : Female	Male : Female
Post-cricoid	1.9 : 1	0.4 : 1
Upper one-third	3.4 : 1	1.3 : 1
Middle one-third	2.5 : 1	0.7 : 1
Lower one-third	2.0 : 1	0.6 : 1

oesophagus than males in the absence of these habits. The higher incidence in women could also be due to the preponderance of cancer in the post-cricoid region. When the effect of chewing and smoking were eliminated, the crude incidence rates of Greater Bombay became — males (3.1) and females (3.3) per 100,000 population. Similarly, the age adjusted (adjusted to world population) rates became males (6.6) and females (7.3) per 100,000 and the truncated adjusted rates became males (10.7) and females (13.6) per 100,000 population (see appendix).

It may also be mentioned that certain iron and vitamin deficiencies have been suspected to be associated with post-cricoid cancers especially in the female, and these may be present in our population too. The equality of sex ratios (or an excess in females) after the elimination of the chewing and smoking habit calls for more research into aetiological factors and further studies are necessary. The factors could be those which would influence both male and female. Certain food habits may be of importance in this connection. Drinking hot tea is quite common especially with the people of Gujarat, who also consume large amounts of milk and other dairy products. For cooking, considerable quantities of oil (especially peanut oil) is used by the people of Gujarat. The significance of all these habits is not yet clear and would require further studies.

Acknowledgement

We are grateful to Dr. A.J. Tuyns for his valuable suggestions.

References

Jussawalla, D.J. and Deshpande, V.A. (1971): Cancer, 28/1, 244.
Mantel, N. and Haenszel, W. (1959): J. nat. Cancer Inst., 22/4, 719.
Paymaster, J.C. (1964): Cancer, 17/8, 1026.
Paymaster, J.C. (1967): In: Progress in Clinical Cancer, Vol. III, pp. 107-124. Editor: Irwing Ariel. Grune and Stratton, New York, N.Y.
Paymaster, J.C., Sanghvi, L.D. and Gangadharan, P. (1968): Cancer, 21/2, 279.
Paymaster, J.C. and Gangadharan, P. (1970): Int. J. Cancer, 5/3, 426.
Paymaster, J.C. and Gangadharan, P. (1971): J. Indian med. Ass., 57/2, 63.
Paymaster, J.C., Potdar, G.G., De Souza, L. and Gangadharan, P. (1973): Indian J. Cancer, 10, 1.
Sanghvi, L.D., Rao, K.C.M. and Khanolkar, V.R. (1955): Brit. med. J., 1, 1111.
Tuyns, A.J. (1970): Int. J. Cancer, 5/1, 152.
U.I.C.C. (1970): Cancer Incidence in Five Continents, Vol. II. Editors: R. Doll, C.S. Muir and J. Waterhouse. U.I.C.C.

Appendix

Note on calculation of incidence of cancer of the oesophagus after eliminating the effect of chewing and smoking habits:

Risk in the no-habit group of people = 1.
The relative risk in the presence of chewing and smoking (calculated for the data presented) in males = 2.2
in females = 2.4

Let X be the incidence of cancer of the oesophagus among those without habits of chewing and smoking.
Among the general male population, 20% were without the habits and 80% had some of the habits. Hence the number of cases per 100,000 population would be

$$\frac{X \times 20,000}{100,000} + \frac{2.2 \times X \times 80,000}{100,000} = 1.96 \ X$$

The crude incidence of cancer of the oesophagus in Greater Bombay is 6.1/100,000, i.e.: 1.96 X = 6.1
or   X = 3.1

Similarly the age adjusted (world population) rates become 6.6 and the truncated rates become 10.7/100,000. Among females, 61% were without habits and 39% were with habits. The 3 rates calculated similarly would become 3.3, 7.3 and 13.6/100,000.

Modern X-ray diagnosis of carcinoma of the colon and rectum

J. Altaras

Wilhelm-Conrad-Röntgen-Klinik, University of Giessen, Giessen, Federal Republic of Germany

Colonic and rectal-carcinomas are no longer a surgical, but a diagnostic problem. Whereas a 98% survival-rate can be achieved with surgical treatment in the early stages, only a 20% survival-rate can be expected with the same treatment at late stages.

Prior to a surgical operation on the colon and the rectum, an exact radiological examination of these organs should be performed. However, it is bad practice to operate on local lesions, for instance hemorrhoids, cystocele, retrocele etc, or without knowledge of the entire state of the colon.

Changes of the large bowel are often multicentric. Frequently, polyps or other precancerous lesions are combined with changes in the more proximal, or the more distal intestinal segments. In patients with disturbances of the colon, the diagnosis is based on a radiological examination with a contrast medium, in addition to history, palpation, rectal examination and procto-sigmoidoscopy. The responsibility of the radiologist is very high for the following reason: only by X-rays is it possible to visualize the entire colon: manual examination and endoscopy are limited to the rectum and the sigmoid colon. The best method of examination is the double-contrast-method. All segments of the intestines are first wholly filled with a positive contrast medium and then, by filling with air, the intestines become, in effect, an unfolded, transparent tube.

The German worker Fischer in 1923 introduced the double-contrast-method, in which a substance opaque to X-rays, combined with air, was used. The method was also used later by Weber (1931) in America. During the last few years, Welin (1955, 1958) in Sweden has perfected this method, as a result of which its diagnostic value for colonic abnormalities has greatly increased. Once optimum results had been obtained my Zürich School adopted this method for routine examination of the colon.

With the double-contrast-method, the technique of radiological examination of the colon (preparation of the patient, contrast medium, simplification of the administration of contrast medium and air) has been brought to a high level during the last decade. It has proved its efficacy and has always been highly valued. However, the double-contrast-method is but one possible method among others, which may or may not be used as desired. It offers definite advantages which can be readily confirmed by the statistics of precancerous lesions and their demonstrable malignant changes. Thus this method, at the present time, should no longer be witheld from the patient. The double-contrast-method remains the only usable, effective examination procedure. However, even this method can fail if it is not carefully prepared, if the necessary instruments are lacking, if an inadequate number of radiograms are obtained, and unless all segments of the bowel have already been screened by fluoroscopy. Obviously, the caecum poses particular problems to many examiners, and thus they prefer to leave the caecum filled with barium. The sigmoid colon frequently is also difficult to evaluate because many loops of bowel are superimposed on one another. In the rectosigmoid colon, free projections of the terminal bowel can be achieved by special views (Chassard-Lapinée).

Because of the overshadowing intestinal loops, it is difficult to visualize the transition of the rectum into the sigmoid. This, unfortunately, is where about 70% of all pathological findings are made. The problem is to examine a tube of 70 cm length. This tube is fixed by two points, at one end by the mesenterium near to the apertura superior of the pelvis, and at the other, at the rectum. These points are only 15 cm apart. Because of this, there are many chances of possible movement of the sigma with superpositions. In view of the anatomical circumstances, the radiological examination of the recto-sigmoid should be carried out with the patient in a ventricumbent and supine position; the examination table being in a declining position at the top end (15-20°), thus guaranteeing free projection of the recto-sigmoid (Altaras, 1968). The application of this system represents a great step forward in the early diagnosis of cancer (Fig. 1).

Pathological findings are frequently visualized directly in a plastic manner due to the high clarity of detail and the decreased visualization of marginal contours at various depths. If a polyp is detected during the digital or sigmoidoscopic examination, the double-contrast-colon-examination should be performed. Experience indicates that frequently other polyps may exist higher in the colon. Polyps may well escape detection at the time of laparatomy because palpation is an unreliable method of detecting individual polyps in the colon. On the radiographs, polyps present a characteristic appearance. If

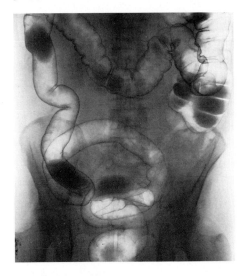

FIG. 1   *An accurate view of the colon and recto-sigmoid walls wetted by the contrast medium, and the lumen extended by the air.*

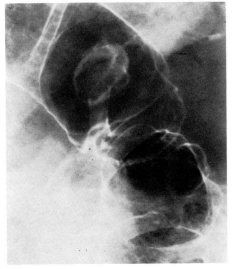

FIG. 2   *The double-contrast study of the colon shows the adenomatous polyp and its long pedicle.*

pedunculated, the stalk appears as double parallel lines (Fig. 2). In the axial view, the stalk projects itself inside the polyp and is seen as an internal concentric figure.

Broad-based polyps are seen in the anterior-posterior radiographs as concentric figures and in the side view — as in the lumen — protruding processes. In ulcerative colitis the so-called pseudopolyps are inflammatory polyps and can be easily differentiated from polyposis. The sharp marginal contours coupled with the examination of the mucosa in a direct view make it possible to obtain a comprehensive survey of the extent of the changes.

Papillary or villous adenomas are mostly found in the rectum and lower sigmoid. The tumor surface is made up of innumerable papillary folds that are so soft that they often escape detection by the examining finger. Double-contrast-visualization very beautifully and almost plastically demonstrates the villous adenoma. Villous adenomas are soft, and because of this, they show characteristic size and form variations during the examination, depending on the amount of air insufflation. Despite a negative histological result from the surface of the tumor, a radiologically demonstrable invagination of the intestinal wall on the base allows proof of an early malignancy (Fig. 3).

All other forms of tumor can almost plastically be demonstrated. Malignant tumors show in the initial stages a rigidity of the contours and the intestinal wall loses its elasticity in this segment. Later, it shortens the intestinal segment and at a still later stage infiltrates the wall with circular stenosis. The cauliflower-like growing tumor which does not cause stenosis but ulcerates, gives a projection with wavy contours and can be mistaken for normal haustra (Figs. 4 and 5).

In patients with stenosis of the large bowel the double-contrast-method may produce excellent results because, even in cases with extreme stenosis, air can enter the proximal segment, and thus the entire length of the stenosis can be visualized. Only the double-contrast-method permits visualization of the typical changes in the bowel wall and mucosa in patients with intestinal complications after gynecological radiotherapy. It makes possible the differentiation between radiological stenosis and relapse. The double-contrast-method with new pictures of the rectum and sigmoid answers the following questions: single or multiple, isolated or in groups, with a stalk or broad basis, smooth or

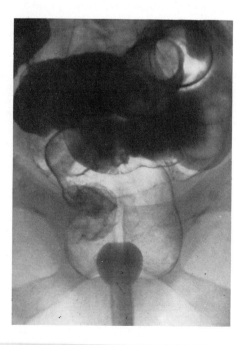

FIG. 3   *Villoma of the rectum with invagination at the base. Histology: malignant.*

villous or both, benign or malignant, infiltrative or not? It is therefore advisable to perform a radiological examination before a proctoscopy, for the benefit of the surgeon.

Discussion of, for example, contradictory statistics on the malignant transformations of various excrescences of the colon and rectum prior to operation, are useless unless the clinician is armed with the best radiogram of the colon. Only then can we establish an objective basis for the analysis and planning of operations.

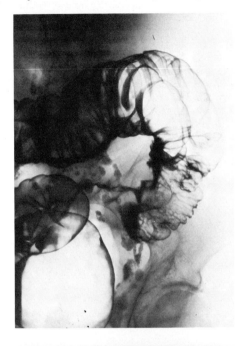

FIG. 4   *Carcinoma of the caecum. Irregular tumor structure in the caecum and terminal ileum.*

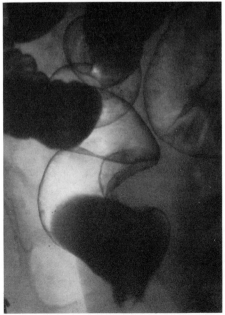

FIG. 5   *Plaque-like rectal carcinoma.*

Summary

The best procedure for early cancer detection is the double-contrast-method. The author describes application of the double-contrast-method to examination of the colon. The technique utilises Clysodrast for improved flushing of the bowel, and Barotrast as a positive contrast medium. Some cases, in which the value of the method is apparent for the whole pathology of the colon are described. Because of the overlapping intestinal loops it is difficult to visualize the transition of the rectum into the sigmoid; but this is where about 70% of all pathological findings are made.

The newly developed method of sigma examination is a particularly useful tool for the early diagnosis of cancer as it renders possible the detection of precancerous lesions. The method answers the following questions: single or multiple, isolated or in groups, with a stalk or broad basis, smooth or villous or both, benign or malignant, infiltrative or not? — All other forms of tumors can be demonstrated in a near plastic form. It is therefore advisable to perform a radiological examination before a proctoscopy, for the benefit of the surgeon.

References

Altaras, J. (1967): Med. Welt (Berl.), 40, 2392.
Altaras, J. (1968): Röntgen-Bl., 8, 376.
Altaras, J. (1969): Actual. hépatogastro-entérol. Hôtel-Dieu, 5/3, B-95.
Altaras, J. (1971): Röntgenbrief 'Du Pont', 10,1.
Andren, L., Freiberg, S. and Welin, S. (1955): Acta radiol. (Stockh.), 45, 201.
Bell, J. C. and Douglas, J. B. (1948): Radiology, 51, 279.
Bell, J. C. (1950): Radiology., 55, 20.
Del Buono, M. S. (1961): Riv. Radiol., 1/3, 455.
Deucher, F. and Cotar, Z. (1967): Schweiz. med. Wschr., 16, 501.
Ettinger, A. and Elkin, M. (1954): Amer. J. Roentgenol., 72, 199.
Gianturco, C. A. and Miller, G. A. (1953): Radiology, 60, 496.
Hoch, A. P. and Forster, S. E. (1958): Schweiz. med. Wschr., 88, 730.
Ledoux-Lebard, R. and Garcis-Calceron, J. (1933): J. Radiol. Electrol., 17, 429.
Levene, G. and Kaufmann, S. A. (1967): Amer. J. Roentgenol., 78, 685.
Moreton, R. D. (1953): Radiology, 60, 510.
Moreton, R. D. Cooper, E. M. and Foegelle, E. F. (1951): Radiology, 56, 214.
Robinson, J. M. (1957): Amer. J. Roentgenol., 77, 700.
Rüttimann, A. (1961): Bibl. Radiol. (Basel.), 2, 77.
Rüttimann, A. (1960): Schweiz. med. Wschr., 90, 807.
Swenson, P. C. and Wigh, R. (1948): Amer. J. Roentgenol., 59, 108.
Weber, H. M. (1931): Amer. J. Roentgenol., 25, 577.
Welin, S. (1955): Fortschr. Röntgenstr., 82, 341.
Welin, S. (1958): Münch. med. Wschr., 100, 1142.
Young, A. C. (1969): In: Diseases of the Colon, Rectum and Anus, p. 38. Editor: Basil C. Morson. William Heinemann Medical Books, Ltd. London.

Antecedents of colorectal cancer: Ulcerative colitis

J. Altaras

Wilhelm-Conrad-Röntgen-Klinik, University of Giessen, Giessen, Federal Republic of Germany

The most serious complication of ulcerative colitis is malignant degeneration. In some English speaking countries a prophylactic proctocolectomy is being recommended in view of the frequency of the phenomenon, the speedy, continued and metastatic spreading of the tumor, and the resulting unfavorable prognosis.

A relationship between chronic ulcerative colitis and the subsequent development of carcinoma of the colon has been well established, although substantial differences of opinion on its frequency remain.

The carcinoma does not show a homogeneous distribution. It seems to depend a great deal on the extension, degree, development, timing and duration of the colitis. It has been emphasized that onset of ulcerative colitis in childhood, duration of activity of the colitis and the severity of symptoms all appear to be factors that predispose to neoplastic change.

Malignant degeneration does not seem to be related to the progressive or regressive course of the inflammatory changes. Thus, a malignant tumor may occur during a remission when the patient is almost free from symptoms and roentgenologically much improved. Cancer of the colon or rectum may superimpose on chronic ulcerative colitis any time after onset of colitis. Also, the two diseases may begin simultaneously, or the cancer may precede ulcerative colitis. Special attention is needed to demonstrate the simultaneous presence of true adenomatous polyps which, unlike the 'pseudo-polyps' of inflammation, represent a precancerous condition.

Investigation shows no constant characteristic in the roentgenologic appearance of the colon with ulcerative inflammatory changes which developes carcinoma. Configurations of these inflammatory lesions, as demonstrated by barium enema, are frequently indistinguishable from malignancy. The correct diagnosis is frequently overlooked or made too late to achieve an encouraging number of cures.

The detection of such neoplasms requires a formal double-contrast enema. A short, poorly defined stricture in ulcerative colitis is more likely to be malignant than benign. Hence, careful periodic radiological (double-contrast) examination is advised of patients who have had ulcerative colitis in its severe and destructive form. The sharp marginal contours, coupled with the examination of the mucosa in a direct view, makes it possible to obtain a comprehensive survey of the extent of the changes. When this is done, carcinoma may be detected during the stage of operability.

The estimated frequency of the malignant degeneration of ulcerative colitis ranges from 0 to 65% and an average of 10%. There are great differences of opinion among surgeons, internists and pathologists as well as between one country or town or even clinic and another (Tables 1 and 2). We attempted to clarify the conflicting information on malignant degeneration in ulcerative colitis. By questioning numerous clinics in different countries and by studying the relevant world literature, we concluded that the frequency of ulcerative colitis itself in West Germany and other Central European countries — 6 to 8 cases per 10,000 patients — is considerably lower than in the U.S.A. (Table 3). It seems prevalent in highly civilized countries in which psychosomatic factors play a more important role than here, and where different living and feeding habits exist.

TABLE 1   *Reported incidence of carcinoma in ulcerative colitis up to 1961*

Author	Year	No. of colitis cases	No. of carcinoma cases	Proportion (%)
Lynn	1945	1467	28	1.9
Jackmann et al.	1940	871		3.2
by that under 16 years by outbreak of colitis		95		6.3
Ricketts and Palmer	1946	206	3	1.4
Cattell and Boehme	1947	450	10	2.2
Johnson and Orr	1948	164	2	1.2
Kasich et al.	1949	143	7	4.9
Felsen and Wolarsky	1949	855	0	0
Glecker and Brown	1950	316	12	3.8
Sloan et al.	1950	2000		5.0
Lyons and Garlock	1951	226	9	3.9
by that more than 12 years sick		16		43.0
Counsell and Dukes	1952	63	7	11.1
Weckmesser and Chinn	1953	118	4	3.4
Bargen et al.	1954	1564	98	6.3
Wheelock and Warren	1955	483	31	6.2
Bacon et al.	1956	402	12	2.9
by that treated operatively		84	12	14.2
Dukes and Lockhart-Mummery	1957	153	8	5.2
Goldgraber et al.	1958	792	22	2.7
Dawson et al.	1959	663	19	2.9
Slaney et al.	1959	222	15	6.7
Dennis et al.	1961	267	16	7.4

With advances in world communication our European life is much influenced by American customs which are widely reflected in our dietary habits as well as in our daily life. This will cause an increase of ulcerative colitis throughout Europe. We believe that ulcerative colitis will be seen more frequently in Europe in future than today. Malignant development increases with the frequency of colitis patients. This is supported by the available statistics in the U.S.A., which show a 10-fold higher colitis morbidity.

The frequency of malignant degeneration of ulcerative colitis is low in the statistics for Germany and Central Europe, and prophylactic proctocolectomy is therefore not justified solely by the potential for malignant degeneration. According to our findings, colitis-induced carcinoma represents a true rarity in Germany and Central Europe. Improved colitis therapy with azulfidine and corticosteroid will surely inhibit the development of carcinoma in spite of future improvement in the standard of living.

One study of carcinoma in ulcerative colitis by Bargen et al. (1954) shows that the typical patient with chronic ulcerative colitis was 31 years old at the time of his clinic visit and that he has a more than 50% chance of living 25 years. For that reason, Bargen opposes early removal of the colon.

The simultaneous presence of multiple adenomatous polyps and colitis, and the

TABLE 2   *Reported incidence of carcinoma in ulcerative colitis up to 1973*

Author	Year	No. of colitis cases	No. of carcinoma cases	Proportion (%)
Edwards and Truelove	1964	624	22	3.5
Mörl	1964	137		0.2
Welch et al.	1965	750	25	3.3
Fahrländer	1966	172	1	0.4
Feiereis	1966	139	0	0
Henning	1967		0	0
Maratka and Nedbal	1968	645	3	0.5
Demling et al.	1969	277	4	1.4
Deucher et al.	1971	42	2	4.9
Matsunaga	1972	259	1	0.4
Maratka	1972	761	3	0.4
Hafter	1973	113	4	3.5
Dombrowski and Martini	1973	202	2	1.0
Franchini	1973	100	0	0

TABLE 3   *Incidence of ulcerative colitis*

Country	Rate of incidence per 10,000 hospital admissions
Sweden	3.5 – 15.0
Switzerland	5.8
Poland	6.6
Finland	7.0
Denmark	7.8
Belgium	10.8
Czechoslovakia	10.0
Scotland	6.9
England	10.9 – 50.9
U.S.A.	10.0 – 100.0
Germany	7.0

connexion between the two diseases prompted Deucher et al. (1971) to propose the idea of a *Colitis-polypoid-tumor-syndrome*. In theory, the syndrome could arise as a result of ulcerative proctocolitis leading to the development of polypoid tumors, or in the reverse manner, namely, polypoid tumors leading to the appearance of ulcerative proctocolitis. However, most of the authors I know experienced on this subject deny the existence of essential relations between colitis and cancer.

References

Bargen, J. A. (1961): Dis. Colon Rect., 4, 1.
Bargen, J.A., Sauer, W. G., Sloan, W. P. and Gage, R.P. (1954): Gastroenterology, 26, 32.
Counsell, P. B. and Dukes, C. E. (1952): Brit. J. Surg., 39, 485.
Dawson, I. M. P. and Price-Davies, J. (1959): Brit. J. Surg., 47, 113.
Deucher, F. (1955): Ergebn. Chir. Orthop., 39, 66.
Deucher, F., Widmer, A. and Dippon, R. (1971): Schweiz. med. Wschr., 101, 707.
Demling, L., Hegemann, G., Classen, M. and Emde, J.V.D. (1969): Dtsch. med. Wschr., 6, 247.
Edling, N. P. G. and Eklof, O. A. (1961): Gastroenterology, 41, 465.
Edwards, F. C. and Truelove, S. C. (1964): Gut, 5, 15.
Fahrländer, H. (1966): Dtsch. med. Wschr., 44, 1953.
Farmer, R. G. and Brown, C. H. (1964): Arch. art. Med., 113, 153.
Finkelstein, S. S., Finkelstein, A. and Stein, G. B. (1960): West. J. Surg., 68, 112.
Gallart-Mones, F. and Gallart-Esqerdo, A. (1956): Gastroenterologia, 86, 632.
Girard, M., Bertrand, P., Pouyet, M., Chabanon, R. and Lombard-Platet (1961): Monde méd., 37, 11.
Goldgraber, M. B. and Kirsner, J. B. (1964): Cancer (Philad.), 17, 657.
Ilefti, M. L. (1967): Schweiz. med. Wschr., 97, 1324.
Hickey, R. C. and Tidrick, R. T. (1958): Cancer (Philad.), 11, 35.
Hinton, J. M. (1966): Gut, 7, 427.
Kühn, H. A. and Nägele, E. (1967): In: Ergebnisse der inneren Medizin und Kinderheilkunde, Vol. 25.
    Editors: L. Heimeyer, A.-F. Muller, A. Prader and R. Schoen. Springer-Verlag, Berlin-Göttingen-
    Heidelberg-New York.
Lyons, A. S. and Garlock, J. H. (1951): Gastroenterology, 18, 170.
Miller, B. and Martini, G. A. (1970): Lebensversicher.-Med., 5, 97.
Henning, N. (1967): Dtsch. med. Wschr., 15, 721.
Müller-Wieland, J. (1972): In: Colitis Ulcerosa und Granulomatosa, p. 228. Editors: C. Krauspe,
    K. Müller-Wieland and F. Stelzner. Urban & Schwarzenberg, Munich-Berlin.
Morson, B. C. (1966): Gut 7, 425.
Morson, B. C. and Pang, L. S. C. (1967): Gut 8, 423.
Prèvot, R. (1972): In: Colitis Ulcerosa and Granulomatosa, p. 343. Editors: C. Krauspe, K. Müller-Wie-
    land and F. Stelzner. Urban & Schwarzenberg, Munich-Berlin.
Reifenscheid, M. (1960): Langenbecks Arch. klin. Chir., 293, 558.
Slaney, G. and Brooke, B. N. (1959): Lancet, 2, 694.
Theisinger, W. (1969): Münch. med. Wschr., 22, 1252.
Welch, C. E. and Hedbeng, S. E. (1965): J. Amer. med. Ass., 191, 815.

6. *Organizations of mass screening campaigns*

A new approach to cancer detection*

Alton I. Sutnick, Daniel G. Miller and John W. Yarbro**

*The Institute for Cancer Research and American Oncologic Hospital, The Fox
Chase Center for Cancer and Medical Sciences, Philadelphia, Penn., and
The Preventive Medicine Institute–Strang Clinic, New York, N.Y., U.S.A.*

When cancer detection is part of a concerted effort rather than an incidental part of a general examination, it is more likely that:
1. Cancer will be detected at an earlier stage.
2. A more intensive effort will be made to educate patients with regard to avoidance of agents likely to cause cancer and to instruct them in preventive medicine practice.
3. There will be greater emphasis on research in improved cancer detection techniques.
4. There will be uniform policies for managing suspicious lesions.
5. Risk factors will be analyzed and more intensive diagnostic efforts made when characteristic risk patterns become apparent.

New approaches

The approach to cancer detection might be thought of in terms of programs for malaria control, diabetes detection, and tuberculosis detection programs in the past. All of these have been very specifically aimed toward individual diseases, and have been very successful in accomplishing their goals.

Our proposed examination will be disease-oriented, directed towards specific signs and symptoms of cancer (and some other diseases) in a systematic way. It has been designed to be instituted simultaneously at the Preventive Medicine Institute-Strang Clinic in New York City and the Fox Chase Center for Cancer and Medical Sciences in Philadelphia. It will be aimed principally at a population without complaints; the content of the examination will be determined by each patient's cancer risk factors (Miller, 1972). Following this principle, each patient will be specifically asked about symptoms for each of the diseases for which he is being examined. He will not be asked to describe symptoms which do not relate to these diseases. In addition, we shall have the opportunity for a patient education program in early signs of cancer. For example, each woman will be instructed to perform routine self examination of the breast. The program will provide: (1) a demonstration of the feasibility of providing a high quality cancer screening program at a reasonable cost; (2) a pilot training program for paramedical personnel in techniques of cancer detection; (3) a demonstration of the development of a program in two major institutions in different large cities as an indication of the feasibility of multi-center collaboration; (4) a shared data base permitting information on both groups of patients to be used

* This work was supported by U.S.P.H.S. Grants No. CA-06551, CA-06927 and RR-05539 from the National Institutes of Health and by an appropriation from the Commonwealth of Pennsylvania.

** Present address: National Cancer Institute, National Institutes of Health, Bethesda, Md.

for evaluation of new techniques, results in improved longevity, etc. by both centers; (5) a valuable resource for research on cancer detection and fundamental aspects of the cancer problem; and (6) the development of techniques and an approach that can be applied to other types of programs in health maintenance and disease prevention.

The cancer detection program will be directed principally toward specific malignant tumors against which early treatment is likely to be effective. These include cancer of the skin, larynx, thyroid, breast, large intestine, kidney, prostate, testis, ovary, uterine cervix, and lymphomas. Studies for bronchogenic carcinoma and other tumors may also be included, but these will be principally for research purposes.

The standard examination will include skin, lymph nodes, head and neck, breast, abdomen, pelvic and Pap smear, male genitalia, digital rectal examination, hematocrit, occult blood in stools and urine and, when indicated, proctosigmoidoscopy, indirect laryngoscopy, and mammography. Additional studies will be recommended on the basis of the automated decision logic described below.

Use of paramedical personnel

We plan to utilize paramedical personnel to conduct most aspects of the examination. These personnel will have had previous education in medical services and most will be registered nurses. Paramedical personnel will be instructed in the techniques of physical examination and other examination procedures. Training will include formal courses in anatomy, pathology and diagnostic techniques, examination of patients in the hospital with known tumors, and on-the-job examination of outpatients in the cancer detection program. When the paramedics have demonstrated proficiency in identifying tumors in selected patients they will be given the full responsibility of examining patients, with spot-checking only by physicians.

We intend to compare the efficacy of paramedical examiners with that of physician examiners in the detection of any lesions. Prior to and during the training period of the first group of paramedics, the examinations will have been performed by physicians. Testing of paramedics will be done by using an appropriate control group of patients which will continue to be regularly examined by physicians so that a comparison can be made between these examiners in their effectiveness in detecting malignant and premalignant lesions, as well as non-malignant lesions. This controlled study should allow us to determine the proper role of paramedics in such examinations.

There is currently in progress at the Straub Clinic in Hawaii a program in which the performance of physicians' assistants in proctosigmoidoscopic examinations is being evaluated. There is evidence that nurses with 6 months' additional training can perform pelvic examinations as well and as reliably as fully trained Ob-Gyn residents (Copher, 1971). Preliminary data at PMI-Strang Clinic also indicate that nurses detect breast lesions with an effectiveness equal to that of doctors.

Decision logic

The tests to be performed in screening an individual for a specific tumor will be selected by a computer program based on factors in each patient's history that are associated with a risk of developing that tumor. We are currently developing computer programs to automate the determination of the sequences of considerations leading from medical history and physical findings to decisions for recommended studies and the patient's future management. A diagram for decision-making in detection of lymphoma is illustrated in Figure 1. Suspicious clinical symptoms shift the patient to a physician consultant without need to be examined routinely by the paramedical examiner. Abnormal physical findings would also require consultation, and risk factors (in this case age) determine frequency of re-examination. We have constructed similar decision logic diagrams for other cancers and other diseases in which early diagnosis and treatment are instrumental

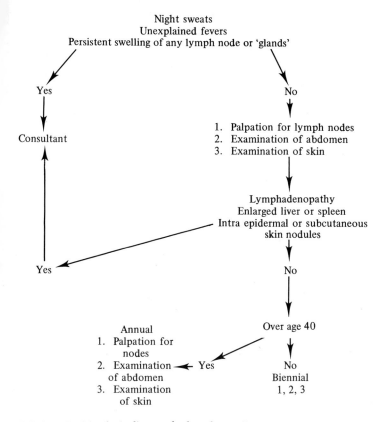

Night sweats
Unexplained fevers
Persistent swelling of any lymph node or 'glands'

Yes   No

Consultant   1. Palpation for lymph nodes
                2. Examination of abdomen
                3. Examination of skin

Lymphadenopathy
Enlarged liver or spleen
Intra epidermal or subcutaneous
skin nodules

Yes   No

Annual   Over age 40
1. Palpation for
    nodes
2. Examination ◄ Yes   No
    of abdomen   Biennial
3. Examination   1, 2, 3
    of skin

FIG. 1   *Decision logic diagram for lymphoma. See text.*

in prolonging survival. The computer integrates the data and generates reports (1) after getting the health history data to indicate what examinations should be performed, and (2) after receiving examination findings to provide recommendations to the patient and an appointment for the next routine visit. Results will be discussed with the patient and a report will be sent to his physician.

Automated data base

The patient's history is self-administered with a standard questionnaire, and is partially automated by use of mark-sense data cards. The data obtained in this history are read into a computer to determine the patient's current status. What examination procedures and laboratory tests should be done on the basis of the history? Can the entire examination be conducted by paramedical personnel or should he be seen by a physician-consultant? These procedures are performed and results are brought back to the same point in the flow diagram. If no additional procedures are indicated, a decision is generated for the disposition of the case. Does the patient need specialized consultation? When should he return for re-examination? Reports of this decision go to the patient, the personal physician of the patient, and to the data base.

    Each patient contributes information to the data base, and the information is under constant surveillance by the control program in the computer. Each day the entire data base may be reviewed and new appointment lists generated. Letters of appointment are sent to each patient whose data indicate that one is necessary; a reply card is sent with the letter. If the reply card does not come back (via the mail input to the system) within a reasonable time, then a sequence of motivating letters are sent until the patient is tracked down. There may be a need for our sending this patient's data to another cancer center and accepting future data on that patient from other centers. When the patient complies with his return appointment instructions, his records are obtained and extracted. The algorithm defining the current status would request a different, usually less extensive history than from a new patient, and fewer tests and examinations may be required. Input from related and compatible data bases will permit periodic revisions of current status and decision algorithms by analysis of risk factors in relation to the development of disease in the patients in the data base.

Research in cancer detection

The research program will include the evaluation of paramedical personnel as mentioned above, and other aspects of applied research. The program would also serve as a laboratory for the evaluation of new techniques of cancer detection, with the hope that simpler, more effective or more economical procedures will be developed. The facility will also be a resource for future, yet unexplored projects. Clinical data, serum and possibly other biological material, will be collected for storage and subsequent analysis, and will provide a basis for clinical and biological research. These data could be valuable in defining the immunologic and genetic characteristics of patients seen in the cancer control program who ultimately develop malignant disease. The combined data would also be useful for environmental and epidemiologic studies when applied to specific populations, and would serve as a data base to which might be added information from other similar clinics.

In conclusion we believe that a system has been devised for cancer detection examinations which can be applied to a large number of people at the lowest cost. This advantage derives from the utilization of computational facilities and trained paramedical personnel. The program has been developed jointly by two institutions in two different cities; thus it may well find broad applications in clinics in many other areas. Furthermore, it provides the opportunity for more meaningful clinical research projects which can be expected to be useful to patients with cancer.

References

Copher, D. E. (1971): Clin. Res., 19/2, 499.
Miller, D. G. (1972): J. Amer. med. Ass., 222/3, 312.

A multiphasic mobile cancer detection unit: Cancer control implications*

J. Lynch, H. T. Lynch, W. Harlan, M. Swartz, J. Marley, L. Meyer, E. Grinnell, C. Kraft, H. Guirgis and A. Krush

Creighton University School of Medicine, Omaha, Neb., U.S.A.

Modern medical practice is oriented toward the patient's presenting complaint and the chief objective is the therapeutic solution of that problem. Early cancer is rarely accompanied by symptoms and for this reason many persons come to medical attention only after they have reached an advanced and often incurable stage. It seems evident that a method for actively seeking out patients before the appearance of early signs and symptoms of malignant disease and bringing those who have positive findings of early disease to treatment is imperative if we are to significantly diminish cancer morbidity and mortality.

We know that the majority of people fail to undergo periodic cancer screening. Their reasons include socioeconomic and educational factors, geographic inaccessibility to a physician's office, transportation problems, and most important, psychological factors, including fear of cancer, denial, fatalism, and misconceptions about cancer such as the fact that many people think that pain is a prerequisite of cancer (Lynch and Krush, 1968). Statistics gathered as part of a joint survey by the American College of Clinical Pathologists and the Cancer Control Division in 1963, revealed that only 15% of American women had ever had a Papanicolaou smear (Leight, 1971). Fortunately, this problem has improved but we are still a long way from the objective of a 'Pap for every woman'.

Carcinoma of the colon is the most frequently occurring visceral cancer among both men and women in the United States with an annual mortality incidence (1972) of 47,000 (American Cancer Society, 1972). No significant improvement in survival has been noted during the past 30 years. Delay is a frequent problem. Most clinical oncologists believe that the best hope at this time rests in *earlier* diagnosis for which we have an extremely simple and effective method for finding up to 70 to 80% of these lesions – namely proctosigmoidoscopy. However, few physicians perform routine, periodic sigmoidoscopic examinations on their asymptomatic patients. Our own preliminary statistics indicate that of 231 individuals questioned only 33 (14%) stated that they had previously been examined by proctosigmoidoscopy.

The establishment of stationary cancer screening clinics (Gilbertsen, 1970) is an important step in motivating the public toward a greater awareness of the importance of the cancer problem. The effectiveness of stationary clinics, however, is diminished as the geographical area which they serve becomes more and more thoroughly screened.

The utility of mobile cancer screening units has already been demonstrated in both England and Japan where a number of mobile cancer screening units are effectively fulfilling a role in screening for cancer of single anatomic sites (uterine cervix or gastric carcinoma but not both in any single unit). Since the fundamental objective of such an endeavor is to induce the patient to present himself for examination, it would seem reasonable to examine him for a number of common malignancies of accessible organs, thus extending the effectiveness of the screening program.

We believe firmly that once people fully accept cancer screening by actually participating in these procedures, they will find it a convenient health maintenance mechanism, and thereafter many will not only avail themselves of these procedures, but will actually ask their family physician to perform them.

* Supported by the Nebraska Regional Medical Program and Nebraska Division, American Society.

This report will pertain primarily to our experiences with a Multiphasic Mobile Cancer Screening Unit which has been funded by the Nebraska Regional Medical Program and administered by Creighton University School of Medicine. So far as we can determine, this mobile unit is the first in the world devoted to screening of *multiple* high-risk cancer target organs.

Description of the unit

Our unit is housed in a 60′ by 12′ custom-built house trailer, with a reception area, a number of examination rooms, lavatories, and X-ray facilities (Figs. 1 and 2). It is hauled to the site by a semi-tractor on a contract basis. A site is chosen which is convenient for the majority of the people residing in the locality. Adequate parking, water, electricity, and sewage facilities are essential. Publicity is coordinated prior to the arrival of the unit by the local physicians and health representatives. Appointments are prescheduled on the basis of 14 to 16 persons per hour, which is the limit of the operating capacity of the unit.

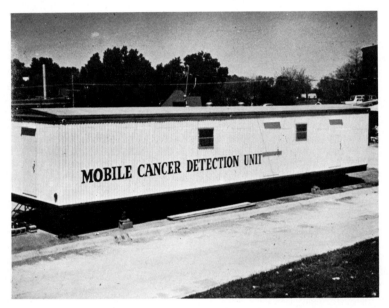

FIG. 1

Procedure

Height, weight, and blood pressure are determined on each patient, after he has completed an automated history form. All patients receive a thorough examination of the oral cavity by a dentist and cytology smears are taken from any suspicious areas. The skin is examined and palpation of the abdomen is performed. All patients over 40 years of age (granting permission) are given a proctosigmoidoscopy examination and all women over age 16 are given both bimanual and speculum pelvic examinations. Papanicolaou smears are taken in each case. Finally, a thorough examination is made of the breasts of each woman and the patient is taught self-breast examination. Mammography is performed on women over 45 years of age, and on younger women if any masses are discovered, if there

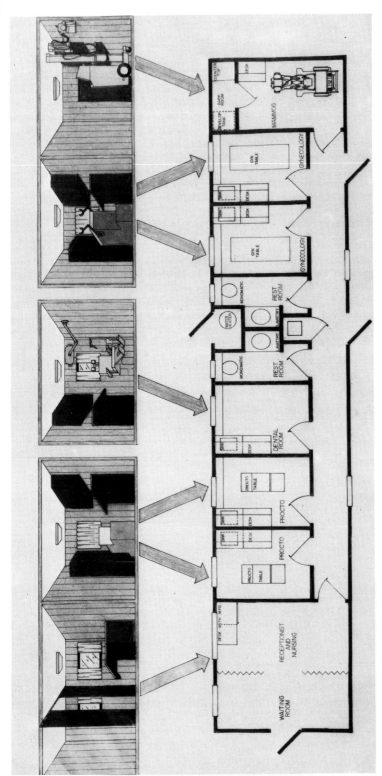

FIG. 2   *Mobile cancer detection unit*

is a past history of breast cancer, chronic cystic mastitis, or if there is a positive family history of breast carcinoma.

A letter summarizing our findings and including pertinent points from the medical history is sent promptly to the patient's family physician. When significant abnormalities are found at the screening examination, the patient is urged to see his physician at once and his physician is called by telephone. Follow-up contacts are made later to determine whether the patient has visited his physician. Unfortunately, sometimes patients refuse to follow through.

Results

Cancer diagnoses

The unit has been in operation approximately 18 months and we have examined about 3,400 patients. These data are shown in Tables 1 and 2. These figures are highly conservative and with respect to visceral cancer are based exclusively on histological diagnoses.

Follow-up is not complete at this time. Nevertheless, we have diagnosed positive visceral cancer in 17 patients (about 1 in every 214 patients screened), and possible skin cancers in 63 patients. Histologic verification is lacking in many cases of skin lesions since the physician often performs curettement or cautery in lieu of obtaining a biopsy. While this number appears to represent an increased incidence of skin cancer over that expected, it

TABLE 1   *Total number screened at each location and number of subjects with abnormal findings*

Town	Total	Male	Female	Total positive	% total positive	Male	Female
Macy	280	78	202	78	27.9	18	60
Winnebago	197	66	131	41	20.8	7	34
Lynch	670	262	408	172	25.7	28	144
Bassett	466	131	335	208	44.6	48	160
South Sioux City	279	84	195	128	45.9	18	110
Tekamah	680	196	484	283	41.6	76	207
Mt. St. Scholastica	306	–	306	136	44.4	–	136
Holdrege	241	62	179	135	56.0	36	99
Omaha	220	66	154	119	54.0	31	88

TABLE 2   *Malignant neoplasms detected at screening examinations: malignant neoplasms confirmed*

	Skin and lymphatics	Penis	Lip	Colon	Prostate	Breast	Lung	Stomach	Thyroid
Males	*	1	1	1	2	–	1	1	–
Females	*	–	–	4	–	5	–	–	1
Total		1	1	5	2	5	1	1	1

Total malignancies – 17

* Many skin cancers (more than 63)

TABLE 3   *Other abnormalities detected through the cancer screening program*

Circulatory system	No. of subjects	Oral cavity and larynx	No. of subjects	Skin	No. of subjects	Colon and rectum	No. of subjects
Elevated casual blood pressure (140/90 or greater)	629	Leukoplakia	72	Actinic keratosis	113	Polyps	55
				Possible skin cancer	63	Ulceration	9
Significant hypertension	145	Irritation and inflammation	70	Papilloma	96	Internal hemorrhoids	50
		Hyperplasia	50	Enlarging moles nevus	57	Proctitis	9
		Fibroma	22				
		Papilloma	17	Possible melanoma	25		
		Mass	21				

is not too surprising when one considers that the population which has been screened was white and of North European and Scandinavian extraction, many of whom were involved in outdoor occupations such as ranching and farming.

The colon cancers were diagnosed on proctosigmoidoscopy. None were within reach of the digital finger on rectal examination. The prostate lesions were diagnosed on digital examination. The breast cancers were found on palpation of the patient's breast. Mammographies were interpreted as negative in each case. False negatives have been a problem with mammography and have pointed out the need to perform thermography concurrently as an adjunctive diagnostic measure.

We have not routinely performed chest X-rays as part of our cancer screening program. However, when a significant history of lung problems or physical findings consistent with broncho-pulmonary disease were found, chest X-rays were performed. One such patient was a '3-pack-a-day' cigarette smoker who gave a history of weight loss and a productive cough with occasional hemoptysis. We performed a chest X-ray which revealed a large mass in the right upper lobe of the lung consistent with bronchogenic carcinoma. A lobectomy was performed on this patient confirming the diagnosis of bronchogenic carcinoma. It should be remembered that our concern is the screening of allegedly *well* patients and in the majority of patients subsequently proven to have cancer symptoms were lacking.

Other diagnoses

While cancer screening is our major mission, many general medical diagnosis have been encountered whose pathology has had no direct relationship to cancer. Among these diagnoses were: hypertension, congestive heart failure, obesity, and diabetes mellitus. Abnormalities which have been detected through our cancer screening and which require further evaluation are presented in Tables 3 and 4.

It is not practicable to attempt to estimate the percentage of the adult population who came for screening examination from all of the communities surrounding the towns in which the mobile unit is placed. However, we were able to obtain this figure for a small community composed of 533 persons (264 males and 269 females), 360 of whom (67.7%) are over age 18. 187 persons from this township were examined in the mobile unit, or 52% of the adult population of this township which contains about one-ninth of the population of the county in which the town is situated.

TABLE 4   *Other abnormalities detected through the cancer screening program*

Male genital organs	No. of subjects	Female genital organs	No. of subjects	Breast	No. of subjects
Significant prostate hypertrophy	42	Possible uterine fibroids	47	Cystic mastitis	136
Prostate nodules	4	Cervical polyps	63	Nodules	245
		Vaginitis	49	Inverted or retracted nipple	34
		Chronic cervical inflammation or erosion	175	Discharge	14
		Enlarged adnexa (ovary)	14		
		Genital prolapse	28		
		Cervical or nabothian cysts	54		

Cost

Cost is a major consideration in any medical screening program. Cancer screening is no exception. Neuberger (1966) estimated that a $9 return is given for every dollar spent in screening programs for cervical cancer. This is reflected by reduced expenditure for medical care, increased patient productivity, and the saving of life itself, as a result of earlier diagnosis.

Estimate of cost for cancer screening operations on a per patient basis is difficult to assess with precision since it involves the initial cost of equipment, staff salaries, and supplies. Therefore, we are presenting our costs roughly by categories (Table 5).

TABLE 5   *Cost accounting*

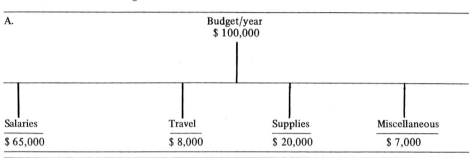

A.			Budget/year $ 100,000		
Salaries		Travel		Supplies	Miscellaneous
$ 65,000		$ 8,000		$ 20,000	$ 7,000

B.	Individual costs
Estimated cost for:	
Males	$ 26.60
Females	30.50
Estimated cost for:	
Mammography	3.25
Proctosigmoidoscopy	1.65
Pelvic examination	0.65
Dental examination	0.20
Stationary supplies	0.50

Education

The educational impact of our unit will be difficult to assess. For example, the number of breast cancers which may later be discovered by women who were taught self-breast examinations, the number who gave up smoking, and those who took precautions from excessive sun exposure may only be realized after many years.

Discussion and summary

We have attempted to give a brief accounting of our 18 months' experience in the screening of some 3,000 patients in a Mobile Cancer Detection Unit. Our follow-up at this time does not permit a critical, detailed analysis of results; however, our preliminary findings indicate that we are able to detect cancer effectively in asymptomatic patients. We firmly believe that Mobile Multiphasic Cancer Detection units provide a positive approach to cancer control and merit trial in other areas of the world. We believe that support for this need is amply demonstrated in a 1969 report of a World Health Organization Expert Committee which concluded that: 'A substantial proportion of cancer patients can be cured and the number being cured at present could be doubled if patients could reach a treatment center earlier than they do; and one of the most effective methods of cancer prevention is the early detection and diagnosis of premalignant conditions, followed by prompt treatment.'

The report emphasizes that programs should consider needs of the inhabitants of the regions being screened and most important, should consider the prevalence of cancer of specific sites (*high risk groups*), the availability of reliable detection techniques, materials, and manpower resources, and the socio-economic education, and cultural level of the population. The application of epidemiological methods has demonstrated that the frequency of different kinds of cancer differs widely from country to country. Moreover, within each country, different sections of the population have been shown at risk in varying degrees. The high risk groups lend themselves ideally to screening programs.

References

American Cancer Society (1972): Cancer Facts and Figures. National Headquarters, American Cancer Society, New York, N.Y.
Gilbertsen, V. A. (1970): Geriatrics, 25/10, 149.
Leight, L. E. (1971): Amer. Fam. Phycn., 4/5, 137.
Lynch, H. T. and Krush, A. J. (1968): Arch. environm. Hlth, 17/8, 204.
Neuberger, M. G. (1966): Detection and Prevention of Chronic Disease Utilizing Multiphasic Health Screening Techniques. A Report of the Subcommittee on the Health of the Elderly of the Special Committee on Aging. Washington, D.C., United States Senate, 89th Congress, 2nd Session. U.S. Government Printing Office.
World Health Organization (1969): Wld Hlth Org. techn. Rep. Ser., No. 422.

Delay deters cancer detection

Anne J. Krush* and Henry T. Lynch

Creighton University School of Medicine, Omaha, Neb., U.S.A.

During the past 10 years our research group has been involved in medical genetic studies of a large number of families with the cancer family syndrome, which is characterized by: (1) increased incidence of adenocarcinoma, predominantly endometrial and colonic adenocarcinoma, (2) increased incidence of multiple primary malignant neoplasms, (3) early age at onset of carcinoma, and (4) autosomal dominant mode of inheritance. In the course of these investigations we have noted repeatedly that even though cancer had occurred in more than 25% of family members, many of those who were at risk for cancer failed to seek medical consultation for signs and symptoms of cancer (Krush et al., 1965; Lynch et al., 1968). This observation led us to a study of the reasons for delay in seeking medical care not only by susceptible members of cancer families, but we also investigated reasons for delay among a group of cancer patients who were receiving therapy for cancer of the breast at a cancer institute. In addition we selected a group of post-menopausal women who had been graduated from a woman's college 30 years previously, to ascertain their attitudes toward health maintenance examinations (Krush, 1971).

Arbitrarily we defined delay as a period of 3 months or longer between the time an individual first noted a sign or symptom of cancer and the time he sought medical advice. We defined physician delay as a period of 3 months or longer from the time a patient sought medical attention and the time that specific treatment for cancer was instituted.

Cancer family 'N'

The proband in Family 'N' was ascertained at the Omaha Veterans Administration Hospital at which time it was learned that many members of his family, including 6 brothers and sisters (of 12) had received diagnoses of cancer. Permission was obtained from interested family members to conduct a genealogical and medical study of the entire family. This study was later reported in the medical literature (Lynch et al., 1966; Lynch and Krush, 1967).

A number of field visits have been made to the northwestern area of Missouri where many of the family members reside in order to interview them, perform physical examinations, and obtain blood and other biological specimens for biochemical and immunological studies. At these visits we have been afforded ample opportunities to evaluate the emotions, attitudes, fears, worries, and misconceptions about the disease cancer, among the family members and to note the persistent refusal of some members of the family ever to attend a field visit. These attitudes, which were directly related to delay in seeking medical care may be summed up as follows:

1. Fear, which includes fear of cancer, fear of pain, fear of death following a prolonged and painful illness, fear of mutilation, fear of an unknown outcome following treatment, and fear that a doctor may consider the individual a hypochondriac.

2. Denial or an unwillingness to believe that one has symptoms of cancer. One member of the family stated that he had frequent abdominal pains, but so long as he could keep on working on his farm, he did not want to take time off to consult his physician.

---

* Present address: The Moore Clinic, Johns Hopkins Hospital, Baltimore, Md., U.S.A.

3.   Fatalism (including hopelessness and depression) was a prevalent attitude in this family. This attitude among family members at risk for cancer appeared to be in direct proportion to the number of their close relatives who had had an unfavorable outcome following treatment for cancer. One member, noting that her aunt had developed breast cancer at age 91, said that 'it will get *all* of us if we live long enough!'.

4.   A constant misconception about the diagnosis of cancer was that pain was a necessary accompaniment of cancer. This was especially true among women with breast cancer. They could feel and see unusual 'lumps and bumps', and note changes in appearance of their breasts, but if they felt no pain, they thought that theirs was a benign condition and therefore did not see their physician often till late in the course of the disease.

5.   Communication problems between the patient and his physician were also related to delay. Some members of this family seemed to think that the doctor should be able to determine the nature of one's illness by a physical examination alone. In a stoical manner, they would submit to the examination but would not tell the physician about their symptoms. Others feared that if they discussed all of their 'aches and pains' with the doctor he would consider them neurotic. They told us that they did not want to take too much of the doctor's time because he was already overloaded with work and patients. Some patients felt that communication was difficult because the doctor spoke in 'medical language', using medical terms which they could not understand, but they were too embarrassed to ask for a clearer definition of their problem or condition. Some physicians gave even the cancer susceptible members of the family the impression that preventive health maintenance examinations either were not necessary or took too much time away from their physically ill patients. Other physicians appeared to share with their patients a feeling of hopelessness about cancer. Therefore it behooves the physician to examine his own feelings about this disease and to work them out in such a way that he can offer positive assistance to his cancer patient (Gibson, 1964).

A series of patients with breast cancer

Two groups of patients who were receiving treatment for breast cancer were interviewed at a cancer institute. Group 1 included women who had received their diagnosis at an early stage of the disease and for whom surgery had been recommended. Group 2 included women who were receiving palliative treatment for breast cancer which had been diagnosed at a later stage. When these 2 groups of women were compared it was found that group 2 delayed much longer than group 1 before seeking medical care for their breast problems. Again, we found the same reasons for delay as we had found among the member of the 'N' cancer family. In addition, the threat of the loss of part of one's body and a part that is intimately connected with one's sexual life (Menainger, 1938) was found to be another potent reason for delay among this group of women.

College educated post-menopausal women

Perhaps the most striking misconception which was found among a group of 216 women college graduates was that 65 members (30%) responding to our questionnaire stated that they began to have regular annual health maintenance examinations at age 40 and 10 women (5%) began at age 50. The age of 40 to 45 was most frequently suggested to these women by their physicians and other paramedical personnel as the proper age at which to begin these examinations, thus overlooking the fact that cervical cancer occurs at younger ages, and that susceptible members of cancer families are likely to develop cancer in their thirties.

Factors which influenced these women to plan for regular health maintenance examinations included: (1) physician reminders (which were used by only 26% of their physicians), (2) increased incidence of cancer in the woman's family (21%), (3) menopause (16%), (4) influence of mass media (14%), (5) already a regular family habit (25%), and (6) medical background in the family (8%).

Fear (44%), denial or attempt to ignore symptoms (20%), fatalism (6%), dislike or distrust of the physician or his method of treatment (3%), modesty, discomfort or repugnance of the type of examination (5%), and apathy, depression, etc. (3%) were the most frequent psychological or emotional reasons given for delay in planning for regular health maintenance examinations. Only 3% of these women thought that pain was a requisite for the diagnosis of cancer; only 9% were unaware of some of the signs and symptoms of cancer, and only 1% had a false sense of security because there was no family history of cancer. Physician delay (4%), finances (5%), and 'too busy to take time for an annual physical examination' (20%), were material or extrinsic reasons given for delay or unwillingness to plan for regular health maintenance examinations.

Although approximately half of the members of this college educated group of women had been taught self breast examination, only a small number practised it, and many of those practised it only infrequently. A few stated that their physicians preferred that they not perform this examination, but that this procedure should be performed once a year by the physician. Other physicians did not teach this procedure unless requested to do so by the patient.

Some women expressed confusion about what kind of a doctor should be consulted for an annual physical examination. During the child-bearing years they consulted obstetricians. Pediatricians cared for their children. Now, with the menopause they wondered if they should consult a general practitioner, a gynecologist, or a physician in internal medicine. They felt that some specialists only examined the part of the body of their specialty. Therefore the expense involved in consulting several specialists was becoming exorbitant. A few women expressed the thought that if cancer screening examination could be included in health insurance plans such as Blue Cross and Blue Shield, then many women would take advantage of this opportunity for a regular checkup.

We noted in our own recent cancer screening program which was funded by the Nebraska Regional Medical Program (Lynch et al., 1972) that women of all socioeconomic levels and of all ages (16-89) came spontaneously for cancer screening tests. Some told us that their own physician did not perform these tests and they hesitated to ask him for them. Others stated that it was less embarrassing to have this checkup when it was performed by an 'outside' group and many other members of their community were having the same tests performed. Again it was noted both in the college group of women and among the persons screened at a cancer screening unit that communication problems often existed between the patient and her own family physician or specialist.

We concluded from these studies that communication is a 2-way street. It is absolutely essential for the patient to communicate not only his physical complaints but also his attitudes and feelings about the disease in his family to his physician, and important also for the physician to explain medical matters to his patient in a empathetic manner and in terms that the patient can understand, so that misconceptions about the disease cancer can be set right, and thus minimize the delay problem.

References

Gibson, R. (1964): Brit. med. J., 2, 965.

Krush, A. J. (1971): In: Cancer and You, pp. 238-259. Editor: H. T. Lynch. Charles C. Thomas Company, Springfield, Ill.

Krush, A. J., Lynch, H. T. and Magnuson, C. W. (1965): Amer. J. med. Sci., 249, 432.

Lynch, H. T., Harlan, W., Swartz, M., Marley, J., Becker, W., Lynch, J., Kraft, C. A. and Krush, A. J. (1972): Cancer (Philad.), 30, 774.

Lynch, H. T. and Krush, A. J. (1967): Gastroenterology, 53, 517.

Lynch, H. T. and Krush, A. J. (1968): Arch. environm. Hlth, 17, 204.

Lynch, H. T., Shaw, M. W., Magnuson, C. W., Larsen, A. L. and Krush, A. J. (1966): Arch. intern. Med., 117, 206.

Menainger, K. (1938): Man Against Himself. Harcourt, Brace and Co., New York, N.Y.

Early detection cancer screening: 8 years incidence and findings in 10 cooperative rural settlements

F. Ch. Izsak, H. J. Brenner and J. Medalie

Detection and Follow-up Clinic, Government Hospital, Jaffa; Department of Oncology, Chaim Sheba Medical Center, Tel Hashomer; and Department of Family Medicine, Medical School, Tel-Aviv University, Tel-Aviv, Israel

By early detection is meant that the growth process is found when it is still asymptomatic and the patient has no complaints, or signs directly referable to the growth (Izsak et al., 1972). On the assumption that early diagnosis of cancer prolongs and even saves lives (Day, 1969; Gilbersten, 1970; Hichcock and Sullivan, 1961; Iszak et al., 1972; Jafarey, 1970; Kessler, 1968), an early detection cancer programme was initiated in 1961 based on a special cancer multiphasic screening clinic attached to the Donolo Hospital in Jaffa.

Population groups of closed rural communities — cooperative settlements (kibbutzim) — were studied. The reasons for selecting these groups were as follows: *(a)* they constituted a relatively stable population; *(b)* their way of life produced a uniformly high socio-economic standard with the exclusion of individual economic problems; *(c)* their high sense of community participation; and *(d)* the curative care of these settlements is uniformly good with comprehensive medical records and information available on all members, so that follow-up of detected and undetected cases would be easy and accurate.

The study was set up with the aim of finding the answers to the following 4 questions:

1. What is the incidence and distribution of cancer in this population and what proportion of these tumours were accessible to the methods employed in their detection?
2. Can a total population be covered by a screening programme for cancer?
3. Do the results of such a programme concerning participation and positive findings, justify the time and effort invested into it?
4. Does a periodic screening programme induce the public and the primary physician to accept the annual (periodic) screening as a routine aspect of their medical care?

The Central Tumour Board responsible for this study consisted of surgeons, pathologists, radiotherapists, chemotherapists, gynaecologists, radiologists, internists, family physicians and other specialists invited as deemed necessary. The examining group visited 10 settlements at least 4 times each during the 8-year period between 1965–1972. Every member of the community above the age of 35 was invited to participate. The clinical examination consisted of inspection and palpation with particular emphasis on the skin, mouth, tongue, lip, neck, throat, breasts, lymph nodes, abdomen, genitals, rectal and vaginal examinations. Abnormal findings were recorded and the patient was referred to the regional specialist for further evaluation. The results of these investigations were then sent to the examining team. In addition, the central team was also notified if any member of the settlements involved was shown to have cancer at any time during the above period, irrespective of whether they had participated in the screening programme or not.

TABLE 1   *Cancer screening in ten settlements*

Settlement	Total No. of population	Max. No. registered for examination	Yearly attendance								Total No. examined
			1965	1966	1967	1968	1969	1970	1971	1972	
E.HA.	700	243	178	180	165	168	160	173	151	153	1328
T.YO.	600	202	158	141	o	101	o	96	88	o	585
KIN.	660	222	o	150	o	o	121	61	104	o	435
DAG.	600	208	133	o	o	143	o	146	120	o	542
E.SH.	640	210	134	150	o	126	143	o	o	83	636
MA.Z	460	210	159	o	178	151	166	99	22	64	840
E.CH.	800	263	o	166	150	113	o	o	113	o	542
G.YA.	300	106	95	73	o	69	82	45	46	50	460
G.CH.	530	210	o	171	117	131	62	93	99	o	673
NGB.	600	180	73	123	119	92	114	115	75	107	818
Total	5890	2054	930	1154	729	1094	848	828	818	457	6859

o = No examinations performed

Results

From Table 1, it can be noted that the total population of the 10 settlements here reviewed was 5,890 with a total of 2,054 individuals participating in the screening. Except for occasional younger people, the vast majority of these 2,054 were adults aged 35 and over at the time of examination.

Participation in screening examinations

Over the 8-year period, the 10 villages were visited 58 times, varying from 4 to 8 visits with an average of 5.8 visits per community. For all practical purposes nearly every adult aged 35 and over was examined at least once. If each of the 2,054 adults would have participated each time the screening was performed at his/her settlement, there would have been 11,688 examinations. In reality there were 6,859, i.e. a participation of 58.7% over the entire period.

TABLE 2   *Results of screening of 2,054 subjects by settlements (1965–1972)*

| | | | | Malignant tumours | | | |
| | | | | Accessible sites | | Non* | |
Settlement	No pathological findings	False positive	Benign tumours	Found	False* negative	accessible sites	Total examinations
E.HA.	1231	20	74	3	2	1	1328
T.YO.	534	6	41	4	0	0	585
KIN.	391	12	30	2	1	1	435
DAG.	501	10	26	5	2	2	542
E.SH.	598	13	22	3	1	1	636
MA.Z.	797	7	34	2	1	3	840
E.CH.	492	15	31	4	2	0	542
G.YA.	427	8	21	4	0	0	460
G.CH.	637	4	30	2	4	2	673
N.GB.	770	10	34	4	1	1	818
Total	6378	105	343	33	14	11	6859

* These figures are included in the column 'No pathological findings' at screening and therefore should not be added to the 'Total examinations'.

Results of the screening examinations (Table 2)

Of the 6,859 examinations performed there was no pathology detected in 6,378 (i.e. 92%). Of the other 8% (481 examinations) positive screenees, 33 were found to have malignant tumour within one year after the screening examination (false negative) while a further 11 developed malignancies in sites that are not accessible on clinical screening examination.

Total community cancer incidence (Table 3)

There were 103 malignant tumours among the 2,054 adults over the 8 years i.e., an

TABLE 3   *Total community cancer by settlements (1965–1972)*

| Settlement | Attenders | | | Non attenders | | Total |
| | Accessible sites | | Non accessible sites | Accessible sites | Non accessible sites | |
	Found	False negative				
E.HA	3	2	1	3	2	11
T.YO.	4	o	o	2	1	7
KIN.	2	1	1	1	1	6
DAG.	5	2	2	2	2	13
E.SH.	3	1	1	4	1	10
MA.Z.	2	1	3	4	2	12
E.CH.	4	2	o	1	1	8
G.YA.	4	o	o	2	1	7
G.CH.	2	4	2	3	9	20
NGB.	4	1	1	2	1	9
Total	33	14	11	24	21	103
Male	19	7	4	14	8	52
Female	14	7	7	10	13	51

incidence of 5% over the entire period or an approximate annual average of 0.6% or 6 malignancies of all types per 1000 adults aged 35 and over per year. The average annual number of malignant tumours found per 1000 adults persons varied widely between kibbutzim from 12/1000 in G. Ch. to 3/1000 in E. Ch.

The approximate average annual incidence of all malignant tumours of the total population (all ages) was 103 found in 5,890 people over 8 years, i.e. an average annual incidence of 2.2 malignancies per 1000 people of all ages.

Malignancies by site

Table 4 shows that 32 (31%) of the 103 carcinomata were growths of the skin with the commonest being 11 malignancies of the breast and 7 of the prostate, with the others spread through a number of different systems.

Of these 103 tumours, 71 occurred in sites that are accessible to a clinical examination. Of these however, 14 occurred within one year after a screening examination (false negative) at which no sign of them had been detected.

24 malignancies in accessible sites were found among non-attenders. The latter are defined as those in whom a cancer was found more than 1 year after their last screening examination or anyone under the age of 35 years. Of these malignancies, 10 were on the skin, 4 in breast, 3 on lip and others spread among various sites.

The sites not accessible to clinical screening examinations produced 32 tumours, of which 21 were in non-attenders as defined here. These 32 included 5 of the lungs, 6 in pancreas/liver area and 4 were miscellaneous sarcomata.

Benign tumours (Table 5)

There was a total of 343 benign tumours recorded of which 135 were operated on. Almost a third of the total were found in the breast while another approximately 20% each were found in the male and female genital (excluding breast) tracts.

TABLE 4   *Total community cancers by site (1965–1972)*

Site	Attenders Accessible site Found	Attenders Accessible site False negative	Attenders Non accessible site	Non attenders Accessible site	Non attenders Non accessible site	Total
Skin	13	9		10		32
Lip				3		3
Buccal mucosa	1					1
Tongue	1					1
Parotid		1				1
Thyroid				1		1
Breast	6	1		4		11
Lung			1		4	5
Oesophagus					2	2
Stomach			2		1	3
Colon	1		1		1	3
Rectum	1	1		1		3
Pancreas–liver			2		4	6
Kidney			1		1	2
Bladder			2		1	3
Prostate	4	1		2		7
Testicle				1		1
Ovary	1	1		1		3
Uterus	2			1		3
Malign. lymphoma	3		1		2	6
Leukaemia			1		1	2
Soft tissue sa					4	4
Total	33	14	11	24	21	103

Looking at Tables 4 and 5 together shows that of the 111 breast lumps detected at screening, 53 were operated on (1 of 2) and 7 turned out to be malignant, i.e. 1 of 16 breast tumours found were malignant and 1 of every 7 biopsies was malignant. There were 75 prostatic hypertrophies deemed abnormal of which 22 were operated on and 5 found to be malignant (1 in 15 of all hypertrophies and 1 in 4 operated cases). The rectum produced 11 tumours (polyps, etc.) of which 10 were operated on and 2 found to be malignant.

The variation of malignancy rates between settlements is quite striking but should be accepted with caution because of the small numbers.

Discussion

Returning to the basic questions we set out to answer, the first one was: What is

TABLE 5   *Benign tumours found in screening of 2054 subjects by site (1965–1972)*

Site	Finding	Operated			No operation			Grand total
		Male	Female	Total	Male	Female	Total	
Skin	Naevus, verruca	2	3	5	5	3	8	
	Fibroma, neurofibroma		2	2	1	2	3	
	Haemangioma	1	1	2		2	2	
	Lipoma	1	3	4	3	2	5	
		4	9	13	9	9	18	31
Lip	Cyst				1	2	3	
	Leukoplakia				3		3	
					4	2	6	6
Tongue	Papilloma	1	1	2	2		2	
		1	1	2	2		2	4
Thyroid	Nodular goitre		2	2		2	2	
			2	2		2	2	4
Breast	Cystadenoma		22	22		4	4	
	Fibroadenoma		16	16		6	6	
	Cystic mastopathy		8	8		48	48	
			46	46		58	58	104
Female genitals	Uterus myomatosus		17	17		25	25	
	Endo/parametritis		13	13		8	8	
	Cervical polyp		5	5		1	1	
			35	35		34	34	69
Male genitals	Hypertrophy of prostate	17		17	53		53	
	Hydrocele	4		4				
		21		21	53		53	74
Lymphatic system	Unspecified lymph node hypertrophy	3	2	5	11	7	18	
		3	2	5	11	7	18	23
Rectum	Polyp	3	5	8	1		1	
	Haemorrhoids	2	4	6	10	3	13	
		5	9	14	11	3	14	28
Total		33	102	135	90	115	205	343

the incidence and distribution of cancer in this population and what part of these tumours were accessible to the methods of examination employed? The average annual incidence found here was 2.2/1000 in the total population and 6.1/1000 among the group screened above the age of 35. It could also be concluded, that 70% of all cancer cases which emerged in this population evolved in organs accessible for diagnosis, by the methods employed here. Our second question was, whether a total population can be covered by a screening programme for cancer? In the present example, where the attendance was voluntary, less than 60% of those eligible participated in the programme, despite the very favourable conditions both on behalf of the settlements and the examining teams highly conducive for the success of such a screening scheme. In view of these data the pertinence of our third question – namely 'do the results of such a programme justify the expenditure in time and effort' – is in the affirmative. Notwithstanding the incomplete attendance noted here and despite the 14 false negative results, it is our strong feeling that the answer to this last question is in the affirmative. The arguments in favour of this answer are as follows: Of the 103 cancers detected, 71 were found in sites accessible by the methods employed here. All the cancer cases uncovered, even in those patients who did not attend the screening programmes regularly, were in stage 1 or 2, hence they were feasible for radical surgery. To our last question — whether a periodic screening programme educates the public and the primary physician towards the acceptance of annual screening as a routine aspect of their medical care — the answer is again a positive one. This conclusion is strongly supported by the observation that the so-called non-attenders came to the physician for advice at a relatively early stage of their disease.

The success of cancer therapy today is largely dependant upon its detection at an early stage of the disease. The present study has served to demonstrate, that this aim can be achieved by schemes similar to those described here. It seems to us that the screening approach by itself is not the real answer to this problem. Under ideal conditions it should be a supplement to the family physician. The latter can himself perform the screening by examining 2 subjects daily, which would not be an undue strain on his daily schedule. This would probably be the ideal method of early detection.

Summary

From 1965–1972 an annual detection screening programme was carried out, as part of the Donolo Hospital Early Detection Clinic, on the over 35-year-old members of a stable agricultural population (kibbuts). The screened individuals were of equal socio-economic status with excellent medical services. 6,859 examinations were carried out in this period. The programme covered all the physically accessible sites (no laboratory assistance), and the examinations took place in the medical centres of the settlements. All adults were examined at least once with the overall coverage being 58.7%. There were 103 cancer cases found over the 8-year period, both by screening and the ordinary medical care service. This gave an approximate incidence of 2.2 malignancies/1000 of all ages and 6.1/1000 adults aged 35 and over. The common cancers were of the skin, breast and prostate while 70% of all cancers over the 8-year period were in sites accessible to a simple clinical screening examination. It is stressed that a screening programme should be an integral part of the medical care services with the participation of the primary or family physician.

References

Day, E. (1969): J. chron. Dis., 16, 397.
Gilbersten, V. A. (1970): Geriatrics, 25, 149.
Hichcock, C. R. and Sullivan, W. H. (1961): Surgery, 39, 54.
Izsak, F. Ch., Brenner, H. J. and Cohen-Haddad, R. (1972): Israel J. med. Sci., 8, 972.
Jafarey, N. A. (1970): J. Pak. med. Ass., 20, 101.
Kessler, E. (1968): Med. Klin., 63, 1854.

Cancer control in the People's Republic of China

Haitung King

National Cancer Institute, Bethesda, Md. and Georgetown University, Washington, D.C., U.S.A.

Since the formation of the People's Republic, the Chinese government has been determined to 'Give Cancer Its Death Blow.' Reviewed briefly below are reports of China's achievements in cancer prevention, therapy, and research, supplemented by selected epidemiologic findings. Hopefully, this report, despite its incompleteness, can contribute to our knowledge about the control in the People's Republic of a significant chronic disease, which was reportedly the number one killer in Shanghai (Sidel, 1972).

The 'Anti-Cancer Shock Brigade' model

As with most other Chinese public health programs, the reported success of the anti-cancer campaign was primarily attributable to the operational model adopted, i.e., mass social mobilization. As early as the mid-1950's, a Youth Anti-Cancer Shock Brigade was organized. The Brigade was sponsored by the Second Communist Youth League Branch of the preclinical departments in the Academy of Medical Sciences (Peking), and its members came mainly from the pathology department. The organization of the Brigade led to the establishment of the Committee for Cancer Research in the Academy and similar committees in several cities, as well as the formulation of an extensive 5-year plan for the conquest of cancer.

The Brigade's major contribution was the analysis of data from microscopic examinations. In 1958 the Brigade examined 27,000 tumors among 150,000 surgical specimens. These came largely from the former Peking Union Medical College and spanned a 40-year period. Motivated by patriotism, Brigade members worked for 8 days around the clock to complete the examinations and tabulations. Several other medical colleges followed suit, including the First Shanghai Medical College whose students completed in 20 days a similar analysis of 47,922 tumor cases from 220,650 specimens. These specimens spanned a 30-year period. The number of tumor cases examined at these colleges was estimated to be over 100,000.

The analytical findings have added much to our knowledge of cancer morphology in China to date and are particularly useful for epidemiologic research. Published reports give frequency distribution of broad cancer sites and/or histologic types by sex, with limited tabulations by age and other characteristics. A summary of morphologic types from Peking data appears elswhere (King, 1972). An apparently low frequency of Hodgkin's disease was found in both Peking and Shanghai data, as shown in Table 1 which presents the proportionate distribution of examined cases.

Screening, survey and registration programs

In accordance with the Chinese government's announced determination to eliminate cancer, screening and survey programs were carried out feverishly. During 1958-1960, mass examinations for cervical cancer were launched in 20 cities from coast to inland, and in

TABLE 1   *Frequency distribution by sex of primary cancer sites, Peking and Shanghai*

Primary site	Peking 1917–1957		Shanghai 1927–1957	
	Male	Female	Male	Female
Cancer, all sites	N = 7,446	N = 9,996	N = 10,000	N = 18,824
Buccal cavity and pharynx	9.6	2.8	16.6	2.0
Esophagus	7.1	1.1	5.6	0.8
Stomach	5.2	1.0	9.2	1.7
Intestines	4.5	1.5	7.7	3.1
Liver, primary	1.2	0.2	3.2	0.6
Lung	0.6	0.2	1.8	0.3
Breast	0.7	14.3	0.2	11.5
Cervix uteri	i.a.	44.5	i.a.	52.8
Corpus uteri	i.a.	2.0	i.a.	3.9
Ovary	i.a.	2.0	i.a.	2.4
Prostate	0.4	i.a.	0.2	i.a.
Penis	12.1	i.a.	4.3	i.a.
Hodgkin's Disease	0.9	0.2	1.4	0.2

i.a. Inapplicable
Source: Adopted from King (unpublished data)

2 cities in Inner Mongolia. Preceded by an extensive educational campaign, the examinations were conducted in factories, schools, and neighborhood hospitals, or at people's homes in the evening. It was reported that 1,693 cases were detected among 1,169,949 examinees and that detected cases per 100,000 examinees ranged from 18 for Canton to 100 for Shanghai, 290 for Tianjin, 612 for Changsha and 1,382 for Sining. The detected cases per 100,000 examinees for 51 in situ and 248 invasive cases were, respectively, 72.8 and 302.1 (under age 40), 129.6 and 604.7 (age 40-49), and 117.1 and 729.6 (age 50 and over).

A survey of the prevalence of esophageal cancer was conducted in selected areas in 4 northern provinces (Honan, Shansi, Hopei, Shantung) during 1958-1960 and covered a population of 17 million. All persons over age 30 were interviewed in both urban areas and rural communes. Special attention was directed to persons who complained of difficulty in swallowing. Roentgenologic examination with barium meal was given to individuals suspected of having the disease. Annual follow-up surveys in 2 consecutive years were initiated in Yangch'uan County, Shansi and for an indefinite period in Lin County, Honan. An extremely high frequency was reported for Lin County during the period 1959-1970.

It is not possible to estimate for any time-period the total number of persons covered under various screening and survey programs in the entire country. The size must be enormously large considering the four million figure reported for four provinces and eight cities alone during 1958-1959.

Cancer registries are known to have been established in several areas, notably the Shanghai Tumor Registry of 1958. Published data on 19,000 registered malignancies in Shanghai include frequency distribution and/or incidence rates by primary site and sex. The incidence figures for selected sites are reported under epidemiologic findings.

A special registry for gynecological malignancies was inaugurated in 1957 in the Nanking area which has a population of some 1,500,000. In contrast to previous findings on Asian populations, the ratios for choriocarcinoma and malignant mole to live births were low for this area, according to the authors. They were 1 to 21,957 and 1 to 43,914, respectively.

Research and clinical activities

The importance of cancer research in the People's Republic of China was clearly indicated in the national 12-year plan for scientific development proclaimed in 1956. The proliferation of agencies devoted to cancer studies showed the impact of the program. In experimental tumor research alone there were about 24 agencies engaged in research activities until 1959. These were the Tumor Institute, the Research Institute of Experimental Biology, the Research Institute of Pharmacology, and the Research Institute of Experimental Medicine, all in the Academy of Medical Sciences. Research in epidemiology of cancer was conducted mainly by the various medical colleges throughout the country.

Reports of research findings generally appear in the Chinese Journals of Pathology, Obstetrics and Gynecology, Surgery, and Radiology (all in Chinese, with an occasional abstract in English), and in the Chinese Medical Journal (English and Chinese editions, articles non-duplicating). There is no journal specializing in cancer. A review of a 1962 monograph consisting of 33 papers submitted to the Eighth International Cancer Congress indicate a wide range of interest in both experimental and clinical oncology. These include biology of cancerous cells, induced carcinogenesis, histopathologic types, antitumor drugs, surgery, radiotherapy and chemotherapy. Several papers reported findings of population surveys (Chinese Academy of Medical Sciences, 1962).

Tumor chemotherapy has been strongly emphasized throughout the years. A notable experiment is the use of *actinomycin K*, which was isolated in 1957 from *Streptomyces melanochromogenes*, obtained from the soil in South China. When used experimentally with nitrogen mustard, the drug was said to show a marked inhibitory effect on animal tumors. The drug was reportedly tried on Hodgkin's disease patients with encouraging results.

Recently, the use of *kengshenmycin* (a variation of *actinomycin K;* since shown to be *actinomycin D* (Shanghai Municipal Tumor Hospital, 1971; Li, unpublished data)) along with other therapeutic agents commonly reported in Western literature was claimed to be effective in the treatment of malignant trophoblastic tumors. As shown in Table 2, the mortality figures of choriocarcinoma decreased from 89 to 57% during 1949-1965, and that of chorioadenoma, decreased from 25 to 13%. Since 1965, the mortality figures have decreased to 39 and 5%, respectively.

Furthermore, the new antitumor agent N-formyl-sarcolysine (N-F) reportedly was effective in treating malignant lymphomas and, particularly, seminoma of the testis and multiple myeloma (Table 3). Clinical trials also indicated that the toxic effect of N-F was relatively mild, compared to other alkylating agents of similar nature (Institute of Material Medica and Oncology, 1967).

It has also been reported that in experimentation of short-term explant cultures of human cancer, bladder papillocarcinoma was very sensitive to bis-thiosemicarbozone of β-ethoxy-a-oxo-butyraldehyde (C-6323) (Institute of Material Medica, 1967).

Other statistics on therapy indicated that the 5-year survival rates for patients in all stages of cervical cancer receiving radiation therapy at the Peking Union Hospital during 1952-1953 was reported to be 53% (Yu and Ko, 1959). While this is similar to a 51% rate for U.S. registered cases for the years 1950-1954, the two sets of figures are not strictly comparable. Differences between the countries with respect to selection of patients and other factors must be considered.

In the case of cancer of the esophagus, the 5-year survival rate following resection at Fu Wai Hospital, Peking, 1940-1960 was 23.7% (Wu et al., 1962).

Since 1955 cancer studies directed to the *materia medica* of China have been greatly intensified. In that year, the Institute of Epidemiology in the Academy of Medical Sciences began to screen anti-tumor herb drugs of simple formula. Subsequently, intracor-

TABLE 2 Therapeutic results of treatment of malignant trophoblastic tumors, Fanti Hospital, Peking, 1949–1968

Period	Type of treatment	Total		Choriocarcinoma		Chorioadenoma	
		Number of cases	Deaths (%)	Number of cases	Deaths (%)	Number of cases	Deaths (%)
1949–July 1958	Surgery**	64	62.5	37	89.2	27	25.9
August 1958–1965	Combined chemotherapy and surgery***	238	37.4	131	57.3	107	13.1
1966–1968*	Combined chemotherapy and surgery****	279	20.4	126	38.9	153	5.2

* Includes deaths up to November, 1970

** Some patients received deep X-ray irradiation and/or chemotherapy (nitrogen mustard and nitromin)

*** The main chemotherapeutic agent was 6 – Mercaptopurine (6MP), with occasional use of Methotrexate (MTX). Since 1964, 5 – Fluorauracil (5 Fu) and Kengshenmycin (KSM) were used in a few cases

**** The chief therapeutic agents were 5Fu and KSM; 6MP and MTX were used occasionally
Source: Fanti Hospital, Peking (1971)

TABLE 3   *Clinical efficacy of N-formyl-sarcolysine*

Type of tumor	Total patients	Patients evaluated	Response of patients evaluated*		
			Strong	Fair	None
Total	193	147	53	36	58
Seminoma	41	26	22	4	–
Multiple myeloma	8	7	3	3	1
Hodgkin's disease	29	25	9	11	5
Lymphosarcoma	36	23	9	6	8
Recticulum cell sarcoma	29	23	9	7	7
Giant follicular lymphoma	1	1	–	1	–
Malignant ovarian tumor	8	3	1	1	1
Bronchogenic carcinoma	7	7	–	–	7
Mammary carcinoma	5	5	–	2	3
Primary carcinoma of liver	5	5	–	–	5
Carcinoma of gastro-intestinal tract	4	3	–	–	3
Malignant melanoma	4	4	–	–	4
Osteogenic sarcoma	3	2	–	–	2
Other malignancies	13	13	–	1	12

* Strong = Tumor either totally regressed or the original diameter was reduced by one-half or more

Fair = Tumor definitely regressed but the residual diameter was at least half the original dimensions

None = No change in the tumor size

Source: Institute of Material Medica and Oncology (1967)

poreal screening in experimental tumors of anti-tumor compound and simple traditional formulae was initiated in the Research Institute of Experimental Medicine, the Research Institute of Pharmacology (both in the Academy of Medical Sciences), and several medical colleges.

Reportedly great progress was made in the treatment of cancers of esophagus, stomach, colon and breast as a result of a combination of traditional and Western medicine. In patients with cervical malignancy, reports said that some traditional drugs reduced cyclical changes in a manner similar to radiation therapy. The drugs were said to promote substantial relief of pain and distress in many advanced cases. Two drugs, *lithospermum officinale* and *pei yao* (produced in Yunan province), were said to be beneficial in treatment of choriocarcinoma.

Several known tumor hospitals had played a major role in clinical studies. One is the Tumor Institute (300 beds) in the Academy of Medical Sciences. The tumor hospital at the Shanghai First Medical College was inaugurated about 1950. The Huanan (South China) Tumor Hospital (140 beds) in Canton, established in 1964, has the formal Departments of Radiology, Internal Medicine, Gynecology, Chest and Abdomen, and Head and Neck. Two other tumor hospitals are located in Hangchow (Chekiang Province) and Taiyuan (Shansi Province). The Tumor Department at Tianjin Hospital has the status of a hospital.

Selected epidemiologic findings

Epidemiologic research has been greatly facilitated by the availability of voluminous amounts of clinical materials, and by accumulation of massive statistical information from extensive analyses of microscopically examined materials. The results of cancer survey, registration, and screening programs further open new avenues of inquiry. A detailed analysis of the epidemiologically relevant results will be reported separately (King, unpublished data). Some selected findings are presented below.

In the city of Shanghai, for which 1960 registration data are available, crude incidence rates per 100,000 *general population* for all cancers combined were reported to be 71.0 for males and 114.5 for females, in contrast to 197.2 and 189.0 for selected U.S. Chinese populations (Table 4). The corresponding figures for U.S. whites in Connecticut, 1963-1965 were 300.1 and 281.7. For more meaningful comparison, the Shanghai data were age-adjusted to the 'World Population' to obtain standardized incidence rates (Doll et al., 1970). These were 112.8 and 146.5 per 100,000 males and females, respectively, compared to 208.9 and 218.4 for selected U.S. Chinese populations, and 256.9 and 205.7 for Connecticut.

TABLE 4   *Crude and standardized incidence rates per 100,000 for all cancers by sex, Shanghai, 1960, U.S. Chinese, 1960–64, and Connecticut, 1963–65.*

Area	Crude		Standardized**	
	Male	Female	Male	Female
Shanghai	71.0	114.5	112.8	146.5
U.S. Chinese*	197.2	189.0	208.9	218.4
Connecticut	300.1	281.7	256.9	205.7

 * Alameda County, California and Hawaii

** Adjusted to World Population. Doll et al. (1970)

Published data on other areas are confined to frequency distribution. For our general reference Table 5 is presented below, indicating rough variations for selected sites by region.

Three cancer sites are known to have high risks among the Chinese, namely, esophagus, liver and particularly, nasopharynx. For cancer of the nasopharynx, crude incidence rates of 4.8 (male) and 2.2 (female) per 100,000 *general population* were reported for Shanghai, in contrast to 12.6 and 4.8 for selected U.S. Chinese populations, and 0.6 and 0.1 for Connecticut. Of particular interest is the apparently higher relative frequency of nasopharyngeal cancer in South China than in North or East and the striking Kwantung-Fukien (provinces) disparity shown for southern Chinese. Consider the latter: the proportions of this site among all cancers combined (confirmed autopsy cases) were 26 to 6% for capitals of Canton (Kwangtung) and Foochow (Fukien), respectively. Such a disparity seems to support the biogenetic predisposition hypothesis, but the influence of ecologic and sociocultural intervention can not be ruled out (King, unpublished data).

In contrast to nasopharynx, esophageal cancer appears to have a slightly higher frequency in the North than in the South. Consumption of vodka-like *pei kan* (made of *kao liang*, a sorghum plant grown in the North) is generally considered to be associated with this malignancy. The reported crude incidence rates for Shanghai were 10.9 for males and 4.9 for females, and corresponding figures for males in selected U.S. Chinese males (no female cases) and Connecticut counterparts were 7.4 and 6.6, respectively.

Liver is another highly susceptible cancer site among Chinese. It was reported that out of 2,424 autopsies on Chinese at the Chinese Union Medical College, 1917-1942 and 1947-1950, 19 or 0.8% of the cases were diagnosed as primary cancer of the liver. The

TABLE 5   Percent distribution by sex of six most frequently reported cancers in two provinces and six cities, The People's Republic of China

Sex and site	North				South			East
	Peking	Tianjin	Tsinan	Sian	Canton	Fukien*	Kwangsi*	Shanghai
Males								
All cancers	5137	1562	2738	879	3010	1010	672	9521
Buccal cavity 140–145	2.5	7.9**	5.1	6.7***	—	8.3	—	—
Nasopharynx 146	4.0	12.9	24.5	16.0	56.9	16.2	31.1	6.4
Esophagus 150	10.3	11.3	8.5	6.3	—	10.6	—	9.0
Stomach 151	6.6	9.6	—	—	6.0	15.0	4.8	11.0
Intestines 152, 153	—	—	5.8	9.0	—	—	7.3	—
Colon	—	—	—	—	—	—	—	8.9
Liver, primary 155	—	5.3	—	—	4.9	12.0	11.2	—
Nose 160	3.4	—	—	5.7	—	—	—	—
Larynx 161	—	—	4.0	—	—	—	—	—
Penis 179	17.5	14.7	12.4	6.5	5.7	—	7.4	—
Bladder 181	—	—	—	—	—	—	—	5.8
Skin 190, 191	—	—	—	—	9.7	5.4	9.7	5.8
Females								
All cancers	8151	4202	3797	2615	4026	1068	748	18829
Buccal cavity 140–144	—	—	—	—	—	—	—	—
Nasopharynx 146	—	—	—	—	17.4	4.7	10.0	—
Esophagus 150	—	—	3.0	—	—	3.8	—	—
Stomach 151	—	1.4	—	—	—	—	—	—
Intestines 152, 153	1.9	2.1	2.2	2.1	—	—	—	—
Colon 153	—	—	—	—	—	—	—	3.4
Maxillary sinus 160.2	—	—	—	—	—	—	—	—
Breast	17.4	7.3	14.6	7.0	17.1	15.6	12.9	11.9
Cervix 171	5.4	72.6	56.0	69.9	35.3	37.2	31.4	55.8
Corpus uteri 172	2.4	3.1	—	2.7	—	9.9	8.6	1.9
Other uterus 173	—	—	—	—	—	—	—	—
Ovary 175	2.5	—	3.3	2.5	3.5	3.6	5.6	2.6
Vulva 176	1.9	2.3	2.1	2.3	—	—	—	—
Vagina 176.1	—	—	—	—	—	—	—	—
Skin 190, 191	—	—	—	—	5.1	—	7.0	2.0

Source: Adopted from King (unpublished data)

*   Province
**   Includes nose
*** Includes larynx

earliest known age at diagnosis of this malignancy is 38 days after birth. Diagnosis in males rises from that age up to the sixth decade of life. Several theories seek to account for the high risk of the liver cancer, including schistosome or clonorchis sinensis infection and liver cirrhosis. Consumption of raw fish is thought to be a major source of clonorchis infection in South China.

Among Shanghai females, a high incidence rate of 49.6 was reported for cervical cancer, compared to 18.2 for selected U.S. Chinese populations and 12.2 for Connecticut.

Several cancer sites seem to be relatively infrequent among Chinese, notably the prostate and the female breast. A low crude incidence rate of lung cancer was also reported for Shanghai, being 6.7 and 3.7 for males and females, respectively, in contrast to 26.6 and 10.4 for selected U.S. Chinese populations, and 50.6 and 10.0 for Connecticut. This is interesting in view of recent observations of visitors to China who noted a rather high prevalence of smoking among the Chinese. For leukemia, reported low crude incidence rates for Shanghai were 1.5 (males) and 0.9 (females). The corresponding figures were 8.1 and 7.1 for selected U.S. Chinese populations, and 10.7 and 7.5 for Connecticut.

Other malignancies of interest include colonic cancer. This disease appears to be higher in East China than in the North. The reason is thought to be related to the endemic prevalence of schistosomaisis over vast areas south of the Yangtze River, where mild climate, abundant rainfall, extensive irrigation, and fertile soil are favorable for the breeding of a possible intermediate host and spreading of an infection.

Another is choriocarcinoma, the relative frequency of which led to the formation of a special study section of this malignancy in the Academy of Medical Sciences in 1958.

Another is the skin cancer which has strikingly high frequency in North China. One possible correlate could be the wide and prolonged use in the winter in this area of the 'kang', or heated brick bed.

To sum up, epidemiologic studies, as with clinical morphologic investigations, largely deal with cancers of the nasopharynx, esophagus, colon, liver, and cervix. Other sites that are generally affected by physical environmental factors such as the lung and leukemia are neglected.

Conclusion

This cursory review of anti-cancer campaign in the People's Republic clearly indicates that the reported achievements are largely attributable to the model of mass social organization adopted. Evidently, many of the published studies are well-designed and credibly present findings drawn from large amounts of clinical materials. In view of the fact that there are fewer than half a dozen exclusively tumor-oriented hospitals in the United States, the 6 known tumor hospitals established in China apparently reflects its determination to conquer this disease.

The limited epidemiologic findings unmistakably reveal that the Chinese present a distinctive site profile which necessitates further investigations. The relatively few known studies on cancer of the lung and leukemia are in keeping with the pattern prevalent in countries in the process of industrialization. In these countries physical environmental carcinogens may play a less crucial role.

Finally, we must emphasize that an objective evaluation of the reported achievement in New China's cancer research, prevention, and therapy should take into consideration all the socioeconomic, technological, and personnel limitations inherent in various programs. Further, there is a lack of complete knowledge of the development in the above areas in the recent past, particularly since the 1966 Cultural Revolution when nearly all professional publications ceased. It is encouraging to note, however, the resumption of publication in January, 1973 of the Chinese Medical Journal. We look forward to comprehensive up-to-date information through exchange between cancer scientists, both medical and non-medical, in future years.

Summary

The reported success in cancer control in the People's Republic of China was mainly attributable to the 'mass social mobilization' model adopted. An example is the organization of the Anti-Cancer Shock Brigade. The total number of persons covered under various screening and survey programs in the entire country must be large considering the four million figure reported for 4 provinces and 8 cities alone during 1958-1959. The number of tumor cases examined at various medical colleges was estimated to be over 100,000, spanning a 30-year period.

Reported research studies indicate a wide range of interest in experimental and clinical oncology. Chemotherapy seems to be strongly emphasized. Among the drugs known to be effective in the treatment of tumors include actinomycin K (Hodgkin's disease), Keng-shenmycin (trophoblastic tumors), and N-F (seminome of the testis and myeloma). Two Chinese herbs, *lithospermum officinale* and *pei yao* were reported to be beneficial in treatment of choriocarcinoma. There are 6 cancer hospitals.

Epidemiologic findings indicate that esophagus, liver and particularly, nasopharynx are the 3 cancer sites with high risks. Cancers of the prostate and female breast seem to be relatively infrequent. Regional variations are reported. In Shanghai, 1960 age-adjusted incidence rates per 100,000 for all cancers combined were reported to be 112.8 for males and 146.5 for females, compared to 208.9 and 218.4, respectively, for selected Chinese populations in the United States, 1960-64, and 256.9 and 205.7 for Connecticut, 1963-65. The distinctive incidence pattern among the Chinese suggests further investigation.

References

Chinese Academy of Medical Sciences (1962): Selected Papers on Cancer Research. Scientific and Technical Publications, Shanghai.

Doll, R., Muir, C. and Waterhouse, J. (Editors) (1970): Cancer Incidence in Five Continents. UICC Technical Report No. II. Springer-Verlag, Berlin.

Fanti Hospital, Peking (1971): Progress in the Treatment of Malignant Trophoblastic Tumors During the Last Two Decades in the Peking Fanti Hospital, Paper presented to the Bi-annual Conference of the Nepal Medical Association, February 1971.

Institute of Material Medica and Oncology, Chinese Academy of Medical Sciences, Peking (1967): China's Medicine, No. 8, 606.

Institute of Material Medica, Chinese Academy of Medical Sciences, Peking (1967): China's Medicine, No. 12, 879.

King, H. (1972): In: Medicine and Public Health in the People's Republic of China, pp. 72-97. Editor: J. R. Quinn. Fogarty International Center, NIH, DHEW Publication No. (NIH) 72-67.

Shanghai Municipal Tumor Hospital (1971): In: Prevention and Treatment of Tumors, p. 250. Commercial Press, Hongkong. In Chinese.

Sidel, V. W. (1972): The Participation of People in Health Care in the People's Republic of China, Paper presented at the annual meeting of the American Public Health Association, November 13-16, Atlantic City, New Jersey.

Wu, Y. K., Huang, K. C. and Chang, W. (1962): In: Selected Papers on Cancer Research, pp. 194-198. Editor: The Chinese Academy of Medical Sciences. Scientific and Technical Publications, Shanghai.

Yu, A. F. and Ko, T. K. (1959): Chin. J. Obstet. Gynec., 7, 374.

Health education activities in Hungary

A. Nagy and J. Métneki

National Cancer Institute and Health Education Centre, Ministry of Health, Budapest, Hungary

With the voluntary work in 1948 of the Hungarian gynecologists, a cancer screening activity was started in the country. This activity, based on the Eötvös Lóránd Radium and Roentgen Institute, was the starting point for the creation of the National Cancer Institute and of its oncological network. The Institute, which has been active since 1952, is leading the fight against cancer in Hungary, as well as the efforts for cancer prevention and early diagnosis.

The Hungarian screening activity was initiated by gynecologists. This, and because malignancies of the female genitals and to a lesser degree cancer of the breast can be detected at an early phase, are the reasons why mass screenings in Hungary are associated with these cancer sites. In this paper, when we refer to screenings, we mean gynecological screenings, including breast palpation, which are completed with the examinations of the skin, visible mucous membranes and rectum. The annual compulsory chest X-ray screen test can be regarded also as a mass-screening in Hungary, and within recognised limits, provides an early diagnosis.

TABLE 1   *The number and effectiveness of screening examinations (1964–1972)*

Year	No. of screening examinations	No. of detected cancer cases	Detected cancer cases as per cent of the screening examinations
1964	454,466	1,386	0.30
1967	496,646	1,481	0.30
1970	480,548	1,426	0.30
1971	480,064	1,441	0.30
1972	516,365		

Table 1 shows that the population screened involves about half a million women annually. As can be seen from the table, the number and effectiveness of the screening examinations has hardly changed since 1964. About 1,400 women are sent to hospitals annually, which is 0.3% (three per thousand) of all examinations. It is scarcely necessary to add that the screening examinations detect other oncological and non-oncological diseases, which must be cared for by the screening doctor.

The obligatory reports on all cancer cases make it possible to compare the cases detected by screening with the others registered by the reports of the health institutions. From Table 2 we see that more than half of the screened uterine cervix carcinoma cases are in stages 0-I, while not even one quarter of the cases detected by other means go to treatment at the same early phase.

With cancer of the breast the difference is less marked. 78% of the cases from screen-

TABLE 2   *Cervical cancer cases, registered in 1970, according to the stage-distribution*

Stage	Total cases		Detected by screening		Detected without screening	
	No.	%	No.	%	No.	%
0 – I	412	31.8	199	50.3	213	23.7
II	428	33.1	140	35.4	288	32.1
III – IV	380	29.4	51	12.8	329	36.6
Not cleared up	74	5.7	6	1.5	68	7.6
Total	1,294	100.0	396	100.0	898	100.0

TABLE 3   *Breast cancer cases, registered in 1970, according to the stage-distribution*

Stage	Total cases		Detected by screening		Detected without screening	
	No.	%	No.	%	No.	%
I – II	1,266	62.9	398	78.0	868	57.8
III – IV	511	25.4	105	20.6	406	27.0
Not cleared up	235	11.7	7	1.4	228	15.2
Total	2,012	100.0	510	100.0	1,502	100.0

TABLE 4   *Stage-distribution of cervical and breast cancer cases detected by screening in 1955–1971*

Year	Uterine cervix			Breast	
	0–Ia – I	II	III – IV	I – II	III – IV
1955	23.9	31.5	44.6	70.2	29.8
1960	35.4	22.5	42.1	59.4	40.6
1964	47.8	27.4	24.8	76.0	24.0
1969	46.3	30.5	23.2	78.6	21.4
1971	53.4	25.3	21.3	78.6	21.4

ing are diagnosed in I-II stage by Steinthal, and 52.8% of the non-screened cases are in the same stages. This difference cannot be easily evaluated because 15.2% of registered cases are not staged (the stage is not given on the report form) (Table 3).

Table 4 demonstrates the changes of effectiveness of the screenings. The most important warning is that effectiveness has increased only slightly. Drawing a lesson from this, we are trying to strengthen the cytological basis of the screenings. For this purpose, we started a course for pre-screening and increased the number of histopathological laboratories doing routine cytological examinations.

An unfortunate accompaniment of the screenings is the lack of interest in the population. Often 10-20 women appear in response to requests sent to 100. To improve the position we have, with the aid of the Health Education Centre, made effective films, books, 4 kinds of posters, 5 kinds of leaflets, a series of slides and travelling exhibitions. One of the films made this year was presented at the symposium with English commentary. The films deal not so much with screening, but with the warning signs of cancer. In that film, 7 cured patients (8-30 years tumor-free) speak about their lives and diseases.

Four further short films have been made to support lectures, if possible at the time of screening examinations. Their subject is the prevention and early detection of cancer.

The text of the posters is generally simple and easy to understand: they appeal for participation in population screenings, and describe the successful treatment and cure of the early-diagnosed cancer. One series directs attention to the 7 warning signs of cancer: one poster for each indication. The point of interest in these bills is that they do not call attention directly to cancer, but send the patient to the doctor on noticing certain complaints. The title of the series appears only in small letters at the bottom of the poster. Figure 1 gives examples of two of our best posters against smoking, but it is difficult to say anything about their influence.

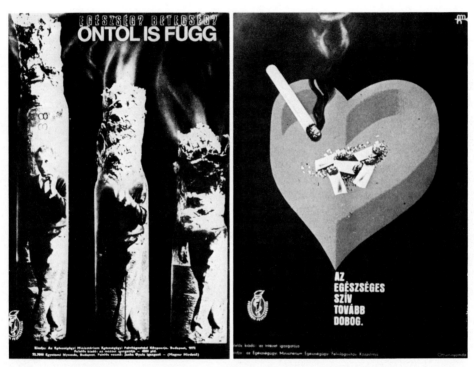

FIG. 1   *Examples of two of the best posters designed to campaign against smoking.*

In this short paper we have described our mass screening with its great tradition, and the methods and tools used in health inquiry. We have to emphasize that the preparation of inquiry material is much easier than its adequate use. We must improve our methods, and in future we hope to report on the effective use of this propaganda material.

The significance of team work in the early detection of breast cancer in women

P. Bagović, M. Bolanča, Ž. Maričić, P. Nola, M. Ribarič and
I. Vodopija

Gynecological Clinical Hospital, Zagreb, Yugoslavia

Introduction

A breast cancer detection program on a large scale was recently started in Zagreb. However, surgeons and other specialists had different views regarding the organization of the program. At the same time, mortality-rates from breast cancer showed a relatively high increase in Zagreb, over the last 8 years. This is seen in Table 1.

This table compares the death-rates and their trends, for 4 types of gynecological cancer in Zagreb, over a period extending from 1963 to the end of 1971. Breast cancer shows a definite increase. Ovarian cancer appears to increasing only slowly, while corpus uteri cancer remains at about the same level. Only cervical cancer is declining, which is substantiated by the campaign for early detection of that type of cancer in Zagreb (Audy et al., 1971). The average age of death from breast cancer is 59 years. In our Central Institute for Tumors and Allied Diseases, where the majority of cases are treated, nearly 20% of the women coming for breast cancer treatment have distant metastases at the time of surgical intervention.

Confronted with these facts, it was decided to try and organize a campaign for the detection of breast cancer. However, we had to keep in mind that such a campaign had to be acceptable to the women in our area.

TABLE 1   *Trends of death-rates from gynecological cancers in the City of Zagreb, 1963-1971*

WHO code number	Localization	Trend
174	Breast	$y = 49.1 + 5.1 x$
182	Corpus uteri	$y = 39.6 + 1.1 x$
183	Ovaries	$y = 20.2 + 0.7 x$
180	Cervix uteri	$y = 26.7 - 1.8 x$

Basic principles

Results from our campaign for the early detection of cervical cancer indicated that the campaign was accepted by our women. Now that they appreciate the privilege of better health, they are individually promoting the issue of cancer detection in this part of the country (Bačić et al., 1967). Consequently, these women have become a decisive factor in influencing various bodies to provide money for preventive activities and measures.

The gynecologists have been the key to the success of the cervical cancer detection campaign and are inevitably involved in the movement for the detection of breast cancer. The reasons are as follows:

1.   Gynecologists assist in the delivery of children, providing mothers with pre-natal examinations and consultation.

2.   The same specialists, because of the doctor-patient relationship, are later frequently consulted for various gynecological problems, including contraception.

3.   Furthermore, these specialists have been individually conducting examinations for cervical cancer for years and have saved many lives.

Confidence in the doctor has been established through these contacts and thus only a small step is involved in giving the patient a breast check every time she comes for her gynecological examination. This idea and this approach have been fully accepted. The gynecologists are excellently placed for detecting this type of cancer. Having the woman's medical history, age, number of births, abortions, and information about the heredity of breast conditions in her family (mother and sisters), it is not difficult for gynecologists to screen women at high risk for breast abnormalities. Among such high risk groups, are particularly those women aged 40 and above and those with 3 and more births and/or abortions. High risk groups include those women who have a history of breast cancer in the family.

If there are any skin changes or a lump on the breast, then the gynecologist sends the woman to have more detailed check-up and examination. A whole team of specialists, surgeons, radiologists, cytologists, and endocrinologists take over the selected women and perform the necessary examinations.

This is the basic structure of our organization for the detection of breast cancer in Zagreb. In this way, breast cancer detection is included as a part of the general gynecological cancer detection activities.

This autumn, we are starting a campaign to provide the entire city with available resources and personnel in order to examine 26,000 women each year. Gynecological dispensaries will send the selected women for detailed examinations to one of the 6 centers for breast diseases organized in the General Hospitals. A standard and detailed procedural examination is to be used and the same applies for data collection and follow-up (Ribarić, 1972).

Discussion

The adoption of this campaign is urgent because, as mentioned earlier, 20% of the women coming to the Central Institute for Tumors and Allied Diseases for surgical treatment of breast cancer already have distant metastases. The interval between the average age of death from breast cancer and the age when we detect most of our cases with breast cancer is too short. At the moment, this period is only 3-4 years because most of the women we detect are in the age-group of around 55-56 years.

TABLE 2   *Number of women examined for breast diseases and findings*

No. of women examined	Diagnosis			
	Cysts	Abscess	Fibroadenoma	Breast cancer
23,238	43	5	21	67

To obtain more detailed information regarding the structure of the campaign we began work in 3 pilot areas in 1972. Such breast campaign screening examinations were performed in the Gynecological Dispensary in Medveščak, the Gynecological Clinical Hospital and in the Central Institute for Tumors and Allied Diseases. The result of this work in the pilot areas is presented in Table 2.

Perhaps the number of detected breast cancers are not as high and do not correspond to the figures in other countries (Strax, 1971). That remains to be seen. Our examinations which checked for breast conditions were made on women aged 18 years and above.

Conclusion

The principle of having the gynecologists in the forefront of the detection of gynecological and breast cancer was whole-heartedly accepted by women in Zagreb. After the experience gained from 3 pilot areas, we are now embarking on a larger campaign to cover the entire area of Zagreb. The detailed results of this effort will be presented in due course.

References

Audy, S., Bačić, M., Bagović, P., Bolanča, M., Urbanke, A. and Vodopija, I. (1971): Minerva ginec., 23/1, 20.
Bačić, M., Bagović, P., Bolanča, M., Karačić, M. and Vodopija, I. (1967): Zdrav. novine, 20/3-4, 105.
Ribarić, M. (1972): In: Akcija za Masovno rano Otkrivanje raka Genitala i raka Dojke u Žena, pp. 13-44. Editor: Z. Pavlić. Zavod za Taštitu Zdravlja Grada, Zagreb.
Strax, P. (1971): Practical Mass Screening for Breast Cancer. Guttman Institute, New York, N.Y.

Evaluation of publicity and self-detection procedures for breast cancer

D. J. Hill

Anti-Cancer Council of Victoria, Melbourne, Australia

Introduction

A field study was undertaken in the State of Victoria, Australia, to identify variables relating to the presentation of women with medical breast problems, including breast cancer. The study was designed as a field experiment in which television publicity was manipulated for certain time periods and in certain geographical areas. General Practitioners (GPs) were recruited to keep a daily record of patients presenting with breast problems.

Materials and methods

Commercial television stations made time available free of charge over a period of several months. Publicity advocated the regular practice of breast self-examination (BSE). The campaign was launched with a well-publicised afternoon screening of a 14 min film 'The Life in Your Hands'. This includes some basic cancer biology, and stresses BSE and cervical cytology as important cancer safeguards for women. In the 8 weeks following the launching, a 30 sec advertisement advocating and demonstrating BSE was screened at least 31 times on commercial TV, including some at peak viewing times. Less intensive TV publicity continued to the end of the study period.

To record baseline rates for breast problems in general practice and to assess the influence of publicity upon such rates, 425 volunteer GPs throughout Victoria were provided with appropriate pads of stationery on which to notify relevant patient details.

Any female patient who initiated discussion with the doctor about a breast problem was listed and a note made of:the date seen; her age; whether it was a breast lump she complained of; nature and duration of breast signs and symptoms; and whether the doctor confirmed the presence of a breast problem.

If an objective problem was present, the following data were obtained — marital status, parity, how problem was discovered, GPs' first impression of problem, GPs' decision about treatment or referral (if any), definitive diagnosis of the condition, plus summary of clinical and treatment details. Annual follow-up for survival data is planned.

Results

Overall findings

From October, 1972 to March, 1973, a total of 1,598 breast problem enquiries were reported by participating GPs. In 53% of these the doctor confirmed the existence of a problem. 41% of the confirmed breast problems were found by patients reported as 'doing self-examination'. Of the breast signs confirmed by a doctor, 83% were lumps. Of the others, pain was the most common but in only half of the cases where patients complained of breast pain was the doctor able to find a problem. This contrasts with patients complaining of a lump — 75% of these were confirmed by the doctor. There were 62 breast malignancies (7.2% of the confirmed breast problems) and the mean age of these cancer patients was 59 years. In 44% of the confirmed problems, the GPs' decision was to take no action or to observe; 40% were referred to specialists or hospitals and 16% were treated by the GPs.

Publicity effects

The problem of manipulating (even defining) publicity exposure on breast cancer proved difficult (see Discussion). In the following analysis, patients have been allocated to 'high publicity' and 'low publicity' categories according to whether or not they attended a doctor practising in a TV reception area at a time when the special breast cancer publicity campaign was being run. In the second category, the term 'low' rather than 'no' publicity is used because there was unavoidable overflow of the publicity campaign and because there was presumably a residual effect of years of less intensive prior breast cancer education.

Figure 1 presents the weekly number of patients recorded as complaining of a breast lump up to the 17th week of the study. The upper curve plots the tally of breast lump patients reporting to doctors in the 'high publicity' areas. The lower curve plots the lump-reporting rate for the areas outside the range of T.V. publicity. As this 'low publicity' area was considerably less populated than the 'high publicity' area it had a much lower baseline rate during Weeks 1 and 2 (before any special publicity began), as well as afterwards.

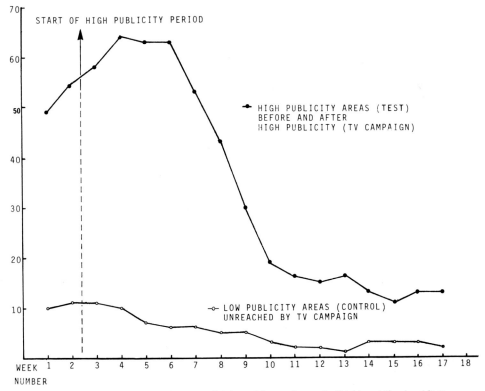

FIG. 1   *Weekly number of patients complaining of breast lumps in 'high' and 'low' publicity areas. (3 week running average).*

Since the general rate of lump reporting to GPs is presumably fairly stable over time (if special publicity effects are absent), the declining report rate for the 'low publicity' area must be explained — probably by an inevitable decrement in the efficiency of data recording. No doubt such factors as forgetfulness, waning enthusiasm, and intervening vacations, among the GPs, contributed to this trend. These factors must also have affected the reporting rate in 'high publicity' areas.

In 'low publicity' areas, the reporting rate was stable for 4 weeks, after which it started to decline until levelling off at about Week 11. In the 'high publicity' area, the rate climbed after the start of publicity and did not decline to its baseline rate until the eighth week. Part of this decline is presumably artefactual due to the abovementioned decline in reporting efficiency. However, the slope between Weeks 6 and 10 is steeper in the 'high' than 'low publicity' areas — even after adjusting for the artefactual effects as estimated on the 'low publicity' controls.

Table 1 provides evidence which explains the steep decline in reporting rate after the peak associated with the introduction of publicity. There is a significant relationship between the duration of breast lump signs and the level of publicity. Women in the 'high publicity' area were more likely to report breast lumps within a week than were woman from 'low publicity' areas. Obviously publicity itself cannot *create* lumps. Thus when publicity induces an excess of early breast lump reports,those lumps which would have appeared in later weeks will be counted in the early and not the later weeks. The steepness of the decline in weekly breast lump reporting is thus predictable from the data in Table 1. It appears that the TV campaign was successful in improving the early reporting rate.

TABLE 1   *Exposure to publicity and duration of breast problem signs**

	Duration of signs		
	< 1 week	1–4 weeks	> 4 weeks
High publicity	118 (101)**	176 (180)	114 (127)
Low publicity	32 (49)	90 (86)	73 (60)
	$\chi^2 = 12.41, p < .01, 2$ df		

* 603 patients who complained of lumps which were medically confirmed and for whom duration of signs was provided

** ( ) expected frequencies if publicity had no effect

Since the publicity advocated that women adopt the practice of breast self-examination, an increase in the proportion of women reporting lumps discovered while doing BSE was expected to be associated with 'high publicity'. Although this expected trend was found, it was slight and did not reach statistical significance. The failure of publicity to significantly increase the number of patients reporting lumps following BSE could be due to a fault in the wording of the form doctors were asked to fill out, as well as to the inherent difficulties doctors found in differentiating patients who inadvertently discovered a lump from those who, unsuspecting of any problem, set out to examine their breasts systematically.

Breast cancers found

Of the 62 breast cancers found, 52 patients had first come to their doctors complaining of a breast lump. 24% found the problem while 'doing self-examination'; most of the remainder found the problem inadvertently but two cases were detected at routine examination and two during medical breast examination done at the request of the patient.

Significant publicity effects on such variables as smaller lumps, with less node involvement were *not* found.

Table 2 presents data for breast cancer patients relating mean duration of signs to publicity. Mean duration of signs before seeking medical advice was less for the high publicity group — a finding which reflects the overall results presented above. However, the difference is not significant at the 90% confidence level.

TABLE 2   *Exposure to publicity and duration of breast problem signs (48 breast cancer patients)* *

	N	Mean duration (weeks)**
High publicity	32	10.9
Low publicity	16	20.1

 * Duration of signs not available for 14 patients

** Difference between means: P > .10

Discussion

Problems were encountered in this study which make it difficult to draw definite conclusions. The value of publicity in promoting the practice of breast self-examination, let alone its effect on prognosis, is not proven here. However, a publicity effect was demonstrated for the number of patients with breast lumps attending doctors, particularly quickly-reported lumps. Although the persuasiveness of the film itself and/or the inherent persuasibility of women on the subject of BSE should be questioned and investigated, greater audience penetration of the publicity might considerably improve the response.

Compared with commercial campaigns, this breast cancer TV campaign was not large and so perhaps the number of women who saw the advertisements a sufficient number of times to be spurred to action was not large. As well as the relative lack of audience penetration, a further methodological problem in relying on TV stations' charity was the stations' inability to specify in advance exactly when and how much publicity could be given. Thus, the definition of 'high publicity' was, of necessity, crude.

A pleasing result was that no negative effects were found. Publicity did not keep more women away from their doctors than it brought in. This is important, for it can plausibly be speculated that drawing attention to breast cancer signs might activate 'head-in-the-sand' (denial) reactions that actually deter women from seeking medical advice. Nor is there any evidence that cancer-phobia was induced. The proportion of medically unconfirmed breast 'lumps' was the same for the 'high' and 'low' publicity groups suggesting that publicity has little or no effect on producing imagined complaints.

Although inconclusive, the results do indicate a potentially useful publicity effect among some women in the short term. If this is so, the campaign has probably influenced a larger number of women who have not yet, but will in future, develop breast lumps and act with alacrity when they appear. Presumably, continued publicity will be needed to recruit women to the practice of BSE and to maintain the gains made in the initial campaign.

Psychopathological profile of the population attending a cancer detection clinic

Y. Fassin, G. Van Hemelrijck and P. Ch. Van Reeth

Centre de Dépistage du Cancer de l'Institut J. Bordet et Service de Psychologie Médicale du Centre de Santé de l'Université Libre de Bruxelles, Brussels, Belgium

Anxiety, psychosomatic complaints and psychopathological disorders seem frequent among the population attending the Bordet Institute Cancer Detection Clinic. This impression comes from the clinical interviews and also from the multiplicity and varieties of complaints described by the applicants when they answer the cancer detection questionnaire. *The aim of this study* is to measure the prevalence of this psychopathological morbidity.

Method

A short screening test was used: the Langner questionnaire (22-item screening score of psychiatric symptoms indicating impairment), followed by a clinical interview with a psychiatrist. Other questions were added in connection with educational and professional level, motivations to apply and other items related to cancer detection strategy. Moreover, the 'lie' scale from the Eysenck Personality Inventory was used in order to evaluate a distortion factor and a tendency to falsify the answers.

The clinic is situated in an urban Preventive Health Center. Only females attend it. Some apply on their own initiative, others through the initiative of their employer (office or factory) who spreads the information about the detection center and facilitates the visit without making it compulsory. 107 women attending the clinic for the first time were studied. The great majority were in the age group 25-50 years.

The test items had been selected by Langner from larger questionnaires on the basis of their discriminating power between known 'well' groups and 'ill' groups (i. e., in psychiatric treatment); and on their correlation with a judgment of impairment based on psychiatric interviews. The items mainly cover psychophysiological symptoms, anxiety and depression. Thus, this screening procedure does not provide a psychiatric diagnosis; it simply indicates the position of people on a continuum of impairment in life-functioning.

The test provides a screening score. A score equal or superior to 8 indicates severe

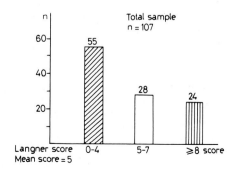

FIG. 1   *This histogram shows the importance of psychopathological impairment: 24 + 28 cases out of 107.*

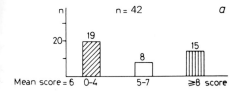

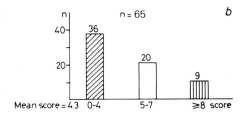

FIG. 2 *Difference of psychopathological scores between own request attenders and employer's initiative. (a) Group of attenders applying on their own request; (b) group of attenders applying on their employer's initiative.*

impairment (at the level of patients under psychiatric treatment, as in- or out-patients). The mildly or moderately impaired range from 5-7. A score below 5 is indicative of presumed good mental health.

Results

Figure 1 indicates the high prevalence of psychopathological impairment in the total population sample. Figure 2 shows different psychopathological profiles when 2 sub-populations are considered separately: (1) The attenders applying on their own initiative have a higher mean score (6) and 15 (out of 42) have a score of 8 or more. (2) Those who apply at their employer's suggestion have a lower mean score (4.3) and only 9 (out of 65) have a pathological score of 8 or more. In this group, the applicants who had received from their employer the first information about the detection clinic do not seem to differ in level of psychopathology from those who had received previous information from other sources (Fig. 3). The same group (employer's request attenders) seem to present the same profile as a control sample of the whole population at work in a similar type of work (Fig. 4) (Bertoux, 1971).

It may be concluded that attenders coming on their own initiative have a higher score of psychopathological impairment. On the other hand, the applicants coming at their

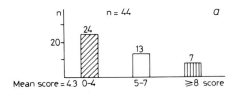

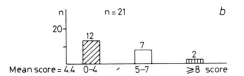

FIG. 3 *No difference exists according to the source of information in the group attending on the employer's initiative. (a) First information given by the employer; (b) first information previous to employer's information.*

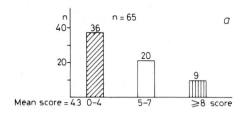

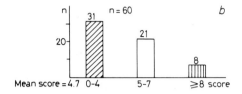

FIG. 4 *No difference according to attenders applying on their employer's initiative and a sample of population in similar type of work. (a) Attenders applying on their employer's initiative; (b) sample of population in similar type of work.*

employer's request do not differ from the general population from the same type of firm.

As the source of information does not seem to be relevant, the main determinant of higher psychopathological level seems to be the personal *motivation* to apply at the center. In the motivation questionnaire the most frequents answers were:

1. fear of cancer (64 cases)
2. a recent case of cancer among relatives (58 cases)
3. bodily complaints (47 cases)
4. belief in the heredity of cancer.

In the questionnaire, as well as in the psychiatric interviews, depressive symptoms were very frequent, even in the low score group (under 5). This depressive mood seems to enhance the receptivity to a latent fear of cancer. This would account for the great number of patients who come on their own initiative to the cancer detection clinic in a depressed state. It is generaly stated that attenders are anxious because they believe they might have a cancer; the psychiatric interviews showed, rather, that they believe they have a cancer because they are anxious and depressed.

This study shows that if the persons examined in a cancer detection clinic apply mainly on their own initiative, the rate of psychopathology will be high and a psychosomatic approach is indicated.

References

Langner, Th. S. (1962): J. Hlth hum. Behav., 3, 269.
Amiel, R. and Lebigre, F. (1970): Ann. méd.-psychol., 1/128, 565.
Bertoux, Cl. (1971): Etude Comparative des Troubles Psychosomatiques chez les Jeunes Travailleuses. Mémoire de Licence en Médecine du Travail. Université Libre de Bruxelles.

7. Paraneoplastic manifestations and malignancy associated changes

Cell alterations related to cancer (MAC according to Nieburgs)

M. Martuzzi, D. Amadori, A. Ravaioli and F. Padovani

Clinical Pathology and Oncologic Center, G.B. Morgagni Hospital, Forli, Italy

Some alterations can be detected in epithelial or stromal cells from tissue either in proximity to or at a distance from, a neoplastic focus. According to Nieburgs (Nieburgs et al., 1959, 1962; Nieburgs, 1967, 1968) they are named Malignancy Associated Changes

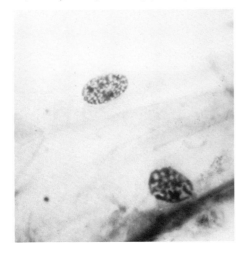

FIG. 1 *Buccal mucosa smear. Mature corni-fied cells with telophase nucleus (MAC I or A) (left top) and prophase nucleus (MAC II or C) (right lower). (Papanicolaou-Nieburgs stain; original magnification 1000X). Reduced for reproduction 25%.*

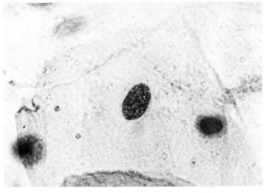

FIG. 2 *Buccal mucosa smear. Mature cornified cell with telophase nucleus (MAC I or A) – (Papa-nicolaou-Nieburgs stain; original magnification 1000X). Reduced for reproduction 40%.*

(MAC) and consist of telophase (MAC I) or prophase (MAC II) arrangements of the nuclei (Figs. 1 and 2) in completely mature cells with a high N/C ratio and an increased nuclear chromatin (Nieburgs, 1967). Evidence of MAC-type findings is frequent in neoplastic patients and much more rare in non-neoplastic ones (Nieburgs, 1967, 1968; Meisels, 1969; Martuzzi et al., 1969a,b; Martuzzi, 1970; Finch and Von Haam, 1971; Martuzzi et al., 1971). MAC can be detected in some subjects before there is clinical evidence of cancer, or after surgical removal of a neoplastic focus (Nieburgs, 1967; Martuzzi et al., 1971).

A relation between MAC-type findings and a systemic disturbance of the process of the cellular differentiation or maturation has been assumed by Nieburgs (1967).

In spite of the high rate of MAC findings in neoplastic patients, its diagnostic usefulness cannot be considered great (Finch and Von Haam, 1971). Microscopic investigation involves some difficulties in revealing the typical features of MAC (Martuzzi, 1971), which are best detected only at the highest magnifications of the optical microscope, using oil-immersion (Nieburgs, 1967). Besides, doubts can be put forward, related to

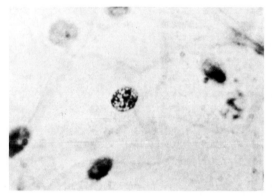

FIG. 3   *Buccal mucosa smear. Mature cornified cell with initially pyknotic nucleus resembling MAC feature – (Papanicolaou-Nieburgs stain; original magnification 1000X). Reduced for reproduction 40%.*

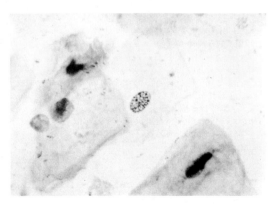

FIG. 4   *Buccal mucosa smear. Mature cornified cell with nucleus in initial karyorrexis simulating MAC feature – (Papanicolaou-Nieburgs stain; original magnification 1000X). Reduced for reproduction 40%.*

technical artefacts (fixing and dyeing), or with degenerative processes [pyknosis (Fig. 3), karyorrhexis (Fig. 4)], or with questionable interpretation (Fig. 5) of the nuclear structure (Finch and Von Haam, 1971), or with intermediate features (BA cells, that is cells with nuclear chromatin structure partially interphase, partially telophase (Fig. 6) and BC cells, that is partially interphase, partially prophase type). Routine smears and sections can be inadequate to the needs of this delicate investigation which must evaluate either structure or chromasia of the nuclear chromatin. Nevertheless, the biological significance of the topic has to be considered sufficiently important to justify careful study.

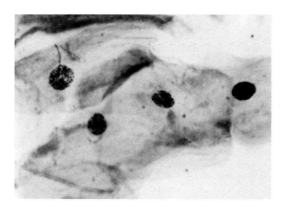

FIG. 5   *Buccal mucosa smear. Mature cornified cells with nuclei showing incomplete and dubious features of MAC – (Papanicolaou-Nieburgs stain; original magnification 1000X). Reduced for reproduction 40%.*

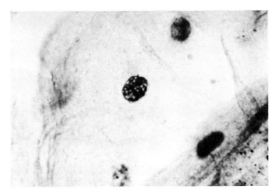

FIG. 6   *Buccal mucosa smear. Mature cornified cell with nucleus showing a nucleolus (interphase feature) and clear round areas (telophase features) – (Papanicolaou-Nieburgs stain; original magnification 1000X). Reduced for reproduction 40%.*

Material and methods

Diagnostic description of all cases was always based on histological examination. The choice of each case depended only on the availability of smears and histological sections of a good technical standard.

In order to detect MAC, at least 10 microscopical fields were examined in each section or smear, at the highest magnification (1000 x) of the optical microscope.

A 'MAC' statement about the cells was always based upon Nieburgs' original description. We avoided assessing a case as MAC-positive when only one cell had been detected, but we continued with the investigation to find more than one.

At least two observers, who had no knowledge of the clinical condition, performed independent examinations.

TABLE 1   *MAC-cells detected in buccal mucosa smears*

	No. of cases	MAC	% incidence
Neoplastic cases (from various sites)	50	36	72
Non-neoplastic cases	50	6	12

	Cancer	Non-cancer	Total	% accuracy
MAC	36	6	42	86
Non-MAC	14	44	58	76

Results

Tables 1–4 show the incidence of MAC in the cases we were able to study and the ability of MAC to assess or exclude cancer. These data are broadly in accordance with our previous presentation and that of Nieburgs.

In addition, some qualitative comments can be made about some particular findings. Some cells rarely show a nuclear MAC-type pattern, although this is very frequently detected in some other cells, such as breast ductal epithelium. For example, our findings of MAC in bronchial epithelium are rare even in proximity to a neoplastic focus. Nevertheless, bronchial epithelium shows some distinct nuclear patterns when cancer is present: the nucleus is enlarged, with an increased content of chromatin and with a chromatin arrangement which is not always of A (telophasic) or C (prophasic) type: chromocenters are few and large; chromatin bands are rare, straight and thin; the nuclear membrane is thick and sometimes indented; but a nucleolus can be detected although it is never a big one.

Even though the above mentioned features do not allow these cells to be properly

TABLE 2   *MAC-cells detected in uterine cervix sections and smears*

	No. of cases	MAC	% incidence
Neoplastic cases (uterine cancer)	52	34	64
Non-neoplastic cases	52	11	21

	Cancer	Non-cancer	Total	% accuracy
MAC	34	11	45	75.5
Non-MAC	18	51	69	74

TABLE 3   *MAC-cells detected in bronchial mucosa (histological sections and smears from sputum or washing)*

	No. of cases	MAC	% incidence
Neoplastic cases (lung cancer)	54	27	50
Non-neoplastic cases (other lung diseases)	54	6	11

	Cancer	Non-cancer	Total	% accuracy
MAC	27	6	33	82
Non−MAC	27	48	75	64

TABLE 4   *MAC-cells detected in gastric mucosa (histological sections and washing smears)*

	No. of cases	MAC	% incidence
Neoplastic cases (gastric cancer)	44	29	66
Non-neoplastic cases (other gastric diseases)	44	6	13

	Cancer	Non-cancer	Total	% accuracy
MAC	29	6	35	83
Non-MAC	15	38	53	72

TABLE 5   *Retrospective and follow-up study*

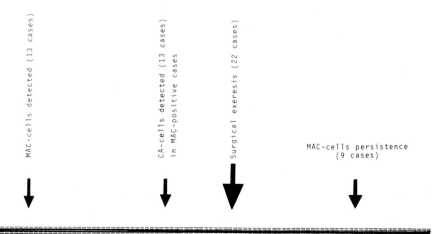

assigned to MAC, it seems obvious they imply a similar impairment of the cell's maturation processes, which can be related to tumor growth.

Another example of an altered pattern of nuclear chromatin of epithelial cells related to cancer, but outside the classical concept of MAC, can be found in gastric mucosa, where the surface and/or glandular epithelium show large nucleoli, an increased RNA chromatin content and a thick nuclear membrane.

This pattern is similar to the findings that are very frequently detected in fields of gastric mucosa in proximity to an ulcer, but differs from it, either by the increased RNA chromatin content, or by the variable size of the nuclei (Amadori et al., 1973).

A small group of cases could be studied on the basis of a retrospective and follow-up analysis (Table 5):

22 cases had a neoplastic focus removed. In 13 of them, MAC-cell detection was possible in a period of from 6 months to 5 years before cancer cells could be detected. MAC-cell persistence was observed in 9 cases for a period of from 2–3 months to 3 years.

The results of the present research confirm and emphasize the role of MAC in the study of the natural history and morphogenetic processes of malignant tumors. MAC detection can substantially improve the accuracy of routine diagnostic processes, but it requires considerable competence and application.

Summary

Cell nuclei were examined at the highest magnification of the optical microscope in smears and histological sections from 200 cases of malignant tumors and 200 non-neoplastic cases. The present data confirm the previous observations of Nieburgs and our own: the average incidence of MAC is about 65% in neoplastic cases and about 16% in non-neoplastic ones.

MAC was occasionally detected in some individuals in whom a tumor was later revealed and in others in whom a tumor had been previously removed. Some other morphological features of the nuclei were observed which are probably related to MAC; they support the hypothesis of a systemic impairment of cell maturation related to the growth of the tumor and its morphological appearance.

References

Amadori, D., Martuzzi, M. and Ravaioli, A. (1973): In: Abstracts, Second International Symposium on Cancer Detection and Prevention, Bologna 1973, p. 165. Editors: C. Maltoni, M. Crespi and P. R. J. Burch. Excerpta Medica, Amsterdam.

Finch, R. R. and Von Haam, E. (1971): Acta cytol. (Philad.), 15, 46.

Martuzzi, M. (1970): In: Biological Seminar of the Faculty of Medicine and Surgery of the Catholic University, p. 116. Rome, January, 1970. Editor: A. Giordano. Ist. Diffusione Opere Scient., Milano.

Martuzzi, M., Amadori, D. and Saragoni, A. (1969): In: Proceedings, XI Congress of the Italian Society on Pathology, p. 629. Rome, October, 1969. Editors: T. Terranova and T. Galeotti. Vita e Pensiero, Milano.

Martuzzi, M., Amadori, D. and Saragoni, A. (1969): In: Proceedings, XI Congress of the Italian Society on Pathology, p. 637. Rome, October, 1969. Editors: T. Terranova and T. Galeotti. Vita e Pensiero, Milano.

Martuzzi, M., Amadori, D. and Saragoni, A. (1971): Minerva ginec., 23, 198.

Meisels, A. (1969): Acta cytol. (Philad.), 13, 473.

Nieburgs, H. E. (1967): Diagnostic Cell Pathology in Tissue and Smears. Grune and Stratton, New York, N. Y.

Nieburgs, H. E. (1968): Acta cytol. (Philad.), 12, 445.

Nieburgs, H. E., Herman, B. F. and Reisman, H. (1962): Lab. Invest., 11, 80.

Nieburgs, H. E., Zak, F. G., Allen, D. C., Reisman, H. and Clardy, T. (1959): In: Transactions of the Seventh Annual Meeting of the International Society Cytology Council, 1959, p. 137.

Cytological features of squamous metaplasia and nuclear structures of the cylindrical bronchial cells in patients with lung cancer

M. Martuzzi, A. Saragoni and L. Lazzari

Clinical Pathology and Oncologic Center, 'G.B. Morgagni' Hospital, Forli, Italy

The association of squamous metaplasia of the bronchial mucosa with lung cancer has been studied by many authors (Valentine, 1957; Kierszenbaum, 1965; Nasiell, 1966; Maltoni et al., 1966, 1968; Mason and Jordan, 1969). Except for a more frequent detection in cancer patients than in other bronchial and pulmonary diseases, a specific role for squamous metaplasia as a pre-cancerous change cannot be affirmed at present, although experimental evidence and studies of smoker's (Auerbach et al., 1951, 1957; Hamilton et al., 1957; Ide et al., 1959; Plamenac et al., 1973), and of occupational cancers (Saccomanno et al., 1965; Maltoni et al., 1966) support the idea. However, some authors (Carrol, 1961) regard the association of squamous metaplasia and squamous carcinoma as coincidental.

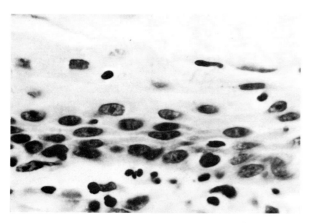

FIG. 1   *Squamous metaplasia in bronchial wall – (Hematoxylin-eosin; original magnification 400X). Reduced for reproduction 33%.*

In spontaneous human pathology, the cell alterations described as 'atypical metaplasia' (Nasiell, 1966), or 'dysplasia' (Kierszenbaum, 1965), can be considered as signs of a coexistent neoplastic focus, but these lesions must undoubtedly be regarded as more advanced than simple squamous metaplasia.

For these reasons, the diagnostic usefulness of squamous metaplasia in smears and histological sections from patients affected by lung or bronchial diseases, is not great.

This is why a more detailed analysis of the cytological features of squamous metaplasia can be considered important. Identification of squamous metaplasia can be obvious in histological sections (Fig. 1) of the bronchial tree, but it must be considered as difficult in smears from sputum because of the mixing with buccal squamous cells (Koss, 1961).

Squamous cells in smears can be regarded as metaplastic when they are larger than basal cells, but smaller than squamous cells of oral origin (Nasiell, 1966), and when they are mixed with columnar cells (Kierszenbaum, 1965), or with bronchial macrophages.

Material and methods

Specimens were drawn from patients affected either with lung cancer (80 cases) or with other lung diseases (100 cases). Each cancer case was supported by at least one biopsy specimen. Each cancer and non-cancer case was frequently supported by many cytological and cyto-histological specimens either from sputum or from bronchial washings.

Smears were stained by Papanicolaou-Boshann or Papanicolaou-Nieburgs methods. Histological sections were coloured with hematoxylin-eosin, Van Gieson, or Mallory stains.

TABLE 1   *Squamous metaplasia (in smears and histological sections)*

	No. of cases	Squamous metaplasia
Lung cancer patients	80	65 (81%)
Other lung diseases	100	23 (23%)

Results

The main data from the present study (Table 1) confirm the different rate of findings of squamous metaplasia in cancer and non-cancer patients.

In a general sense, a squamous metaplastic cell can be more or less mature (Fig. 2); its degree of maturation should affect the nuclear parameters only, by way of nuclear regression, until complete pyknosis take place.

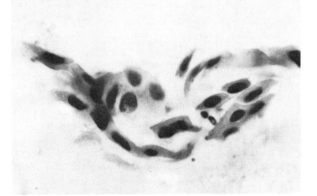

FIG. 2   *Squamous metaplastic cells in a bronchial washing showing different degrees of evolution (Cytohistological specimen; hematoxylin-eosin; original magnification 400X). Reduced for reproduction 33%.*

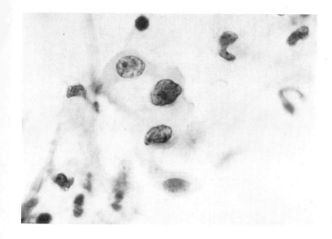

3

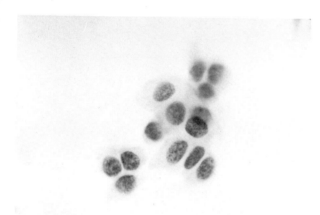

4

FIGS. 3 and 4 *Squamous metaplastic cells in bronchial washings from lung cancer patients. Cytoplasmic cornification and nuclei unregressed – (Smears; Papanicolaou-Nieburgs stain; original magnification 1000X). Reduced for reproduction 33%.*

    This process seems to be frequently altered in cancer patients and only seldom and partially in non-cancerous ones: cytoplasmic maturation goes on towards complete evolution, with a frequent pattern of a well-defined cornification while the nucleus remains unregressed (Figs. 3 and 4) and shows, on the contrary, the chromatin arrangements of telophase- (Fig. 5) and prophase-type (Figs. 6 and 7) with hyperchromasia and an altered N/C ratio. The contrast between the nuclear and cytoplasmic features can reach an advanced stage in cancer patients, until complete atypia takes place (Fig. 8), while a normal ratio, as in epidermal epithelium, is usual in non-cancer patients. The findings of these features are summarized in Table 2.

    The ciliated columnar epithelium of the bronchial tree shows alterations at some distance from the neoplastic focus. They have long been well known, mostly as cytoplasmic changes [Ciliocytophtoria and degenerative changes; 'Pap' cells (Papanicolaou, 1954; Papanicolaou et al., 1961); koilocytotic atypia (Kierszenbaum, 1965)], but many

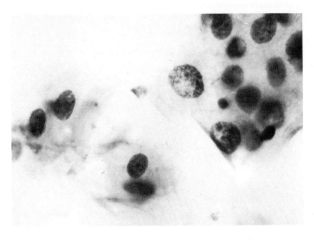

5

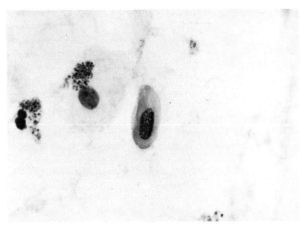

6

FIGS. 5 and 6   *Chromatin arrangements of telophase type in squamous metaplastic cells from lung cancer patients – (Sputum smears; Papanicolaou-Nieburgs stain; original magnification 1000X). Reduced for reproduction 33%.*

authors have emphasized the increased and variable size and also the hyperchromatic nuclei, mainly associated with basal cell hyperplasia (Umiker, 1961; Carrol, 1961; Lanza, 1968).

By the highest magnifications of the optical microscope (1000 diameters and more), and by well standardized technical processes (fixing and dying), the nuclear features can be studied, and they provide a more objective evaluation of the cellular pattern related to cancer development.

In comparison with non-cancerous patients, the bronchial columnar cells from cancer patients show a more variable but always increased size and chromasia (Fig. 9) of the nuclei and a higher proportion of telophase and prophase arrangements (A and C cells) (Table 3, Fig. 10).

Similar changes affect also the nuclei of the buccal squamous cells when they are examined in sputum smears or in directly-drawn smears. The contrast between a mature cytoplasmic pattern and a nucleus which is enlarged, hyperchromatic, unregressed and characterized by telophase or prophase arrangements, is prominent and frequent.

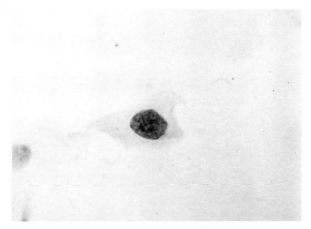

FIG. 7   *Chromatin arrangements of prophase type in squamous metaplastic cells from lung cancer patients — (Sputum smears; Papanicolaou-Nieburgs stain; original magnification 1000X). Reduced for reproduction 33%.*

TABLE 2   *Nuclear features in bronchial squamous metaplastic cells*

	No. of cases	Rate of pyknotic nuclei	High N/C	High chromatin	Rate in non-pyknotic nuclei	
					A-cells (telophase)	C-cells (prophase)
Neoplastic cases (lung cancer)	65	52%	74%	85%	frequent	frequent
Non-neoplastic cases (other lung diseases)	23	60%	60%	30%	very rare	rare

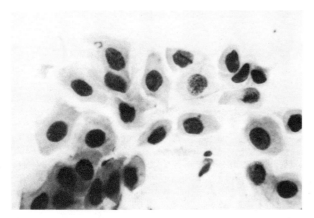

FIG. 8   *Various degrees of nuclear alterations up to complete atypia in squamous metaplastic cells from lung cancer patients — (Sputum smears; Papanicolaou-Nieburgs stain; original magnification 1000X). Reduced for reproduction 33%.*

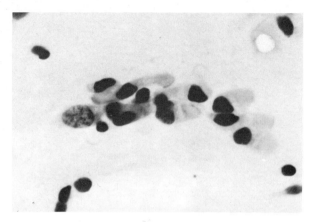

FIG. 9   *Columnar cells with various degrees of nuclear alterations in a lung cancer patient – (Bronchial washing; Papanicolaou-Nieburgs stain; original magnification 1000X). Reduced for reproduction 33%.*

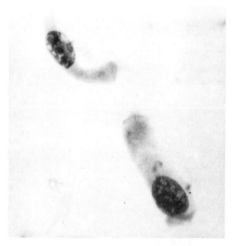

FIG. 10   *Columnar cells with prophase-type nuclei and increased chromatin in a lung cancer patient – (Bronchial washing; Papanicolaou-Nieburgs stain; original magnification 1000X). Reduced for reproduction 25%.*

A highly differentiate cell which shows telophasic hyperchromatic nuclei, comes into the concept of MAC (Malignancy Associated Changes) according to Nieburgs (Nieburgs et al., 1959) and may be considered as a sign of a systemic disturbance of the processes of cellular maturation, which is related to the morphogenesis of cancer.

The present cytological features can help to improve the diagnostic accuracy of the cytological and cyto-histological examinations of sputum and bronchial washings from lung cancer patients, because the nuclear alterations may represent several aspects of the disturbance of cellular maturation and division related to cancer morphogenesis.

Summary

Squamous metaplastic cells are very frequently detected (81.2%) in sputum smears and bronchial mucosa from patients with lung tumors (80 cases examined). They may be

TABLE 3   *Nuclear features in bronchial columnar epithelium*

	No. of cases	Various size	High N/C	High chromatin	Rate of cell-types	
					A-cells (telophase)	C-cells (prophase)
Neoplastic cases (lung cancer)	71	74%	86%	67%	frequent	frequent
Non-neoplastic cases (other lung diseases)	24	25%	45%	25%	rare	rare

* Unsuitable cases, with smears and/or sections not properly processed for nuclear investigation, had to be excluded.

found also (23%) in patients with other lung diseases (100 cases examined). These cells show a small, overmature cytoplasm and a very hyperchromatic, large, but not pyknotic nucleus. In neoplastic patients they frequently show (at ×1000 magnification) chromatin arrangements of a telophasic and prophasic kind. Also, bronchial columnar cells show nuclear changes even at a distance from the tumor: variable size, increased N/C ratio, hyperchromatin and prophasic and telophasic arrangements. Similar nuclear alterations are observed also in squamous cells from oral mucosa, at high frequency in patients with lung carcinoma, but very rarely in non-neoplastic subjects.

References

Auerbach, O., Gere, J. B., Forman, J. B., Petterick, T. G., Smolin, H. J., Muehsam, G. E., Kassouny, D. Y. and Stout, A. P. (1957): New Engl. J. Med., 256, 104.
Auerbach, O., Stout, A. P., Hammond, E. C. and Garfinkel, L. (1951): New Engl. J. Med., 265, 253.
Carrol, R. (1961): Brit. J. Cancer, 15, 215.
Hamilton, J. D., Sepp, A., Brown, T. C. and MacDonald, F. W. (1957): Canad. med. Ass. J., 77, 177.
Ide, G., Suntzeff, V. and Cowdry, E. V. (1959): Cancer (Philad.), 12, 478.
Kierszenbaum, A. L. (1965): Acta cytol. (Philad.), 9, 365.
Koss, L. G. (1961): Diagnostic Cytology and its Histopathologic Bases, pp. 204 – 205. J. B. Lippincott Co., Philadelphia, Pa. 1961.
Lanza, G. (1968): Riv. Pat. clin. sper., 9, 953.
Maltoni, C., Carretti, D. and Perretti, S. (1966): Arch. Ostet. Ginec. (Suppl.), 71, 364.
Maltoni, C., Carretti, D., Canepari, C., Ghetti, G. (1968): Cancro, 4, 349.
Mason, M. K. and Jordan, J. W. (1969): Thorax, 24, 461.
Nasiell, M. (1966): Acta cytol. (Philad.), 10, 421.
Nieburgs, H. E., Zak, F. G., Allen, D. C., Reisman, H. and Claroy, T. (1959): In: Transactions of the Seventh Annual Meeting of the International Society Cytology Council, 1959, p. 137.
Papanicolaou, G. M. (1954): Atlas of Exfoliated Cytology. Harvard University Press, Cambridge, Mass., 1954.
Papanicolaou, G. M., Bridges, E. L. and Railey, C. (1961): Amer. Rev. resp. Dis., 83, 641.
Plamenac, P., Nikulin, A. and Pikula, B. (1973): Acta cytol., (Philad.), 17, 241.
Saccomanno, G., Saunders, R. P., Archer, V. E., Auerbach, O., Kuschner, M. and Beckler, P. A. (1965): Acta cytol. (Philad.), 9, 413.
Umiker, W. O. (1961): Dis. Chest, 40, 154.
Valentine, E. H. (1957): Cancer (Philad.), 10, 272.

Nuclear cell structures in mastopathy and related lesions concomitant with cancer

D. Amadori, M. Martuzzi and M. Savoia

Clinical Pathology and Oncologic Center, 'G.B. Morgagni' Hospital, Forli, Italy

The suggestion of a morphopathogenetic role of mastopathy (M.) and above all of ductal hyperplasia (D.H.), ductal papillomatosis (D.P.) and lobular hyperplasia (L.H.) towards carcinoma, has been supported by many authors (Warren, 1940; Levinson and Lyons, 1953; Haagensen, 1956; Humphrey and Swerdlow 1962; Tellem et al., 1962, 1965; Rush and Kramer, 1963; Davis et al., 1964; Karpas et al., 1965; Evans, 1966; Shah and Mathur, 1967; Stein 1967; Bauer, 1967; Humphrey and Swerdlow, 1968; Berndt and Marwitz, 1968; Veronesi and Pizzocaro, 1968; Kern and Brooks, 1969; Gallager and Martin, 1969; Martuzzi, 1972; Haagensen, 1971; etc.).

As is well known, D.H., D.P. and L.H. ('mastopathy related changes' or lesions) are regarded as morphologic changes related with mastopathy (Haagensen, 1971); they frequently coexist with it and represent a dysplastic type of pathologic process, like mastopathy. They can indeed be considered as single elementary alterations in the whole complex picture of mastopathy together with duct cysts, apocrine cysts, adenosis and stromal fibrosis (Haagensen, 1971).

Some statistical or follow-up studies showed a rather more pronounced tendency for these changes to progress towards mammary cancer than simple mastopathy. Accordingly, a 'precancerous' significance has been proposed by some authors (Evans, 1966; Humphrey and Swerdlow, 1968; Bassler, 1969; Gallager and Martin, 1969; etc.).

Nevertheless, the evidence for this progression cannot be regarded as properly defined either in terms of the frequency of cases or in relation to time. On the other hand, the structural studies failed to show features that could unquestionably be regarded as being related to cancer morphogenesis, even if certain suggestions could be made (Gallager and Martin, 1969; Martuzzi, 1972).

A deeper analysis of the above-mentioned changes by taking account of the cell and nuclear parameters in fields of M.; D. H.; L. H.; and D. P., associated or not associated with breast cancer, seemed to be an useful approach to the problem of evaluating the possible stages of progression.

Material and methods

210 cases of breast cancer and 195 cases of fibrocystic mastopathy were reviewed. The only selection criterion was the availability of more than one histological section, from different quadrants of the same mammary gland, surgically excised or biopsied. Several cases were also concerned with smears from spontaneous duct secretion or needle aspirates.

Smears were stained by the Papanicolaou method as modified by Boshann, or by Nieburgs. Histological sections were processed with routine hematoxylin-eosin, Van Gieson, Mallory and Silver-methenamine methods. Randomized smears and sections were examined separately by two observers at least, without any clinical or pathological records. 200 cells were recorded in each specimen for the classical parameters: nuclear-cytoplasmic ratio (N/C); and chromasia. In addition the same cells were classified according to Nieburgs' concepts into 3 main types: A or telophase cell; B or interphase cell; C or prophase cell (Fig. 1) (Nieburgs et al., 1970).

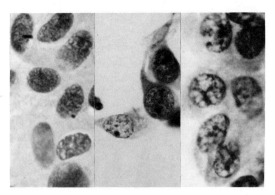

FIG. 1   *Cell types according to Nieburgs (from left) A-cell (telophase nucleus), B-cell (interphase nucleus), C-cell (prophase nucleus) – (Original magnification 1000X). Reduced for reproduction 41%.*

A cell (telophase): chromatin structure consists of numerous small, uniform chromocenters, of curved chromatin bands of uniform length and thickness attached around the chromocenters and surrounding little clear circular areas of equal size. Nucleolus is absent.

B cell (interphase): nucleus always shows an obvious nucleolus; perinucleolar chromatin may be absent or arranged in small uniform chromocenters connected by thin chromatin bands.

C cell (prophase): chromatin structure is characterized by chromocenters of different size and shape connected by straight chromatin bands of various length and thickness. Clear areas surrounded by chromatin bands are of different size and shape. Nucleolus is absent.

TABLE 1   *Nuclear features in histological fields of pure mastopathy* from breast cancer and non-cancer patients*

	Cancer (71 cases)		Non-cancer (62 cases)	
	No.	%	No.	%
High N/C ratio	60	85	17	27
High chromasia	56	79	17	27
A-cells (telophase)	detected in 35% cases: rate 4%		detected in 22% cases: rate 3%	
C-cells (prophase)	detected in all cases: rate 27%		detected in all cases: rate 18%	

* 139 cases of the cancer series and 133 cases of the mastopathy series showed associated changes.

Results

The histological fields of pure mastopathy (Table 1) show cytological changes in neoplastic cases: the nuclei of the epithelial cells present a high N/C ratio in 85% of the cases and high chromasia in 79%. A-cells (telophase) have been detected in 35% of the cases with a rate of 4% of the other cytotypes (undamaged mammary tissue usually contains only very infrequent A-cells in our experience). C-cells (prophase) have been detected in all cases with a rate of 27% (this rate is much higher than in undamaged tissue). The same

TABLE 2   *Nuclear features in histological fields of mastopathy-related changes from breast cancer and non-cancer patients*

	Neoplastic patients (139 cases)		Non-neoplastic patients (133 cases)	
	No.	%	No.	%
High N/C ratio	139	100	91	68
High chromasia	139	100	66	50
A-cells (telophase)	detected in 42% cases: rate 5%		detected in 34% cases: rate 4%	
C-cells (prophase)	detected in all cases: rate 30%		detected in all cases: rate 23%	

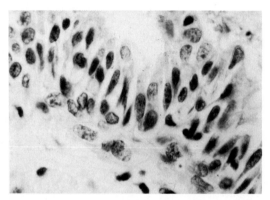

FIG. 2   *Mammary duct hyperplasia in non-cancer patient – (Histological section – Hematoxylin-eosin; original magnification 1000X). Reduced for reproduction 41%.*

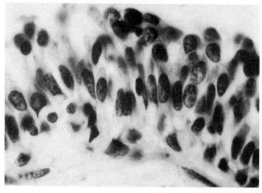

FIG. 3   *Mammary duct hyperplasia in cancer patient – (Histological section – Hematoxylin-eosin; original magnification 1000X). Reduced for reproduction 41%.*

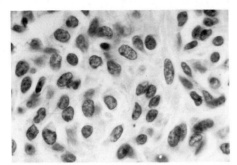

FIG. 4   *Mammary lobular hyperplasia in non-cancer patient – (Histological section – Hematoxylin-eosin; original magnification 1000X). Reduced for reproduction 41%.*

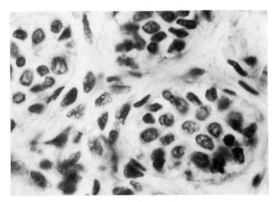

FIG. 5   *Mammary lobular hyperplasia in cancer patient – (Histological section – Hematoxylin-eosin; original magnification 1000X). Reduced for reproduction 41%.*

nuclear features have been detected in less than 1/3 of the cases of pure mastopathy not associated with cancer.

Histological fields of *mastopathy-related changes* (D. H., L. H., D. P.) associated with carcinoma (Table 2) show clear-cut alterations of the nuclear parameters: a high N/C ratio and chromasia have been detected in 100% of the cases; A-cells have been detected in all cases, with a frequency of 30%. The same nuclear features have been detected in a little more than half the cases of mastopathy-related changes not associated with cancer (Figs. 2 to 7). Incidentally, the nuclear changes appear more frequently and prominently in the multiple association of D. H., L. H. and D. P.

Discussion

Prominent nuclear changes can be detected in patients with pure mastopathy associated with carcinoma of the same mammary gland and in patients with 'masthopathy-related changes' associated with carcinoma of the same mammary gland. These alterations consist of an increased N/C ratio, nuclear chromasia and a higher frequency of A (telophase) and C (prophase) cell-types. Similar alterations can be observed in patients with pure mastopathy or 'mastopathy-related changes' not associated with breast carcinoma, but their frequency and prominence are less evident.

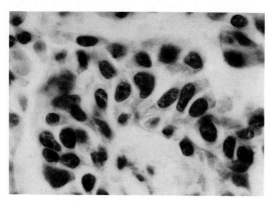

FIG. 6   *Mammary duct papillomatosis in non-cancer patient – (Histological section – Hematoxylin-eosin; original magnification 1000X). Reduced for reproduction 41%.*

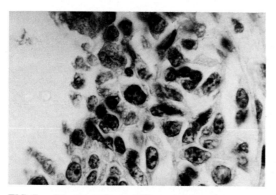

FIG. 7   *Mammary duct papillomatosis in cancer patient – (Histological section – Hematoxylin-eosin; original magnification 1000X). Reduced for reproduction 41%.*

A morphopathogenetic role of these features towards carcinoma can be assumed, either on the morphologic basis, or on account of the well-known high frequency of clinical evolution of mastopathy cases into carcinoma, according to reports in the literature.

The finding of these alterations in the cases in which a breast carcinoma has not been revealed in the same mammary gland, can be regarded either as indicative of a cancer focus in the contralateral breast or in other organs, or alternatively, as support for the hypothesis that they signify pre-cancerous changes.

Summary

The present study, using a cytological method, considers the nuclear appearance of epithelial cells in areas of mammary tissue affected by mastopathy, ductal hyperplasia, ductal papillomatosis and lobular hyperplasia in association with breast cancer (210 cases), or not associated with breast cancer (195 cases).

The alterations observed in the cases in which carcinoma is concomitant are fairly systematic and consist of an increased N/C ratio and chromasia, as well as an increased frequency of cells with a telophasic or prophasic nuclear arrangement.

References

Bassler, R. (1969): Dtsch. med. Wschr., 94, 108.

Bauer, W. (1967): Zbl. Chir., 92, 2322.

Berndt, H. and Marwitz, S. (1968): Arch. Geschwulstforsch., 32, 137.

Davis, H. H., Simons, M. and Davis, J. B. (1964): Cancer (Philad.), 17, 957.

Evans, R. W. (1966): Histological Appearances of Tumours. E. and S. Livingstone Ltd., Edinburgh-London.

Gallager, H. S. and Martin, J. E. (1969): Cancer (Philad.), 24, 1170.

Haagensen, C. D. (1956): Diseases of the Breast. W. B. Saunders Co., Philadelphia – London.

Haagensen, C. D. (1971): Diseases of the Breast. W. B. Saunders Co., Philadelphia – London – Toronto.

Humphrey, L. and Swerdlow, M. (1962): Surgery, 52, 841.

Humphrey, L. J. and Swerdlow, M. (1968): Arch. Surg., 97, 592.

Karpas, C. M., Leis, H. P., Oppenheim, A. and Mersheimer, L. (1965): Ann. Surg., 162, 1.

Kern, W. H. and Brooks, M. D. (1969): Cancer (Philad.), 24, 668.

Lewison, E. F. and Lyons Jr, J. G. (1953): Arch. Surg., 66, 94.

Martuzzi, M. (1972): Acta Ginec., 23, 131.

Nieburgs, H. E., Levis, F. and Cappa, A. P. M. (1970): Minerva med., 61, 4926.

Rush, B. F. and Kramer, W. M. (1963): Surg. Gynec. Obstet. 117, 425.

Shah, H. S. and Mathur, B. B. C. (1967): Indian J. Path. Bact., 10, 197.

Stein, A. A. (1967): In: Pathology Annual 1967, p. 47. Butterworth, London.

Tellem, M., Prive, I. and Meranze, D. (1962): Cancer (Philad.), 15, 10.

Tellem, M., Shane, J. J. and Imbriglia, J. E. (1965): Surg. Gynec. Obstet., 120, 17.

Veronesi, V. and Pizzocaro, G. (1968): Surg. Gynec. Obstet., 126, 529.

Warren, S. (1940): Surg. Gynec. Obstet., 71, 257.

Morphological features of ductal hyperplasia, ductal papillomatosis and lobular hyperplasia associated with breast cancer

M. Martuzzi, A. Saragoni, A. Ravaioli and M. Savoia

Clinical Pathology and Oncologic Center 'G.B. Morgagni' Hospital, Forli, Italy

The relationship between fibrocystic mastopathy and breast carcinoma had been studied by many authors (Warren, 1940; Levison and Lyons, 1953; Haagensen, 1956; Davis et al., 1964; Evans, 1966; Shah and Mathur, 1967; Stein, 1967; Bauer, 1967; Berndt and Marwitz, 1968; Veronesi and Pizzocaro, 1968; Haagensen, 1971; etc.).

Some morphopathogenetic relations were assumed and confirmed by more recent studies (Haagensen, 1971), but others have strongly denied this relation (Devitt, 1972).

Other studies emphasized a more pertinent connection between breast cancer and some other alterations, related with mastopathy, such as ductal hyperplasia (D. H.) (Fig. 1), lobular hyperplasia (L. H.) (Fig. 2) and ductal papillomatosis (D. P.) (Fig. 3) (Humphrey and Swerdlow, 1962; Tellem et al., 1962; Rush and Kramer, 1963; Tellem et al., 1965; Karpas et al., 1965; Stein, 1967; Humphrey, 1968; Kern and Brooks, 1969; Orcel et al., 1969; Gallager and Martin, 1969; Martuzzi, 1972; Haagensen, 1971; etc.).

A morphopathogenetic role of these alterations towards carcinoma, like a precancerosis, is affirmed by some (Evans, 1966; Humphrey and Swerdlow, 1968; Bassler, 1969; Gallager and Martin, 1969; etc.), but the rate and time of this evolution have been evaluated in very different ways. The lack of a uniform terminology and classification of benign breast diseases is held responsible for these different evaluations (Haagensen, 1971; Perzin and Lattes, 1972; Devitt, 1972). Concurrent and multiple association of these alterations with cancer in the same mammary gland can be regarded as an additional cause.

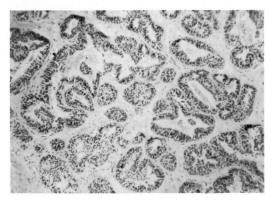

FIG. 1   *Ductal hyperplasia of mammary gland (Hematoxylin-eosin; original magnification 250X). Reduced for reproduction 39%.*

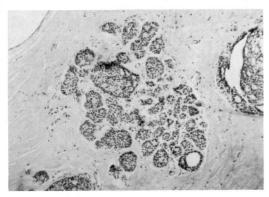

FIG. 2   *Lobular hyperplasia of mammary gland (Hematoxylin-eosin; original magnification 100X). Reduced for reproduction 39%.*

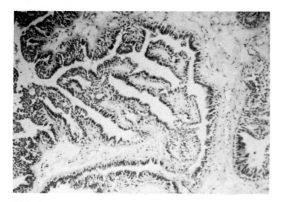

FIG. 3   *Ductal papillomatosis of mammary gland (Hematoxylin-eosin; original magnification 250X). Reduced for reproduction 39%.*

The terms 'lobular in situ carcinoma' (Foote and Stewart, 1941; Hutter and Foote, 1969) and 'lobular neoplasia' (see Haagensen, 1971) seem to refer to pathological entities which may represent additional links in the possible chain of the morphogenetic changes from epithelial hyperplastic or dysplastic lesions, towards carcinoma. But a definite role of precursor of mammary cancer cannot be assigned even to lobular in situ carcinoma (Kaufmann et al., 1971).

A perspective study of the morphologic features related to the growth of breast cancer must be considered a difficult task because of the anatomical characteristics of the breast and the obvious risk of missing minute foci of cancer when histology is performed on sections from tissue (Haagensen, 1971).

The study of the histological peculiarities and the differences between mastopathy, ductal and lobular hyperplasia, and ductal papillomatosis genuinely associated with cancer from the same lesions not associated with cancer, can be considered a useful approach to the problem, until we have at our disposal a large series of cases in which pathological changes classified according to the most detailed and accepted criteria, are supported by good histological evidence and a prolonged follow-up.

Material and methods

The only selective criterion for the cases to be examined was the availability of some histological sections from different fields of the mammary gland. The histological sections to be examined from the neoplastic cases were to be taken remote from the neoplastic focus, in the same mammary gland. These specimens must be accepted as representative of the whole gland, because of the lack of a complete histological examination. We know that at a good standard level of work, this assumption can be accepted.

Tissue preparation followed the usual routine: formol or alcohol fixing, paraffin embedding, microtome sections at 4-7μ, hematoxylin-eosin, Van Gieson, Mallory, Silver-methanamine dying.

313 cases of mammary carcinoma and 195 cases of mastopathy were examined. A randomization of all histological sections was performed, so that the nosographic decision in each case was unknown. Mastopathic changes were detected in 210 cancer cases. A comparison was therefore possible between histological features of 195 'pure' mastopathies and 210 cancer-associated mastopathies.

Histopathological definition of the lesions (either associated, or not associated with cancer) to be examined was done according to classical and well-defined concepts (Stewart, 1950; McDivitt et al., 1968; Haagensen, 1971; Black et al., 1972). No distinction was made between mastopathy with objective clinical signs and that with purely histological evidence. Papillary adenoma (Haagensen, 1971) as a unique focal lesion either in the nipple, or elsewhere, was not taken into consideration. Cancer diagnosis was never made without evidence of a broken epithelial-stromal membrane and a very disordered pattern of the epithelial layers into the ducts and acini. 'Lobular hyperplasia' was only diagnosed when a clearly benign proliferation of the acinar epithelium was present without any cellular atypia or breaking of the basal membrane.

TABLE 1   *Histological breast changes associated with cancer and mastopathy*

	Mastopathy (195 cases)		Cancer plus mastopathy (210 cases)*	
	No.	%	No.	%
Ductal hyperplasia	49	25	63	30
Lobular hyperplasia	32	16	8	4
Ductal papillomatosis	58	30	115	55
2 or 3 changes together	19	10	115	55
No other changes	62	32	71	34

* 103 of 313 cancer cases showed no mastopathic associated changes

Results

The main numerical data as given in Table 1, show that ductal hyperplasia and ductal papillomatosis are more frequently detected in mastopathic tissue from cancer patients than in non-cancer patients. Lobular hyperplasia is less frequently detected than other alterations, but its rate is higher in non-neoplastic patients than in neoplastic ones. Multiple associations are much more frequently detected in cancer patients than in non-cancer ones.

In a general sense, and from a morphopathogenetic point of view, the above mentioned data can be considered indicative and they give support to similar findings from many other authors. However, for diagnostic purposes, certain morphological details should be apparent.

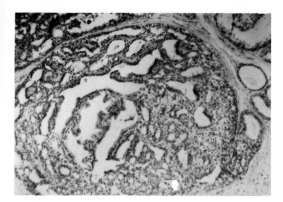

FIG. 4   *Cribriform pattern of the ductal proliferation (Hematoxylin-eosin; original magnification 250X). Reduced for reproduction 39%.*

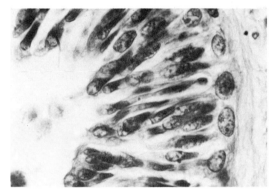

FIG. 5   *Hyperplastic pattern of the myoepithelial layer in a mammary duct (Hematoxylin-eosin; original magnification 1000X). Reduced for reproduction 39%.*

All the material was reviewed for an evaluation of the following histological features which have been regarded as indicative of neoplastic evolution by some authors: the cribriform pattern of the ductal proliferation (Fig. 4), (Evans, 1966; Haagensen, 1971; Fechner and Houston, 1972); myoepithelial proliferation (Fig. 5), or disordered layers in the fields of ductal or lobular hyperplasia associated with cancer (Kuzma, 1943; Black et al., 1972; Fechner and Houston, 1972; Von Haam and Murad, 1973); and the multiple and disordered layering of the epithelial ductal hyperplastic cells (Fig. 6) (Evans, 1966; Black et al., 1972; Fechner, 1972).

Numerical data of this investigation (Table 2) cannot be considered as indicative: crybriform patterns of ductal hyperplasia were detected in 6% of the neoplastic cases as well as non-neoplastic ones. Findings of a hyperplastic or proliferating myoepithelial component were revealed in 10% of non-neoplastic cases and in 9% of neoplastic ones. Irregular lining of the duct epithelial cells could be seen in 4% of non-neoplastic cases and in 5% of neoplastic ones.

Apart from the low frequency of these alterations, they failed to show any significantly different features between neoplastic and non-neoplastic subjects. We can only point to

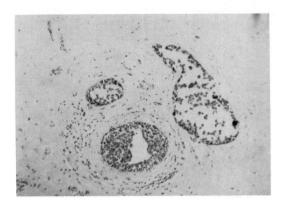

FIG. 6   *Multiple and disordered layering of the epithelial ductal cells (Hematoxylin-eosin; original magnification 100X). Reduced for reproduction 39%.*

TABLE 2   *Histological features of the changes associated with breast cancer and mastopathy*

	Mastopathy (195 cases)		Cancer plus mastopathy (210 cases)*	
	No.	%	No.	%
Cribriform ductal hyperplasia	12	6	13	6
Proliferating myoepithelial cells	19	10	19	9
Non-regular lining of the duct epithelial cells	8	4	10	5

* 103 of 313 cancer cases showed no mastopathic associated changes

a somewhat more extensive manifestation of the above-mentioned changes in cancer patients than in non-neoplastic ones; but this is a rather subjective evaluation.

On the other hand, a deeper study of cellular features in histological fields of mastopathy and related lesion in cancer and non-cancer patients, revealed some different patterns of the cell parameters (nuclear-cytoplasmic ratio, nucleolo-nuclear ratio, chromasia, etc.) and the frequency of cell-types. As these observations come from cytological investigation, they were considered in another study.

Summary

The study is based on 313 cases of mammary carcinoma and on 195 cases of mastopathy.

In 210 of the cancer cases, mastopathy changes were detectable.

The frequency of ductal hyperplasia, lobular hyperplasia and ductal papillomatosis is higher in mastopathic tissues from cancer patients than from non-cancer ones.

Mastopathy, ductal hyperplasia, lobular hyperplasia, and ductal papillomatosis associated with carcinoma did not distinguish structural histological differences from those not associated with carcinoma.

References

Aschkari, R., Hatder, S. I. and Robbins, G. F. (1971): Cancer (Philad.), 28, 1182.
Bassler, R. (1969): Dtsch. med. Wschr., 94, 108.
Bauer, W. (1967): Zbl. Chir., 92, 2322.
Berndt, H. and Marwitz, S. (1968): Arch. Geschwülstforsch., 32, 137.
Black, M. M., Ballay, T. H. C., Cutler, S. J., Hankey, B. F. and Asire, A. J. (1972): Cancer (Philad.), 29, 338.
Davis, H. H., Simons, M. and Davis, J. B. (1964): Cancer (Philad.), 17, 957.
Devitt, J. E.(1972): Surg. Ginec. Obstet., 134, 803.
Evans, R. W. (1966): Histological Appearance of Tumours. E. and S. Livingstone Ltd., Edinburgh — London.
Fechner, R. E. (1972): Cancer (Philad.), 29, 1539.
Fechner, R. E. and Houston, M. D. (1972): Arch. Path., 93, 164.
Foote, F. W. and Stewart, F. W. (1941): Amer. J. Path., 17, 491.
Gallager, H. S. and Martin, J. E. (1969): Cancer (Philad.), 24, 1170.
Haagensen, C. D. (1956): Diseases of the Breast. W. B. Saunders Co., Philadelphia — London.
Haagensen, C. D. (1971): Diseases of the Breast. W. B. Saunders Co., Philadelphia — London — Toronto.
Humphrey, L. J. and Swerdlow, M. (1962): Surgery, 52, 841.
Humphrey, L. J. and Swerdlow, M. A. (1968): Arch. Surg., 97, 592.
Hutter, R. V. P., and Foote, F. W. (1969): Cancer (Philad.), 24, 1081.
Karpas, C. M., Leis, H. P., Oppenheim, A. and Mersheimer, L. (1965): Ann. Surg., 162, 1.
Kaufmann, C., Hamperl, H., Baldus, F. and Ki, B.D. (1971): Dtsch. med. Wschr., 41, 1581.
Kern, W. H. and Brooks, M. D. (1969): Cancer (Philad.), 24, 668.
Kuzma, J. F. (1943): Amer. J. Path., 19, 473.
Lewison, E. F. and Lyons Jr, J. G. (1953): Arch. Surg., 66, 94.
Martuzzi, M. (1972): Acta Ginec. (Madr.), 23, 131.
McDivitt, R. W., Stewart, F. W. and Berg, J. W. (1968): In: Atlas of Tumor Pathology, Second Series, Fascicle 2. Armed Forces Institute of Pathology, Washington D.C.
Orcel, L., Delcour, M., Grynbeat, A. and Marsan, C. (1969): Ann. Anat. path., 14, 353.
Perzin, K. H. and Lattes, R. (1972): Cancer (Philad.), 29, 996.
Rush, B. F. and Kramer, W. M. (1963): Surg. Gynec. Obstet., 117, 425.
Shah, H. S. and Mathur, B. B. C. (1967): Indian J. Path. Bact., 10, 197.
Stein, A. A. (1967): In: Pathology Annual 1967. Butterworth, London.
Stewart, F. W. (1950): In: Atlas of Tumor Pathology, section IX, Fascicle 34. Armed Forces Institute of Pathology, Washington, D.C.
Tellem, M., Prive, L. and Meranze, D. (1962): Cancer (Philad.), 15, 10.
Tellem, M., Shane, J. J. and Imbriglia, J. E. (1965): Surg. Gynec. Obstet., 120, 17.
Veronesi, V. and Pizzocaro, G. (1968): Surg. Gynec. Obstet., 126, 529.
Von Haam, E. and Murad, T. (1973): In: Abstracts, Second International Symposium on Cancer Detection and Prevention, Bologna, 1973, p. 124. Excerpta Medica, Amsterdam.
Warren, S. (1940): Surg. Gynec. Obstet., 71, 257.

Blood cell types associated with bovine lymphosarcoma*

The occurrence and significance of nuclear malignancy associated changes in the blood of normal and leucotic cattle

V. E. O. Valli, B. J. McSherry, J. H. Lumsden, M. E. Smart,
H. H. Grenn and B. Heath

Ontario Veterinary College, Guelph, Canada

Introduction

Bovine lymphosarcoma is endemic in the domestic cattle of Europe and North America (Bendixen 1963; Theilen et al., 1968). The disease is associated with an RNA leukovirus (Dutcher et al., 1964; Miller et al., 1969) and is believed to be horizontally transmitted to neonatal calves (Larson et al., 1970). The disease is of significance to man because the causative agent is apparently associated with leukocytes shed in milk (Yilmazer et al., 1970). Epidemiologic studies on the correlative incidence of human and bovine lymphosarcoma have generally been negative; however a positive correlation was shown by Aleksandrowicz et al. (1965) in Poland. Efforts to eradicate bovine lymphosarcoma on the basis of a persistent lymphocytosis (Bendixen, 1964) have been criticized because of the inability of this method to identify the subclinical disease in an individual animal (Abt et al., 1970; Lax and Hofirek, 1970). Nieburgs and Goldberg (1968) reported malignancy associated changes (MAC) occurring in the neutrophils of human patients with lymphosarcoma. In addition, Nieburgs (1971a) described a nuclear chromatin pattern with closely aggregated lightly stained circular areas (CALSCA) in cells from tumors and from tumor distant sites in patients with cancer. We have identified this same chromatin pattern (CALSCA) in cells of animals with spontaneous tumors. The object of this study was to determine if MAC in neutrophils and the CALSCA pattern in lymphocytes occurred in bovine lymphosarcoma, and if these changes could be used to increase the efficiency of detection of this tumor.

Materials and methods

Wright's stained blood smears were examined from 4 groups of 25 animals with these diagnoses:
1. Cows with lymphosarcoma proven at necropsy;
2. Cows with non neoplastic diseases proven at necropsy;
3. Cows with (persistent) lymphocytosis and believed to have subclinical lymphosarcoma according to the Bendixen test;
4. Normal, mature cows at an abattoir.

* This work was supported by the Ontario Ministry of Agriculture and Food and the National Research Council of Canada.

The blood smears were screened for quality, randomized and numbered 1 to 100 by a technician. These slides were examined by the senior author to photograph the various cell types and develop the criteria of cellular classification. The slides were then relabeled and examined blindly by 5 of the authors (V.E.V., J.H.L., M.E.S., H.H.G., B.H.). Fifty granulocytes and 50 mononuclear cells were differentially classified into 4 cell types each on all slides. Cellular examinations were carried out using 100 x plan objectives and 16 x oculars.

The results of these examinations were rearranged into their respective groups and the mean count of each cell type determined, and the significance of their differences determined by the use of the Student 't' test (Steel and Torrie, 1960).

Criteria for cellular identification

The terms heterochromatin, chromocenter and euchromatin are used here as defined by Nieburgs (1967) and by Koss (1968). All figures are x 2,500.

Granulocytes

The chromatin pattern in basophils is too obscured by granules to be evaluated. Eosinophils can be evaluated, and because they segment less fully than neutrophils their chromatin distribution is usually more flat and diffuse than neutrophil chromatin.

Type 0 (Fig. 1): This cell type is indicative of homeostasis. The chromatin pattern is flat and uniform with broad areas (an entire lobe) in which there is no internal nuclear detail visible. There may be folds and wrinkles in the nuclear membrane which causes some coarse and indistinct chromatin banding. Unstained areas (holes) may be present, but lightly stained areas (CALSCA) are not present.

Type 1 A (Fig. 2): This type of cell is indicative of a subacute or chronic inflammation. The nuclear chromatin is flat and stains uniformly. Poorly defined chromocenters may be present, but the euchromatin areas are only slightly lighter than chromocenters and have an irregular pattern of unstained areas (holes) which may be circular or irregular, often oval and elongated. The euchromatin is criss-crossed by lightly stained linear or curved slits.

Type 1 B (Fig. 3): A toxic form of type 1 occurs which is indicative of acute inflammation. There is internal nuclear detail discernible consisting of large, often pale chromocenters with a fine sieve-like euchromatin pattern that is fuzzy and indistinct. These cells are usually immature and may be myelocytes, metamyelocytes, bands or segmented cells with large rounded segments joined by a fine chromatin thread. There are often cycloplastic vacuolations and Doehle bodies.

Type 2 (Fig. 4): The presence of this type of cell suggests that (lymphoid) tumor is present. The nucleus is usually well matured with normal segmentation and smaller lobes than in types 0 or 1. There are *no* unstained areas (holes) present in any of the lobes. Some poorly defined large chromocenters may be present, but these are without halos. The euchromatin has a closely aggregated lightly stained circular area pattern (CALSCA) over at least 2/3 of it, and the rest is uniform and lighter than the larger chromocenters.

Type 3 (Fig. 5): The presence of this cell appears to indicate that (lymphoid) tumor is present. The type 3 granulocyte is almost always a neutrophil and differs from the type 2 cell in not having large chromocenters. In addition, there must be CALSCA in a row and quadrant formation *or* 6 or more CALSCA in a single lobe. There can be no unstained areas present (Nieburgs and Goldberg, 1968).

Lymphocytes and monocytes

The criteria are based on a gradation in the development of nuclei with well defined large chromocenters completely surrounded by CALSCA. Monocytes are consistently more suggestive of tumor than the lymphocytes and may appear erroneously positive. Mono-

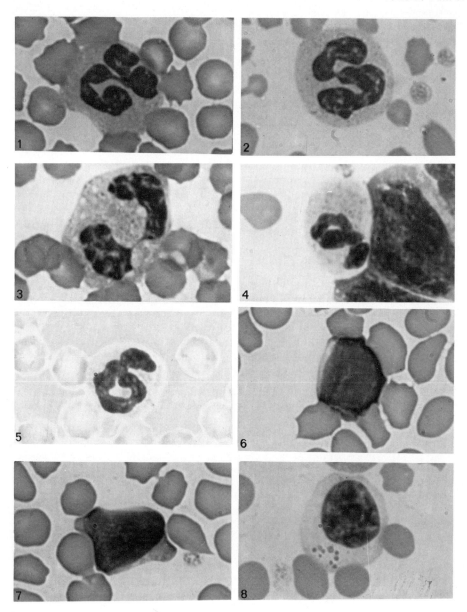

FIGS. 1-8

cytes can be counted in with lymphocytes by judging them on the same criteria as lymphocytes and then placing them in the next category lower than their nuclear morphology would indicate.

Type 0 (Fig. 6): This type of cell is indicative of homeostasis. The chromatin is of uniform density without chromocenters and appears waxy and lacks internal detail similar to a section of amyloid. There may be poorly defined coarse banding due to wrinkles or folds in the nuclear membrane. Nucleoli are usually absent but may be present and the

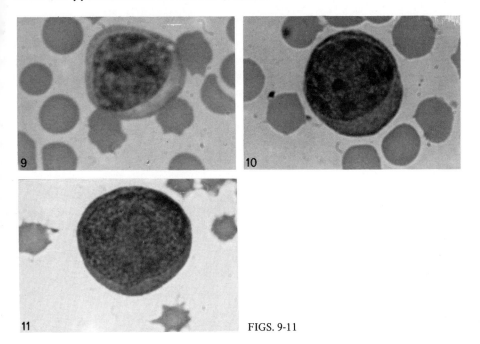

FIGS. 9-11

N/C is low. The cytoplasm is pale and the nuclear outline is irregular and frequently indented by adjacent cells.

Type 1 A (Fig. 7): This type of cell is indicative of an inflammatory state. The chromatin is like that of type 0 with more internal nuclear detail. There may be chromocenters but the euchromatin areas are irregular, granular, and irregular clear areas may be present. The nuclei may be small to large and the N/C is low (for lymphocytes). Nucleoli are rarely present. The cytoplasm is pale and large round azurophilic granules are commonly present.

Type 1 B (Fig. 8): A toxic form of type 1 occurs which has a more basophilic and vacuolated cytoplasm. The chromocenters are exaggerated with a heavily stained rim and a lighter center, and the euchromatin is irregular, light and heavily stained in a patchy distribution without fine chromatin band formation. Azurophilic granules are often present.

Type 2 (Fig. 9): This type of cell suggests that (lymphoid) tumor may be present. The nucleus is usually larger than types 0 and 1 and is usually round or indented. The N/C ratio is high and the cytoplasm is agranular and basophilic. The nucleus has a well developed pattern of chromocenters which are almost completely surrounded by CALSCA. One or two heavy, short chromatin bands may be present and there may be several round unstained areas or irregular not round, lightly stained areas. Nucleoli are small and inconspicuous if present.

Type 3 A (Fig. 10): This type of cell is indicative of lymphoid tumor. The nuclei are large and round, rarely indented. The large chromocenters are multiple (4-10), well defined, of medium size, uniformly stained and completely surrounded by euchromatin with CALSCA pattern. There are no unstained areas or heavy bands. Nucleoli are often present and are small and tend to be multiple. The N/C is high and the cytoplasm agranular and basophilic. The cell tends to correspond to descriptions of prolymphocytes.

Type 3 B (Fig. 11): This cell is apparently a blastic lymphocyte which is either malignant and neoplastic, or has malignancy associated changes (MAC). The nucleus is large and round with a very high N/C and the cytoplasmic rim may be barely visible throughout the circumference of the cell. Large chromocenters are not present and the entire nuclear pattern is made up of CALSCA which is more hyperchromatic than in the 3A cell. Nucleoli are always present, usually multiple and may vary considerably in size and shape. Only the smallest order of chromocenters are present, surrounded on 4 sides by CALSCA, and there are no unstained areas or heavy bands.

TABLE 1   *Levels of blood leukocytes, test groups of cattle*

Diagnosis 25 Cows/group	Total leukocytes/mm³			Total lymphocytes/mm³		
	Mean	Range	SD	Mean	Range	SD
Necropsy lymphosarcoma	46.528	11,000 – 204,000	42,880	41,823	3,318 – 195,000	44,040
Necropsy non neoplastic	14,883	1,600 – 65,000	17,391	4,571	768 – 36,960	7,076
Normals abattoir	6,473	4,500 – 9,100	1,507	3,843	1,920 – 5,460	949
Bendixen + ve and S	12,404	5,500 – 22,000	3,632	8,011	5,150 – 17,140	2,544

Results

The levels of blood leukocytes in the 4 test groups of cattle are given in Table 1. The mean results from differential counts on the 4 test groups of cattle by 5 observers are given in Table 2. These results are the means of the actual counts out of 50 granulocytes and 50 mononuclear cells classified by each observer on each blood smear. The means times two would thus approximate percentage incidence of each cell type. The results of analysis for significance of difference of means between the respective cell types of the 4 test groups are given in Table 3. The overall incidence of type 3 cells (indicative of tumor) tallied by 5 observers are given in Table 4. The *Total entries* in Table 4 is the total number of cases where type 3 cells were recorded by 5 observers successively examining the same group of 25 slides. The *x% incidence* is the *Total entries* ÷ 125 x 100. A computerized analysis of cellular interaction is incomplete and will be reported separately. Results of cellular interaction for one observer showed a very strong interaction between the type 0 neutrophils and lymphocytes with a wide separation of the normal (highest) + lymphosarcoma (intermediate) and non neoplastic (lowest) groups. This interaction overlapped in the type 1 cells and was again strong and well separated in the type 2 and 3 cells with the previous order reversed. It can be seen from the very large standard deviations that there is very wide variability in the individual data.

Discussion

Three of the observers were experienced in examining material of this kind, while two

TABLE 2   *Means* and S.D. of blood cell types from cattle with lymphosarcoma or other diseases*

Diagnosis 25 Cows/group	Granulocytes				Mononuclear			
	Normal 0	Inflammation 1	Inconclusive 2	Cancer 3	Normal 0	Inflammation 1	Inconclusive 2	Cancer 3
Necropsy lymphosarcoma	6.1 ± 9.7	31.8 ± 11.1	11.0 ± 9.1	1.1 ± 2.5	2.0 ± 3.3	20.4 ± 9.5	20.2 ± 9.5	9.9 ± 10.8
Necropsy non neoplastic	14.2 ± 13.3	30.0 ± 12.3	5.6 ± 7.1	0.4 ± 1.4	19.5 ± 12.8	23.4 ± 9.9	6.7 ± 7.4	0.6 ± 7.2
Normals abattoir	23.4 ± 12.6	24.0 ± 11.6	2.0 ± 3.3	0.1 ± 0.3	31.1 ± 9.9	16.7 ± 8.7	1.9 ± 2.2	0.04 ± 0.2
Bendixen + ve and S	10.6 ± 8.7	35.0 ± 8.5	4.0 ± 4.8	0.2 ± 0.8	16.3 ± 11.7	24.7 ± 9.3	7.6 ± 7.9	1.4 ± 3.9

* Means are derived from the number of cells tallied / category out of 50 granulocytes and 50 mononuclear cells counted by each of 5 observers. N = 125

TABLE 3   *Significance of differences between the means of eight cell types from each group of twenty-five cattle*

Means tested	Cell types							
	Granulocytes				Mononuclears			
	0	1	2	3	0	1	2	3
+ PM and − normal	**	**	**	**	**	**	**	**
+ PM and − PM	**	−	**	*	**	*	**	**
+ PM and + Bendixen's	**	**	**	**	**	**	**	**
− PM and + Bendixen's	**	**	*	−	*	−	−	−
− PM and − Normal	**	**	**	**	**	**	**	*
− Normal and + Bendixen's	**	**	**	−	**	**	**	**

**   Differ at the 99% level of significance

*   Differ at the 95% level of significance

+ Bendixen's includes both positive and suspicious cases

TABLE 4   *Incidence of type 3 cells in cattle with and without tumor: Results from five observers on four groups of animals each (N = 125)*

Diagnosis 25 Cows/group	Type 3 granulocytes			Type 3 lymphocytes		
	Total entries	Total cells	x̄ % incidence	Total entries	Total cells	x̄ % incidence
Necropsy lymphosarcoma	42	133	33.6	101	1,233	80.8
Necropsy non neoplastic	15	55	12.0	21	79	16.8
Normals abattoir	11*	12	8.8	4	5	3.2
Bendixen + ve and S	15	28	12.0	33	170	26.4

* 9 entries by 1 observer

had 1-2 years experience. It is interesting that in their individual data the least experienced observers were almost as efficient overall as their colleagues in numbers of false positive and false negative cellular classifications. This would suggest that the cellular criteria described in this work are more easily reproducible and accurate than diagnoses based on 'atypical', 'bizarre' and nucleolated lymphocytes.

There was a very well defined association between the 0 cell types and homeostasis (Table 2). The means of the 4 groups are much closer in the type 1 cells, but both granulocytes and lymphocytes in the normal group are significantly lower than in the other groups (Table 3). Both the type 2 and type 3 cells differ markedly between the cancer and the non cancer groups. As might be expected, the most difficult determination is between animals with tumors and those with serious but non neoplastic disease. It is likely that more experience with the present method would reduce the number of cells judged types 2 and 3 in the diseased but non tumor group. It appears that the most marked abnormalities in the cellular morphology are caused by severe inflammation and not cancer. In fact, the *uniformity* of the closely aggregated and lightly stained circular pattern in the nuclear chromatin is the key to distinguishing tumor from non tumor. In the diseased but non tumor group the chromocenters may be very prominent with 'rimming' of borders, but the euchromatin chromatin pattern is smudged, irregular and focally diffused (Fig. 8). The necropsy non neoplastic group have low means of type 0 cells and high means in the type 1 category (Table 2), as would be expected, since all had serious disease (21 inflammatory, 2 degenerative, 1 traumatic, 1 developmental). The low levels of type 2 and 3 cells seen in this group must be considered false positives. The distinction between a toxic or reactive type 1 cell and a type 2 cell is the most difficult distinction with this system.

The Bendixen group comprised 14 animals judged 'suspicious' (absolute lymphocyte counts of 6,500-8,500/mm^3, with age) and 11 'positive' animals (absolute lymphocyte counts in excess of 8,500/mm^3, with age) (Bendixen, 1959). These samples were collected from animals in a herd with a history of high incidence of lymphosarcoma. The group thus includes animals with subclinical tumors and others with intercurrent infection causing transient lymphocytosis. It is interesting that the group as a whole reflects this mixed status in the present study. Because they are all abnormal for a variety of reasons, the type 0 cells are low and the type 1 cells are high. Because there are animals with tumor in the group, the type 2 and type 3 cells are higher than the normals and less than the tumor positive group. Six of the 11 'positive' animals of the Bendixen group were given high type 2 and some type 3 cell values by all observers. On a recheck of the levels of circulating lymphocytes in these animals, 4 were still 'positive', one had become negative, and one was lost to follow-up. Of the other Bendixen 'positives' on recheck, two reverted to 'suspicious', two to negative, and the other remained 'positive' but was given a low index of suspicion in this study. In the 'suspicious' category, 8 became negative on recheck, 6 remained suspicious, and one was lost. Since it is in the nature of the lymphoid leukemia in cattle to have a fluctuating lymphocyte count, none of these changes in total lymphocyte count are conclusive for or against presence of tumor. The recognition of type 2 and some type 3 (MAC) neutrophils in 6 of the Bendixen positives would seem to lend assurance to a true positive diagnosis in these cases.

The levels of circulating leukocytes in the various groups of cattle from which the test slides were made are given in Table 1. There is undoubtedly some positive bias induced by the recognition of lymphocytosis in the test slides (total and differential counts were not given to the observers). We were aware though that only 1/4 of the animals had proven tumor, and that there would be (benign) lymphocytosis in many of the non neoplastic group and all of the Bendixen group. Because of the total number of cells involved (10,000), each observer rapidly became adjusted to judging the cells on an individual basis without the benefit of intuition. Observers were instructed to scan the slides briefly at low power to ensure that the cells counted were representative of the entire smear, and to give a clinical diagnosis of positive or negative at the end of the differential count. It is interesting and significant that most of the observers were more accurate on a diagnosis arrived at by analysis of their counts than by their intuitive interpretation of the smear based on experience.

The relative incidence of type 3 cells in the various groups (positive and false positive diagnoses) is given in Table 4. It is not surprising that all observers found the interpretation of the granulocytes (MAC incidence) more difficult than the lymphocyte (CALSCA incidence) interpretation. Undoubtedly more experience would decrease the number of type 3 (MAC positive) neutrophils tallied in negative cases. The morphologic appearance of the MAC positive neutrophil is believed to be due to prolongation of telophase (Nieburgs, 1971 *b*). In our experience (Table 4), the most frequent misinterpretation of neutrophils with MAC occurred in the group with non neoplastic but largely infectious diseases. The presence of systemic toxemia is known to cause the release of immature cells from the bone marrow (Valli et al., 1971), and it is likely that some of these cells have either skipped mitosis or are delayed in completing the previous division. Thus the recognition of immaturity, toxic vacuolation and granulation and 'hurried' segmentation should alert the observer to use very conservative application of the criteria for MAC. Nieburgs and Goldberg (1968) have defined the neutrophils with MAC as having a single circular clear (unstained) area usually associated with a quadrant. Since the distinction between neutrophils with MAC and those with non malignant associated changes rests on the recognition of clustered circular lightly stained areas, it was felt that the present investigation would be most informative if no clear (unstained) areas were allowed in the criteria for MAC. This restriction undoubtedly reduced the incidence of type 3 neutrophils recognized, but also reduced the false positives in the same category (Table 4). The types of MAC positive neutrophils recognized in this study were about evenly divided between those with row and quadrant formation and those with 6 or more CALSCA in a single lobule (Fig. 5). Further analysis of our data should indicate the number of type 3 cells (if more than 1) required for a positive diagnosis and the level of type 2 cells alone which indicate lymphoid tumor.

The interaction between the same cell types in the granulocytes and mononuclear categories suggests that neutrophils with MAC occur in cattle with lymphosarcoma. There is likely some tendency to find more type 3 neutrophils in an animal which is obviously leukemic; however there was sufficient overlap in total leukocytes between the groups (Table 1) to ensure that most of the positive tallies were correctly made. There may be some MAC occurring in the mononuclear cells as well, but in a tumor of the lymphoid system it is not possible to distinguish between lymphocytes with MAC and malignant neoplastic lymphocytes. These changes could be tested by looking for the same (CALSCA) changes in lymphocytes of cattle with granulocytic leukemia (which is rare) or in the neutrophils of cattle with other than lymphoid tumors. A useful finding from this study was that nucleoli were frequently present in benign type 0 and type 1 lymphocytes, and that nucleoli per se were not of value in arriving at a diagnosis of lymphosarcoma.

In summary, we feel that there are systemic effects of lymphosarcoma in cattle manifested in the blood granulocytes and likely in some lymphocytes as well. The recognition of the closely aggregated and lightly stained circular area nuclear pattern in mononuclear cells is a useful criterion for cancer detection, and is more reliable and easily mastered than criteria based on 'abnormal' or 'atypical' cells. The system of cellular identification used in this study appeared more accurate in detecting cancer in an individual animal than was the Bendixen key. Future work should concentrate on the quantitative changes occurring in the leukocytes of cattle with lymphosarcoma, so that these changes may be made the basis of a rapid, individually reliable cancer screening test. It is possible that the CALSCA pattern in nuclear morphology could be correlated with quantitative changes in DNA that could be rapidly measured in an automated flow through system.

Acknowledgements

We wish to acknowledge the technical assistance of Mrs. Jean Claxton, R. T., and Mr. Edwin Fountain.

References

Abt, D. A., Marshak, R. R., Kulp, H. W. and Pollock Jr, R. J. (1970): In: Comparative Leukemia Research, Bibliographica Haematologica No. 36, pp. 527-536. Editor: R. M. Dutcher. Karger, Basel, Switzerland.
Aleksandrowicz, J., Halecki, J. and Janicki, K. (1965): Med. Weteryn., 11, 666.
Bendixen, H. J. (1959): Nord. Vet.-Med., 11, 733.
Bendixen, H. J. (1963): Ann. N. Y. Acad. Sci., 108, 1241.
Bendixen, H. J. (1964): In: Reports, III International Meeting on Diseases of Cattle, Copenhagen, p. 420.
Dutcher, R. M., Larkin, E. P. and Marshak, R. R. (1964): J. nat. Cancer Inst., 33, 1055.
Koss, L. K. (1968): Diagnostic Cytology and Its Histopathologic Bases, 2nd ed., Chapter 7, pp. 76-90. J. B. Lippincott Company, Philadelphia, U.S.A.

Larson, V. L., Sorensen, D. K., Anderson, R. K. and Perman, V. (1970): Amer. J. vet. Res., 31/9, 1533.

Lax, T. and Hofirek, B. (1970): In: Comparative Leukemia Research, Bibliographica Haematologica No. 36, pp. 544-547. Editor: R. M. Dutcher, Karger, Basel, Switzerland.

Miller, J. M., Miller, L. D., Olson, C. and Gillette, K. G. (1969): J. nat. Cancer Inst., 43, 1297.

Nieburgs, H. E. (1967): In: Diagnostic Cell Pathology in Tissue and Smears, Chapter 2, pp. 8-46. Grune and Stratton, New York, N. Y.

Nieburgs, H. E. and Goldberg, A. F. (1968): Cancer (Philad.), 22/1, 35.

Nieburgs, H. E. (1971a): Gazz. Sanit., 20/1,3.

Nieburgs, H. E. (1971b): Acta cytol. (Philad.), 15/6, 513.

Steel, R. G. D. and Torrie, J. H. (1960): Principles and Procedures of Statistics. McGraw-Hill, New York, N. Y.

Theilen, G. H., Dungworth, D. L. and Kawakami, T. G. (1968): Calif. Med., 108, 14.

Valli, V. E. O., Hulland, T. J., McSherry, B. J., Robinson, G. A. and Gilman, J. P. W. (1971): Res. Vet. Sci., 12/6, 535.

Yilmazer, S. K., Kmetz, M., Schultz, R. D. and Dunne, H. W. (1970): Amer. J. Vet. Res., 31/4, 619.

8. Tumour specific antigens

The carcinoembryonic antigen (CEA) and a normal colonic mucosa antigen (NC) in neoplastic and non-neoplastic disorders of the gastrointestinal tract

Gerhard Tappeiner, Helmut Denk and J. Heinrich Holzner

Pathologisch-anatomisches Institut der Universität Wien, Vienna, Austria

The carcinoembryonic antigen (CEA) was originally isolated by Gold and Freedman (1965*a*) from adenocarcinomas of the large bowel. Later it was found in carcinomas of the stomach, pancreas and liver as well as in the fetal gastrointestinal tract (Gold and Freedman, 1965*b*; Krupey et al., 1968; Martin and Martin, 1970, 1972; Burtin et al., 1972*a*). It has been shown by immunofluorescence and by immuno-electronmicroscopy that the CEA is located on the luminal surface of the tumor cells and that it is probably secreted into the lumina of the tumor glands (Gold et al., 1968, 1970; Von Kleist and Burtin, 1969; Norland et al., 1969; Denk et al., 1972; Trappeiner et al., 1973).

Although Martin and Martin (1970) could not find a correlation between the degree of differentiation of a tumor and its content of CEA by an extraction procedure, Denk et al. (1972) showed by comparison of the histological and immunohistological pattern that the quantity of CEA produced by a tumor depends upon its degree of differentiation. Well-differentiated adenocarcinomas of the gastrointestinal tract contain large amounts of CEA, whereas anaplastic ones contain little or none. In some gastric, pancreatic and colonic carcinomas, CEA could be demonstrated within the cytoplasm of 'signet ring' cells (Denk et al., 1972; Burtin, personal communication).

The organ- and cancer-specificity originally proposed by Gold and Freedman (1965*a*, *b*) was disproved later by several authors. Burtin et al. (1972*a*, *b*) detected CEA by indirect immunofluorescence in benign polyps of the colon, in large bowel mucosa of children, in inflammatory large bowel disease and in apparently normal mucosa surrounding adenocarcinomas of the colon. Martin and Martin (1970), Freed and Taylor (1972), Rosai et al. (1972) and Abeyounis and Milgrom (1972) found a substance immunologically-identical with CEA in extracts of non-cancerous colonic mucosa, whereas Egan et al. (1972) and Coligan et al. (1972) found no CEA in extracts of normal colonic mucosa using a radioimmune assay. Crichlow and White (1970) were unable to demonstrate CEA in perchloric acid extracts of three benign colonic polyps by the Ouchterlony technique.

In the present study, the distribution and localisation of CEA was compared to that of perchloric acid soluble normal colonic mucosa antigen (NC) in neoplastic and non-neoplastic disorders of the gastrointestinal tract using the indirect immunofluorescence method. NC can be regarded as a marker for mucus of intestinal type (Tappeiner et al., 1973). It is always present in the secretory part of the goblet cells (Burtin et al., 1971; Tappeiner et al., 1973) and in the mucus of the large bowel in normal and cancerous colonic mucosa.

Material and methods

48 carcinomas of the stomach, 3 pancreatic carcinomas, 42 carcinomas of the large bowel, 4 benign colonic polyps, 4 cases of ulcerative colitis and 3 of diverticulitis were included in this study. With the exception of 2 of the 3 pancreatic carcinomas (autopsy material) the specimens were obtained within 6 hr after surgical removal, snap-frozen in isopentane cooled with dry ice-acetone and stored at $-80°$ C for one week at the most.

The indirect immunofluorescence method and the optical equipment used have been described (Denk et al., 1972). Antisera against perchloric acid extracts of colonic carcinomas, or of their liver metastases (anti-CEA-serum), and of normal colonic mucosa (anti-NC-serum), respectively, were used (for preparation, see Denk et al., 1972; Tappeiner et al., 1973). The term 'serum' used in this paper refers to the globulin fractions of the sera prepared by ammonium sulphate precipitation. The anti-CEA-serum was compared with a specific anti-CEA-serum kindly provided by Dr. Von Kleist. It gave identical reactions against colonic carcinoma extract. Furthermore, the anti-CEA-serum was kindly tested by Dr. P. Gold and found to contain anti-CEA activity.

Anti-CEA-serum was absorbed with lyophilized perchloric acid (PCA) extract of normal colonic mucosa (30 mg/ml serum), lyophilized pooled human plasma (Hyland, 30 mg/ml serum), lyophilized PCA extract of normal human lung (30 mg/ml serum) and with human blood group AB erythrocytes. Anti-NC-serum was absorbed with lyophilized pooled human plasma (Hyland, 20 mg/ml serum), and with human AB erythrocytes. These sera were used in the first layer of indirect immunofluorescence; FITC-coupled anti-rabbit globulin (Hyland) was used in the second layer. The specifications of the antisera were the same as described previously (Denk et al., 1972).

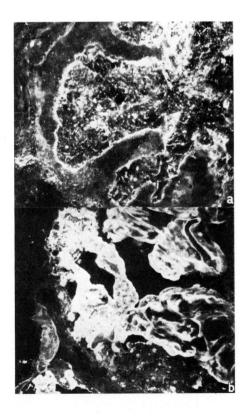

FIG. 1 *Mucoid carcinoma of the colon; 250x. Reduced for reproduction 33%. (a) Specifically stained material (CEA) on luminal surface of tumor cells and in granular form within the lumen of a tumorous gland (mucus). (b) Diffuse staining pattern (NC) of the mucus of a tumorous gland.*

Results

Well-differentiated adenocarcinomas of the colon contained large amounts of CEA on the luminal surface of the tumor cells as well as within the lumina of the tumorous glands (Fig. 1*a*). Detritus or detached cells may be coated with CEA, but did not show CEA-specific fluorescence themselves. Carcinomas with a lower degree of differentiation, with adeno-papillary structures and formation of secondary lumina showed less strong CEA-specific fluorescence in granular form on the luminal surface of the cells and sometimes in secondary lumina. Anaplastic carcinomas contained no demonstrable CEA. The cancer tissue showed, however, a weak diffuse cytoplasmic fluorescence upon staining with anti-CEA, but not with anti-NC that was independent of its degree of differentiation (Figs. 2*a*, *b*). This finding remains to be explained by further studies.

Anti-NC-serum specifically reacts with cell-bound and free mucus of intestinal type. It therefore stains the secretory part of the cytoplasm of the goblet cells of normal colonic mucosa (Fig. 3*a*). In adenocarcinomas, the quantity of NC found depends largely upon the presence of tumor cells closely resembling normal goblet cells. In the mucus of both well- and poorly-differentiated carcinomas, large amounts of NC are seen yielding a diffuse cloudy staining pattern (Fig. 1*b*). The mucus contains CEA in granular or cloudy form when the underlying tumor is well-differentiated (Fig. 1*a*). This shows that secretion of mucus and CEA are not identical functions of tumors.

NC-content of colonic polyps depends upon the presence of goblet cells which are specifically stained; CEA may be found as a superficial linear or granular layer on the

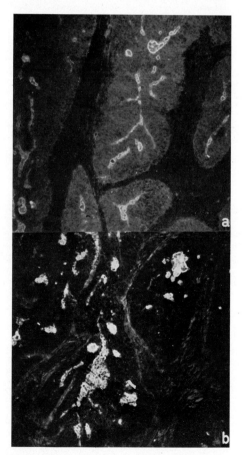

FIG. 2   *Moderately well-differentiated colonic adenocarcinoma; 100x. Reduced for reproduction 20%. (a) Note the staining of the cancer tissue with anti-CEA as compared to the (unstained) connective tissue. (b) No staining of the cancer tissue with anti-NC.*

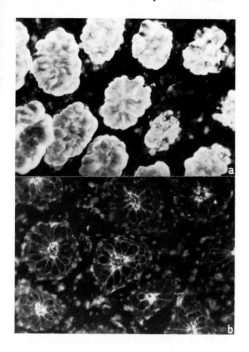

FIG. 3   *400x.   Reduced for reproduction 40%. (a) Staining pattern of normal colonic mucosa (goblet cells) with anti-NC. (b) CEA-specific superficial fluorescence of the goblet cells of peritumoral mucosa.*

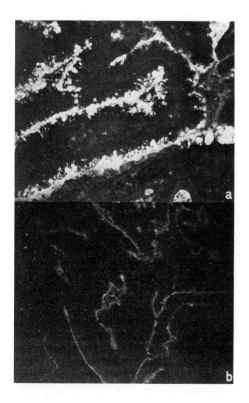

FIG. 4   *Adenomatous colonic polyp; 100x. Reduced for reproduction 30%. (a) Bright staining with anti-NC of the secretions within the lumen and of goblet cells. (b) Weak staining superficial coat of the cells with anti-CEA.*

luminal surface of the cells (Figs. 4*a*, *b*). Morphologically normal peri-tumoral colonic mucosa may exhibit a rather weak CEA-specific fluorescence on the luminal surface of the goblet cells (Fig. 3*b*).

CEA seems to be present in small amounts in inflammatory large bowel disorders like diverticulitis and ulcerative colitis. The dependence of CEA-production upon tumor cell differentiation is even more striking in pancreatic carcinomas. In well-differentiated adenocarcinomas of the pancreas, or in their liver metastases, large amounts of CEA were found in a similar localisation to that in colonic carcinomas. Cells with CEA-specific cytoplasmic fluorescence and with morphology resembling 'signet ring' cells could be detected in liver metastases of a highly-differentiated pancreatic carcinoma (Figs. 5*a*, *b*).

In fairly well-differentiated gastric carcinomas, with adenoid or adeno-papillary structures lined by columnar epithelium, CEA was demonstrated in linear or granular form on the luminal surface of the tumor cells and in the lumina of the glands. It was missing from irregular glands lined with poorly-differentiated cuboidal or squamous epithelium.

In these tumors, NC was present as a superficial lining of the tumor cells, or diffusely in deposits of mucus, irrespective of the degree of differentiation of the tumor. The secretory part of the cytoplasm of tumor cells resembling goblet cells, a carcinoma cell type rarely encountered in gastric carcinomas, was specifically stained with anti-NC-serum. Undifferentiated solid or scirrhous parts of a tumor with cells with darkly-staining oxyphil cytoplasm did not yield any CEA-specific fluorescence. Sometimes, however, NC was present in deposits of varying size between the cells. In 'signet ring' cell carcinomas, CEA could be demonstrated in large amounts as specifically staining granules in the cytoplasm of the 'signet ring' cells and in the mucus surrounding the cells. These cells either infiltrated the wall of the stomach or floated freely in mucus (Fig. 6*a*). With anti-NC-serum, however, mucus usually was stained in a diffuse, cloudy fashion. Intra-

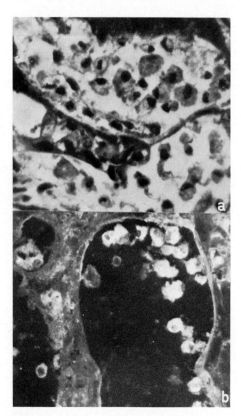

FIG. 5   *Liver metastases of a pancreatic carcinoma; 400x. Reduced for reproduc-
tion 20%. (a) Isolated tumor cells, H
& E. (b) Section parallel to (a).
Bright specific staining of the cytoplasm of these cells with anti-CEA.*

cellular mucus deposits in 'signet ring' cells showed a strong NC-specific fluorescence as well and sometimes were hardly distinguished within the mucus (Fig. 6b). Thus the 'signet ring' cells are similar to a CEA-producing line of colonic carcinoma cells (Goldenberg and Hansen, 1972) in their morphological and immunomorphological aspects.

In areas of intestinal metaplasia surrounding carcinomas of the stomach, variable results were obtained upon staining with anti-CEA-serum. In most cases, a superficial lining of specific fluorescence could be observed independent of the presence or absence of goblet cells (Fig. 7a). With anti-NC-serum, the secretory part of the goblet cells as well as their mucus secretions, showed a specific fluorescence similar to that of the mucosa of normal large bowel. Metaplastic areas without goblet cells showed only a fine specifically-stained superficial line on the luminal surface of the epithelium (Fig. 7b).

Like colonic tumors, all gastric carcinomas studied revealed a weak diffuse cytoplasmic fluorescence of the tumor cells upon staining with anti-CEA but not with anti-NC; this fluorescence dissappeared upon absorption of the anti-CEA-serum with purified CEA. The significance of this finding is not yet clear.

Summary

1. CEA cannot be considered to be cancer-specific because it is present, not only in malignant, but also in non-malignant changes (polyps, inflammation, intestinal metaplasia) of the gastro-intestinal mucosa.

2. The production of CEA depends upon the differentiation of the carcinoma, as shown with different tumors of the gastro-intestinal tract.

3. CEA seems to be a secretion product. However, no intimate relationship exists between the production and secretion of mucus on one hand and of CEA on the other.

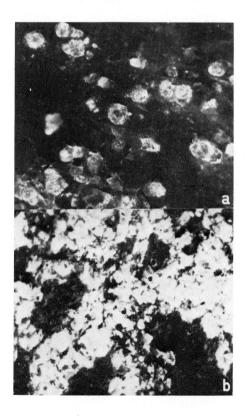

FIG. 6 *'Signet ring' cell carcinoma of the stomach; 400x. Reduced for reproduction 15%. (a) Tumor cells infiltrating the wall of the stomach. Specific granular staining of the cytoplasm with anti-CEA. (b) Cytoplasmic fluorescence of the tumor cells upon staining with anti-NC.*

4. 'Signet ring' cells are considered to be fairly-well-differentiated tumor cells (as judged by their content of CEA), with a defect in their secretion mechanism. Striking similarities exist between 'signet ring' cells and cultured colonic carcinoma cells with respect to CEA-content and morphological appearance.

5. The faint, but possibly specific cytoplasmic fluorescence observed in all carcinomas of the digestive tract may be interpreted in the sense that even anaplastic tumors produce CEA but lack secretory capacity. This assumption, however, awaits experimental proof.

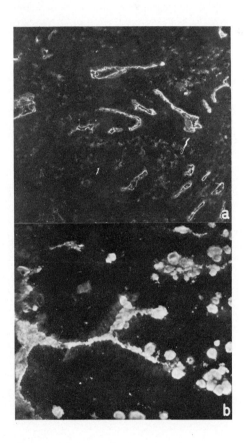

FIG. 7   *Intestinal metaplasia of the stomach. 250x. Reduced for reproduction 15%. (a) Superficial lining of the metaplastic mucosa with CEA-positive material. (b) Bright staining of the goblet cells and their secretions with anti-NC-serum.*

References

Abeyounis, C. J. and Milgrom, F. (1972): Int. Arch. Allergy, 43, 30.
Burtin, P., Martin, E., Sabine, M. C. and Von Kleist, S. (1972a): J. nat. Cancer Inst., 48, 25.
Burtin, P., Sabine, M. C. and Chavanel, G. (1972b): Int. J. Cancer, 10, 72.
Burtin, P., Von Kleist, S. and Sabine, M. C. (1971): Cancer Res., 31, 1038.
Coligan, J. E., Lautenschleger, J. T., Egan, M. L. and Todd, C. W. (1972): Immunochemistry, 9, 377.
Collatz, E., Von Kleist, S. and Burtin, P. (1971): Int. J. Cancer, 8, 298.
Crichlow, R. W. and White, R. R. (1970): Proc. Amer. Ass. Cancer Res., 11, 18.
Denk, H., Tappeiner, G., Eckerstorfer, R. and Holzner, J. H. (1972): Int. J. Cancer, 10, 262.
Egan, M. L., Lautenschleger, J. T., Coligan, J. E. and Todd, C. W. (1972): Immunochemistry, 9, 289.
Freed, T. L. J. and Taylor, G. (1972): Brit. med. J., 1, 85.
Gold, P. (1967): Cancer (Philad.), 80, 1663.

Gold, P. and Freedman, S. O. (1965a): J. exp. Med.,121, 439.

Gold, P. and Freedman, S. O. (1965b): J. exp. Med., 122, 467.

Gold, P., Gold, M. and Freedman, S. O. (1968): Cancer Res., 28, 1331.

Gold, P., Krupey, J. and Ansari, H. (1970): J. nat. Cancer Inst., 45, 219.

Goldenberg, D. M. and Hansen, H. J. (1972): Science, 175, 1117.

Krupey, J., Gold, P. and Freedman, S. O. (1968): J. exp. Med., 128, 387.

Logerfo, P., Krupey, J. and Hansen, H. J. (1971): New Engl. J. Med., 285, 138.

Mach, J. P. and Pusztaseri, G. (1972): Immunochemistry, 9, 1031.

Martin, F. and Martin, M. S. (1970): Int. J. Cancer., 6, 352.

Martin, F. and Martin, M. S. (1972): Int. J. Cancer, 9, 641.

Moore, T. L., Kupchik, H. Z., Marcon, N. and Zamchek, N. (1971): Amer. J. dig. Dis., 16, 1.

Nairn, R. C., Fothergill, J. E., McEntegard, M. G. and Porteous, I. B. (1962a): Brit. med. J., 1, 1788.

Nairn, R. C., Fothergill, J. E., McEntegard, M. G. and Richmond, H. G. (1962b): Brit. med. J., 1, 1791.

Norland, C. C., Maass, E. G. and Kirszner, J. B. (1969): Cancer, 23, 730.

Rosai, J., Tillack, T. W. and Marchesi, V. T. (1972): Int. J. Cancer, 10, 357.

Tappeiner, C., Denk, H., Eckerstorfer, R. and Holzner, J. H. (1973): Virchows Arch. Abt. A, 360, 129.

Thomson, D. M. P., Krupey, J., Freedman, S. O. and Gold, P. (1969): Proc. nat. Acad. Sci. (Wash.), 64, 161.

Von Kleist, S. and Burtin, P. (1969): Int. J. Cancer, 4, 874.

Further comparisons of separated intestinal cancer, fetal intestinal and normal intestinal soluble membrane antigen and the role of tumor related antigens in the diagnosis and treatment of intestinal cancer*

A. Hollinshead, P. Gold and R. Herberman

*The George Washington University Medical Center, Washington, D.C., U.S.A.,
Division of Clinical Immunology, The Montreal General Hospital, Montreal,
Canada, and Cellular and Tumor Immunology Section, Laboratory of Cell Biology,
National Cancer Institute, Bethesda, Md., U.S.A.*

In previous studies (Hollinshead et al., 1970, 1972) delayed hypersensitivity reactions to intradermal skin tests of specific soluble antigens from human intestinal cancer and fetal intestines were observed, whereas negative reactions were obtained with comparable fractions from normal intestinal cells. The skin reactive fetal intestinal antigen was shown to consist of two polypeptide chains. These antigens, of course, are carcinoembryonic antigens, but for the sake of differentiation with the Gold CEA, we are now calling these antigens: SRA. Another fetal antigen (Gold CEA) used in a current radioimmunoassay (Gold and Freedman, 1965; Krupey et al., 1972) consists of 75% glycoprotein gel and does not elicit a skin reaction (Gold and Freedman, 1965; Krupey et al., 1972).

I would like to start off right away by stating that there are still many problems connected with the use of the Gold CEA in diagnostic testing for cancers of the intestinal tract. Most antigens used in the radioimmunoassay contain both types of CEA in various proportions, that is, the Gold CEA and the Hollinshead SRA. In order for the clinician to understand this work, it will be necessary for me to review rather quickly the most significant work, and I will be necessarily discussing methodology. When Gold first began his studies he chose adenocarcinoma of the human colon because this lesion generally does not extend intramurally for more than 6 to 7 cm either proximal or distal to the site of the grossly visible tumor. Mucosa taken from the surgical specimens beyond these points was therefore available as normal control tissues from the very same donors who supplied the cancer material. This of course somewhat overcomes the problems of allo-antigenetic differences. In his early study he prepared anti-tumor serum in rabbits, absorbed with normal tissue and, by a variety of techniques, demonstrated that all human adenocarcinomata arriving from the entodermally derived epithelium contained these tumor specific antigens. A similar constituent was found in embryonic and fetal gut, pancreas and liver during the first two trimesters of gestation. Because this component could not be detected in any other normal, diseased or neoplastic tissue, nor in the bacterial flora of the bowel, nor in the usually high concentrations of fibrin frequently found in malignant tumors, Gold called it the carcinoembryonic antigen of the human digestive system.

During the same time period, in my laboratory we had been routinely testing first, second and third trimester fetal antigens from tissue which matched the adult tissue of origin for each category of solid tumor. The search in my laboratory was at that time and still is concerned with the membrane and soluble membrane antigens of tumor and

* This work was supported by USPHS Contract No. NIH-NCI-G-69-2176, National Cancer Institute.

control material. We have been separating the HLA antigens, antigens which are virus directed or virus associated, and antigens which produce delayed hypersensitivity reactions in skin tests. Our methods of separating skin reactive antigens from tissues are described elsewhere (Hollinshead et al., 1970, 1972). In brief, the membrane extracts are prepared from select human intestinal cancers and from fetal intestines by a modification of the Davies procedure. The membrane extracts are next subjected to sequential low frequency sonication and the solubilized materials are then separated on Sephadex G-200. To make a long story short, we isolated a specific soluble fraction of membranes prepared either from autologous or allogeneic tumor cells which produced highly specific reactions, and this skin reactive antigen was also detected in soluble cell membrane fractions from first and second trimester fetal intestines.

In 1968, Dr. Gold and I discussed our pre-publication data at a privileged conference, and decided to cooperate. Dr. Gold's radioimmunoassay involves three main components; the patient's own blood, purified CEA which is radio-iodinated and goat blood which has CEA antibody. The goats were originally immunized with live colon cancer cells, and for some experiments were immunized with purified CEA. Now how does this assay work? To put it simply, if there is antigen in the patient's blood, it will compete for link-up with the radio-iodinated CEA. If it is not present, then the goat sera antibodies will react with the CEA in a standardized test. It is a relatively simple measurement. After the three elements are combined in the test tubes and centrifuged, the antigen and antibody will unite and collect in the bottom of the tube. The test tube is then placed in the Geiger counter and scanned. If all of the tagged radioactive CEA originally put in the tube collects at the bottom, it seems that there were no antigens in the patient's blood sample to compete for link-up with the available antibodies. However, if the counter finds only a portion of the radioactive antigens in the antigen-antibody pairs at the bottom, then the non-radioactive antigen there must have come from the patient's blood. This test has been used extensively in the United States and elsewhere, and the results from various groups have been very confusing. Many groups reported positive results in benign as well as malignant disorders. When one examines these reports in detail, it becomes clear that the background noise in these assays varies from laboratory to laboratory. Indeed, most of the laboratories use a much shorter version of the Gold test, and employ different types of reagents. This led many doctors to conclude that the differences were quantitative rather than qualitative, and that this CEA assay while useful, would have to be an adjunct to other methods.

Our efforts and our contributions are not meant to either confirm or deny the conclusion made at present. Rather, our contributions are meant to perfect, and to explore scientifically, the various parameters of such studies. We have found that most antigens used in the radioimmunoassay contain both the CEA and the two SRA antigens in various proportions. This includes CEA preparations which are just as good, if not better, than the original preparations by Gold. I refer to the very elegant work of Coligan et al. (1972). Very recently, Dr. Coligan further separated the material prepared as previously described (Coligan et al., 1972), by the additional use of separations of the semi-purified material using isoelectric focusing. He subjected his samples to extensive dialysis to remove ampholytes, and sent these to us for testing (Herberman and Hollinshead, in preparation). This further separation resulted in bands which were easily stained for glycoprotein, and which were free of other protein bands detected in the previous preparations. It will be of interest to know whether or not CEA separated by isoelectric focusing, and therefore subjected to rather harsh chemicals, will produce strong enough antisera. If these antigens are proven to be intact for immunologic purposes, this will be a step forward (see Fig. 2).

To complicate things even further, antibody to another polypeptide present in some normal intestinal cells and also in fetal intestinal cells (Von Kleist et al., 1972) and shared in many of the CEA preparations used throughout the world, may interfere with specific radioimmunoassays. We studied this antigen preparation several times, including the alpha- and beta-migrating components of the preparation (Herberman and Hollinshead, in preparation). These alpha and beta preparations failed to elicit positive skin reaction. The majority of the proteins in the alpha preparation migrated further into the gels, and these did not contain SRA. The beta preparation contained some normal colon polypeptides and in addition, a polypeptide which we have also seen in fetal intestinal preparations. In order to understand this relationship, it is necessary to study the pattern of protein distribution with our carefully separated and purified material, by further fractionation of the materials using polyacrylamide gel electrophoresis (Hollinshead et al., 1972) (Fig 1). CEA migrates into the region 1, or 4.75% gel preparation. SRA migrates into the 10% gel region 3 and gel region 4. These two polypeptide bands are always associated with a third polypeptide band which migrates along with the SRA. This polypeptide band is present in region 2. The region 2 polypeptide band from our gently extracted antigens does not give a skin reaction, nor does it give a positive test for CEA. However, using the perchloric acid extracted materials (Gold and Freedman, 1965; Krupey et al., 1972; Von Kleist et al., 1972), this region 2 band gives a partial CEA positive reaction (Hollinshead et al., 1972). We further tested the bands produced by the beta antigen by immuno-diffusion tests (Herberman and Hollinshead, in preparation), and found that this beta preparation had a second band in region 1 which gave a very light arc against CEA antisera. The region 2 bands did not react with the antisera, indicating that whatever this component in region 2 might be, it was not immunogenic. It is possible that this material is a breakdown product of part of the CEA antigen. Conversely, it may be a normal fetal antigen containing within it some of the peptide sequences present in the CEA, loosened by perchloric acid treatment (see Fig. 2).

One of the major problems in the CEA radioimmunoassays has probably been the lack of a highly specific antisera. Even under the best conditions, with the finest antigens, there is often a lack of specificity of antisera prepared in goat and in rabbit. It will be of interest to see how specific tests can be using highly specific antisera prepared in inbred guinea pigs or other animals. Another problem is the manner in which the CEA is

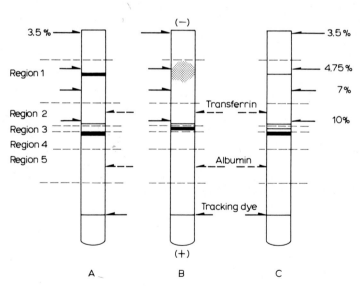

FIG. 1   *The partially purified CEA preparation (B) and the skin reactive Sephadex G-200 (C) fractions of the intestinal cancer and the fetal intestinal membrane extract (A) were fractionated by gradient polyacrylamide-gel electrophoresis (3.5 to 10% gel). A tracking dye (bromphenol blue) was used in each preparation. Albumin (67,000 molecular weight) and transferrin (approximately 90,000 molecular weight) were run on separate gels. On each of the 4 gels was placed 13 μg of protein of the membrane-extracted materials and 15 μg of CEA. One gel of each preparation was stained with Coomassie brilliant blue. The others were sliced into 5 parts as indicated by the dashed lines and the proteins were eluted and concentrated by ultrafiltration for testing. The diffuse zone of glycoprotein is indicated by the hatching. (From Hollinshead et al., 1972. By courtesy of the Editors.)*

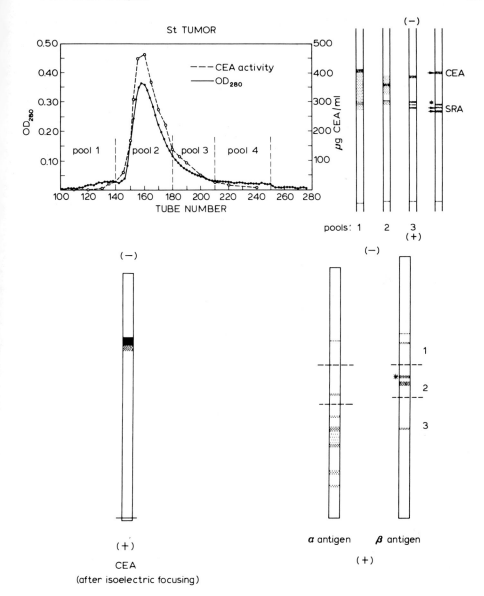

FIG. 2   *Separation by Dr. Coligan of tumor from patient (St) by his described method (Coligan et al., 1972): Upper left shows Sephadex separation of first peak (which contains most of the CEA). Upper right shows our analysis of the indicated pools 1, 2 and 3 using our method of gel electrophoresis. On the far right is shown a gel electrophoretic analysis of the cancer antigens separated by our methods (Hollinshead et al., 1970, 1972). Such gels may be sliced for elution of specific antigens. Another method is that of isoelectric focusing: a further separation of the St pools by Dr. Coligan was analyzed by our gel electrophoretic technique. This is shown in the lower left of the figure, and is a cleaner preparation of CEA. On the lower right: analysis of the α- and β-antigens from Dr. Von Kleist. These are antigens of normal colonic tissues (Von Kleist et al., 1972). The upper band of β region 2 is a fetal antigen* which migrates with SRA in our cancer preparations, but has no known activity.*

prepared, and that it might be useful for serodiagnostic measurement, but some of the constituents which might be necessary for a good immuno-reaction may be absent. We trust that this careful assessment of various antigens may be useful in improving the serologic studies undertaken by various laboratories.

Of greater interest to us are the use of the SRA antigens for immunotherapy regimes. We have undertaken large scale cooperative skin test studies of intestinal cancer patients and matched control patients with other types of cancer, in order to better understand the cell mediated immunity to these antigens. The results of these tests as well as other in vitro studies will aid our decision.

Acknowledgements

We are grateful for the excellent technical assistance of O.B. Lee, K. Tanner, P. Jones, M. Dannbeck and P. Pugh.

References

Coligan, J. E., Lautenshleger, J. T., Egan, M. and Todd, C. W. (1972): Immunochemistry, 658, 1.
Gold, P. and Freedman, S. (1965): J. exp. Med., 122, 467.
Herberman, R. and Hollinshead, A., In preparation.
Hollinshead, A., Glew, D. and Bunnag, B. (1970): Lancet, 1, 1191.
Hollinshead, A., McWright, C. G., Alford, T. C. and Glew, D. H. (1972): Science, 177, 887.
Krupey, J., Wilson, T., Freedman, S. O. and Gold, P. (1972): Immunochemistry, 9, 617.
Von Kleist, S., Chavanel, G. and Burton, P. (1972): Proc. nat. Acad. Sci. (Wash.), 69, 2492.

Evaluation of specific antibodies in human sera by a CEA antigen isolated with a modified method

E. Sega, F. Isabella, M. Crespi and G. Citro

Regina Elena Cancer Institute, Rome, Italy

During the last few years the specificity of CEA, one of the best characterized onco-fetal antigens (OFA), has been challenged. The use of radioimmunoassay methods for detecting antigens with CEA activity in normal and cancer tissue extracts, and in sera of healthy persons and of patients with neoplastic and non-neoplastic diseases has given false-positive and false-negative results (Lo Gerfo et al., 1972; Zamchek et al., 1972).

Recently, the demonstration of a partial identity between CEA and a normal glyco-protein of a smaller size, extracted from a normal adult tissue, raises not only theoretical questions but also practical implications (Mach and Pusztaszeri, 1972). We can present the problem of CEA in the form of two propositions:

(*a*) CEA is an antigen produced both in normal and in cancer cells; the difference is only quantitative.

(*b*) If we could purify CEA sufficiently we would obtain a specific cancer antigen. It is only a question of performing more sophisticated methods of extraction and separation and of removing the normal fraction.

With the aim of pursuing (*b*) we have tried to devise a better method of separation and purification and a more careful immunological absorption of normal constituents from the perchloric acid soluble extracts.

The detection of antibodies in the sera of patients with large bowel cancer or with other malignant tumours is a controversial question. Hemagglutinating activity was found in the sera of 70% of patients with non-metastatic cancer of the digestive system (Gold, 1967); no antibodies were detected by Collatz et al. (1971) and Lo Gerfo et al. (1972). A very sensitive radioimmunoelectrophoresis method was used by Gold et al. (1972) and antibodies were detected with a possible cross-reactivity with blood group substance A.

Materials and methods

Preparation of normal and tumour tissue extracts

Tumour and normal tissue extracts were derived from colon carcinomas and from sections of colon more than 7 cm distant from the visible edges of the tumour; and from a colon adenocarcinoma liver metastasis at autopsy. Cancer tissue was carefully separated from normal tissue and minced into small pieces. Then the material was put in an Omni Mixer Sorval and homogenized at $7,000 \times g$ for 20 min. A second homogenization was performed in a Potter homogenizer in buffer distilled water. An equal volume of 1.2 M perchloric acid solution was added to the homogenate and the mixture was stirred for 30 min at room temperature. The suspension was then centrifuged at 2,000 rpm at $4°C$ for 15 min. The sediment was discarded and the supernatant was dialyzed for 3 days against distilled water, centrifuged again at $35,000 \times g$ at $4°C$ for 30 min, concentrated in Aquacide and finally lyophilized.

Purification of tumour specific antigens

Antisera were prepared by injecting rabbits and sheep with perchloric acid extracts of normal gut and normal colon tissue, following the schedule adopted in our laboratory. The lyophilized perchloric soluble extracts of cancer tissue were absorbed against these antisera according to the method of Avrameas and Ternynck (1969).

The supernatants were compared before and after immunoadsorption by immuno-diffusion, Sephadex G-200 gel filtration and polyacrylamide gel electrophoresis (PAGE), to demonstrate the efficiency of the absorption of normal components.

The immunopurified perchloric acid extract was chromatographed by gel filtration with Sephadex G-200 (columns of 1 x 50) in 0.05 M phosphate buffer pH 7.5. The elution was done with the same buffer. The eluate with CEA activity was further chromatographed with DEAE cellulose, equilibrated with a sodium phosphate buffer 0.01 M pH 8.0. The column 1 x 10 was packed and eluted with the same buffer. The most purified fraction with CEA activity was labelled by iodination according to the chloramine-T method: 2.5 g of protein, 1 ml of ^{125}I and 20 g of chloramine-T were used. For the detection of antibodies, sera were obtained from 25 patients with cancer of the rectum and colon, from 12 lung carcinoma patients and the normal sera of 5 blood donors. Initially, we used radioimmunoelectrophoresis (R.I.E.P.) according to Gold et al. (1972). ^{125}I conjugated CEA, prepared with our method, was incubated with 20 μl of serum for 48 hr at 37°C. Five microliters of the mixture were electrophoresed in a Hyland apparatus using agar 0.8% in phosphate buffer pH 8.6. Precipitin lines were developed for 48 hr with monospecific rabbit antisera directed against human IgG, IgM, IgA. After washing, autoradiographs of the agar plates were developed on Kodak X-ray film N.S. Non-precipitin lines were demonstrated in the film, even after 20 days of exposure.

A radio-immunoassay was also performed in the liquid phase. After contact with the second antibody, the mixture was centrifuged to separate free from antibody-bound ^{125}I-CEA. Before labelling for R.I.E.P., purified CEA was absorbed against sera containing anti-A antibodies. A pool of blood type AO sera and commercially available anti-A antisera were used according to Avrameas and Ternynk. The 25 sera tested with R.I.E.P. were absorbed with a pool of group A erythrocytes.

Results

The total protein content of perchloric acid extracts of liver metastasis before absorption with anti-normal liver tissue serum was 25 mg/ml. After absorption it was 10 mg/ml. Immunoabsorption was carried out until the disappearance of the precipitin line between the cancer perchloric acid extract and normal liver tissue antiserum. The elution profile of the Sephadex G-200 chromatography of cancer tissue perchloric acid extracts before absorption showed three peaks (Fig. 1). The CEA activity was detectable in the first peak. After absorption, only the first peak was evident in the chromatographic pattern (Fig. 2).

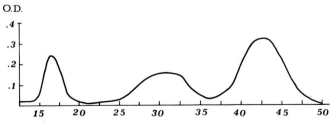

FIG. 1   *Elution of the Sephadex G-200 chromatography of cancer tissue perchloric acid extracts before absorption, showed three peaks.*

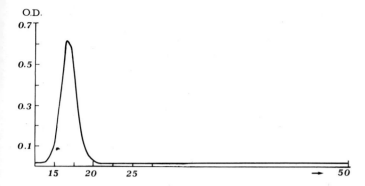

FIG. 2   *After absorption, only the first peak was evident in chromatographic patterns.*

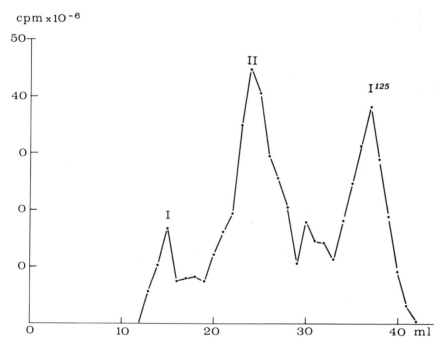

FIG. 3   *After iodination of the immuno-purified material, two protein peaks were separated from unbound iodine. The first peak reacted with the absorbed antiserum, the second should represent damaged material produced during the iodination, because it failed to react with both absorbed and unabsorbed antiserum against pathological liver extracts.*

After iodination of the immuno-purified material, two protein peaks were separated from unbound iodine (Fig. 3). The percentage of labelling was 40.4%. The first protein peak reacted with the absorbed antiserum, the second one should represent damaged material, produced during the iodination, since it failed to react with both absorbed and unabsorbed antiserum against pathological liver extracts. We set up a radioimmunoassay by using as specific antiserum, anti-pathological liver extract (at a working dilution of

1 : 2000), and the first peak of the iodinated protein as a tracer (about 10,000 cpm/ tube). Inhibition of binding was done with 0.2 ml of serial dilution of various materials. The complex was precipitated with the addition of anti-rabbit gammaglobulin serum.

With this technique, we checked the immunopotency, as CEA activity, of the normal liver extracts. We found that it was only about 1% of the cancer liver extract in terms of weight. This confirms the value of the absorption procedure. Afterwards, gel filtration on Sephadex G-200 of the normal and liver cancer metastasis extracts, immunologically purified, was performed in order to separate the more active fraction with CEA activity.

The pattern of the Sephadex G-200 chromatography of the purified extract of liver cancer metastasis showed four peaks. The fractions were assayed in the radio-immunoassay system described above, using the starting material as a 'standard'.

As illustrated by the height of the column in the second peak, this was found to be 8 times more active than the crude extract (Fig. 4). The second fraction was chromatographed on DEAE-C and the fractions we obtained were checked as described above. In this case also, a fraction 6 times more active was eluted with the sodium potassium phosphate buffer 0.01 M pH 8.0 containing 0.1 M NaCl (Fig. 5).

After absorption of purified CEA with erythrocytes of group A and absorption of tested sera with anti-A antibodies, we did not find antibodies in the sera of 18 patients with malignant neoplasias.

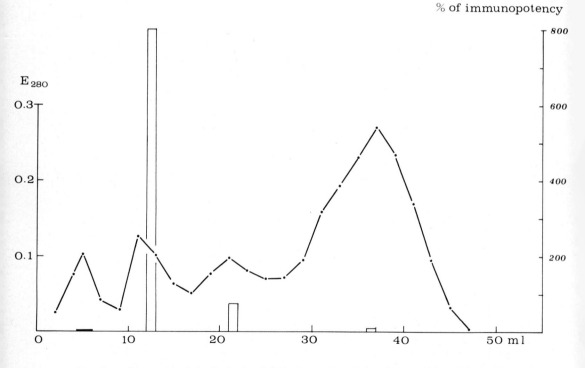

FIG. 4   *The pattern of the Sephadex G-200 chromatography of the purified extract of liver cancer metastasis showed four peaks. The fractions were assayed in the radio-immunoassay system using the starting material as a 'standard'. As illustrated by the height of the column in the second peak, this was found to be 8 times more active than the crude extract.*

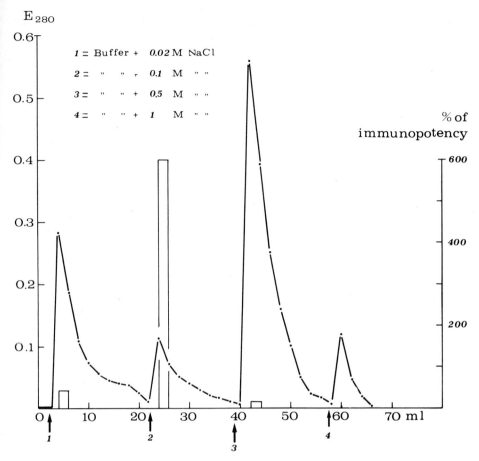

FIG. 5   *The second fraction was chromatographed on DEAE-C and it showed a CEA-activity 6 times greater than the second peak previously separated.*

Discussion

The problem of the presence of antibodies against CEA in the sera of patients with carcinoma has not yet been solved. CEA separated by us from a liver metastasis of cancer of the colon, and absorbed with normal liver tissue antiserum and with anti-A substances, did not reveal antibodies in the sera of patients with colon carcinoma. Radio-immuno-electrophoresis and a radio-immunoassay in liquid medium was employed.

These results may be explained in the following way:

(*a*) The titer of antibodies in cancer sera is very low and even with a very sensitive method it is impossible to find them.

(*b*) The presence of antibodies in cancer patients may be transient and hence a large number of cases would have to be tested before getting significant results.

(*c*) CEA is not an antigen and the host does not recognize it as 'not-self'. Therefore antibodies are not produced by the host. Autoantigenicity of CEA is not demonstrated.

The last hypothesis does not exclude the possibility of using CEA-detection in the sera of cancer patients as a method for cancer diagnosis. The use of radio-immunoassay for detecting CEA in sera has allowed the detection of nanograms of this antigen. The high sensitivity of the method challenged its cancer specificity and levels of CEA higher than normal were found not only in carcinoma of the gastro-intestinal tract but also in carcinomas of other organs and in non-malignant disease.

Investigation of circulating antibodies, directed against CEA, in sera of patients with intestinal cancer, or with neoplasias of other organs, gave variable and controversial results. The disappointments may be due to the presence of common antigenic determinants between CEA and proteins, which could be present in normal tissue of the system, or of other normal organs. Only sophisticated and careful absorption of the purified CEA, or specific antisera with normal tissue components, or with the related antisera is reliable. Our attempts to purify CEA by immunological means may be worth considering.

We have concentrated our efforts on obtaining the most purified fraction that may have CEA activity in extracts of colon carcinoma tissue. We believe that, in order to avoid the pitfalls and disappointments so common in the field of tumour antigens, it will be necessary to make additional investigations as indicated in the introduction. It will be useful to purify to a greater extent the cancer tissue extracts and to absorb the antigen and the antisera with all the means we have at our disposal. This must be done before we can deal with the immunological reaction in human sera and before definite conclusions can be reached. We believe that in the field of CEA we have passed too quickly from theoretical investigation to practical and clinical application.

Acknowledgements

We are grateful to Dr. Donini and Dr. Olivieri for their help and cooperation in radio-immunoassay methods and Mr. Luigi Dall'Oco for his technical assistance.

References

Avrameas, S. and Ternynck, T. (1969): Immunochemistry, 6, 53.
Collatz, E., Von Kleist, S. and Burtin, P. (1971): Int. J. Cancer, 8, 298.
Egan, M. L., Lautenschleger, J. T., Coligan, J. E. and Todd, C. W. (1972): Immunochemistry, 9, 289.
Gold, J. M., Freedman, S. O. and Gold, P. (1972): Nature New Biol., 239/13, 60.
Gold, P. (1967): Cancer (Philad.), 10, 1663.
Lo Gerfo, P., Lo Gerfo, F., Herter, F., Barker, G. and Hansen, H. J. (1972): Amer. J. Surg., 123/2, 127.
Mach, J. P. and Pusztaszeri, G. (1972): Immunochemistry, 9, 1031.
Moore, T. L., Kupchik, H. Z., Marcon, N. and Zamcheck, N. (1971): Amer. J. dig. Dis., 16/1, 1.
Zamcheck, N., Moore, T. L., Dhar, P. and Kupchik, H. (1972): New Engl. J. Med., 286, 83.

Serum alpha-fetoproteins in chronic liver diseases and primary cancer of the liver in children and adults

J. Milosavljević, M. Stajić, D. Filipović, N. Vilhar and J. Teodorović

Mother and Child Health Institute, and Department of Medicine, General Hospital in Zemun, Belgrade, Yugoslavia

The synthesis of alpha-fetoprotein (AFP) which takes place in proliferating liver cells, probably hepatoblasts, starts very early: its presence can be demonstrated in the fetal serum as early as the sixth week of intrauterine life. With further development of the fetus, the AFP concentration increases to reach its highest level between the twelfth and sixteenth week (Houstek et al., 1968; Van Furth and Adinolfi, 1969). Two to four weeks before birth, this protein fraction shows a rapid decrease and at birth its concentration is 1-3% of the highest value reached during fetal life. AFP synthesis stops after birth and AFP therefore disappears from the serum of the newborn baby at the end of the first month of life.

Outside the embryonal phase, AFP was first observed in experimentally induced liver cancer in mice (Abelev et al., 1963) and rats (Stanislawski-Birenswaig et al., 1967). In view of the fact that the presence of AFP was also demonstrated in the sera of adults with primary liver cancer (Tatarinov, 1964), this finding has been considered to be a reliable test in the diagnosis of hepatocellular cancer (Leblanc et al., 1967; Abelev et al., 1967). However, the presence of AFP was also demonstrated in the sera of patients with malignant undifferentiated teratomas, liver cancer of the mixed type and in patients with cancer metastases in the liver from a primary cancer in the pancreas, or from gastric adenocarcinoma (Tatarinov and Nogaller, 1966; Houstek et al., 1968; Bourreille et al., 1970; Geffroy et al., 1970a; Geffroy et al., 1970b; Alpert et al., 1968; Bernades et al., 1971). By means of very sensitive radio-immunological methods it has been possible to demonstrate the presence of AFP also in a small number of pregnant women (Foy et al., 1970), in patients with regenerative processes in the liver and in healthy individuals. In all these cases, AFP was present in very small concentrations which were undetectable by the usual immunological methods. Although it has been proved that this protein is synthesized in proliferating liver cells (Abelov, 1970; Gitlin and Boesman, 1967), their biological properties are not yet known. The results obtained in the existing studies on the incidence of positive findings in patients with primary liver cancer are very variable and range between 27 and 87%.

However, Masopust and co-workers (Masopust et al., 1968) have found AFP in children up to the age of 12 months if they have had hepatitis or other liver lesions.

Material and methods

Sera were examined from 666 persons aged between 4 days and 73 years. Controls consisted of 100 sera of which 50 were obtained from pregnant women in the second half of pregnancy and 50 from school children 17-18 years old. The remaining 566 sera were divided into two groups. The first group included sera from adults with a chronic liver disease, or liver cancer (Table 1), and the second group included sera from children with a chronic liver disease or other illnesses (Tables 2 and 3). Diagnosis was established on the

TABLE 1   *Alpha–fetoprotein in sera of examined patients*

Diagnosis	No. of patients	A F P	
		No. of positive cases	%
Normal persons	50	–	–
Pregnant women	50	–	–
Cirrhosis } compensated	5	–	–
Hepatis } uncompensated	17	–	–
Hepatitis acuta	2	–	–
Hepatitis } agressiva	5	–	–
Chronica } persistens	5	–	–
Steatosis hepatis	10	–	–
Hepatopathia secundaria	4	–	–
Icterus obstructivus	3	–	–
Echinococcus hepatis	1	–	–
Carcinoma hepatis metastasis	1	–	–
Carcinoma hepatis primaria	5	2	40

basis of clinical and biochemical criteria, and in the majority, liver biopsy was also performed, except in adult cases with uncompensated liver cirrhosis in whom laparoscopy was carried out.

Unless the analyses were done immediately the sera were stored at -20°C. Three immunological techniques were used for the demonstration of AFP: Kohn's modification of Pesendorfer's method of immuno-precipitation (Kohn, 1970), immunodiffusion after

TABLE 2   *Alpha-fetoprotein in sera of children with a chronic liver disease or other illnesses*

Diagnosis	No. of patients			No. of alpha-fetoprotein positive cases	
	Total	Less than 1 year	1 year and above	Less than 1 year	1 year and above
Cirrhosis hepatis	33	1	32	1	–
Hepatitis acuta	18	6	12	1	–
Hepatitis chronica	13	–	13	–	–
Icterus neonatorum	9	9	–	7	–
Icterus prolongatus	12	12	–	3	–
Other liver diseases	7	3	4	3	–
Leucosis lymphoblastomata acuta	77	1	76	–	–
Lymphogranulomatosis	5	–	5	–	–
Collagenosis	64	–	64	–	–
Neuroblastoma	4	–	4	–	–
Reticulosarcomatosis	3	–	3	–	–
Anemia	32	6	26	1	–
Sepsis; Status febrilis	225	74	151	5	–

TABLE 3   *Alpha-fetoprotein in sera of children with a chronic liver disease or other illnesses*

Diagnosis	No. of patients			No. of alpha-fetoprotein positive cases	
	Total	Less than 1 month	1 month- 1 year	Less than 1 month	1 month- 1 year
Cirrhosis hepatis	1	–	1	–	1
Hepatitis acuta	6	–	6	–	1
Icterus neonatorum	9	9	–	7	–
Icterus prolongatus	12	5	7	2	1
Other liver diseases	3	1	2	1	2
Leucosis lymphoblastomata acuta	1	–	1	–	–
Anemia	6	3	3	1	–
Sepsis: St. febrillis	74	8	66	5	–

Ouchterlony, and commercially available Partigen plates (Behringwerke AG) for the quantitative determination of this fraction.

Results

Of the total number of 666 sera which were analyzed, 100 sera represented samples from the control group in which AFP was not found.

Of 566 patients under study, 64 were adults and 502 children. Among the adults (Table 1) 22 patients had liver cirrhosis, and of these 5 were in the compensated and 17 in the uncompensated phase of disease. Two patients had acute hepatitis and 10 had chronic hepatitis. Among the latter, 5 persons had the aggressive form and the other 5 the persistent form of chronic hepatitis. The next group of 10 consisted of patients with liver steatosis of different etiology. Only one patient had echinococcus of the liver. Three sera belonged to persons with obstructive jaundice subsequent to choledocholithiasis. Four patients suffered from secondary hepatopathy. Metastatic liver cancer was present in 7 patients: in 4, the primary was in the stomach, 2 had primary cancer of the colon, and 1 female patient had cancer of the ovaries. AFP was not found in the serum of any of these patients.

Of the 5 patients with primary liver cancer AFP was found in 2 cases. The first positive finding of AFP was in the serum of a 23-year-old patient with hypernephroma hepatis prim. – adrenal rest carcinoma (verified surgically and by autopsy). The concentrations of AFP ranged between 26.4 and 88.0 mg/100 ml.

The second serum with the positive finding, at a concentration of 6.6 mg/100 ml, belonged to a 68-year-old patient with a primary hepatocellular cancer of the liver and liver cirrhosis.

Negative findings in the sera of patients with liver cancer were obtained in the following cases:

1. Carcinoma hepatis prim. hepatocellulare (verified by laparoscopy and biopsy) in a 72-year-old patient.

2. Carcinoma hepatis prim. hepatocellulare (verified by surgery and autopsy) in a 47-year-old female patient.

3. Lymphosarcoma hepatis in a 65-year-old patient.

The group of children under study included 502 patients between 4 days and 14 years of age. This group was further divided into two sub-groups: children below, and those over 12 months of age. The following pathological findings were recorded in these children;

liver cirrhosis, acute and chronic hepatitis, neonatal and prolonged jaundice, inadequately defined diseases of the liver (thyroxinemia or hemorrhagic disease of the newborn), acute lymphoblastic leukemia, anemia of different etiologies as well as sepsis and febrile states.

AFP was not found in any sera from children over 12 months of age. Of the total number of 112 children below 12 months, AFP was found to be present in the sera of 21 children (18.7%).

AFP was also present in 5 of 86 sera from the newborn babies (5.8%). The oldest child was 10 months and suffered from thyroxinemia with hepatosplenomegaly. A 4-month-old child had acute hepatitis. Prolonged jaundice was present in a child of 2.5 months, in whom AFP was found at a concentration of 23.0 mg/100 ml. In a 60-day-old child with a congenital abnormality of the biliary tract complicated with liver cirrhosis, AFP was present both before, and 14 days after, the operation. In the youngest patient, who was only 34 days old, and who suffered from neonatal M. hemorrhage, AFP persisted in the serum for 30 days at a concentration of 1 mg/100 ml. Of the 26 children aged under 30 days, AFP was found in the sera of 16 (62.5%). Among the children with positive AFP (6, 7 or 8 days old) 7 had neonatal jaundice. Two children with prolonged jaundice were 20 days old, while the oldest child from this group was 25 days old and had an abnormality of the biliary tract.

Severe anemia accompanied by a positive AFP was found in a 25-day-old newborn baby. In 5 newborn babies (3, 4, 5 or 6 days old) who had sepsis. AFP was present in concentrations from 1.1 to 6.5 mg/100 ml.

Discussion

It has been shown in various studies that AFP may be present in the serum of patients with hepatocellular cancer and undifferentiated teratomas as well as in those with cancer metastases in the liver.

In view of the fact that AFP is synthesized by undifferentiated embryonic liver cells, the appearance of this protein in the serum of adult persons may be explained on the basis of pathological regression of the liver tissue, viz the reappearance of undifferentiated cells of embryonic type. The failure to find AFP in the serum of some patients with primary liver cancer may be the sign of inadequate regression of the liver tissue, which is thus unable to synthesize this protein. If the lack of AFP synthesis outside the embryonic phase is due to a mechanism of inhibition in hepatocytes, the reappearance of AFP in the serum of adults could be explained by the phenomenon of 'derepression' (Uriel, 1970).

The presence of this protein in the blood of newborn babies during the first 30 days after birth has been considered normal. However, according to our findings, AFP is present only in those cases in which the other clinical and biochemical findings indicated the existence of abnormal liver function. The problems of the prevalence and significance of this protein fraction in the serum of the newborn are not clear on the basis of the existing studies. The finding of AFP in the newborn was always associated with severe impairment of liver function.

Summary

The presence of alpha-fetoprotein (AFP) in the sera of 566 patients (from 4 days to 73 years of age) was studied by the following methods: Kohn's modification of Pesendorfer's method of immunoprecipitation, immunodiffusion after Ouchterlony, and commercially available Partigen plates (Behringwerke AG). In our experience, all three methods proved equally sensitive.

The control group consisted of 100 sera (50 from pregnant women and 50 from school children aged 17-18 years). AFP was not detected in any of the control sera.

AFP was not found in children over 12 months old and in adults suffering from the following diseases: liver cirrhosis, acute and chronic hepatitis, liver steatosis, secondary hepatopathies and metastatic cancer of the liver.

Of 5 patients with primary cancer of the liver, AFP was found to be present in 2 patients. Alpha-fetoprotein was found in concentrations from 26.4 to 88.0 mg% in a patient with hypernephroma hepatis prim. – adrenal rest carcinoma. The other positive finding of AFP in the concentration of 6.6 mg% was in a patient with carcinoma hepatis prim. et cirrhosis hepatis.

Among 86 newborn babies, AFP was found to be present in the sera of 5 (thyroxinemia, acute hepatitis, prolonged jaundice, congenital abnormality of the biliary tract and hemorrhagic disease of the newborn).

AFP was found in 16 of 26 newborn babies (neonatal and prolonged jaundice and abnormalities of the biliary tract).

References

Abelev, G. I. (1970): In: Protides of the Biological Fluids. Proceedings of the XVIIIth Ann. Colloquium, Bruges. Elsevier Publ. Co., Amsterdam.

Abelev, G. I., Perova, S. D., Kharamkova, N. I., Postnikova, Z. A. and Irlin, I. S. (1963): Transplantation, 1, 174.

Abelev, G. I., Assecritova, L. V., Kraevsky, N. A., Perova, S. D. and Perevodchikova, N. I. (1967): Int. J. Cancer, 2, 551.

Alpert, M. E., Pinn, V. W. and Isselbacher, K. J. (1971): New Engl. J. Med., 285, 1058.

Alpert, M. E., Uriel, J. and Nechand, B. (1968): New Engl. J. Med., 278, 984.

Bernades, P., Smadja, M., Rueff, B., Bonnefond, A., Tursz, T., Martin, E., Bognel, C., Barge, J. and Uriel, J. (1971): Presse méd., 79, 1585.

Bourreille, J., Metayes, P. and Sanger, F. (1970): Presse méd., 78, 1277.

Foy, H., Kondi, A., Parker, A. M., Stanley, R. and Venning, C. D. (1970): Lancet, 2, 1336.

Geffroy, Y., Denis, P. and Colin, R. (1970a): Presse méd., 78, 1107.

Geffroy, Y., Metayer, P. and Denis, P. (1970b): Presse méd., 78, 1096.

Gitlin, D. and Boesman, M. (1966): J. clin. Invest., 45, 1826.

Gitlin, D. and Boesman, M. (1967): Comp. Biochem. Physiol., 21, 327.

Houstek, J., Masopust, J., Kithier, K. and Radl, J. (1968): J. Pediat., 72, 186.

Kohn, J. (1970): J. clin. Path., 23, 733.

Leblanc, L., Quenum, C., Loisillier, F. and Grabar, P. (1967): C.R.Acad.Sci.(Paris), 265, 75.

Masopust, J., Kithier, K., Rádl, J., Kontecký, J. and Kotál, L. (1968): Int. J. Cancer, 3, 364.

Stanislawski-Birenswaig, M., Uriel, J. and Grabar, P. (1967): Cancer Res., 27, 1990.

Tatarinov, I. S. (1964): Vop.med.Khim., 10, 90.

Tatarinov, S. Y. and Nogaller, M. A. (1966): Vop.Onkol., 12, 26.

Uriel, J. (1970): In: Protides of the Biological Fluids. Proceedings of the XVIIIth Ann. Colloquium, Bruges. Elsevier Publ. Co., Amsterdam.

Van Furth, R. and Adinolfi, M. (1969): Nature (Lond.), 222, 1296.

Immunochemical studies on a tumour-associated antigen in human lung cancer

E. Sega, P. G. Natali and G. Citro

Regina Elena Cancer Institute, Rome, Italy

In the last two decades the detection of cancer specific antigens in tumours of experimental animals has stimulated a similar intense investigation in human oncology. Along these lines of studies several reports have appeared in the literature dealing with the presence of abnormal components in human tumour tissue which do not have their counterpart in the normal organ. They have been named 'tumour specific antigens' or 'neoantigens' or 'oncofetal antigens' because it was either possible to prepare specific hetero-antisera, or because antibodies and/or specific immune lymphocytes could be found in patients with carcinoma – see references in Southam (1971); Alexander, (1972).

Yachi et al. (1968) described the presence of human lung-cancer-associated-antigens which are soluble in 50% saturated ammonium sulphate. Two tumour-tissue components were found and named 'X' and 'Y'. The two antigens were larger in molecular size than 7 S, and the 'X' component was larger than the 'Y' antigen. No subsequent report from these authors has appeared.

The present study deals with the preliminary description and partial isolation of a tumour-associated-antigen which appears to be present in human lung cancer tissue. Such attempts are justified by the fact that in this pathological condition no laboratory or radiological test allows early detection of this malignancy.

Materials and methods

For this study, cancer and normal tissue material were obtained after surgery and either immediately processed or quickly frozen at -80°C. The neoplastic tissues included samples from 10 patients with lung carcinoma. Histological types were as follows: epidermoid carcinoma, adenocarcinoma and undifferentiated carcinoma ('oat cell' carcinoma). Normal tissue was also obtained after surgery from the normal lung of the same patient. All tissues were kept at -80°C until use.

Preparation of extracts

All procedures were carried out at -4°C in a sterile box. Two main methods were employed:

1. Homogenization method

The neoplastic tissue of all cases of lung carcinoma was separated from normal tissue: connective tissue and blood vessels were removed. The tissue was then minced and washed at least three times in cold PBS at pH 7.2. The homogenate was prepared in PBS (ratio: tissue/PBS $-1/2$) in a Mini Mixer Homogenizer at 6,500 rpm for 20 min. This procedure was completed in a Potter-Elvejhem homogenizer. The homogenate was centrifuged at

4,000 rpm (23,000 g) for 20 min and the supernatant decanted and dialysed against PBS for 24 hr. The dialysed supernatant was concentrated with Aquacide (CalBio-chemical, Los Angeles) to obtain a final concentration of 30 ml; tested by Folin's method. This material was kept at $-80°C$ until use.

2. Cell suspension method

Tumour tissue of one carcinoma (a case of epidermoid carcinoma) was separated from normal tissue under histological observation and minced as mentioned above (see lyophilization method). The fragments were quick-frozen and sliced in 8 nm-thick sections in an International cryostat. The sections were pooled and dispersed at room temperature in PBS. The cell suspension, washed 3 times in cold PBS, was used for immunization procedures.

Immunization of animals and preparation of antisera

White New Zealand rabbits (weight about 6— 7 pounds) were used throughout the experiments. Cell suspensions freshly prepared from frozen tumour tissue stored at $-80°C$, were injected intracutaneously at multiple sites and in foot pads, according to the following schedule: First injection of 3 ml of a cell suspension (5×10^7 to 1×10^8 cells per ml) plus 3 ml of complete Freund-adjuvant. The second and third injections were given with the same number of cells once a week for two consecutive weeks. A fourth injection was repeated without adjuvant. The animals were bled 8 to 10 days after the last booster injection.

Absorption of antisera

The rabbit antisera were successively absorbed with:
  (i)   human red blood cells AB Rh+ group
  (ii) pooled normal human plasma insolubilized according to Avrameas and Ternynk
  (iii) normal lung tissue extracts insolubilized by the same method.

Immunochemical methods

The identification of the presence of abnormal protein fractions, related to tumour tissue, was performed by double immunodiffusion in 0.5% agarose, dissolved in phosphate buffered saline (PBS), 0.01 M phosphate, 0.15 M NaCl, pH 7.2 containing 0.1 sodium azide. Precipitin reactions were obtained with wells of 8 mm in diameter, placed 4 mm apart. Precipitin reactions were allowed to develop at room temperature and were examined for at least 48 hr.

Separation and characterization of fractions

Separation was performed with electro-focusing in sucrose gradient (pH-3-10). A column for electro-focusing (LKB 8101, 110 ml) was filled with a linear density gradient prepared by mixing a light solution of sucrose with a dense solution by a gradient mixer (LKB 8121). The light solution contained distilled water, 1/4 of the Carrier Ampholytes and the sample, the dense solution contained 3/4 of the Carrier Ampholytes and 28 g of sucrose in 42 ml of distilled water. The anode was surrounded with a dilute acid solution and the cathode with a dilute alkaline solution. The pH gradient is formed when a voltage (300 to 600 V) is applied across the mixture. (Normally the current for one column does not exceed 10 mA, the power dissipated being 3 to 6 W.) To avoid heat convection, the column was thermostatically controlled during operation. Elution was performed with a faction collector and the eluted proteins were analyzed by a recording absorption meter, operating at a wavelength of 280 nm.

Results

Reaction of the heteroantiserum with tissue extract is shown in Figure 1. Here the precipitating activity of the rabbit antiserum was compared with saline extracts from normal (peripheral well n°1), tumour (n°2) lung tissue and sera from normal (n°3) and lung cancer patients (n°4). Multiple common precipitin lines were observed, but rabbit antiserum appeared to develop a precipitin line with lung cancer saline extract, which was not detectable in normal tissue saline extract and with sera from normal persons and cancer patients (see Fig. 1).

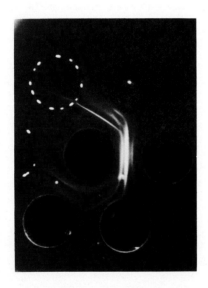

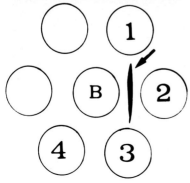

FIG. 1   *B Central well: rabbit antiserum to tumour cell suspension. Peripheral wells: (1) Saline extract from a pool of normal lung tissue; (2) saline extract from a pool of cancer tissue; (3) pool of cancer patients' sera; and (4) pool of normal sera.*
The rabbit antiserum appears to detect an extra component in the tumour tissue extract which is not present, either in normal tissue extract, or in sera from normal and cancer individuals.

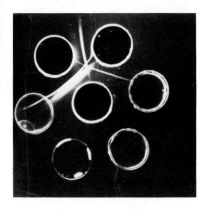

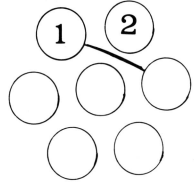

FIG. 2 *Central well: saline extract from pooled cancer tissue. Peripheral wells: (1) Anti-whole-human-serum; and (2) Lung cancer tissue antiserum repeatedly absorbed with NHS and normal lung tissue.*
No common antigens are recognised by the two antisera. The antigen detected by the absorbed antiserum to lung cancer appeared completely unrelated to serum proteins.

When the rabbit antiserum was absorbed as previously described, only one precipitin line could be observed with the lung tumour extract, as is shown in Figure 2. From the same experiment, this tissue component seems to be completely unrelated to normal human serum antigens which contaminate the tumour-tissue extracts.

To obtain a further characterization of the components detected by rabbit antiserum in the tumour-tissue saline extracts, homogenates from cancer and normal tissues were submitted to fractionation by the electro-focusing method in a pH gradient of 3 to 10. The results of this separation, performed with tumour saline extract, are shown in Figure 3. The method allowed the separation of 5 major components. Among these, only the second (P.I. 4.3) and the fifth (P.I. 7.2) fractions appeared to contain the antigen recognized by rabbit antiserum in the whole tumour-tissue extract (see Fig. 3).

Although the 2 components showed a quite different mobility in the pH gradient used, they appeared to be antigenically identical. The reason and the significance of such a phenomenon has not yet been further investigated. When the normal lung tissue extract was analyzed by the same method, only 3 fractions were present in the chromatographic pattern and none of them reacted with the rabbit antiserum (Fig. 4).

Discussion

Early diagnosis of the disease appears to be of primary importance for the treatment of cancer until such a time as neoplastic patients can be cured by efficient single or combined therapy that will allow a complete and definitive recovery from illness.

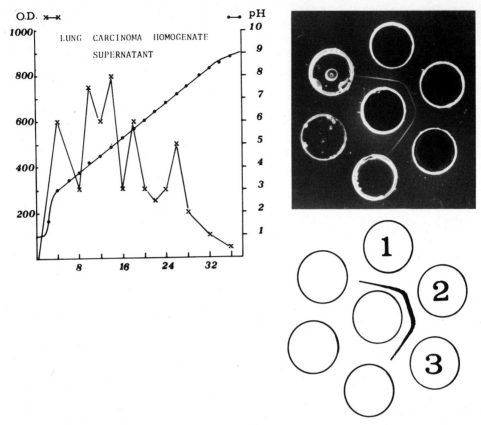

FIG. 3   *Separation of a pool of lung cancer tissue supernatant by electro-focusing. Central well: rabbit anti-lung-tumour-tissue repeatedly absorbed with NHS and normal lung tissue. Peripheral wells: (1) Saline extract of pooled cancer tissue; (2) Fraction II, P. I. 4.3; and (3) Fraction V, P.I. 7.2.*
                The antigen detected by rabbit antiserum appears to be present in the electro-focusing fractions II and V.

    Recently, it has become clear that almost any neoplastic disease is able to elicit a specific immune reponse in the host. Therefore, the studies on the presence of specific antigens, or on the production of antibodies or immune lymphocytes represent an ideal biological condition to gain more insight into the tumour-host relationship and to provide specific diagnostic methods.

    In view of such considerations, intense investigation of the antigenic properties of human tumours seems to be justified from the theoretical and practical points of view. Due to its subtle nature, early detection of lung cancer requires special interest on the part of the investigators.

    Immuno-diffusion was used all through our study and it is known that this method is not very sensitive. Therefore, the lack of reactivity of the rabbit antitumour serum with normal lung tissue saline extract does not allow the exclusion, at this point of our investigation, of the abnormal component detected in cancer tissue being present at a low concentration in the normal lung. Such phenomena have been observed lately in other tumour-associated antigens, and in particular in CEA.

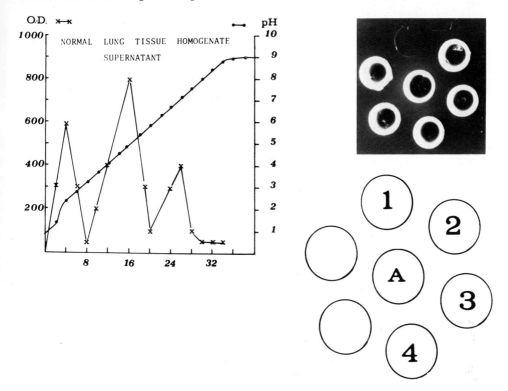

FIG . 4   *Separation of a pool of normal lung tissue supernatant by electro-focusing. Central well:*
rabbit anti-lung-cancer-tissue repeatedly absorbed with NHS and normal lung tissue. Peri-
pheral wells: (1) Fraction I, P. I. 2 .4; (2) fraction II, P .I. 4 .5; (3) fraction III, P .I. 6 .8:
and (4) Saline extract of normal lung tissue pool.

Further separation and purification of this antigen is in progress to obtain more suitable immunoreactive components to be used in more sensitive methods. It may be possible
to obtain by radio-immunoassay quantitative evaluation of the presence of the antigen in
normal and cancer tissue. Once such tests are available, it will be of extreme interest to
check the possibility of either this antigen, or specific antibodies detectable in the sera of
lung cancer patients.

References

Alexander P. (1972): Nature (Lond.), 235, 137.
Yachi, A., Matsura, Y., Carpenter, C. M. and Hyde, L. (1968): J. nat. Cancer Inst., 40, 663.
Southam, C. M. (1971): In: Immunological Disease, 2nd ed., Vol. 1., Chapter 42, pp. 743-764.
    Editors: M. Samter, D. W. Talmage, B. Rose, W. D. Sherman and Y. H. Vaughan. Little, Brown &
    Co. Boston, Mass.

Soluble membrane antigens of human malignant lung cells

T.H.M. Stewart, Ariel C. Hollinshead and R.B. Herberman

Ottawa General Hospital, University of Ottawa, Faculty of Medicine, Ottawa, Canada; Laboratory for Virus and Cancer Research, Department of Medicine, The George Washington University, Washington, D. C.; and Cell and Tumor Immunology Section, National Cancer Institute, National Institute of Health, Bethesda, Md., U.S.A.

The importance of cellular mediated host defence against lung cancer was suggested in a study of the brief effectiveness of methotrexate in cases of carcinoma of the lung (Stewart et al., 1969). The present study was initiated so that the specificity of delayed hypersensitivity reactions toward lung tumour could be assessed. If specific anti-tumour activity could be shown toward cell membrane material derived from human lung cancer it would suggest a logical choice of antigens (Hollinshead et al., 1972; Prager et al., 1974) for use in a controlled clinical programme of immunochemotherapy.

Materials and methods

The cancer tissue was separated from the fresh surgical specimen by the pathologist at the Ottawa General or Ottawa Civic Hospital. Uninvolved lung (normal) was also removed at the same time. The fresh tissue was immediately minced, washed several times, and the cells separated by the use of 60 mesh stainless steel sieves and by aspiration through a 5ml bore pipette. The cells were then frozen at $-80\,^\circ$C and shipped by air the same day to Washington, D. C. The sterility of the cell suspension and of the material in the subsequent procedures was monitored by cultures in blood agar plates and in thioglycollate broth. The preparation of the cells required about 2 hr. The viable cell count using trypan blue and neutral red was used as a base for the calculations of the active antigen protein content. On arrival in Washington 24 hr later the frozen cell suspension was thawed quickly and stepwise isotonic to hypotonic saline extraction conducted and the membranes pelleted from the extracts by centrifugation at 100,000g for 1 hr, without brake. The membrane pellets were then subjected to sequential low frequency sonication for 3-time intervals (Table I) with centrifugation for 1 hr after each interval. The total combined soluble membrane sonicate, the membrane preparation, and the viable cell preparation samples were evaluated for protein content, and Sephadex G-200 columns were prepared to accommodate the amount of protein obtained. The columns were washed for several hours and the flow rate determined using Dextran blue. The next day the soluble sonicates were separated over Sephadex gels and the protein profile recorded. Appropriate cuts were made of the fractions collected which make up a single protein peak, and these tubes, each of which contained 2ml, were combined, and the pooled fraction concentrated by Diaflo ultrafiltration. In all of these steps, the materials were kept cold, except for the column separation, which was conducted at room temperature, with collection of eluates in the cold in an automatic fraction collector. The following day, any concentrations which were not accomplished the previous day were completed, and all of the material tested by the Lowry procedure for protein content. A record of each separation was recorded in the laboratory, and a separate summary record was written up for further

TABLE 1

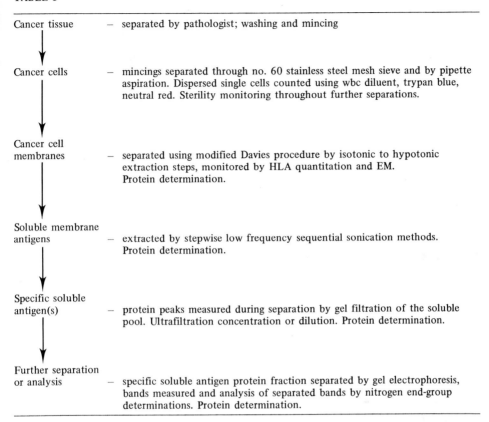

Cancer tissue	— separated by pathologist; washing and mincing
Cancer cells	— mincings separated through no. 60 stainless steel mesh sieve and by pipette aspiration. Dispersed single cells counted using wbc diluent, trypan blue, neutral red. Sterility monitoring throughout further separations.
Cancer cell membranes	— separated using modified Davies procedure by isotonic to hypotonic extraction steps, monitored by HLA quantitation and EM. Protein determination.
Soluble membrane antigens	— extracted by stepwise low frequency sequential sonication methods. Protein determination.
Specific soluble antigen(s)	— protein peaks measured during separation by gel filtration of the soluble pool. Ultrafiltration concentration or dilution. Protein determination.
Further separation or analysis	— specific soluble antigen protein fraction separated by gel electrophoresis, bands measured and analysis of separated bands by nitrogen end-group determinations. Protein determination.

experiments and for forms used in the skin testing procedure. After the protein content of the various fractions was determined, each fraction was either diluted or further concentrated in order to have fractions of similar protein content for skin testing. Each of these fractions was then Millipore-filtered in a syringe (Swinney), and sterility tests were checked for several days. This material was then provided for skin testing, if it met with the required standards. In general, normal counterpart tissues and cancer tissues were handled, using separate equipment and separate hoods, during the same time period.

Theoretically, injection of cell extracts could produce local irritation as well as fever. However, in the patients tested, this was not observed. There was, however, pain at the injection site at the time the material was administered intradermally, which lasted for 20 to 30 sec. An injection of Demerol 75 mg, 30 min before skin testing lessens this discomfort.

After the initial tests of this partially separated material, tests were made of further separated material. These methods of gradient gel electrophoresis are described in detail elsewhere (McWright, 1970; McWright et al., 1971). The number of columns run at one time was generally 6, and 5 unstained gels were kept at 4°C until the location of the bands was seen in the stained gel. The remaining 5 gels were then sliced for precise regions, comparable regions pooled, and eluted with sterile saline at 4°C for 50 hr, concentrated by ultrafiltration, rediluted 100 fold, and reconcentrated. The eluates were divided into appropriate aliquots, passed through Millipore Swinney filters, sterility tests made, and materials drawn up into sterile syringes for skin testing.

The material was placed in labeled small screw-cap vials in plastic packets and sent to Ottawa on dry ice in polystyrofoam boxes. The materials were drawn up in tuberculin syringes with No. 26 needles for skin testing. The recipient was tested with 0.1 ml of each preparation intradermally into the skin of the back. The area injected was marked appropriately at each site. The tests were read for immediate reactions and at 24 and 48 hr. At these time intervals the injection sites were measured for induration and erythema, pictures were taken and biopsies made for pathologic evaluation. The results were recorded on a protocol sheet. 5ml of clotted blood was sometimes drawn at the time of testing and at appropriate intervals thereafter.

Each patient was clinically staged and all stages of malignancy were studied. No patient was included who had received chemotherapy or extensive irradiation in the previous 14 days. If possible, skin tests in post-operative patients were avoided until at least 24 hr following surgery. Prior to testing with the separated antigens, each patient was evaluated for the ability to produce a delayed hypersensitivity reaction by skin testing with candida, mumps and streptokinase-streptodornase (SKSD). Those that were anergic are excluded. Mumps or SKSD (SK40:SD10 units) usually were positive at 48 hr and were the most useful in determining anergy by a single test.

TABLE 2   *The range and mean of protein concentration in 0.1 ml of each fraction*

Stage	Patient		Membranes**	I*	II*	III*	IV*	V	
1	Goud.	Cancer	0	+	+	0			Epid.
		Normal	0	+	0	0			
1	Lam.	Cancer	. 0	+	+	+	0		Epid.
		Normal	0	0	0	0	0		
2	Rad.	Cancer	0	+	+	0	0		Epid.
		Normal	0	0	0	0	0		
2	McC.	Cancer	0	+	+	0	0		Adeno.
		Normal	0	+	+	0	0		
3	Que.	Cancer	0	+	+	+	0		Alveolar
		Normal	0	0	+	+	0		
3	Joh.	Cancer	0	0	0	0			Oat
		Normal	0	0	+	0			
4	Duv.	Cancer	0	+	0	0	0	0	Adeno.
		Normal	0	0	0	0	0	0	
4	Big.	Cancer	0	0	0	0	0		Epid.
		Normal	0	0	0	0	0		

** Membrane protein injected

Ca	Normal
Range 49–325	17–1232
mean 166	mean 291

* Soluble fractions	I	II	III	IV
Ca Range	13–90	15–95	3–28	1–12
	mean 62	mean 65	mean 10	mean 4
Normal	10–45	16–58	3–11	1–7
	mean 24	mean 35	mean 7	mean 4

+ = 5 mm of induration or more at 48 hr

Results

Eight patients were tested with their autologous membranes and soluble membrane fractions from their cancer tissue and from lung taken distal to the tumour – 'normal'. Six patients reacted to one or more of the soluble cancer fractions and of these 6, 3 reacted to fractions derived from 'normal' autologous lung. The frequency of this reaction is greatest in patients with Stage 1 and 2 disease. Table 2 summarizes these results in autologous skin tests. It will be noted that a greater protein concentration was injected in the membrane material, that was non-reactive, then with the soluble reactive material. Figure 1 shows the characteristic histology of positive reactors biopsied at 48 hr. Eighteen patients were tested with allogeneic material, derived from epidermoid carcinoma, adenocarcinoma and oat cell carcinoma. Fourteen reacted to soluble cancer antigen, 11 to 'normal' lung. In these tests there was no clear association with the stage of the patient being tested. Thus, Stage 1; 2/2 reacted. Stage 2; 3/6. Stage 3; 2/3 and Stage 4; 7/8 reacted. The source of the material giving a positive reaction was not related to a lack of reaction. Thus soluble antigen derived from a Stage 4 epidermoid carcinoma gave positive reactions in 4 patients with epidermoid carcinoma, two Stage 4; one Stage 3 and one Stage 2. Only one patient reacted to the cancer membrane but not to 'normal' lung membrane.

It was of interest to see which soluble fractions gave the most frequent positive skin reactions and to see if antigens from histologically different tumour types gave a cross reaction when tested. The frequency of reactions to normal lung were also noted. These tests are summarized in Tables 3 and 4. Lung cancer antigens gave a positive reaction

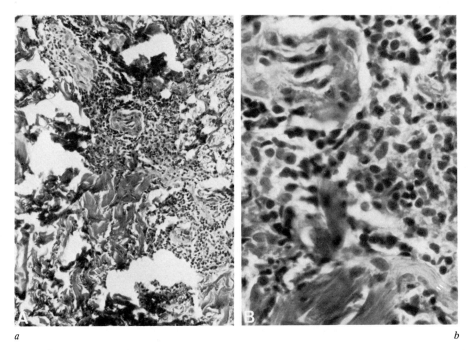

a   *b*

FIG. 1a,b *This shows the reaction at 48 hr on autologous testing with Fraction I derived from epidermoid cancer of lung. (Patient Rad. Table 2) The vascular spaces show marked endothelial swelling and proliferation. Their walls are thickened and their lamina narrow. There is no necrosis of the wall. There is a marked perivascular mononuclear infiltrate made up of lymphocytes and histiocytes. Only an occasional polymorphonuclear is encountered. H.P.S.: (a) × 250 (b) × 998. Reduced for reproduction 47%.*

TABLE 3   *This shows the results of allogeneic skin testing with fractions derived from epidermoid carcinoma*

Fractions	Epidermoid to epidermoid (10 cases)			
	I	II	III	IV
Ca	6	7	7	1
N	3	2	3	0
	Epidermoid to oat			
Ca	0	1	1	
N	0	0	0	
	Epidermoid to carcinoma (no tissue)			
Ca	1	1	1	
	0	0	1	
Total				
Ca	7/12	9/12	9/12	1/12
N	3/12	2/12	4/12	

TABLE 4   *This shows the results of allogeneic skin testing with fractions derived from adeno-carcinoma*

Fractions	Adenocarcinoma to adenocarcinoma			
	I	II	III	IV
Ca	1/3	3/3	1/3	0/3
N	1/3	2/3	0/3	0/3
	Adenocarcinoma to epidermoid			
Ca	0/2	0/2	0/2	0/2
N	0/2	0/2	0/2	0/2
	Adenocarcinoma to oat			
Ca	1	1	1	
N	–	1	–	
Total for adenocarcinoma				
Ca	1/6	4/6	2/6	0/6
N	1/6	3/6	0/6	0/6
Total for allogeneic*				
Ca	8/18	13/18	11/18	1/18
N	4/18	5/18	4/18	0/18

* This shows the combined distribution of positive fractions in allogeneic testing with epidermoid and adenocarcinoma material

twice as frequently as normal lung antigens and the cancer fractions 2 and 3 gave a greater frequency of positive reaction, compared to the situation in autologous testing where fraction 1 gave the highest incidence. Thus Sephadex preparations do not show specific cancer reactions or more than one set of proteins are involved in producing delayed hypersensitivity reactions. In Table 5 we see the comparison of skin tests in one patient with epidermoid cancer of lung tested with allogeneic lung cancer antigens and these derived from two tumours growing, but not originating, in lung. It is apparent that there is cross reactivity between epidermoid carcinoma of cervix and epidermoid carcinoma of lung.

TABLE 5   *Comparison of soluble antigens from allogeneic epidermoid lung cancer cells with those derived from two tumours growing, but not originating, in the lung. Patient tested was Mr. Wes., stage 3 mucoepidermoid carcinoma of the lung. Allogeneic testing*

Stage		Soluble Fractions						
		I		II		III		
		μg	SR	μg	SR	μg	SR	
3	Goud. Ca	76	+	95	+	12	0	Ca lung epid.
	N	20	0	36	0	6	0	
	Len. Ca	26	0	37	0	18	0	Ca sigmoid
	Biaz Ca	44	0	40	+	10	0	Ca cervix epid.

Further separation of soluble membrane antigens. We decided to study the patterns of separation of the different types of lung cancer, the counterpart tumour-free tissues of the same patients, and to contrast these patterns with the pattern of separation of the soluble membrane antigens from normal lung tissue from a normal individual.

Five tumours from 5 different patients were used to prepare the separated and eluted gradient gel regions; 3 epidermoid carcinomas, one adenocarcinoma and one oat cell carcinoma. A 17 year old male victim of a traffic accident provided fresh lung at the time his kidneys were removed for transplantation, following cerebral death. This material will be referred to as 'normal normal', to distinguish it from 'normal' lung taken distal to the tumour at the time of surgery. The details of the donors of this material are shown in Table 6.

TABLE 6   *Description of donors whose tumour or normal lung were used to prepare the gradient gel electrophoretic fractions*

Donor	Sex	Age	Tumour
Mel	M	46	oat cell carcinoma
McC	M	61	epidermoid carcinoma
AH	M	69	epidermoid carcinoma
LB	M	60	epidermoid carcinoma
BH	F	58	adenocarcinoma
G	M	17	normal normal lung – accident victim

TABLE 7　　*Allogeneic skin tests using soluble cell membrane antigens further separated by gradient gel electrophoresis*

Stage			Regions* I	II	III	IV
	Source:					
	Mel	allogeneic oat				
3	Trem	Ca	+	o	++	++
	epid	N	++	++	+	+
4	Sara	Ca	0	0	+	0
	oat	N	0	0	0	0
	Source:					
	McC	allogeneic epid				
3	Trem	Ca	+	0	0	0
	epid N		0	0	0	0
1	Lam	Ca	+	+	0	0
	epid	N	0	0	0	0
	Source:					
	BH	allogeneic adenocarcinoma				
3	Gal	Ca	+	++	++	+
	epid	N	+	+	+	±
		N.N.	+	+	0	0**
3	Vi	Ca	+	+	0	0
	epid	N	+	+	0	0
		N.N.	±	±	0	0**
	Source:					
	BH	allogeneic adenocarcinoma				
3	Laf	Ca	+	+	0	0
	oat	N	0	+	0	0
	Source:					
	L B	allogeneic epidermoid				
3	Vi	Ca	+	0	+	0
	epid					
3	Por	Ca	0	0	0	0
	oat					
2	Pell	Ca	0	0	0	0
	epid	N	0	0	0	0

TABLE 7   *(continued)*

Stage			Regions I	II	III	IV
	Source:					
	AH	allogeneic epidermoid				
3	Vi Ca		0	+	++	0
	epid					
3	Pot Ca		0	0	0	0
	epid					
4	Ben Ca		0	0	0	0
	epid					
2	Pell Ca		0	0	0	0
	epid N		0	0	0	0

*   0 < 4.5 mm induration

±   4.5 – 5.5

+ > 5.5

++ > 12

**   Note the absence of reactions to regions 3 and 4 derived from healthy lung (Normal-Normal - NN).

A third patient with epidermoid carcinoma stage III reacted to allogeneic epidermoid fractions 1, 2, and 3 prepared by Sephadex separation. A weak reaction to gel region I, negative to II and III, was seen to normal normal lung antigens.

TABLE 8

Stage	Patient	Age	Tumour	Tested with:	Gel 1 2 3 4
2	Barc.	74	Breast Ca	Epid. Ca	0 0 0 0
				N.N.	0 0 0 0
1	St P.	72	Lymphosarcoma	Epid. Ca	0 0 0 0
				N.N.	0 0 0 0
3	Ch.	50	Breast Ca	Epid. Ca	0 0 0
2	Mart.	66	Breast Ca	Epid. Ca	0 0 0
3	Charb.	80	Breast Ca	Epid. Ca	0 0 0
3	Vill.	65	Rectum Ca	Epid. Ca	0 0 0
3	Leg.	54	Prostate Ca	Epid. Ca	0 0 0
3	Pa.	60	Prostate Ca	Epid. Ca	0 0 0
3	Fil.	62	Angiosarc. Breast	Epid. Ca	0 0 0

All patients had shown good delayed hypersensitivity to one or more of the bacterial antigen PPD, Mumps, Varidase or Dermatophytin

Fourteen tests were performed in 9 patients. These results are shown in Table 7. It can be seen that no reaction was seen to 'normal normal' lung antigens, fraction 3 and 4, compared to 7/16 reactions to cancer and 4/11 to normal lung to these fractions. No reaction to 'normal normal' lung was seen when tested in two patients with cancer other than lung, (Table 8). These patients were not anergic, having good reactivity to bacterial extracts. A further 7 patients gave no reaction when tested with gel regions of epidermoid cancer of lung. The details of these patients are given in Table 8. The gel patterns for 5 different oat electrophoresis separations were remarkably similar. The patterns for 4 of 6 adenocarcinomas parelleled but 2 had certain bands which were not the same. The epidermoid cancer separations gave varied patterns for 6 separations and similar patterns for 3 separations.

Conclusion

It is apparent that epidermoid carcinoma, oat cell, and adenocarcinoma of the lung are associated with antigens that are present on healthy normal lung. Reactivity is also seen toward soluble fractions derived from cancers but not to comparable fractions derived from healthy lung. Extracts of lung adjacent to the tumour appear to have reactivity that lie between that given by healthy and malignant lung.

Summary

Eight patients have been skin tested with autologous preparations derived from lung cancer cells and cells from adjacent lung ('Normal'). Eighteen patients were tested with allogeneic material. No reactivity was seen directed toward membranes of lung cancer or adjacent normal lung in either group. Positive reactions were seen when these same membrane preparations were subjected to sequential low frequency sonification, and the soluble portions of the membranes were partially separated into high and low molecular weight protein fractions. Reactions to soluble antigen from cancer cells were seen twice as often as to soluble antigen derived from adjacent 'normal' lung cells. Further separations were made of soluble antigens by special gradient gel electrophoresis and elution of sliced regions of the gels. Nine patients with oat cell, epidermoid and adenocarcinomas were tested with antigens derived from 5 tumours, 5 adjacent lungs and one healthy lung from an accident victim. Positive skin reactions to antigen from adjacent lung and healthy lung were mainly from regions 1 and 2. Positive reactions to antigens from epidermoid carcinomas were mainly from regions 1,2 and 3. The strongest positive reactions were to oat cell and adenocarcinoma antigens from regions 3 and 4. Negative reactions were seen in 9 non-anergic patients with other cancers when tested with antigens from gel regions of epidermoid lung cancer preparations. Two gave a negative reaction to a healthy lung preparation. Thus, skin tests using separated lung cancer soluble antigens produce delayed hypersensitive responses in lung cancer patients. We conclude that this reactivity is directed to certain antigens also present in some normal lung preparations as well as to certain antigens in lung cancer preparations which appear to differ from the normal antigens, thus suggesting some tumour specificity.

References

Hollinshead, A., McCammon, J. R. and Yohn, D. S. (1972): Canad. J. Microbiol., 18, 1365.
McWright, C. G. (1970): Thesis. George Washington University, Washington, D. C.
McWright, C. G., Farrel, K. B. and Roberts, D. B. (1971): Clin. chim. Acta., 32, 285.
Prager, M. D., Hollinshead, A. C., Ribble, R. J. and Derr, I. (1973): J. nat. Cancer Inst., 54, 1603.
Stewart, T. H. M., Klassen, D. and Crook, A. F. (1969): Canad. med. Ass. J., 101, 191.

Specific soluble membrane antigen of malignant and normal breast cells: Delayed hypersensitive skin reactions in cancer patients*

A. Hollinshead[1] , W. Jaffurs[2] , L. Alpert[1] and R. Herberman[3]

[1] *The George Washington University Medical Center, Washington, D.C.,*
[2] *Columbia Hospital for Women, Washington, D.C., and* [3] *Cellular and Tumor Immunology Section, Laboratory of Cell Biology, National Cancer Institute, Bethesda, Md., U.S.A.*

General introduction

At an international symposium of this nature, it is sometimes refreshing if we depart from the formalized presentation of data, in order to consider what advances we have made in improving old concepts and old hypotheses and in defining other objectives and goals for the detection and treatment of the specific type of cancer. There is a great demand for those scientists who are bright, informed and critical enough to adopt a multi-disciplinary approach and to apply to their own area of research all that they can learn from the other fields in their discipline. This depth of thought only serves to focus, sharpen and enhance a concentrated effort on one problem. I would like to paint with the broad brush strokes and to place in perspective the approaches and thinking in 1973 with regard to chemotherapy, surgery, radiation, immunology, virology, genetic and environmental effects on breast cancer.

The mechanisms of anti-cancer agents vary widely. Some agents inhibit tumors by blocking specific biosynthetic pathways in the production of cellular DNA, and others act by inhibiting the replication and mitosis in existing cancer cells. In theory, if all agents could be combined to work at every known site, the most potent therapy would result, but the additive drug toxicities preclude this. However, sophisticated methods of manipulating specific drug toxicities have led to clinically effective combinations of many anti-tumor agents. Antibiotics like Adriamycin and Dactinomycin are used. Dactinomycin blocks DNA synthesis by inhibiting the enzymes needed for transfer RNA synthesis. Nitrogen mustard disrupts the DNA cycle by binding guanine in the base. Mitotic inhibitors such as colchicines, vinblastine and vincristine arrest cells during mitoses. When used in conjunction with or immediately after drugs that inhibit DNA synthesis, the mitotic inhibitors add to the therapeutic value of the other drugs by limiting the population of cells they are intended to attack. Thus, the anti-tumor effect is concentrated on a smaller target. Methotrexate activity depends on its similarity to the DNA precursor folic acid. Combined therapy of children with acute leukemia has increased the median survival time after diagnosis from 2 months to as long as 5 or 6 years. This type of combination chemotherapy is also used in breast cancer, and there are encouraging reports from various groups, using various drug combinations, with regard to increasing the length of time before recurrence of cancer.

* This research was supported by USPHS Contract number NIH-NCI-G-69-2176, from the National Cancer Institute, National Institutes of Health, U.S.A.

However, we must constantly recall the fact that approximately 85% of human malignancies are not significantly affected by available therapeutic agents. Even if this percentage were to change over the next few years, it is quite obvious that many other factors must be studied and researched, and other approaches utilized. Lest the more sophisticated in our audience be offended by the simplicity of this presentation, I would like to remark that some of the best scientists I know are those who keep repeating to themselves the very simple, fundamental knowledge, the facts about the particular system which they are studying, and they sort this knowledge away from the body of *information* which accumulates year by year in their field, and which may or may not be relevant. So let us proceed with our fundamental lesson. In breast cancer, most frequently the lesions arise from the peripheral ducts and there is no special structural arrangement. There are different growth patterns which involve either directly the ducts or one or more of the 15-20 separate lobes which make up the breast. There are mucogenic forms and medullary forms of breast cancer. More rarely, the tumor might be specifically epidermoid involving the skin only or the sweat glands of the breast. The spread of this cancer most commonly goes to the regional lymph nodes but there can also be metastasis to the bone, usually the spine, skin, the lungs, the liver, and the brain in that order. Patients with medullary carcinoma of the breast have good prognoses, and it is suggested that the increased lymphoid tissue in these cancers is concerned with immunologic reactions which permits a strong host defense mechanism. Unfortunately, this is not the more common form of breast cancer.

The *information* on surgical techniques, at this time, is confusing. Some feel that removal of the regional lymph nodes in patients where the primary tumor is small and the nodes are not affected, increases the incidence of metastasis, and that later, during metastasis or spread, the nodes can be removed without lowering the host's resistance. Other bodies of *information* do not contain this point of view. The information implies use of radiation in the immediate post-mastectomy might lower host resistance, and it is suggested that radiation be used after metastasis has occurred. Again there is another body of *information* which maintains the opposite point of view.

Now what about age? Age of course has to do with the level of hormones in the early and late menopause period, and doctors take this into consideration in their choice of androgens or estrogens used in conjunction with other drugs. The incidence of breast cancer is 60 per 100,000 females and this incidence exceeds 300 per 100,000 females after the age of 75. As to genetics, patients commonly have a family history of cancer of the breast and other sites. We need to know much more of the how's and the why's of these data. We know even less about the effect of environmental factors on breast cancer. An early study of mice with mammary cancers showed that a 50% reduction in calories reduced the incidence of mammary tumors from 97% to about 15%. We have not really looked at this factor in human beings. One environmental factor we do know something about is iodine deficiency. In geographic areas where there is profound deficiency in the iodine content of the diet, there is increased incidence of breast cancer.

There have been many advances in the field of immunology, particularly transplantation and tumor immunology, which suggest that immunotherapeutic approaches might be helpful and have at least limited effectiveness in combination with other therapeutic approaches for cancer in man. The cell membrane has a trilaminar structure which, theoretically, is a double layer of lipid molecules covered with a protein layer on each side. On the normal cell there are many major and minor histocompatibility antigens. When the cell becomes cancerous, new antigens appear on the cell surface and perhaps behave as minor histocompatibility antigens. In our laboratory we have conclusively demonstrated the existence of such antigens for several cancers, and were the first to successfully isolate and characterize such antigens. Some of these surface antigens are capable of stimulating immune responses. It has been our approach for some time to study the whole cell, and then to further separate the cell membranes of normal and tumor cells away from the rest of the cell, and then to identify and separate these components on the membranes. If these components are semi-soluble or separable, then one has an advantage, since the special purified soluble or semi-soluble membrane antigen can be diluted or concentrated and regulated for comparison with antigens from other cells, and with such standardized, characterized preparations it is possible to have a very careful survey of the cancer patient's reactions at different stages of disease, and to assess such reactions to antigenic stimulation. At first we pioneered in this work using animal systems and have continued to the point where this field appears to be a critical area for exploration for understanding of the immune responses in human cancer patients.

In skin tests of these components in breast cancer patients we have found that breast cancer is associated with a state of cellular hypersensitivity against components not only from the breast cancers but also from benign breast lesions and from the non-cancerous cells of the breast cancer patient.

The paper

The procedures we have used have been described in detail elsewhere. Briefly, material is obtained fresh from the operating room, and portions of the tissue are carefully character-ized by pathologists, the entire cell population is separated and the viable and non-viable cells counted singly, the membranes extracted, a portion of the membrane subjected to sequential low-frequency sonication by special method. The sonicates then are separated by various procedures. The breast cell membrane sonicates are separated using Sephadex G-200 into peak protein fractions. All of these procedures are monitored by several meth-ods for sterility, and only those materials which are bacteria free and pyrogen free are used for our test. Because of the precision of our procedure, very few cell membrane separations are contaminated. However, if there are any bacteria products, they always elute over Sephadex G-200 in the very early, heavy molecular weight fraction 1.

Before any further separation of the membrane and soluble antigens, these materials are used in initial skin tests of breast cancer and control cancer patients. In contrast to the striking specificity of studies with certain other types of cancers, such as intestinal cancer, the skin tests of breast cancer patients with membrane and Sephadex soluble membrane fractions were quite disappointing. As shown in Table 1, breast cancer patients were tested according to histologic type, and it may be seen that the cell membrane produced very few skin reactions. These delayed hypersensitive skin reactions are measured at various time intervals, and the erythema and induration recorded. Reactions are not considered positive unless the induration at 48 hr is greater than 5 mm diameter; in addition, biopsies of the test site are carefully assessed for true delayed hypersensitivity. Soluble fractions 1 and 3 of breast cancer materials, of benign breast lesions, and of the non-cancerous breast of the breast cancer patient produced no skin reactivity, with the exception of fractions 1 and 3 from medullary breast carcinoma. As shown in Table 1, cell membrane soluble fraction 2 produced positive skin reactions in 8 of 12 breast cancer patients tested. However, fraction 2 prepared from the cell membrane of the non-cancerous breast tissue of the breast cancer patient also produced positive reactions in 4 of 8 breast cancer patients tested. In addition, fraction 2 prepared from cell membranes of the benign breast lesions also produced positive reactions in 2 of 3 breast cancer patients tested. Some of these preparations were also tested in 2 or 3 other patients with cancers other than breast cancer and were negative.

These results were quite discouraging. We made the tentative conclusion that there were probably no tumor specific antigens on the surface of breast cancer cells. However, we had been unable to obtain a normal breast. In order to complete these series of observations, we felt it might be important to obtain normal breast from an accident victim in order to compare it with our studies of so-called non-cancerous breast tissue from the breast cancer patient, and also with antigens present in the benign breast lesions. When this normal material was obtained, we decided to compare the patterns of the Sephadex fraction 2 of fresh specimens of infiltrating ductal breast carcinoma with fresh specimens of benign breast regions and the normal breast cells of a normal individual.

We, therefore, conducted further separations of these 3 Sephadex fractions 2 soluble membrane components by using polyacrylamide gel electrophoresis. We have been suc-

TABLE 1 *Delayed hypersensitive skin tests with membrane and soluble membrane fractions after separation over Sephadex*

Breast cancer patients tested	Breast cancer		Non-cancerous breast of breast cancer patient		Benign breast lesions	
	Cell membrane	Fraction II	Cell membrane	Fraction II	Cell membrane	Fraction II
1. Infiltrating ductal breast carcinoma with fibrosis	2/6	5/9	0/6	3/5	0/1	1/2
2. Infiltrating ductal breast carcinoma (comedo type)	1/1					
3. Infiltrating ductal breast carcinoma, with lobular carcinoma	0/1	1/1	0/1	0/1		
4. Mucinous breast carcinoma		1/1	0/1	1/1	0/1	1/1
5. Medullary breast carcinoma		1/1 (also positive to 2 other fractions)		0/1		
6. Benign breast fibroadenoma and epithelial hyperplasia of terminal ducts	0/1	0/1	0/1	0/1	1/1	1/1
7. Other cancer patients	0/3	0/3	0/2	0/2	0/2	0/2
Total in breast cancer patients:	3/8	8/12	0/8	4/8	0/2	2/3

TABLE 2 *Further separation of Sephadex fractions II of breast cancer, benign breast and normal breast soluble membrane components by gel electrophoresis*

I. Results when fraction II is separated by gel electrophoresis and the proteins are eluted from top (region 1), middle (region 2) and lower (region 3) portions of the gels. Skin tests of non-anergic patients.

Skin test reactions at 48 hr

	Breast cancer Stage I	Breast cancer Stage II	Genital cancer Stage III	Ovarian cancer Stage IV
Breast cancer gel regions: 1	0	0	0	
2	+	+	+	
3	0	0	0	
Benign breast gel regions: 1	0 0	0 0	0 0	0 0
2	+ +	0 0	0 0	0 0
3	0 0	0 0	0 0	0
Normal breast gel regions: 1	0	0		0
2	0	0		0
3	0	0		0

II. Results when gel region 2 is further separated into upper (region 2a) and lower (region 2b) regions. Skin tests of non-anergic patients.

Skin test reactions at 48 hr

	Breast cancer Stage I	Breast cancer Stage IV	Ovarian cancer Stage I
Breast cancer gel regions: 2a	+	0 0	+
2b	±	+ +	0
Benign breast gel regions: 2a	+	0	0
2b	0	0	0
Normal breast gel regions: 2a	0		0
2b	0		0

cessful using this advanced method of gel electrophoresis employing 4 stacked gels (10%, 7%, 4.75% and 3.5%), a method which permitted discrete separation of the peptide band in studies of other types of human cancer. The distribution of protein bands of each of the 3 materials was markedly different. In addition, preliminary tests of the membranes and Sephadex fractions of the normal breast cancer cells were negative when tested in a non-anergic breast cancer patient. We were therefore encouraged to further skin test materials from fraction 2 as further separated by gel electrophoresis. The gels were precisely sliced (see Fig. 1) into 3 separate regions, the proteins eluted, dialysed and concentrated for skin testing. As shown in Table 2, stage 1 breast cancer patient gave positive reaction to the center region 2 both from the breast cancer material and from the benign breast material but not to the normal breast material. The tests in another breast cancer stage 1 patient were repeated for the benign breast gel regions, and, again, gel region 2 of the benign breast material gave a positive test. These 3 gel regions of the breast cancer material were also tested in a stage 4 breast cancer patient and, again, gel region 2 further gave positive skin tests. We were surprised to see that gel regions from the benign breast and normal breast produced negative reactions in the same patient. We repeated the test of the benign breast gel regions in another stage 4 cancer patient, and, again, the reactions were negative. In order to determine whether or not the reactions to the breast cancer and benign breast gel regions in stage 1 breast cancer patients were specific, we selected a non-anergic patient with genital cancer for skin testing. The patient with stage 1 genital cancer registered a positive reaction to breast cancer gel region 2. This reaction was not seen with the benign breast gel regions (see Table 2). Tests with the benign breast gel regions and with the normal breast gel regions were conducted in an ovarian cancer stage 1 and, again, the reactions were negative.

In view of the differences between stage 1 and stage 4 breast cancer skin tests, we decided to further separate gel region 2 into an upper gel region 2a and lower gel region 2b (Fig. 1). As shown in Table 2, reactivity to breast cancer gel regions 2a and 2b was seen in breast cancer stage 1 skin tests. The same patient also reacted to benign breast gel region 2a but not gel region 2b. In addition, neither normal breast gel region 2a nor 2b produced skin reactivity. A non-anergic breast cancer patient with stage IV malignancy was tested with breast cancer gel region and it was of interest to note that gel region 2a produced no positive skin reaction whereas gel region 2b produced a positive skin reaction. The benign breast gel regions 2a and 2b were negative in the same patient. The tests of breast cancer gel regions were repeated in another breast cancer stage IV and again, only breast cancer gel region 2b produced a positive skin reaction. In order to ascertain whether or not the breast cancer gel regions 2a and 2b contained material specific as well as non-specific for breast cancer, the ovarian cancer patient stage I was tested with regions 2a and 2b from breast cancer, from benign breast and from normal breast gel regions. As shown in Table 2, only breast cancer gel region 2a produced a positive response.

While further studies must be conducted, and, especially with other types of breast cancer besides infiltrating ductal carcinoma, it would appear from these preliminary tests that the breast cancer patient, during the earlier stages of malignancy, is reacting both to the cancer antigens and other antigens present on the cell surfaces. It would also appear that stage IV breast cancer patients differentiate in favor of an antigen present only on the breast cancer tissue, and, therefore, a tentative conclusion might be that breast cancer patients are able to give tumor specific skin reaction when they are developing metastatic tumors. While other parameters must be considered, it would appear that some of the results of this investigation may be useful in interpreting immune responses of the breast cancer patient.

I would like to turn your attention now to a different area of consideration, in this brief survey of the various factors which may or may not influence the development of breast cancer. There are a number of agents which are implicated as possible viruses associated with breast cancer. One of these viruses has been found frequently in human milk samples, and resembles the mouse mammary tumor RNA virus. These particles have been found to contain a reverse transcriptase, and, in addition, the length of the poly-adenylic acid region in the 60 s to 70 s RNA molecule of the human milk virus particle

(−)

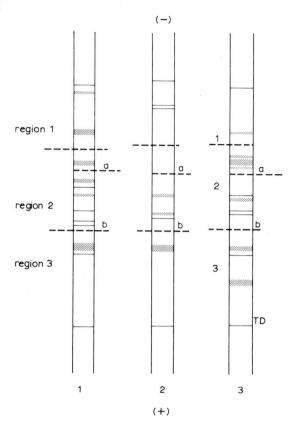

region 1

region 2

region 3

1   2   3

(+)

FIG. 1   *Further separation of Sephadex fraction 2 soluble membrane components by polyacrylamide gel electrophoresis using 4 stacked gels (10%, 7%, 4.75% and 3.5%). Approximately 50 µg protein each of fractions 2 prepared from (1) infiltrating ductal breast carcinoma, (2) normal breast of normal individual, and (3) benign breast tissue were further separated. The gels were sliced and proteins eluted and prepared by ultrafiltration dialysis from regions 1, 2 or 2a and 2b and 3 for various tests. Tracking dye (TD) was bromphenol blue.*

appeared to be the same as the polyadenylic acid region in the mouse mammary tumor virus as well as in the Mason-Pfizer monkey virus RNA molecule. Mason-Pfizer monkey virus particles are those which have been isolated from spontaneous mammary tumors in Rhesus monkeys, and such particles can be grown in monkey and human cell cultures. It was of interest that we found complement-fixing activity in the soluble breast cancer gel regions 1 and 3 when tested with absorbed anti-Mason-Pfizer virus monkey serum. We also found similar CF reactivity in gel regions 1 and 3 from the so-called normal breast from the breast cancer patient; positive reactivity was not seen with the normal breast cells from the normal individual. This suggests that there are present on the breast cell surface certain virus-induced or virus-related antigens which may be expressions of the genetic information present in such cells. It would be of interest to explore the immunogenetic aspects of breast cancers to determine whether the virus genetic information corresponds to the presence of surface antigens. In conclusion, if we are to have a well-coordinated, extensive search of the cause and prevention of human breast cancer, we must understand how to put together and utilize what we know about effective drugs, controlled environment, genetic manipulation, use of the body's own defense mechanisms, and environmental factors.

Acknowledgements

We thank O.B. Lee, K. Tanner, P. Jones, P. Pugh and M. Dannbeck for technical assistance.

References

Ahmed, M., Mayyasi, S. A. and Chopra , H. C. (1971): J. nat. Cancer Inst., 46, 1325.
Alaasarraf, M., Wong, P. and Sardesai, S. (1970): Cancer (Philad.), 26, 262.
Alford, C., Hollinshead, A. and Herberman, R. (1973): Ann. Surg., 178, 20.
Anderson, D. E. (1971): Cancer (Philad.), 28, 1500.
Anderson, V., Bendixen, B. and Schiodt, T. (1969): Acta med. scand., 186, 101.
Bloom, H. J. G., Richardson, W. W. and Field, J. R. (1970): Brit. med. J., 3, 181.
Chopra, H. C. and Mason, M. M. (1970): Cancer Res., 30, 2081.
Chopra, H. C., Zelljadt, I. and Jensen, E. M. (1971): J. nat. Cancer Inst., 46, 127.
Crile Jr, G. (1969): Cancer (Philad.), 24, 1283.
Eskin, B. A. (1970): Trans. N. Y. Acad. Sci., 32, 911.
Feller, W. F., Chopra, H. and Bepko, F. (1967): Surgery, 62, 750.
Feller, W. F. and Chopra, H. C. (1971): Cancer (Philad.), 28, 1425.
Fisher, B. (1971): Amer. J. Roentgenol., 111, 123.
Hollinshead, A. C., Jaffurs, W. T., Alpert, L. K. and Herberman, R. B. (1974): In press.
Hollinshead, A. C., Stewart, T. H. M. and Herberman, R. B. (1974): J. nat. Cancer Inst., 52, 372.
Mackay, W. D., Dulbrook, R. D. and Want, D. (1971): Brit. J. Surg., 57, 386.
MacLellan, E. (1969): Brit. J. Surg., 56, 850.
Melandez, M. D., Daniel, F. G. and Garcia F. C. (1969): Lab. Animal Care, 19, 378.
Meyer, K. K. (1970): Arch. Surg., 101, 114.
Potolsky, A. I., Heath Jr, C. W. and Buckley, C. E. (1970): Amer. J. Med., 50, 42.
Richters, S. A. and Sherwin, R. P. (1971): Cancer (Philad.) 27, 274.
Roberts, M. and Williams, W. J. (1968): Brit. J. Surg., 55, 869.
Roberts, M. M. (1971): Brit. J. Surg., 57, 381.
Schlom, J., Colcher, D. and Spiegelman, S. (1973): Science,179, 696.
Schlom, J., Spiegelman, S. and Moore, D. H. (1972): Science, 175, 542.
Schneider, R. (1970): Cancer (Philad.), 26, 419.
Solowey, A. C. and Rapaport, F. T. (1965): Surg. Gynec. Obstet., 121, 756.
Tannenbaum, M. and Lattimer, J.K. (1970): J. Urol. (Baltimore), 103, 471.
Truscott, B. McN. and Bond, W. H. (1969): Brit. J. Surg., 56, 789.

Application of serum alpha feto-protein assay in mass survey of primary carcinoma of liver

The Co-ordinating Group For The Research of Liver Cancer, China

In recent years, serum alpha feto-protein (AFP) assay has been widely used in the clinical diagnosis of primary hepatocellular carcinoma (Abelev, 1971). Its clinical value has been studied in this country since 1970. Up to Oct. 1972, serum samples from 4,621 cases were assayed in Shanghai (Shanghai Collaborative Group for the Study, Prevention and Treatment of Cancer, 1973). In 797 cases of clinical primary carcinoma of liver, the positive rate was 75.65%. 139 of the 797 cases were histologically confirmed as hepatocellular carcinomas and among them, the positive rate was 76.3%. There were 6 'false positive' cases in 52 patients with metastatic liver cancer, whereas all of the 147 cases with tumors other than liver cancers and teratomas were negative. All but two of the 2,342 cases with non-neoplastic liver and biliary diseases as well as 791 healthy donors were also negative.

Since 1972, AFP assay has been used as a means for mass survey of primary liver cancer in some factories in Shanghai and communes in Kiang-su Province. A number of primary liver cancer cases were detected; some of them were presumably at early stages.

Materials and methods

Persons being screened

1. All of the workers and part of the retired ones from some factories in Shanghai, with a total of 277,167 persons
2. General population (above 16 years of age) from some communes in Kiang-su Province, with a total of 28,176 persons.
3. Persons (above 16 years of age) with liver diseases or history of liver diseases from some other communes in Kiang-su Province, with a total of 38,656 cases.

Antisera used

Antisera were obtained by immunization of rabbits or sheep with pooled sera from 4-6 months fetuses, AFP-rich sera from patients with primary hepatocellular carcinoma, or partially purified AFP prepared from saline extracts of whole fetuses. Rabbit and sheep antisera used were absorbed with equal volume of pooled normal human sera.

Assay methods

Identification of AFP was carried out by Ouchterlony double diffusion method and/or counter current electrophoresis. Some of the dubious positive samples were checked by radioimmunoassay (Shanghai Institute of Experimental Biology, Jui-king Hospital of Shanghai Second Medical College, in press).

Results

Results of AFP screening are shown in Table 1.

TABLE 1   *Results of AFP screening*

	No. of persons examined	No. of AFP (+) cases	Incidence (per 100,000)
Shanghai	277,167	31	11.18
Kiang-su Province (from general population)	28,176	14	49.69
Kiang-su Province (persons with liver diseases or history of liver diseases)	38,656	102	263.87

Results of follow-up

Of the 147 AFP positive cases detected by screening 129 cases (88.4%) were finally diagnosed to be primary carcinoma of liver by physical examination, other diagnostic procedures and tests, laparotomy, pathological examination or 2-10 months of clinical follow-up. Histological examinations were performed in 21 cases, of which 20 were proved to be primary hepatocellular carcinomas, and one was cholangiocellular carcinoma. The other 18 AFP positive cases were followed up for 3-10 months with an average of 6.9 months, yet there were still no obvious clinical features of primary carcinoma of liver. During this follow-up period, AFP assays were repeated 1-6 times with an average of 3.8 times, and most of them were persistently positive. Further investigations are needed for these patients.

Time relation between AFP screening and appearance of obvious signs of primary liver cancer

Table 2 shows the time from AFP positive to the appearance of obvious signs of primary liver cancer (liver enlarged to 5 cm or more below costal margin or 7 cm or more below xyphoid process, hard and nodular; liver enlarged and hard, with obvious nodules; liver enlarged progressively without undue cause) in 53 cases. Of these, only 20 cases had these signs while AFP screening was positive, and the remaining 33 cases showed these signs 1-10 months, averaging 3.1 months, later than AFP screening. This shows that AFP screening can detect primary liver cancer before the appearance of obvious clinical signs.

TABLE 2   *Time from AFP positive to the appearance of obvious signs of primary liver cancer*

Months	At the time of AFP screening	1	2	3	4	5	6	7	8	9	10
No. of cases	20	14	3	5	2	4	2	0	1	0	2

Results of other forms of examination at the time of AFP screening

Table 3 shows the results of other examinations performed within 1-2 weeks after AFP screening in 26 AFP positive cases; all of these 26 cases were diagnosed clinically or confirmed histologically as primary carcinoma of liver. At the time when AFP was positive by screening, the results of other examinations were largely negative. This shows that AFP screening can give positive results earlier than other examinations.

TABLE 3   *Results of other forms of examination at the time of AFP screening*

	AKP	$\gamma-GT$	AKP and LDH iso- enzymes	Ultrasonic detection	Radioactive isotope scanning
No. of cases examined	17	7	8	23	21
No. of positive cases	8	5	4	8	10

Case illustrations

Case 1: L. Y. Sun, a female cotton-mill worker of 49, was found to be AFP positive by screening on Nov. 3, 1972. There were no subjective symptoms and physical examination showed an enlarged liver 2.5 cm below right costal margin, of moderate consistency and with no nodules. Ultrasonic detection and radioactive isotope scanning gave negative results. AFP was repeatedly positive. Operation was performed on Nov. 22, and a cancer nodule with a diameter of 4 cm was found at the upper part of right posterior lobe. Right hemi-hepatectomy was done. AFP turned to be negative after operation. Patient recovered well. Primary hepatocellular carcinoma was confirmed by histological examination.

Case 2: S. K. Yang, a male peasant of 45, was found to be AFP positive on Sept. 15, 1972 through mass screening. There were no subjective symptoms and physical examination showed a slightly enlarged liver 1.5 cm below right costal margin and 3 cm below xyphoid process, soft in consistency, and a nodule of peanut size was palpated. Operation was done on Oct. 6, and a cancer nodule of 4x3.5 cm was found at the left lateral aspect of liver. The left lateral lobe was resected. AFP turned to be negative after operation. Patient recovered smoothly. Pathological examination proved to be primary hepatocellular carcinoma.

Discussion

The usefulness of AFP screening in mass survey of primary liver cancer

Hull et al. (1970) have noted that there are marked regional differences in the AFP positive rate of primary hepatocellular carcinoma. Among 37 cases of histologically proved primary hepatocellular carcinoma yet with AFP negative findings by Ouchterlony double diffusion method and counter current electrophoresis, 14 were randomly tested by radioimmunoassay, and 12 of these were proved to be AFP positive (with an AFP level of 52-933 ng/ml) (Shanghai Collaborative Group for the Study, Prevention and Treatment of Cancer, 1973, Shanghai Institute of Experimental Biology et al., 1973). On that account, the AFP positive rate of hepatocellular carcinoma in Shanghai should be around 95%. As most of the primary liver cancer cases in Shanghai and Kiang-su Province are of hepatocellular type, it is advisable to apply AFP screening as a means for mass survey. If some more sensitive methods such as radioimmunoassay are used in screening, higher rate of positive results can be obtained, but then, the specificity of AFP test will be lowered.

For the convenience of carrying out AFP screening in remote regions, the procedures of assay should be simplified. More simplified methods such as whole blood double diffusion method and filter paper blood sampling method have already been put into practice in this country.

The necessity of repeated AFP screenings in mass survey of primary liver cancer

There are various types of AFP dynamics in primary hepatocellular carcinoma. In one type, the serum AFP level is very low at the beginning and increases gradually in parallel with the progress of disease. Another type is of saddle-shaped curve similar to that noted by Watabe (1971) in animal experiments. If AFP screening is performed only once, those with low AFP level at the beginning or just at the bottom of saddle-shaped curve while screening will be missed. For instance, of 11,004 persons screened as AFP negative in our series, there was one case of AFP positive hepatoma in the 3rd, 4th, 5th, 6th, 7th month respectively and there were two cases in the 8th month after screening. Accordingly, it is essential to carry out repeated AFP screenings in endemic areas of primary liver cancer.

Summary

1.   The results of AFP screening by Ouchterlony double diffusion method and counter current electrophoresis in 343,999 persons for mass survey of primary liver cancer are presented.

2.   Through the observation that while AFP was positive, the results of other examinations were largely negative, and the appearance of obvious signs was found later than AFP screening, it is suggested that AFP screening has some significance in early detection of primary liver cancer.

3.   In endemic areas of primary liver cancer, repeated AFP screenings are recommended.

References

Abelev, G. I. (1971): Advanc. Cancer Res., 14, 295.
Hull, E. W., Carbone, P. P., Moertel, C. G. et al. (1970): Lancet, 1, 779.
Shanghai Collaborative Group for the Study, Prevention and Treatment of Cancer (1973): Chin. med.
     J., 8, 454.
Shanghai Institute of Experimental Biology et al. (1973): Chin. med. J., 8, 463.
Watabe, H. (1971): Cancer Res., 31, 1192.

Index of authors

ED BELOW

UNIVERSITY
San Francisco
THIS BOOK IS DUE ON THE LAST DATE S

7 DAY LOAN

14 7

7 DAY LOAN

RETURNED

7 DAY RETURNED JAN 1 5 1981

AUG 1 5 1975 JAN 1 5 1981
RETURNED

AUG 8 1975

14 DAY

RETURNED

SEP -1 1977

14 DAY
FEB 2 1 1978
RETURNED

14 DAY 5/8
JAN 2 8 1981

15m—6,'78 (C